Brendan T. Finucane · Ban C.H. Tsui
Albert H. Santora

Principles of Airway Management

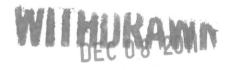

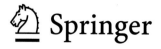 Springer

Brendan T. Finucane, MBBCh, FRCPC
Professor Emeritus
Department of Anesthesiology and Pain
Medicine
University of Alberta
Director of Anesthesia Services Cross
Cancer Institute
Edmonton, Alberta, Canada
Staff Anesthesiologist Leduc Community
Hospital
Leduc, Alberta, Canada

Ban C.H. Tsui, Dip Eng, BSc(Math),
B Pharm, MD, MSc, FRCPC
Professor
Department of Anesthesiology
	and Pain Medicine
Director, Regional Anesthesia
	and Acute Pain Service
Stollery Children's Hospital
University of Alberta Hospital
Edmonton, Alberta, Canada

Albert H. Santora, MD
Athens, GA USA

ISBN 978-0-387-09557-8   e-ISBN 978-0-387-09558-5
DOI 10.1007/978-0-387-09558-5
Springer New York Dordrecht Heidelberg London

Printed on acid-free paper

Springer is part of Springer Science+Business Media (www.springer.com)

Preface

By the time this edition is published, close to 23 years will have passed since *Principles of Airway Management* was first published. A lot of water has passed under the bridge since 1988. Airway groups have been formed in many countries. Several books on the topic of airway management have been published. We now have several algorithms to choose from when confronted with airway challenges. A vast array of airway devices have been invented and the number of publications on airway-related topics has increased exponentially. In 1988, none of us believed that laryngoscopy and endotracheal intubation would be obsolete in 25 years, and of course we were correct. However, that may not be true 25 years from now, and the discussions about that issue are already taking place.

We have seen a decrease in the incidence of airway tragedies in the United States in recent years, judging by the declining number of *Closed Claims* cases involving the airway. Perhaps this decline occurred because we have better equipment and better ways of detecting and managing airway problems. Perhaps the introduction of the LMA and other supraglottic devices has had some influence on these numbers. However, despite the advances we have made, we continue to have our problems, and there is no room for complacency.

When we first published this book, our intended audience was medical students. We have since expanded the scope of the book to provide a reference for a much broader readership. This book should now appeal to any physician or nonphysician who has a primary interest in airway management.

What is so special about this edition? We have made a number of changes, many of which were based on the critiques of the previous edition. Most of the illustrations in this edition have been redrawn and are in color. We have also added two new chapters, making this edition more comprehensive. This edition will also be presented in both hard and soft cover. Last, but not the least, we have recruited Ban Tsui MD, a known expert in pediatric airway management, to join us as a new coauthor and share with us his knowledge of the airway.

Each of the three authors has written five chapters of the book. Below is a summary of how each author contributed to enhance this edition. Dr. Finucane updated the opening chapters entitled "Anatomy of the Airway and Evaluation of the Airway," to both of which he added new and colorized illustrations and improved content. Dr. Finucane also wrote the chapters on "Indications and

Preparation," and "Techniques of Intubation," and finally he wrote the closing chapter, entitled "Complications of Airway Management," which includes statistics on airway complications from around the world. All of these chapters were rewritten in some fashion, have many new illustrations, and have updated bibliographies.

Dr. Tsui wrote the chapters on "Basic Emergency Airway Management and Cardiopulmonary Resuscitation (CPR)" and "Basic Airway Equipment," incorporating many components of the previous edition, but placing stronger emphasis on the importance of bag/valve/mask ventilation technique and maintaining sterility of equipment. Dr. Tsui also wrote the chapter on "Advanced Airway Devices." In that chapter he provides a comprehensive overview, using the most up-to-date information on numerous airway devices now available for use, embellishing his descriptions with numerous illustrations. For "The Difficult Airway" chapter, Dr. Tsui not only updated the practice guidelines from the American Society of Anesthesiologists, but also greatly expanded the scope of the chapter to discuss the circumstances and management of the difficult airway in the emergency room, the intensive care unit, and the operating room. He also stresses the importance of airway management in obese patients and in those with obstructive sleep apnea syndrome. Finally, Dr. Tsui has completed a major revision of the chapter dedicated to "Pediatric Airway Management." He divided this chapter into two sections A and B. In section A, Dr. Tsui updated information from the previous edition on basic and advanced airway management in the child and added some information on intubation trauma and the use of heliox in pediatric airway management. Dr. Tsui also discusses the important interplay between the larynx, the pharynx, and the tongue in pediatric airway obstruction. For section B, Dr. Tsui invited Dr. Hamdy El-Hakim [MD, FRCS(ORL-HNS), Divisions of Otolaryngology and Pediatric Surgery, Department of Surgery, University of Alberta, Edmonton, Alberta, Canada] as a primary author to share his expertise on surgical aspects of pediatric airway management. Drs. Tsui and El-Hakim highlight important considerations for the anesthesiologist and surgeon during otolaryngological (primarily endoscopic) procedures. We are grateful for Dr. El-Hakim's important contribution to this chapter. This contribution by Dr. El-Hakim is an excellent example of the importance of collaboration between anesthesiologists and surgeons when dealing with some of the most challenging airway issues in medicine

Dr. Santora updated chapters on "Fibroptically Guided Airway Intubation Techniques," "Mechanical Ventilation and Respiratory Care," and the "Surgical Options in Airway Management." A new chapter, "Extubation Strategies: The Extubation Algorithm," addresses an area of airway management hitherto relegated to secondary concern. Finally, the chapter entitled "The Laryngeal Mask Airway (LMA™) and other Extraglottic (Supraglottic) Airway Devices" summarizes many new considerations of this revolutionary airway tool. To address valid criticisms leveled at this chapter in the 3rd Edition, extensive thought has been given to the question: Is the extraglottic airway device interchangeable with the endotracheal tube in the practice of anesthesia?

It is evident that we have completed a major revision of *Principles of Airway Management* and have every hope that this edition represents the most up-to-date information on this rapidly advancing discipline.

Edmonton, AB	Brendan T. Finucane
Edmonton, AB	Ban C.H. Tsui
Athens, GA	Albert H. Santora

Acknowledgements

The authors wish to acknowledge Donna Finucane's valuable contribution as we prepared to submit the final edition to the Publisher. We would also like to give credit to Jennifer Pillay for her contributions towards editing a portion of this book. We would also like to thank Brian Belval for helping us get started and Catherine Paduani for helping us finish this important edition. We are grateful to Portia Bridges for centrally coordinating all aspects of this work at a very early stage. We would like to thank the graphic artist Alice Chen for her excellent drawings and for the color version of some of our old drawings. Adam Dryden helped by taking many of the pictures of equipment and devices, and Nicole Stalker helped obtain numerous images for the Advanced Airway Devices chapter. Finally, we would like to acknowledge Jenkin Tsui's drawings which helped the graphic artist interpret what was required in some of the illustrations.

Contents

2 Evaluation of the Airway.. 27
Introduction... 28
The Normal/Abnormal Airway.. 29
Predictive Tests for Difficult Intubation... 29
Elective Intubation 32
   History Pertinent to Elective Airway Management............................. 32
   Diabetes Mellitus.. 32
   NPO Status 33
   Physical Examination 34
Structured Approach 49
Bag/Valve/Mask Ventilation 50
Additional Information 52
   Arterial Blood Gases 52
   ENT Consultation... 53
   Radiologic Studies.. 53
   Pulmonary Function Studies... 53
   Flow-Volume Loops 54
   Difficult Airway Clinic... 54
   The "Awake Look" 55
Summary.. 56
References.. 56
Suggested Reading.. 58

**3 Basic Emergency Airway Management
and Cardiopulmonary Resuscitation (CPR)** 59
Emergency Airway Management... 60
Importance of Basic Life Support... 60
Adult Basic Life Support (BLS) 61
   Chain of Survival.. 62
   Changes in the 2005 and 2010 AHA Recommendations 62
   The AHA Algorithm and Recommendations for Rescue Breaths,
   a Universal Compression-Ventilation Ratio, and Defibrillation............. 63
   Techniques of CPR 68
   Limitations and Complications of CPR... 80
Airway Obstruction... 80
   Etiology of Upper Airway Obstruction 80
   The Tongue as a Cause of Airway Obstruction................................... 81
   Foreign Body Airway Obstruction 82
CPR and Precautions Against the Transmission of Disease 87
   Transmission of Disease from CPR Mannequins................................. 88
Summary.. 89
References.. 89

Chapter 1
Anatomy of the Airway

Contents

B.T. Finucane et al., *Principles of Airway Management*,
DOI 10.1007/978-0-387-09558-5_1, © Springer Science+Business Media, LLC 2011

Introduction

Knowledge of anatomy is essential to the study of airway management. First, anatomical considerations are helpful in diagnosing certain problems, such as the position of a foreign body in a patient with airway obstruction. Second, since some procedures involved in establishing and maintaining an airway are performed under emergency conditions, little if any time may be available for reviewing anatomy. Third, in many procedures involving the airway, such as tracheal intubation, anatomical structures are only partially visible. As a result, one must recognize not only the structures in view but also their spatial relationship to the surrounding structures. This chapter reviews basic airway anatomy, discusses some clinical correlates, and includes a comparison of the pediatric and adult airway.

The Nose

The nose is a pyramidal-shaped structure projecting from the midface made up of bone, cartilage, fibrofatty tissue, mucous membrane, and skin. It contains the peripheral organ of smell and is the proximal portion of the respiratory tract. The nose is divided into right and left nasal cavities by the nasal septum. The inferior portion of the nose contains two apertures called the anterior nares. Each naris is bounded laterally by an ala, or wing. The posterior portions of the nares open into the nasopharynx and are referred to as choanae. One or both of these apertures are absent in the congenital anomaly choanal atresia.[1] Infants born with this condition are at risk of suffocation as they are compulsive nose breathers at birth. Urgent surgical correction of choanal atresia is required soon after birth in these cases.

The nose has a number of important functions, including: respiration, olefaction, filtration, humidification, and is a reservoir for secretions from the paranasal sinuses and the nasolacrimal ducts.

Anatomically, each side of the nose consists of a floor, a roof, and medial and lateral walls. The septum forms the medial wall of each nostril and is made up of perpendicular plates of ethmoid and vomer bones and the septal cartilage (Fig. 1.1). The bony plate forming the superior aspect of the septum is very thin and descends from the cribriform plate of the ethmoid bone. The cribriform plate may be fractured following trauma. Head injury victims should be questioned about nasal discharge, which may be cerebrospinal fluid (CSF). Nasotracheal intubation and the passage of nasogastric tubes are relatively contraindicated in the presence of basal skull fractures.[2] The lateral walls have a bony framework attached to which are three bony projections referred to as conchae or turbinates (Fig. 1.2). The upper and middle conchae are derived from the medial aspect of the ethmoid; the inferior concha is a separate structure. There are a number of openings in the lateral nasal walls that communicate with the paranasal sinuses and the nasolacrimal duct.

A coronal section of the nose and mouth shows the location and relationships of the nasal structures more clearly (Fig. 1.3). Considerable damage can be inflicted

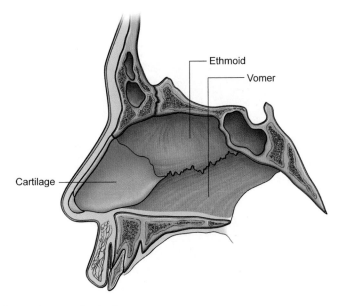

Fig. 1.1 The nasal septum (sagittal)

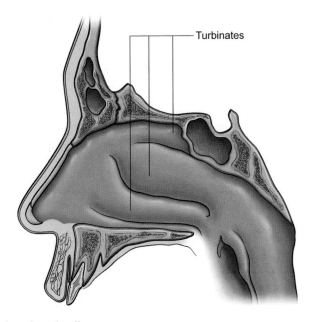

Fig. 1.2 The lateral nasal wall

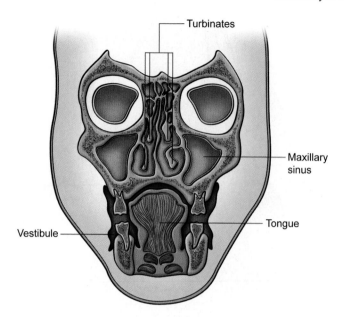

Fig. 1.3 Coronal section through the nose and mouth

on the lateral walls of the nose by forcing endotracheal tubes into the nasal cavity in the presence of an obstruction.

Nasal endotracheal tubes and nasal airways should be well lubricated, and vasoconstricting solutions should be applied to the nasal mucosa before instrumentation. When introducing a nasal endotracheal tube into the nostril, the bevel of the tube should be parallel to the nasal septum to avoid disruption of the conchae (Fig. 8.18, Chap. 8).

Oral Cavity

The mouth or oral cavity (Fig. 1.4), is divided into two parts: the vestibule and the oral cavity proper. The vestibule is the space between the lips and the cheeks externally and the gums and teeth internally (see Fig. 1.3). The oral cavity proper is bounded anterolaterally by the alveolar arch, teeth, and gums; superiorly by the hard and soft palates; and inferiorly by the tongue. Posteriorly, the oral cavity communicates with the palatal arches and pharynx.

Uvula

In the posterior aspect of the mouth, the soft palate is shaped like the letter *M*, with the uvula as the centerpiece. This structure is a useful landmark for practitioners assessing the ease or difficulty of mask ventilation or tracheal intubation.

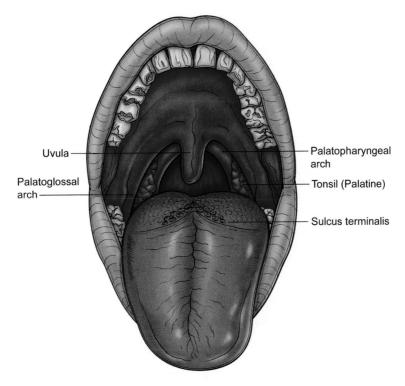

Uvula

Palatopharyngeal
arch

Palatoglossal
arch

Tonsil (Palatine)

Sulcus terminalis

Fig. 1.4 The oral cavity

Tonsils

The tonsils that we see when we look in the mouth are formally known as the palatine tonsils which are collections of lymphoid tissue engulfed by two soft tissue folds, the "pillars of the fauces." The anterior fold is called the palatoglossal arch, and the posterior, the palatopharyngeal arch (see Fig. 1.4). However, tonsillar tissue is far more extensive than that. There is a collection of lymphoid tissue called the "tonsillar ring" which is situated in an incomplete circular ring around the pharynx. It is made up of the palatine tonsils (between the pillars of the fauces), the pharyngeal tonsil, (adenoids), tubular tonsils (which extend bilaterally into the eustachian tubes), and the lingual tonsil (which is a collection of lymphoid tissue on the posterior aspect of the tongue). The lingual tonsil is situated behind the sulcus terminalis and has a cobblestone appearance (Fig. 1.5). Hypertrophy of the pharyngeal tonsil (adenoids) can obstruct the nasal airway, necessitating mouth breathing. Hearing may be impaired when the tubular tonsils become infected. Hypertrophy of the lingual tonsil may cause airway obstruction, difficult mask ventilation, and difficult tracheal intubation.[3]

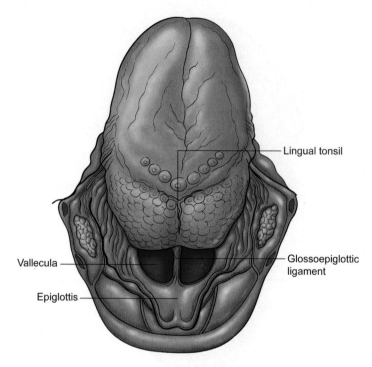

Lingual tonsil

Vallecula

Glossoepiglottic
ligament

Epiglottis

Fig. 1.5 Posterior view of the tongue showing the lingual tonsil and the epiglottis

Tongue

The tongue is a muscular organ used for speech, taste, deglutition, and oral cleansing. It is divided into three parts: the *root,* the *body,* and the *tip*. The posterior aspect of the tongue is divided into two parts by a fibrous ridge called the *sulcus terminalis* (see Fig. 1.4). The tongue is attached to the hyoid bone, mandible, styloid processes, soft palate, and walls of the pharynx. In an unconscious patient, the oropharyngeal musculature tends to relax and the tongue is displaced posteriorly, occluding the airway. Since the tongue is a major cause of airway obstruction, it is an important anatomical consideration in airway management. Its size in relation to the oropharyngeal space is an important determinant of the ease or difficulty of tracheal intubation.

Nerve Supply to the Tongue

The sensory and motor innervation of the tongue is quite diverse and includes fibers from a number of different sources.

Sensory fibers for the anterior two thirds are provided by the lingual nerve. Taste fibers are furnished by the chorda tympani branch of the nervus intermedius (from the facial nerve [VII]). Sensory fibers for the posterior third come from the glossopharyngeal nerve (IX) (Fig. 1.6).

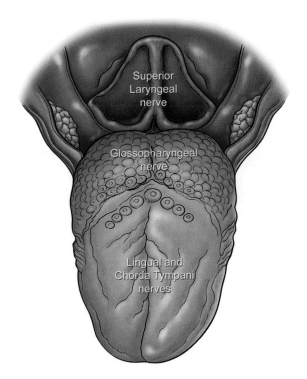

Fig. 1.6 Sensory innervation of the tongue

The Macintosh laryngoscope is inserted into the vallecula during laryngoscopy and theoretically, at least, is less likely to elicit a vagal response because the innervation of the vallecula is provided by the glossopharyngeal nerve. When straight blades are used for laryngoscopy they are inserted with the intention of exposing the laryngeal opening by placing the blade beneath the inferior surface of the epiglottis. The inferior surface of the epiglottis is innervated by the superior laryngeal nerve. Therefore, one is more likely to encounter vagal stimulation during laryngoscopy with a straight blade (Miller or Henderson).

The major motor nerve supply of the tongue is from the hypoglossal nerve (XII) (Fig. 1.7) which passes above the hyoid bone and is distributed to the lingual muscles. Since this nerve is very superficial at the angle of the mandible, it is prone to injury during vigorous manual manipulation of the airway (see Chap. 15).

Pharynx

The pharynx is a musculo-membranous passage between the choanae, the posterior oral cavity, the larynx, and esophagus. It extends from the base of the skull to the inferior border of the cricoid cartilage anteriorly and the lower border of C6 posteriorly. It is approximately 15 cm long. Its widest point is at the level of the hyoid bone and the narrowest at the lower end where it joins the esophagus. Figures 1.8 and 1.9 show

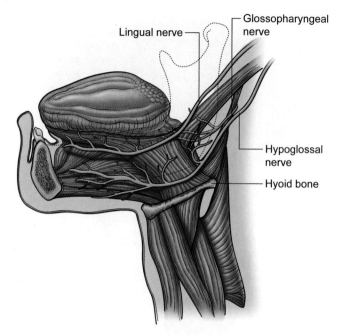

Fig. 1.7 Motor innervation of the tongue

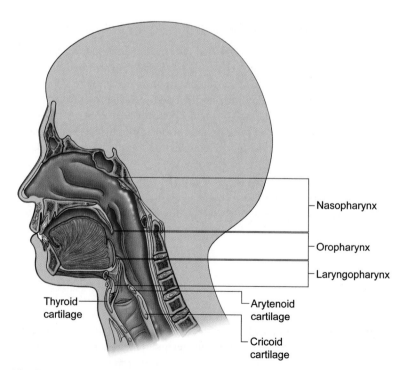

Fig. 1.8 The pharynx (sagittal)

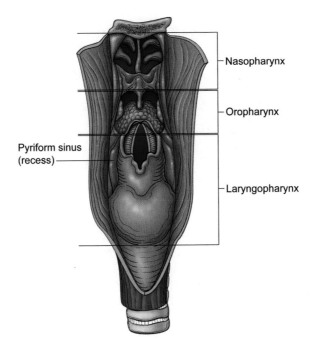

Pyriform sinus
(recess)

Nasopharynx

Oropharynx

Laryngopharynx

Fig. 1.9 The pharynx (posterior)

sagittal and posterior views of the pharynx and should make it easier to visualize this structure. In a normal conscious patient, the gag reflex may be elicited by stimulating the posterior pharyngeal wall. The afferent and efferent limbs of this reflex are mediated through the glossopharyngeal (IX) and vagus (X) nerves.

Prevertebral Fascia

The prevertebral fascia extends from the base of the skull down to the third thoracic vertebra, where it continues as the anterior longitudinal ligament. It also extends laterally as the axillary sheath (Fig. 1.10). Abscess formation, hemorrhage following trauma, or tumor growth may cause swelling in this area and lead to symptoms of airway obstruction.

Retropharyngeal Space

The retropharyngeal space (RPS) is a potential space lying between the prevertebral fascia and the buccopharyngeal fascia, posterior to the pharynx in the midline (see Fig. 1.10). It is confined above by the base of the skull and inferiorly by the superior mediastinum. The normal contents of the RPS are lymph nodes and fat.

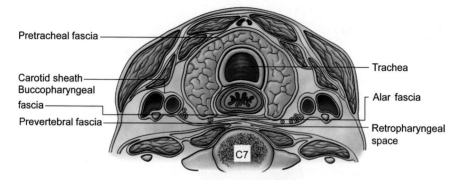

Pretracheal fascia

Carotid sheath
Buccopharyngeal
fascia
Prevertebral fascia

Trachea

Alar fascia

Retropharyngeal
space

C7

Fig. 1.10 Transection of the neck at the level of C.7

Pus from infected teeth can enter this space and reach the thorax. Infectious material may penetrate the prevertebral fascia and enter the RPS causing difficulty swallowing and airway obstruction. Tumors may also invade this space and compromise the airway. It is very difficult to access the RPS clinically; therefore, we are very dependent on imaging techniques (CT and MR) to make a diagnosis of airway obstruction caused by infection or tumor in this space.[4]

Larynx

The larynx is a boxlike structure situated in the anterior portion of the neck and lies between C3 and C6 in the adult. The larynx is shorter in women and children and is situated at a slightly higher level. It occupies a volume of 4–5 cc in adults and is made up of cartilages, ligaments, muscles, mucous membranes, nerves, blood vessels, and lymphatics. The average length of the larynx is 44 mm in the male and 36 mm in the female. The average antero-posterior diameter is 36 mm in the male and 26 in the female and the average transverse diameter is 36 mm in the male and 26 mm in the female.

   The larynx is one of the most powerful sphincters in the body and is an important component of the airway. Functionally, the larynx was designed as a protective valve to prevent food and other foreign substances from entering the respiratory tract. With evolution, the larynx became a highly sophisticated organ of speech when used in combination with the lips, the tongue and the mouth and is one of the distinguishing features of mankind separating us from other primates. The voice change in males occurs at puberty in most cases when the cartilages become larger. The "adam's apple" is more prominent in males following puberty because the angle made between the thyroid laminae is smaller in males and the antero-posterior diameter of the laminae is greater. This gender difference is usually evident by the 16th year.

   Fractures of the larynx may occur during various sporting activities including boxing, karate, kick boxing, and other major contact sports. This injury may also occur in ice hockey, baseball, or cricket and during attempted strangulation from any cause. It may also occur from compression by a seat belt following motor vehicle accidents.

The symptoms and signs of a fractured larynx include: laryngeal distortion, hoarseness, aphonia, aberrant vocalization, airway obstruction, choking, cyanosis, and death.

Laryngeal Cartilages

The larynx consists of three single cartilages (the epiglottis, the thyroid, and the cricoid); and three paired cartilages (the arytenoids, the corniculates, and the cuneiforms).

Single Cartilages

Epiglottis

The epiglottis, a well-known landmark to those performing tracheal intubation, is shaped like a leaf (see Fig. 1.5). At its lower end, it is attached to the thyroid carti-lage by the thyroepiglottic ligament. Its upper, rounded part is free and lies poste-rior to the tongue, and is attached by the median glossoepiglottic ligament. The epiglottis is attached to the hyoid bone anteriorly by the hyoepiglottic ligament. Small depressions on either side of this ligament are referred to as the valleculae. There is a recognizable bulge in the midportion of the posterior aspect of the epi-glottis called the tubercle (Fig. 1.11). During swallowing, as the laryngeal muscles contract, the downward movement of the epiglottis and the closure and upward movement of the glottis prevent food from entering the larynx. When the epiglottis becomes acutely inflamed and swollen (in association with acute epiglottitis), life-threatening airway obstruction may occur. The epiglottis has no function in the process of swallowing, breathing or phonation.

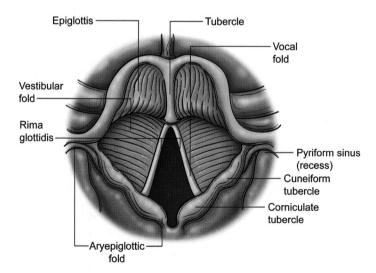

Fig. 1.11 The Larynx (superior)

Thyroid Cartilage

The thyroid cartilage (Fig. 1.12) is a shieldlike structure best visualized diagram-matically. Anteriorly, the two plates come together to form a notch that is more prominent in men than in women. At the posterior aspect of each lamina there are horns on the superior and inferior aspects. The inferior horn has a circular facet that allows it to articulate with the cricoid cartilage.

Cricoid Cartilage

The cricoid cartilage is shaped like a signet ring, with the bulky portion placed posteriorly (Fig. 1.13). It has articular facets for its attachment with the thyroid cartilage and the arytenoids. It is separated from the thyroid cartilage by the crico-thyroid ligament, or membrane.

    The inferior portion of the thyroid cartilage is connected to the superior border of the cricoid cartilage by the cricothyroid ligament. In acute airway obstruction,

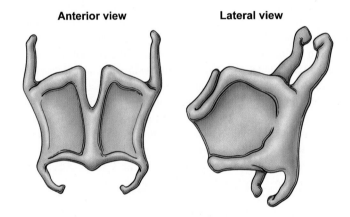

Fig. 1.12 Thyroid cartilage

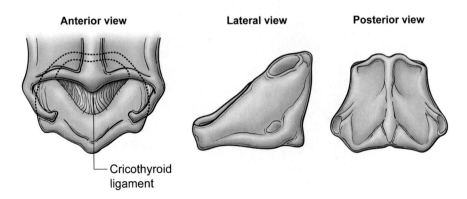

Fig. 1.13 The cricoid cartilage and cricothyroid ligament (membrane)

the cricothyroid membrane may be penetrated with a needle, knife, or tube and connected to an oxygen source. This procedure is called cricothyrotomy and is usually the first surgical procedure performed to relieve asphyxiation. Downward pressure on the cricoid cartilage is required to prevent passive regurgitation of gastric contents during induction of anesthesia in nonfasting patients and in emergency situations. This is also known as Sellick's maneuver.[5]

The Paired Cartilages

Arytenoids, Corniculates and the Cuneiforms

The paired cartilages include: the arytenoids, the corniculates, and the cuneiform cartilages. The arytenoids are triangular structures (Fig. 1.14) located on the postero-superior aspect of the cricoid cartilage. The corniculate cartilages articulate with the superior aspect of the arytenoids (Fig. 1.15). The cuneiform cartilages are small round shaped structures and are embedded in the aryepiglottic fold or ligament bilaterally (see Fig. 1.11).

The Hyoid Bone

The hyoid bone, which is not part of the larynx proper, is a horseshoe shaped structure located in the central part of the neck and lies between the floor of the mouth and the thyroid cartilage (Fig. 1.16). It has no bony articulation. It is connected to the thyroid cartilage by the thyrohyoid ligament anterolaterally. The greater horn or cornu of the hyoid bone articulates with the superior horn of the thyroid cartilage posteriorly (Figs. 1.15. and 1.17). It is connected to the floor of the mouth, the base of the skull and the cervical spine by a series of muscles and ligaments. Calcification of the stylohyoid ligaments bilaterally has been associated with difficult tracheal intubation.[6] The hyoid bone is not easily fractured and when fractures occur strangulation is usually suspected. The hyoid bone is an important structure in relation to airway management.

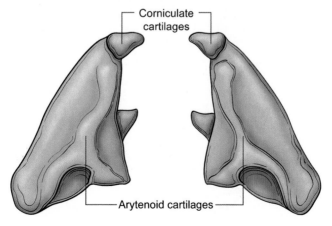

Fig. 1.14 The arytenoids and corniculates

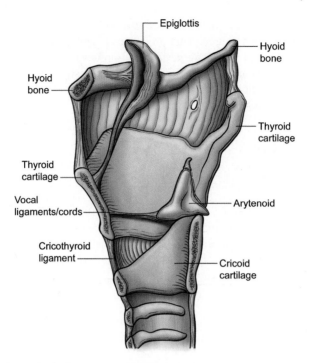

Fig. 1.15 The larynx (sagittal)

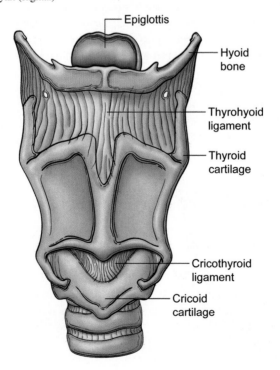

Fig. 1.16 The larynx (anterior)

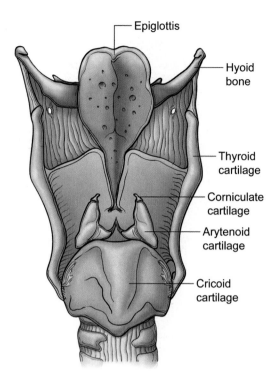

Fig. 1.17 The larynx (posterior)

Laryngeal Cavity

The space between the true vocal cords and the arytenoid cartilages is referred to as the rima glottidis. This landmark divides the larynx into two parts: the upper compartment extends from the laryngeal outlet to the vocal cords and contains the vestibular folds and the sinus of the larynx; the lower compartment extends from the vocal cords to the upper portion of the trachea. The terms *glottis* and *rima glottidis* are often used interchangeably. The difference is that the *glottis* is an all encompassing term which includes the vocal and vestibular folds including the opening into the larynx. The actual space between the true vocal cords is the *rima glottidis* (Fig. 1.18).

Piriform Sinus (Recess or Fossa)

There is a space between the epiglottis and the aryepiglottic folds medially, and the hyoid bone, thyrohyoid ligament, and thyroid cartilage laterally, referred to as the piriform sinus, recess, or fossa (see Figs. 1.9 and 1.11). Occasionally, fish bones and other organic material may be entrapped in this space, giving rise to symptoms of dysphagia. Local anesthetic soaked pledgets may be inserted into the piriform sinus on each side to block the internal branch of the superior laryngeal nerve, using an angled forceps (Krause forceps).

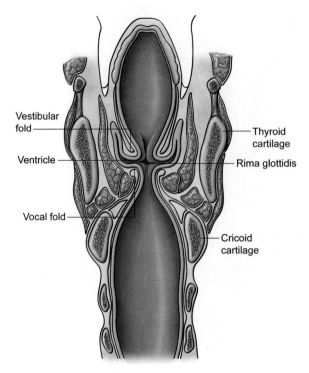

Fig. 1.18 The larynx (coronal)

Nerve Supply to the Larynx

The larynx is innervated by two branches of the vagus: the superior laryngeal and the recurrent laryngeal nerves.

Superior Laryngeal Nerve

The superior laryngeal nerve arises from the ganglion nodosum and descends inferiorly and medially to reach the internal side of the larynx. It communicates with the cervical sympathetics, passing between the greater horn of the hyoid bone and the superior horn of the thyroid cartilage, and divides into an external (motor) branch that descends to supply the cricothyroid muscle (Fig. 1.19) and an internal (sensory) branch that pierces the thyrohyoid membrane; it then divides into upper and lower branches that supply the mucous membrane of the base of the tongue, pharynx, epiglottis, and larynx.

Recurrent Laryngeal Nerve

The recurrent laryngeal nerve arises from the vagus nerve and loops around the subclavian artery on the right side and the aortic arch on the left side behind the ligamentum arteriosum. After ascending between the trachea and esophagus,

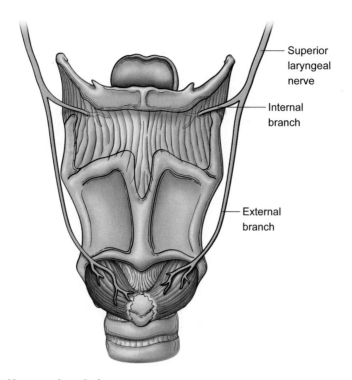

Superior
laryngeal
nerve

Internal
branch

External
branch

Fig. 1.19 Nerve supply to the larynx

it passes behind the thyroid gland and innervates all of the intrinsic muscles of the larynx except the cricothyroid. In addition, it supplies sensory branches to the mucous membrane of the larynx below the vocal cords.

In the event of bilateral recurrent laryngeal nerve damage (secondary to thyroidectomy, neoplasm, or trauma), the action of the superior laryngeal nerve is unopposed leading to varying degrees of airway obstruction. Complete paralysis of the recurrent laryngeal and superior laryngeal nerves simultaneously is characterized by a midway positioning of the vocal cords, often referred to as the cadaveric position, and frequently seen following the administration of neuromuscular blocking drugs. A reflexive, forceful contraction of all the laryngeal muscles, as commonly occurs when a foreign body lodges in the larynx is referred to as laryngospasm. Although laryngospasm normally serves a protective function, in such cases it may exacerbate an existing airway obstruction.

Action of the Cricothyroid Muscle and the Intrinsic Muscles of the Larynx

This will not be a complete description of the actions of the intrinsic muscles of the larynx. For a complete review refer to an otolaryngology text. Contraction of the

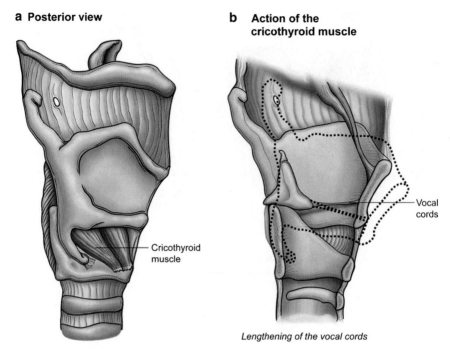

a Posterior view

b Action of the cricothyroid muscle

Cricothyroid muscle

Vocal cords

Lengthening of the vocal cords

Fig. 1.20 Anatomy (**a**) and action (**b**) of the cricothyroid muscle on the vocal cords

cricothyroid muscles results in a forward tilting of the thyroid cartilage on the cricoid, resulting in lengthening and increased tension on the vocal cords (Fig. 1.20a, b).

Contraction of the posterior cricoarytenoid muscle results in *abduction* of the vocal cords (Fig. 1.21a, b). Contraction of the lateral cricoarytenoids results in *adduction* of the vocal ligaments (Fig. 1.22a, b). The transverse and oblique muscles (see Fig. 1.21) also contribute to adduction.

Trachea and Bronchi

The trachea (Fig. 1.23) is a fibrocartilagenous, tubular structure, ranging between 10 and 15 cm long in adults, extending from the cricoid cartilage to the bronchial bifurcation. It has an outer diameter of 2.5 cm. On transverse section, it is shaped like the letter *D,* with the straight portion posterior. Structurally, it consists of 18–24 *C*-shaped cartilages joined by fibroelastic tissue and closed posteriorly by a membranous structure consisting of nonstriated muscle, named the trachealis. Approximately, one third of the trachea lies above the suprasternal notch and one third below. The isthmus of the thyroid gland usually lies over the 2nd and 3rd tracheal ring. Opinions vary about the preferred site of entering the trachea when performing a tracheotomy but the incision is usually made between the 2nd and 3rd or the 3rd and 4th tracheal ring where the isthmus of the thyroid is either displaced

a   Posterior view

**b   Action of the posterior
cricothyroid muscles**

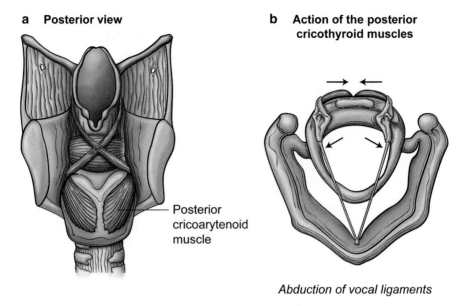

Posterior
cricoarytenoid
muscle

Abduction of vocal ligaments

Fig. 1.21 Anatomy (**a**) and action (**b**) of the posterior cricoarytenoid muscles on the vocal cords

a Lateral dissection

**b   Action of lateral
cricoarytenoid muscles**

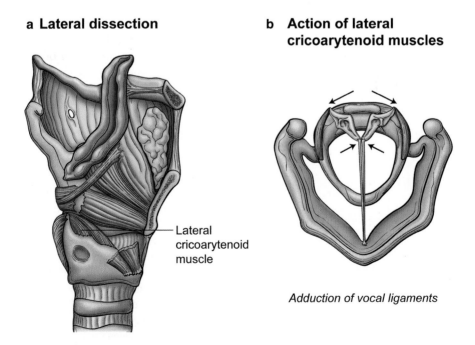

Lateral
cricoarytenoid
muscle

Adduction of vocal ligaments

Fig. 1.22 Anatomy (**a**) and action (**b**) of the lateral cricoarytenoid muscles on the vocal cords

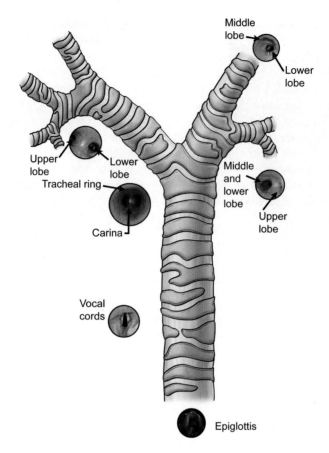

Fig. 1.23 Trachea and upper tracheobronchial tree

or divided at that level. The first ring of the trachea is never cut intentionally as tracheal stricture frequently occurs when incisions are made at that level.

Main Divisions of the Bronchial Tree

At about the level of the fifth thoracic vertebra, the trachea bifurcates into right and left mainstem bronchi. The right mainstem bronchus appears (more than the left) to be a vertical continuation of the trachea; furthermore, the right upper lobe bronchus has its origin about 2 cm from the carina, compared to the left, which arises about 5 cm from the carina. For these reasons, aspiration of food, liquids, or foreign bodies is far more likely to occur on the right side, and right mainstem intubations are far more common than left (see Fig. 1.23). From this illustration, one can see the initial branching-off of the tracheobronchial tree and includes a fiberoptic view of the larynx, trachea, mainstem bronchi and first division of the mainstem bronchi and photographs the entry into the various subdivisions of the bronchi. The right upper lobe bronchus (RUB) leaves the main stem, pointing in a lateral direction (3 o'clock), measures about 2 cm and gives off three branches: anterior, apical, and posterior. Bronchus intermedius extends from the lower end of the origin of the RUB to the take off of the middle lobe orifice which comes off bronchus intermedius, anteriorly (12 o'clock). It has two branches, lateral and medial. The right lower lobe bronchus is the continuation of bronchus intermedius and gives off five branches. The left main stem bronchus exits the trachea at an angle of about 40°. It divides into two main branches, left upper and left lower bronchi. The left upper bronchus divides into three subdivisions, apical, anterior and posterior and the left lower branch divides into superior and inferior lingular branches. The left lower lobe bronchus divides into five separate branches: superior, anterior basal, medial basal, lateral basal and posterior basal.

Comparative Anatomy of the Adult and Infant Airways

Before discussing how the anatomy of the airway varies with age, we should first define what we mean by "adult," "child," and "infant." An adult is an individual aged 16 or older, a child is between the ages of 1 and 8, and an infant is 1 year of

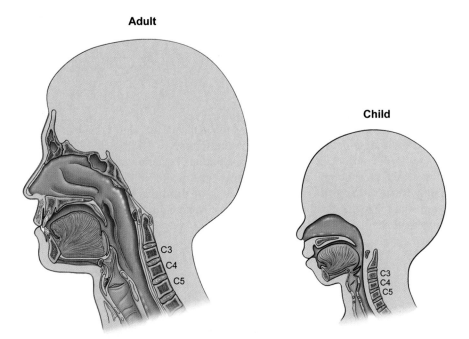

Fig. 1.24 Comparison of the adult and infant airways

age or less. At age 8, the larynx of the child closely resembles that of an adult except in size.

Any clinician involved in the management of airway problems should be cognizant of the infant airway. The differences between the adult and infant airway are not all explained by the age-associated changes in airway diameter (Fig. 1.24). There are differences in structure and function as well as size, involving the head, nose, tongue, epiglottis, larynx, cricoid, trachea, and mainstem bronchi.[7, 8]

Head

In proportion to the rest of the body, the infant's head is much larger than the adult's. This is significant in that, in the absence of muscle tone, the weight of the infant's head forces the cervical spine to assume a more flexed position, which tends to induce airway obstruction.

Nose

The infant's nostrils are smaller in relation to the trachea than are the adult's. It is interesting to note that the infant is a compulsive nose breather during most of the first year of life. However, this is a functional difference rather than an anatomical one.

Tongue

The infant's tongue is proportionately larger than that of the adult's. Lack of muscle tone in the tongue and mandible allow the tongue to "fall back," obstructing the flow of air during inspiration and expiration. Posterior displacement of the tongue is the most common cause of airway obstruction in infants (as well as in adults). Respiratory efforts in the presence of diminished muscle tone tend to pull the tongue in a ball valve-like fashion over the airway, further contributing to obstruction.

Larynx

The larynx is situated at a higher level in relation to the cervical spine in infants (see Fig. 1.24). At birth, the rima glottidis lies at the level of the interspace between the third and fourth cervical vertebrae. Upon reaching adulthood, it lies one vertebra lower. The infant's vocal cords are concave and have an anteroinferior incline. In adults, the vocal cords are less concave and lie more horizontally.

Cricoid Cartilage

The airway of the infant is narrowest at the level of the cricoid cartilage. In contrast, the adult airway is narrowest at the rima glottidis.

Epiglottis

The epiglottis in infants is remarkably different from that in adults. It is relatively longer, more omega shaped (Ω), and less flexible. In infants, the hyoid bone is firmly attached to the thyroid cartilage and tends to push the base of the tongue and epiglottis toward the pharyngeal cavity; consequently, the epiglottis has a much more horizontal lie than in adults.

Trachea and Mainstem Bronchi

The major conducting airways are both narrower and shorter in infants, leaving less room for error in positioning endotracheal tubes. The trachea of a premature infant may be as short as 2.0 cm. In infants, the bifurcation of the trachea (into right and left mainstem bronchi) projects at an angle of about 30° from the tracheal axis, whereas the left mainstem bronchus projects at an angle of about 47°.[9, 10] In adults, the angle between the right mainstem bronchus and tracheal axis is more acute[11] (Fig. 1.25). Therefore, endotracheal tubes inserted too far into the trachea are more likely to enter the right mainstem bronchus than the left in both adults and infants.

   The salient anatomical differences between the infant and adult airways are summarized as follows. The infant's larynx is situated at a much higher level than the adult's. The infant's tongue is relatively larger, and the epiglottis is omega shaped, longer, and stiffer. The narrowest part of the infant's laryngeal airway is at the level of the cricoid cartilage, whereas that of the adult is at the rima glottidis. In infants, the right mainstem bronchus is less vertical than in adults. The most significant difference between the adult larynx and the infant larynx is that the overall diameter of the adult's airway is 10–12 mm wider than that of a newborn. If the internal diameter of a neonate's larynx measures 4 mm at the level of the cricoid cartilage, a 1-mm circumferential reduction in this diameter (caused by either trauma or infection) will reduce the overall cross-sectional area of the

Adult
2.5 cm
10-15 cm
2 cm
5 cm
20-30°
40° male
50° female
Infant
30°
47°

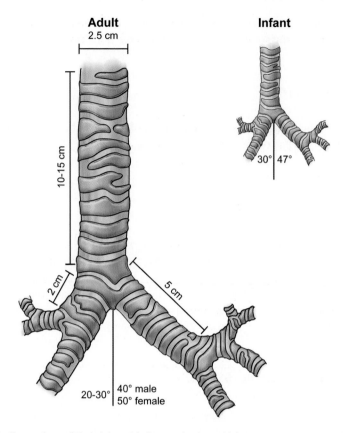

Fig. 1.25 Comparison of the adult and infant tracheobronchial trees

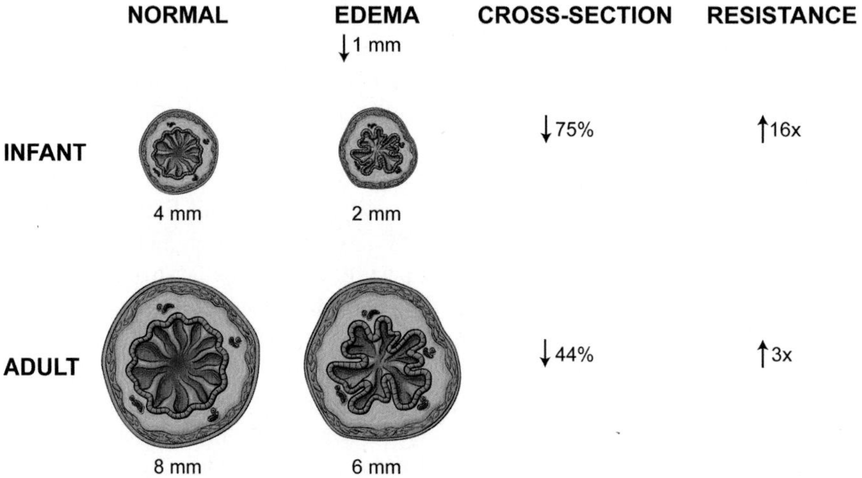

NORMAL
EDEMA
↓1 mm
CROSS-SECTION
RESISTANCE
INFANT
4 mm
2 mm
↓75%
↑16x
ADULT
8 mm
6 mm
↓44%
↑3x

Fig. 1.26 Comparative effects of airway edema in the adult and infant

airway by approximately 75%. A similar reduction in the diameter of the adult airway will reduce the cross-sectional area by about 44% (Fig. 1.26).[12]

Summary

The basics of anatomy presented in this chapter should serve as a foundation for understanding and learning how to manage airway problems.

References

1. Ferguson CF. Pediatric otolaryngology. In: Kendig EL, ed. *Disorders of the Respiratory Tract in Children*. 2nd ed. Philadelphia: WB Saunders; 1972.
2. Benumof JL, Sniderson LJ. *Anesthesia and Perioperative Complications*. 2nd ed. St. Louis: Mosby; 1999:5.
3. Jones DL, Cohle SD. Unanticipated difficult airway secondary to lingual tonsillar hyperplasia. *Anesth Analg*. 1993;77:1285.
4. Davis WL, Harnsberger HR, Smoker WR, et al. Retropharyngeal space: evaluation of normal anatomy and diseases with CT and MR imaging. *Radiology*. 1990;174:59–64.
5. Sellick BA. Cricoid pressure to control regurgitation of stomach contents during induction of anaesthesia. *Lancet*. 1961;2:404.
6. Walls RD, Finucane BT. Difficult intubation associated with calcified stylohyoid ligament. *Anaesth Intensive Care*. 1990;18:110–126.
7. Eckenhoff JE. Some anatomic considerations for the larynx influencing endotracheal anesthesia. *Anesthesiology*. 1951;12:407.
8. Smith RM. *Anesthesiology for infants and children*. 4th ed. St. Louis: CV Mosby; 1980.
9. Kubota Y, Toyoda Y, Nagata N, et al. Tracheobronchial angles in infants and children. *Anesthesiology*. 1986;64:374–376.
10. Brown TCK, Fisk GC. *Anesthesia for Children*. 1st ed. Oxford: Blackwell; 1979:3.
11. Collins VJ. *Principles of Anesthesiology*. Philadelphia: Lea & Febiger; 1966:351.
12. Ryan JF, Todres ID, Cote CJ. *A Practice of Anesthesia for Infants and Children*. New York: Grune & Stratton Inc.; 1986:39.

Suggested Reading

Standring S. *Gray's Anatomy*. 40th ed. Edinburgh, New York: Elsevier, Churchill Livingstone; 2008.
Ellis FH, McLarty M. *Anatomy for Anesthetists*. 2nd ed. Edinburgh: Blackwell; 1969.
Lee JA. *A Synopsis of Anesthesia*. 7th ed. Baltimore: Williams & Wilkins; 1973.
Moore KL, Oriented C. *Anatomy*. 3rd ed. Baltimore: Williams and Wilkins; 1992.
Ovassapian A. *Fiberoptic Airway Endoscopy in Anesthesia and Critical Care*. 1st ed. New York: Rave Press; 1990.
Netter FH. *Atlas of Human Anatomy*. 4th ed. Philadelphia: Saunders, Elsevier; 2006.

Chapter 2
Evaluation of the Airway

Contents

B.T. Finucane et al., *Principles of Airway Management*,
DOI 10.1007/978-0-387-09558-5_2, © Springer Science+Business Media, LLC 2011

Introduction

The safety of anesthesia is predicated on anticipating difficulties in advance instead of reacting to them when they occur. Of course, we do not always have the luxury of time when dealing with unconscious patients. The manner in which we handle the airway is central to the safety of anesthesia because most of the serious problems we encounter in anesthesia usually have an airway component.

What exactly is a "difficult airway"? To many of us a "difficult airway" is one that we cannot tracheally intubate. In reality, a truly difficult airway is one that prevents us from delivering that vital gas, oxygen, to the lungs. So before we even think about difficulties placing an endotracheal tube in the airway, we must ask a more fundamental question. "Will I be able to maintain this patient's airway when he is unconscious and if not can I at least maintain oxygenation?" A thorough evaluation of the airway allows us to estimate that risk in the vast majority of patients, but not all. For example, a patient may have a perfectly normal anatomical airway by assessment and still be very difficult to oxygenate and ventilate because of severe bronchospasm or an undetected foreign body in the airway. Fortunately, these situations are rare, but if they do occur we should be able to make the diagnosis promptly and institute therapy immediately. Therefore, our whole philosophy about airway assessment must change. Before we even render a patient unconscious, we must ask ourselves the following four questions:

1. Will I be able to oxygenate/ventilate this patient using a mask?
2. Will I be able to place a supraglottic device in this patient if required?
3. Will I be able to tracheally intubate this patient should the need arise?
4. Do I have access to this patient's trachea if a surgical airway is required?

The only way we can accurately answer these questions is if we do a thorough assessment of the airway. Even in a dire emergency, we should be able to answer these questions. Fortunately, we will have time to do a proper assessment in most of the cases. Despite the importance of this task, we do not do this very well in many cases and in this text we are appealing to those responsible for airway management to spend more time, not just evaluating the airway, but also recording the findings because quite often in modern practice the person performing the evaluation is not the person assigned to perform the procedure. This unavoidable arrangement results in less careful scrutiny of the airway during the initial evaluation because there is less accountability. We also appreciate that not all airway emergencies involve anesthesia.

Three mechanisms of injury account for most serious airway complications: esophageal intubation, failure to ventilate, and difficult intubation – with difficult intubation playing a role in all three.[1] The vast majority of difficult intubations (98% or more) may be anticipated by performing a thorough evaluation of the airway in advance.[2, 3] Nevertheless, many clinicians pay little attention to this important task and confine their examination of the airway to a cursory examination of the mouth and teeth. The information in this chapter will allow you to anticipate with a reasonable degree of accuracy when airway management may be difficult.

The Normal/Abnormal Airway

There are a number of wide-ranging characteristics and measurements in adults that constitute a "normal airway" (Box 2.1). When patients with these features present for airway management, problems do not usually occur. There are also a number of features that make up the "difficult airway" (Box 2.2), and when patients with these characteristics present for airway management, problems frequently occur.

Predictive Tests for Difficult Intubation

Anesthesiologists are constantly seeking ways to develop a foolproof system for predicting difficult intubation. The Mallampati test has undeserved status as a reliable predictor of difficult intubation. In reality, a Mallampati class III airway only has a positive predictive value of 21% for laryngoscopy grades 3 and 4 combined, and only 4.7% for laryngoscopy grade 4 alone. Therefore, if we relied solely on this test to predict difficult intubation, we would be performing a considerable number of unnecessary

---

Box 2.1 Factors Characterizing the Normal Airway in Adolescents and Adults

1. History of one or more easy intubations without sequelae
2. Normal appearing face with "regular" features
3. Normal clear voice
4. Absence of scars, burns, swelling, infection, tumor, or hematoma; no history of radiation therapy to head or neck
5. Ability to lie supine asymptomatically; no history of snoring or sleep apnea
6. Patent nares
7. Ability to open the mouth widely (minimum of 4 cm or three fingers held vertically in the mouth) with good TMJ function
8. Mallampati/Samsoon class I (i.e., with patient sitting up straight, opening mouth as wide as possible, with protruding tongue; the uvula, posterior pharyngeal wall, entire tonsillar pillars, and fauces can be seen)
9. At least 6.5 cm (three finger-breadths) from tip of mandible to thyroid notch with neck extended
10. At least 9 cm from symphysis of mandible to mandibular angle
11. Slender supple neck without masses; full range of neck motion
12. Larynx movable with swallowing and manually movable laterally (about 1.5 cm on each side)
13. Slender to moderate body build
14. Ability to maximally extend the atlantooccipital joint (normal extension is 35°)
15. Airway appears normal in profile

Box 2.2 Signs Indicative of an Abnormal Airway

 1. Trauma, deformity; burns, radiation therapy, infection, swelling; hema-
    toma of the face, mouth, pharynx, larynx, and/or neck
 2. Stridor or "air hunger"
 3. Hoarseness or "underwater" voice
 4. Intolerance of the supine position
 5. Mandibular abnormality:

    (a) Decreased mobility or inability to open the mouth at least three
        finger-breadths
    (b) Micrognathia, receding chin:

        (i) Treacher Collins, Pierre Robin, other syndromes
        (ii) Less than 6 cm (three finger-breadths) from tip of the mandible
             to thyroid notch with neck in full extension (adolescents and
             adults)

    (c) Less than 9 cm from angle of the jaw to symphysis
    (d) Increased anterior or posterior mandibular depth

 6. Laryngeal abnormalities: fixation of the larynx to other structures of
    neck, hyoid, or floor of mouth
 7. Macroglossia
 8. Deep, narrow, high-arched oropharynx
 9. Protruding teeth
10. Mallampati/Samsoon classes III and IV (see Figs. 5.6 and 5.7); inability
    to visualize the posterior oropharyngeal structures (tonsillar fossae,
    pillars, uvula) on voluntary protrusion of the tongue with mouth wide
    open and the patient seated
11. Neck abnormalities:

    (a) Short and thick
    (b) Decreased range of motion (arthritis, spondylitis, disk disease)
    (c) Fracture (possibility of subluxation)
    (d) Obvious trauma

12. Thoracoabdominal abnormalities:

    (a) Kyphoscoliosis
    (b) Prominent chest or large breasts
    (c) Morbid obesity
    (d) Term or near-term pregnancy

13. Age between 40 and 59 years
14. Gender (male)
15. Snoring and sleep apnea syndrome

awake intubations. It may seem unreasonable to single out this one test; however, in reality anesthesiologists have given enormous credence to this test. The truth, of course, is that most of the other tests we use for this purpose are equally disappointing when positive predictive value is measured, with the exception of a history of difficult intubation.

How reliable is our predictability if we use a combination of tests? Common sense tells us that if we use more than one test to predict difficult intubation, our chances of predicting difficulty increase. However, one of the problems noted is that there is very poor interobservational reliability for many of the tests that we commonly use to predict difficult intubation. A paper by El-Ganzouri et al.[4] demonstrated increased accuracy predicting difficult intubation when one used objective airway risk criteria. They prospectively studied 10,507 patients presenting for intubation under general anesthesia.

Risk factors for difficult intubation include the following:

- Mouth opening less than 4 cm
- Thyromental distance less than 6 cm
- Mallampati Class III or higher
- Neck movement less than 80%
- Inability to advance the mandible (prognathism)
- Body weight greater than 110 kg
- Positive history of difficult intubation

Following induction of anesthesia, the laryngeal view at laryngoscopy was graded. Poor intubating conditions were noted in 107 cases (1%). Logistic regression identified all seven criteria as *independent* predictors of difficulty. A composite airway risk index, as well as a simplified risk weighting system, revealed a higher predictive value for grade 4 laryngoscopy (Table 2.1). While it may be impractical to perform these calculations on all cases, they certainly have potential for the future. The real message here is that multiple abnormal tests predicting difficult intubation are better than any single test.

Table 2.1 Reliability of risk factors in predicting difficult intubation

Risk factor	LG	Sensitivity (%)	Specificity (%)
Mouth opening <4 cm	≥III	26.3	94.8
	IV	46.7	93.9
Thyromental distance <6.0 cm	≥III	7.0	99.2
	IV	16.8	99.0
Mallampati class III	≥III	44.7	89.0
	IV	59.8	87.4
Neck movement <80°	≥III	10.4	98.4
	IV	16.8	97.9
Inability to prognath	≥III	16.5	95.8
	IV	26.2	95.3
Body weight >110 kg	≥III	11.1	94.6
	IV	13.1	94.3
Positive history of difficult intubation	≥III	4.5	99.8
	IV	9.3	99.7

Source: Data from El-Ganzouri[4] LG = Laryngoscopy grade (see figures 2.2 and 2.8)

Elective Intubation

Most elective intubations are performed by anesthetists or anesthesiologists on patients presenting for elective surgery. Occasionally, patients will be tracheally intubated on an elective basis on the ward. In all elective intubations, an assessment of the patient's overall medical status is advised.

The technique of endotracheal intubation depends heavily on the ability to manipulate the cervical spine, the atlantooccipital joint, the mandible, oral soft tissues, neck, and hyoid bone. Therefore, any disease, congenital or acquired, that interferes with the mobility of these structures can create difficulties that prevent one from seeing the larynx during direct laryngoscopy. The same factors apply to successful nasal intubation, but in addition, patency of the nasal passages is required. It should also be remembered that the ability to see the larynx does not always ensure a successful intubation. Occasionally, abnormal dentition or obstruction by other, more proximal, structures may impair one's ability to place an endotracheal tube between the vocal cords. Unrecognized pathology in the vicinity of the larynx may impede the passage of an endotracheal tube large enough to allow adequate ventilation. This background information should be kept in mind when evaluating patients for tracheal intubation.

History Pertinent to Elective Airway Management

Patients should be specifically questioned about:

- Previous airway interventions (review old records whenever possible)
- Dental problems (bridges, caps, fillings, appliances, loose teeth)
- Respiratory disease (snoring, sleep apnea syndrome, smoking, coughing, sputum production, and wheezing)
- Arthritis (temporomandibular joint [TMJ] disease, ankylosing spondylitis, osteoarthritis, and rheumatoid arthritis)
- Clotting abnormalities (especially before nasal intubation)
- A history of gastroesophageal reflux disease (GERD)
- Congenital abnormalities and syndromes (especially those involving the head, face, and neck)
- Type I diabetes mellitus

Diabetes Mellitus

It has been estimated[5] that the incidence of difficult intubation is about ten times higher in patients suffering from long-term diabetes mellitus than in normal healthy patients. The limited joint mobility syndrome occurs in 30–40% of insulin-dependent diabetics and is thought to be due to glycosylation of tissue proteins that occurs in patients with chronic hyperglycemia.[6]

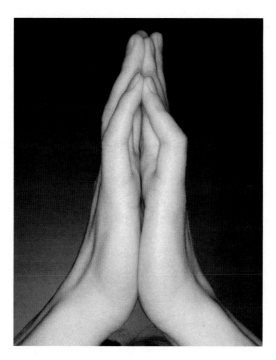

Fig. 2.1 Hands of a young diabetic woman in the "prayer sign" position

Limited joint mobility is best seen when a diabetic patient's hands assume the "prayer sign" position (Fig. 2.1). The patient typically is unable to straighten the interphalangeal joints of the fourth and fifth fingers. Another way of demonstrating this deficiency is to obtain palm print scores on patients with diabetes. To do this, the palm of the hand is stained with black ink and an imprint is made on white paper. Patients with the abnormality have deficient palm prints. It has been postulated that the same process affects the cervical spine, TMJ, and larynx. Nadal et al.[7] recently tested the validity of the palm print test in 83 adult diabetics scheduled for surgery under general anesthesia. They evaluated the airway using the Mallampati test, the thyromental distance, head extension, and the palm print. The sensitivity, specificity, and the positive predictive value were calculated for each test. The palm print test had the highest sensitivity (100%). The other three tests failed to detect 9 out of 13 difficult airways.

NPO Status

Elective intubation of the trachea frequently involves the administration of potent intravenous anesthetic agents and neuromuscular blocking drugs. For this reason, patients who have recently ingested solid food and liquids are at considerable risk when airway intervention is performed in the presence of a full stomach.

Therefore, it is incumbent upon you to ascertain the NPO status of the patient in advance. Elective intubation should not be performed if an *adult* patient has ingested a full meal within an 8 h period or a light meal within a 6 h period.[8] Patients with GERD have an additional risk factor when airway intervention is required.

Physical Examination

General

On first approaching patients presenting for elective intubation, it is advisable to make a general assessment – i.e., the level of consciousness, the facies and body habitus, the presence or absence of cyanosis, the posture, and pregnancy. Rose and Cohen[4] have shown that the incidence of difficult intubation increases: in males, in persons aged 40–59, and in the obese. A recent study from Denmark suggests that a high body mass index (BMI) may be a more appropriate predictor of difficult tracheal intubation than body weight alone.[9]

Facies

Particular attention should be paid to the facial appearance of the patient. A number of syndromes and disease states can make intubation difficult, many of which are associated with abnormal facial features, (e.g., Pierre–Robin, Treacher–Collins, Klippel–Feil, Apert's, Fetal Alcohol syndromes). A comprehensive list of these syndromes can be found in Stewart and Lerman's Manual of Pediatric Anesthesia.[10] Thus, when one encounters a patient with abnormal facial features, one should inquire about specific syndromes or consult a pediatrician. Schmitt et al. recently described a high incidence of difficult intubation in acromegalic patients. They studied 128 patients and reported difficulty in 26% of cases.[11]

Nose

The nose should be carefully examined when nasotracheal intubation is planned, observing the position of the nasal septum and whether or not polyps are present. Nasal intubation should be avoided, if possible, in the presence of a clotting abnormality, CSF leakage, nasal polyps, a history of epistaxis, or a basal skull fracture. The patency of each nostril can be tested by having the patient breathe forcefully through the unoccluded nostril. In many cases, one nostril will be more patent than the other.

Temporomandibular Joint

The ability to open the mouth may be limited by disease of the TMJ or by masseter spasm, or a combination of both. The function of the TMJ is complex, involving

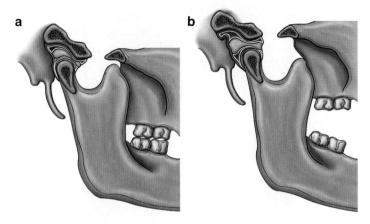

Fig. 2.2 Temporomandibular joint in closed (**a**) and open (**b**) positions. Note the rotation and translation of the condyle

articulation and movement between the mandible and cranium. The mandible may be depressed, elevated, or manipulated anteriorly, posteriorly, or laterally. There are two distinct components to this action, each contributing about 50% to the total. The first is a hinge-like movement of the condyle through the synovial cavity, accounting for the first 20 mm or so of opening, and the second is the forward displacement of the disk and condyle, accounting for an additional 25 mm or so[12] (Fig. 2.2a, b).

A number of conditions can affect TMJ function. Prominent among these are the arthritides (including rheumatoid arthritis, ankylosing spondylitis, psoriatic arthritis) and, most commonly, degenerative joint disease or osteoarthritis. TMJ function should be assessed in all patients presenting for endotracheal intubation. With the middle finger of each hand posterior and inferior to the patient's earlobes, place your index fingers just anterior to the tragus (Fig. 2.3) and instruct the patient to open widely. Two distinct movements should be felt[13]: the first is rotational, and the second involves advancement of the condylar head (Fig. 2.4). Listen and palpate for clicks and crepitus, both of which indicate joint dysfunction.

TMJ function may also be assessed by asking the patient to insert two or three fingers (of their own hand) held vertically, into the oral cavity in the midline (Fig. 2.5). Normal adults are capable of inserting at least three fingers, which corresponds to a range of mandibular opening between 40 and 60 mm.[14] Patients capable of inserting only two or fewer fingers are considered to have major limitations. If the maximal mandibular opening is less than 30 mm in the adult, oral surgeons suggest that significant TMJ dysfunction is present. If less than 25 mm, it is unlikely that the larynx will be visible using conventional laryngoscopy, since exposure of the larynx depends to a great extent upon the ability to move the mandible and soft tissues forward. If mouth opening is 20 mm or less, a Macintosh 3 or 4 blade will not fit in the mouth and therefore alternative methods of intubation are required (e.g., light wand, trach light, or fiberoptic-assisted intubation).

It is important to be able to distinguish between limited mouth opening due to muscle spasm and restriction due to joint disease. The former will respond to

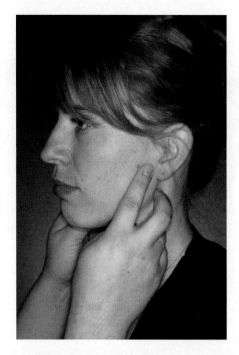

Fig. 2.3 Assessment of temporomandibular joint function

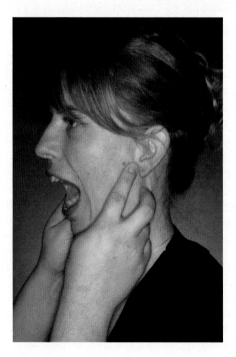

Fig. 2.4 Palpating an advanced condylar head

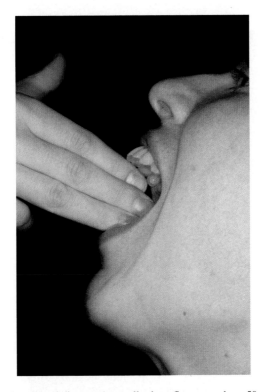

Fig. 2.5 Estimating interdental distance (normally three fingers or about 50 mm)

muscle relaxation, the latter will not. Patients with mandibular fractures have severely limited mouth opening because of trismus. If the fracture does not involve the TMJ, it is safe to induce general anesthesia with muscle relaxation in these patients in preparation for intubation. If there is some doubt, an intravenous or inhalational anesthetic should be administered first without a muscle relaxant, and the ability to open the mouth tested before committing to the use of neuromuscular blocking drugs. Caution should also be exercised when performing laryngoscopy in patients with TMJ disease. Vigorous mouth opening in the presence of profound muscle relaxation may add to existing damage to the TMJ. Avoid direct laryngoscopy in these cases whenever possible.

The *mandibular protrusion test* (Figs. 2.6a–c) can be performed when assessing temporomandibular function. This test is performed by asking the patient to advance the mandible as far as possible and the classification is as follows:

Class A: the lower incisors can be protruded beyond the upper incisors (Fig. 2.6a).
Class B: the lower incisors can be advanced only to the level of the upper incisors (Fig. 2.6b).
Class C: the lower incisors cannot reach the level of the upper incisors (Fig. 2.6c).

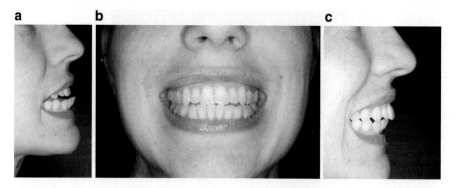

Fig. 2.6 Mandibular protrusion test. (**a**) Shows mandibular advancement beyond the upper teeth. (**b**) Shows that the mandible cannot be advanced beyond the upper teeth. (**c**) Shows that the lower incisors cannot reach the upper teeth

Impaired mandibular protrusion is associated with difficult laryngoscopy and difficult mask ventilation (DMV)[15, 16] Another variation of the *mandibular protrusion test* is the *upper lip bite test* recently mentioned by Khan et al.[17] This test measures the ability to bite (gently) the upper lip with the lower teeth and is another measure of difficult intubation.

Calder et al. stressed the importance of head and neck position when measuring mouth opening. They demonstrated that maximal mouth opening was achieved when craniocervical extension was 26° from the neutral position. This is an important observation because the Mallampati test requires the head to be in the neutral position.[18]

Lips

A cleft lip deformity can present problems during instrumentation of the airway, in that the laryngoscope blade tends to enter the cleft. Absence of the philtrum is a diagnostic feature of Fetal Alcohol syndrome,[19] which is associated with difficult intubation.

Oral Cavity

Before tracheal intubation, the state of oral hygiene should be assessed. Occasionally, foreign bodies, such as candy or chewing gum, may be hidden in the recesses of the oral cavity, especially in children.

Teeth

Upon examining the oral cavity, inspect the teeth. Long, protruding teeth (buck teeth) can restrict visualization of the airway. During direct laryngoscopy, damage is usually caused by excessive pressure on teeth that are already loose or repaired (e.g., fillings, caps, bridges, or other attachments). The incisors and canines are usually at greater risk, because the laryngoscope is generally inserted in close proximity to these teeth.

Experience is a major factor determining the frequency of damage to the teeth. A number of dental accidents occur when teaching novices airway management. Experienced laryngoscopists exert little if any pressure on the upper teeth, unless they are protruding. Teeth can be injured by vigorous manipulation of oral airways. Dental damage occurring in association with anesthesiology procedures accounted for 24.8% of all litigations against St. Paul Fire and Marine Insurance Company between the years 1973 and 1978.[20] More recent data from a New Zealand study[21] confirm earlier observations that dental damage is still one of the most common reasons for complaints against anesthesiologists. A review of files from the Accident Compensation Corporation in New Zealand covering a 2-year period revealed 76 claims. The number of claims made by women was twice that by men. Most injuries occurred to teeth that had already been restored (60%) and, as expected, the upper central incisors were most commonly involved. The most common injury was fracture or displacement of a filling or crown during intubation. However, a significant number of incidents occurred during emergence from anesthesia, and many of these involved biting down on oral airways. A separate survey of dental damage associated with anesthesia in New Zealand revealed an incidence of 10.4 injuries per 1,000 cases, which was much greater than that reported to the Accident Compensation Corporation.

If patients are properly informed of potential dental problems, and reasonable care is taken during the procedure, the clinician is not considered liable if damage occurs. Davies[22] emphasized the importance of careful scrutiny of the dentition and recommended including a schematic diagram of the teeth on the evaluation sheet (Table 2.2). Careful documentation of the intervention is also important not just for medical–legal purposes, but also for subsequent interventions.

Patients presenting with loose or exfoliating teeth are at increased risk for aspiration or ingestion of teeth. Consequently, it is advisable to discuss the potential risks with the patient and seek permission to remove the tooth or teeth prior to intubation. Most patients are agreeable to this approach. Children frequently present for surgery with loose deciduous teeth, and the parents are usually quite willing to consent to a minor dental procedure while the child is anesthetized; also, an

Table 2.2 Dental chart

Right	Left
7,6,5,4,3,2,1	1,2,3,4,5,6,7
7,6,5,4,3,2,1	1,2,3,4,5,6,7

Schematic representation of anterior view of dentition with teeth numbered sequentially from midline. Indicate abnormalities as: *A* appliance; *B* bridge; *C* caps; *L* loose; *M* missing
Source: Modified with permission from Davies.[22]

unheralded visit from the "tooth fairy" tends to lessen the tension surrounding a hospital visit.

Having discussed the implications of the teeth with reference to intubation, it is appropriate to mention that the edentulous state is rarely associated with difficulty visualizing the airway. On the other hand, airway management using bag/valve/mask ventilation is usually more difficult under these circumstances because the normal contour of the face is distorted and collapsed and it is difficult to maintain a mask seal. The insertion of an oral airway usually allows more effective ventilation in the edentulous state.

There is a suggestion that bag/valve/mask ventilation may be facilitated in the presence of dentures. There now are some data supporting the idea that bag/valve/mask airway management is easier when dentures remain in place. Conlon et al.[23] convincingly demonstrated this observation in a clinical trial involving 165 patients. However, most patients are still required to remove dentures before entering the operating suite. Clearly, anything we can do to avoid respiratory embarrassment in our patients is strongly recommended. The removal of dentures preoperatively is the source of significant general embarrassment to most patients and is one of the most disturbing minor concerns patients face when coming to the operating room. We now have some data to support changing this convention, but like many issues in medicine, we are very slow to change our routines.

Tongue

Two features of the tongue may interfere with one's ability to visualize the larynx. One is its size in relation to the oral cavity, and the other is mobility. The tongue may be abnormally large and therefore occupy a greater proportion of the oropharynx or, conversely, be of normal size in an unusually small oropharynx. Mallampati[24] and Mallampati et al.[25] have studied the correlation between the ability to observe intraoral structures and the incidence of subsequent difficult intubation. The patient is instructed to sit erect with the head in neutral position, to open the mouth as widely as possible, and to protrude the tongue maximally. Samsoon and Young[26] modified the Mallampati classification as follows: the examiner sits opposite the patient at eye level and observes various intraoral structures using a flashlight:

Class   I: soft palate, tonsillar fauces, tonsillar pillars, and uvula visualized
Class II: soft palate, tonsillar fauces, and uvula visualized
Class III: soft palate and base of uvula visualized
Class IV: soft palate not visualized (Fig. 2.7)

The results of the Mallampati test vary depending on whether the patient is asked to phonate during the examination or not. The specificity of the test increases with pho-nation, but the number of false negatives also increases.[27] The view of the oropharyn-geal structures improves significantly with phonation.[28] The results of the Mallampati test also vary depending on the position of the patient during the examination, but not consistently. Lewis et al.[29] recommend that the Mallampati test be performed in the sitting position, with the head and neck in full extension and with the tongue

Class 0   Class I   Class II   Class III   Class IV

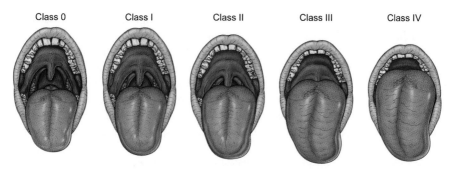

Fig. 2.7 Classification of pharyngeal structures from 0 to IV

Grade I   Grade II   Grade III   Grade IV

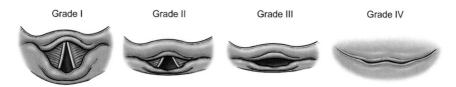

Fig. 2.8 Grading of laryngoscopy view based on Cormack and Lehane's classification[28]

protruded with the patient phonating. A recent publication by Ezri et al. refers to a Class 0 airway.[30] While performing the Mallampati test, it is possible to see the epiglottis in a small percentage of patients. This is not necessarily a predictor of easy laryngoscopy. In some of these cases, the epiglottis is elongated and floppy which may create difficulty when attempting to expose the larynx,[31] especially with the Macintosh blade. In general, exposure of the airway with a Macintosh blade is easy in Class I and II airways, but often difficult in Class III or IV airways. It should be remembered, however, that this classification is only a guideline and cannot be relied upon to be the sole predictor of difficult intubations. Cohen et al.,[32] using Cormack and Lehane's[33] grading system for ease or difficulty of intubation (Fig. 2.8), compared the Mallampati classification with the actual grade observed during attempted laryngoscopy and found a high correlation at the extremes. Pilkington et al. showed that the Mallampati grade increased during pregnancy. They studied 242 pregnant patients. They performed the Mallampati test at 12 and 38 weeks gestation and showed that the number of grade 4 cases had increased by 34%. They speculated that the reason for the change in Mallampati grade was most likely fluid retention.[34] The incidence of failed intubation is reported to be three to ten times greater[24, 35] in obstetric patients compared with the general surgical population and the changing Mallampati score during pregnancy may partially explain this phenomenon.

The diseased tongue may also prevent one from visualizing the larynx – e.g., tumors tend to limit lingular mobility and thus one's ability to expose the larynx. The presence of lingual tonsillar tissue can also create unexpected difficulty with intubation, resulting in catastrophic airway obstruction.[36] Ectopic thyroid tissue can be found at the base of the tongue and may bleed following laryngoscopy, leading to difficulties with the airway. This anomaly is rare, occurring in 1:100,000 cases.[37]

Tongue piercing has become popular among the younger generation. This now established trend may pose problems for those performing any form of airway management. Metal or plastic objects in the tongue may become detached and aspirated or ingested or plainly lost in the course of airway management or anesthesia. Pressure of the laryngoscope or oropharyngeal airway, placement of supraglottic devices, or endotracheal tubes may cause pressure necrosis and there is also a risk of electrocautery burns when metal rings or studs are used. For all of these reasons, it is advisable to remove *all* lingual hardware before any type of airway management. Patients should be informed of the risks and strongly encouraged to remove these objects before arrival in the operating room. Patients express concerns that the opening in the tongue closes in quickly when the tongue ring is removed. It is our understanding that a pierced tongue remains patent for several hours following removal. Epidural catheters have been threaded through the opening in the tongue to maintain patency in some cases. In summary, patients should be encouraged to remove tongue rings or studs before arrival in the operating room.[38, 39]

Mandible and Floor of Mouth

The optimal position for exposure of the larynx when using a Macintosh laryngoscope is attained by flexing the neck and extending the atlantooccipital joint.[40] In individuals with normal anatomy, this aligns the axes of the larynx, pharynx, and mouth so that they are almost parallel (Fig. 2.9). A number of factors may interfere

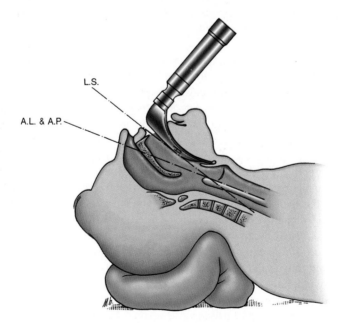

L.S.

A.L. & A.P.

Fig. 2.9 Final exposure

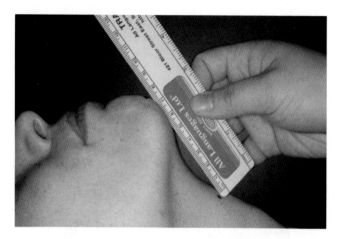

Fig. 2.10 Thyromental distance

with the ability to align these axes, such as a large or tethered tongue, a short mandible, protruding upper incisors, pathology in the floor of the mouth or neck, or reduced size of intra and submandibular space.

Two well-known congenital anomalies associated with mandibular shortening are the Treacher Collins and Pierre Robin syndromes. In these conditions, mandibular shortening is obvious and extreme. A number of individuals, however, will present with less obvious shortening of the mandible. Two very simple measurements that can be made at the bedside are the *thyromental distance*, which should exceed 6.5 cm in adults when the atlantooccipital is fully extended[41] (Fig. 2.10), and the *mandibular angle-mental symphysis distances*, which should be at least 9 cm in adults (Fig. 2.11). Al Ramadhani et al.[42] recently published a report suggesting that the *sternomental distance* was a useful, sole predictor of difficult intubation in obstetric patients. A *sternomental distance* of less than 13.5 cm was a predictor of difficult laryngoscopy in obstetric patients. To our knowledge, this claim has never been validated.

When the above measurements are reduced, one can expect difficulty exposing the larynx with a Macintosh laryngoscope. Few clinicians use a ruler; rather, they estimate the anterior mandibular space by placing their fingers horizontally beneath the patient's chin. In normal adults, the distance from the hyoid bone to the mandibular symphysis is at least three finger-breadths (Fig. 2.12). If it is two finger-breadths or less, the mandible is considered hypoplastic. A number of other measurements may be used, but they are of little practical value.

Neck, Cervical Spine, and Hyoid Bone

The neck and cervical spine should be carefully examined before intubation; the general neck contour should be inspected first. Obese patients with short, muscular, thick necks (which have a limited range of motion) are more difficult to intubate than

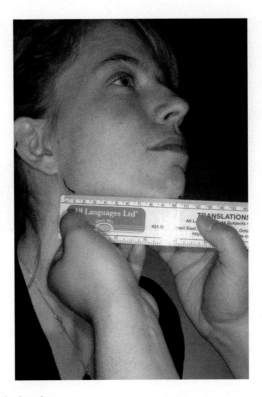

Fig. 2.11 Mandibular length

patients with normal, supple, or elongated necks. Some recent data suggest that neck circumference measurement may be a useful method of predicting difficult tracheal intubation in obese patients. However, on reading these papers the authors of this publication were not convinced that neck circumference measurement by itself was a useful indicator of difficult intubation in morbidly obese patients and so far has not been shown to be an independent risk factor in this group.[43, 44] Patients with Klippel–Feil syndrome (characterized by a reduced number of cervical vertebrae) present problems at intubation, since the neck is shorter and thus has impaired mobility.

During examination of the neck, the skin color should be noted. Pigmentation changes may indicate that a patient has had previous radiotherapy, which could have caused acute inflammatory changes with later scarring and fibrosis in the neck region. Particular attention should be paid to scars or masses in the neck and the overall texture of the neck tissues. Though almost all of these warrant some concern, any due to vascular injuries is particularly ominous because the airway could become occluded without warning when bleeding occurs. Previous tracheostomy scars should lead one to suspect tracheal stenosis and one should then consider selecting a smaller endotracheal tube. Always check for deviation of the trachea and evaluate the degree of tracheal mobility.

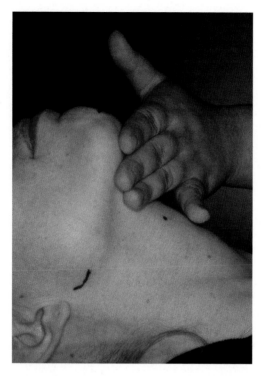

Fig. 2.12 Assessing the mandibular space

What role does the hyoid bone play in facilitating laryngoscopy? Chou et al.[45] radiographically studied the mandibulohyoid distance (MHD) in eleven patients with known difficult airways and compared measurements in 100 patients in the general population (control). They measured the vertical distance between the mandible and hyoid bone and showed that there was considerable variation among the general population, but MHD was significantly longer in those with problem airways compared to the control group and this difference was statistically significant. Mean values in males with difficult airways (rounded) were 34 mm compared to 21 mm in controls. The same was true in the female cohort. Females with difficult airways had a mean MHL of 26 vs. 15 mm in the control group. There was a very large variation in the MHD in both abnormal and control groups. The MHD is another measurement that can be added to an already lengthy list of measurements for predicting difficult laryngoscopy.

A significant number of patients in the general population develop calcification of the stylohyoid ligament, which may interfere with the ability to elevate the epiglottis during laryngoscopy using a Macintosh laryngoscope. There are a limited number of case reports in the literature on this topic.[46–48] The clinical sign that should lead one to suspect this problem is relative immobility of the hyoid bone or larynx. Laryngeal mobility should be routinely checked in all patients presenting for tracheal intubation.

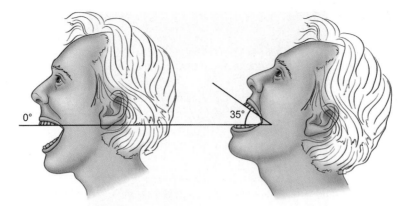

Fig. 2.13 An assessment of atlantooccipital translation can be made by estimating the angle traversed by the maxillary teeth when the neck is extended

Upon palpating the neck, one should assess the degree of mobility of the cervical spine and note any limitation in flexion or extension. The optimal position for endotracheal intubation is flexion of the cervical spine and extension of the head at the atlantooccipital joint. Consequently, flexion or extension deformities of the cervical spine associated with the arthritides may make direct laryngoscopy difficult or impossible. Keenan et al.[49] have reported that problems intubating patients with flexion and extension deformities of the cervical spine are not entirely due to failure to align the axes of the larynx, pharynx, and oral cavity. Rather, an additional factor is present, shortening of the cervical spine, which can cause laryngeal and tracheal deviation or forward buckling of the trachea, and this tends to force the larynx into an anterior position.

Under normal circumstances, 35° of cervical extension is possible at the atlantooccipital joint[50] (Fig. 2.13). This angle can be readily estimated at the bedside by asking the patient to sit straight up, with the head erect and the line of sight parallel to the ground. Then ask the patient to open wide. In this position, the occlusal surfaces of the upper teeth are horizontal to the ground. On extending the atlantooccipital joint, the angle created by moving the occlusal surfaces is estimated. Goniometry may be used to estimate the angle more accurately, but in practice the angle is estimated visually.

Vocal Quality

In listening for vocal quality, try to assess whether stridor is present and, if so, in which phase(s) of respiration it occurs. Stridor at rest in adults indicates that the airway diameter is reduced by about fifty percent. Lesions that are predominantly supraglottic are usually associated with inspiratory stridor, whereas subglottic lesions tend to cause both inspiratory and expiratory stridor.

Cardiorespiratory System

An examination of the airway is incomplete without a review of the cardiac and respiratory systems. This will give some measure of the patient's cardiorespiratory reserve. The minimum information required, even in emergencies, is the vital signs. Time permitting, all patients undergoing endotracheal intubation should have a thorough cardiorespiratory examination that includes a history and physical examination.

Patient History

Every patient should be questioned about coughs and colds and whether they are acute or chronic. A patient presenting with recent cold symptoms is not a good candidate for general anesthesia because inhalation agents tend to irritate the already inflamed mucosa of the larynx, trachea, and bronchi, and this can lead to laryngospasm, bronchospasm, and hypoxemia both intraoperatively and postoperatively.

If sputum is produced, its color and amount should be estimated. Green or yellow sputum or an increased production of sputum suggests acute infection, and elective procedures should be delayed until it has cleared. Each patient should be questioned about smoking and the number of pack-years recorded (the number of packs of cigarettes smoked times the number of years smoking). Smokers are more likely to develop laryngeal spasm during airway interventions. Patients should be questioned about dyspnea, orthopnea, or paroxysmal nocturnal dyspnea and an effort should be made to determine if it is of cardiac or respiratory origin.

Obesity has become a major problem in modern life and is often associated with Sleep Apnea Syndrome. Therefore, it is very important to inquire about snoring and signs of airway obstruction and apneic periods when sleeping. Clearly, this information cannot be gleaned without evidence from a relative or partner, therefore it is very important to include these individuals in the interview.

The patient should also be questioned about asthma; the severity of asthma can be estimated by the number of hospital admissions and the medications required. An asthmatic individual presenting for surgery and requiring steroid therapy has advanced disease and will need supplementation. Patients can usually apprise you of the current status of their asthma and can subjectively rate their chest tightness. Endotracheal intubation in the presence of wheezing often aggravates the situation and elective surgery should be delayed whenever possible. On the other hand, emergency intubation may be required for a patient suffering an acute asthmatic episode. In this case, if the patient presents with a clear history of asthma, they should be pretreated with aerosolized bronchodilators and beta-2 agonists whenever possible.

Information needs to be obtained about the patient's past medical and surgical history pertaining to the respiratory system (e.g., previous thoracotomy, pulmonary aspiration, pneumothorax).

Physical Examination

It is necessary to determine if the patient is cyanotic and, if so, whether the cyanosis is central or peripheral. The degree of cyanosis can be determined by performing pulse oximetry. Does the patient appear dyspneic? Record the respiratory rate and whether retractions are present. The normal adult will breathe 16–20 times per minute. Does the chest expand symmetrically? Is the patient wheezing? Look for scars indicating previous surgery or chest tubes. A patient with a history of chronic bronchitis and emphysema will often have an increased anterior–posterior (AP) diameter (barrel chest).

When palpating the chest, feel the larynx and trachea and determine if they are in the midline, deviated, or mobile. Check for lymph nodes in the supraclavicular fossae and axillae. Feel the apical beat and determine its position. Does the chest expand symmetrically? Percussion may help determine if atelectasis, pneumothorax, consolidation, or pleural effusion is present.

Listen carefully to the breath sounds over both lung fields. Are they normal? Are they equal on both sides? Are there any additional sounds? If rhonchi are present, are they coarse or high pitched, occasional or diffuse, unilateral or bilateral? Crepitations or rales are moist sounds that usually indicate pulmonary edema. They are often present in older patients, but usually clear on coughing. Tubular sounds or bronchial breathing may indicate pulmonary consolidation. Diminished or absent breath sounds may indicate pneumothorax, atelectasis, or pleural effusion, but are frequently due to obesity and emphysema.

Cardiovascular System

Endotracheal intubation may have a profound effect on the cardiovascular system, so a thorough history and physical examination is necessary in elective situations.

Patient History

Ask the patient about chest pain. If present, determine its exact site and radiation. Also try to determine its quality. You may suggest adjectives that assist the patient in identifying the pain (e.g., gripping, stabbing, burning, dull ache, or heartburn). Is it continuous or intermittent? Is it associated with respiration? What relieves the pain? Does it radiate? If so where? Is it associated with exercise? If so, what is the exercise tolerance? What brings it on and what relieves it? Are any medications being taken? Time spent eliciting details about chest pain is most important and should never be rushed.

If dyspnea is present, try to evaluate if it is of cardiac or respiratory origin. Does the patient have orthopnea or paroxysmal nocturnal dyspnea? Does he suffer from palpitations, fainting spells, or ankle edema? Patients with cardiac failure often complain of tiredness and weakness. Pertinent history includes questions about hypertension, previous myocardial infarction (MI), and rheumatic fever. Find out what cardiac medications the patient is taking. Record details about smoking and alcohol intake, both of which can cause serious cardiac disease.

Physical Examination

The physical examination will entail inspection, palpation auscultation, and electrocardiography.

Observe the patient for cyanosis. Look at the neck veins. Jugular venous distention may be an indication of cardiac dysfunction.

Palpate the apical beat and determine its exact location. In normal adults, it is in the fifth left intercostal space 3½ in. from the midline. Determine blood pressure and pulse rate.

Listen for heart sounds. The first heart sound is best heard at the apex, and the second at the base in the aortic area. Also listen for additional sounds. An S_3 gallop indicates left ventricular dysfunction, and an S_4 may be indicative of an atrial abnormality. Mitral murmurs are best heard at the apex, and aortic at the base. If murmurs are present, where are they best heard and do they radiate? Listen for carotid bruits.

A cardiac examination is incomplete unless the ECG is evaluated. Routine ECG is required in all patients with a history of cardiac disease or in patients who are 50 years of age or older.

Structured Approach

In 1991, Davies designed a systematic approach to airway evaluation using the acronym MOUTHS (Table 2.3). It is a quite useful approach and may encourage clinicians to pay more attention to this component of patient evaluation.

Table 2.3 MOUTHS

Components	Descriptors	Assessment activities
Mandible	Length and subluxation	Measure hyomental distance and anterior displacement of mandible
Opening	Base, symmetry, range	Assess and measure mouth opening in centimeters
Uvula	Visibility	Assess pharyngeal structures and classify
Teeth	Dentition	Assess for presence of loose or malpositioned teeth and dental appliances
Head	Flexion, extension, rotation of head/ neck, and cervical spine	Assess all ranges of movement
Silhouette	Upper body abnormalities, both anterior and posterior	Identify potential impact on control of airway of large breasts, buffalo hump, kyphosis, etc.

Source: Modified from Davies,[22] with permission

Bag/Valve/Mask Ventilation

In the process of evaluating the airway, we focus perhaps too much on anticipating difficult intubation and not enough on anticipating DMV. When confronted with difficult intubation, we rely heavily on the ability to perform effective mask ventilation. We must always keep this issue in mind when evaluating the airway. Bag/valve/mask ventilation can be difficult under certain circumstances – for instance, in bearded individuals, the edentulous, and very obese. However, finding a suitable mask fit may be difficult but, more important, the force required to ventilate the lungs may necessitate using two hands and sometimes requires an assistant. It may be difficult to maintain an effective seal in patients with nasogastric tubes. The mouth and nose may be distorted following trauma, preventing maintenance of an adequate seal. Bag/valve/mask ventilation may be impossible when penetrating objects are lodged in the vicinity of the mouth and nose. Patients with mandibular deformities are sometimes more difficult to manage using bag/valve/mask ventilation. Similarly, patients with serious flexion deformities of the cervical spine may not only be impossible to intubate, but also difficult to ventilate using bag/valve/mask ventilation. Tracheostomy may also be very difficult under these circumstances.

Langeron et al.[16] published a study on the topic of DMV. They studied 1,502 patients and reported a 5% incidence of DMV. Using a univariate analysis, risk factors for DMV included: increased BMI, age, macroglossia, the presence of a beard, the edentulous state, a history of snoring, increased Mallampati grade, and a short thyromental distance. They identified five independent factors for DMV in a multivariate analysis and they are listed in order of importance, the odds ratio being greater for the presence of a beard and least for a history of snoring (Table 2.4). The presence of two of these criteria was an accurate predictor of DMV (sensitivity and specificity greater than 70%). The authors also showed that DMV was the harbinger of difficult intubation in up to 30% of cases.

Langeron et al.'s paper sparked further interest in this topic. Kheterpal et al.[51] recently published an additional study involving 22,660 patients. They used a grading system for DMV established by Han et al.[52] Using this system, DMV was graded in the following manner:

Table 2.4 Difficult mask ventilation

Variable
Beard
BMI > 26
Edentulous
Age > 55 years
History of snoring

Parameter listed in order of importance
Source: Data from Langeron et al.[16]

Grade 1 Mask ventilation was readily achieved
Grade 2 Mask ventilation was achieved but required either an airway or muscle relaxant (NMB)
Grade 3 Mask ventilation was difficult requiring additional manual assistance ± NMB
Grade 4 Mask ventilation was impossible

Using this grading system, Kheterpal et al.[51] observed a 1.4% incidence of grade 3 DMV and a 0.16% incidence of grade 4 DMV and a 0.37% incidence of grade 3 or 4 DMV and difficult intubation. The disparity between the two studies on the incidence of DMV can be explained on the basis of the different measuring tools used by the researchers. The risk factors for DMV were comparable in both studies but Kheterpal et al. added an additional factor and modified some of the existing factors reported by Langeron et al.[16] (Table 2.5).The ability to advance the mandible is an important addition to the existing list of independent risk factors for DMV.

Is there any link between DMV and difficult intubation (DI)? Langeron suggested that DMV was linked with DI in 30% of the cases. Kheterpal et al. provided a list of independent risk factors for grade 3 or 4 DMV and difficult intubation which they gleaned from their study (Table 2.6). There were 37 cases of grade 4 DMV in Kheterpal et al.'s original study, one patient required a cricothyrotomy, 10 experienced difficult intubation, and 26 were easily intubated. In Kheterpal's most recent study in which there were 77 cases of IMV, 19 of these cases proved to be difficult intubations (25%).

Table 2.5 Risk factors for DMV

Independent risk factors for grade 3 DMV
BMI $\geq$ 30 kg/m^2
Beard
Mallampati Class III or IV
Age $\geq$ 57
Snoring
Jaw protrusion – very restricted
Independent risk factors for grade 4 DMV
Snoring
Thyromental distance <6 cm

Source: Data from Langeron et al.[16]

Table 2.6 Independent risk factors for grade 3 or 4 mask ventilation and difficult intubation

Jaw protrusion – very restricted
Thick/obese neck
Sleep apnea
Snoring
BMI $\geq$ 30

Source: Data from Kheterpal et al.[51]

Table 2.7 Independent risk factors for impossible mask ventilation include

Previous neck radiation
Male gender
Sleep apnea syndrome
Mallampati Class III or IV
Beard

Source: Kheterpal et al.[53]

Kheterpal et al.[53] have completed yet another study on the topic of DMV recently. This time they included more than 50,000 patients in their study. They reported a 1.5% incidence of grade 3 DMV, which is very similar to that observed in their earlier report. In this most recent study, they accumulated 77 cases of impossible mask ventilation (0.15%) and again the incidence of grade 4 DMV was very similar to that observed in the previous report (0.16%) (Table 2.7).

The most important factor associated with IMV was *previous neck radiation,* which had an odds ratio of greater than 7.

In summary, a considerable amount has been written about DMV in the past 10 years or so, which certainly makes up for the paucity of information on this topic before then. It may be difficult to remember the details of all of these studies. Most of the factors linked with DMV are also associated with DI. Therefore, a complete and thorough examination of the airway will reveal either of these problems or both as they are often linked. In addition to all the usual warning signs of difficult intubation and DMV, we must now add previous *neck radiation* and remember that it is the harbinger of impossible mask ventilation in a significant percentage of cases.

The introduction of the laryngeal mask airway (LMA) has lessened our anxiety about DMV. In a "cannot intubate, cannot ventilate" situation, one should not hesitate to insert an LMA or an alternative supraglottic device. DMV will also be discussed in some detail in Chap. 9.

Additional Information

Arterial Blood Gases

The decision to perform endotracheal intubation in nonoperating room situations often depends upon arterial blood gas results, and so in a hospital setting, this information is usually readily available. Arterial blood gas specimens are not required in healthy patients undergoing intubation for elective surgery. However, if these data are available, record them and use them to assess the success or failure of your subsequent intervention.

ENT Consultation

An ENT consultation is warranted if you suspect pathology in the vicinity of the airway. Indirect laryngoscopy, which is usually performed by an ENT surgeon, involves examination of the larynx by observing its reflection via a laryngeal mirror or fiberoptic laryngoscope. Thus, the airway can be visualized and the nature and extent of any disease assessed before the patient is anesthetized for direct laryngoscopy and intubation. Yamamoto et al.[54] evaluated indirect laryngoscopy as a predictor of difficult intubation in more than 6,000 patients. This test had a specificity of 98.4%, a sensitivity of 69.2%, and a positive predictive value of 31%. The test could not be performed in 15% of patients because of an excessively active gag reflex.

Radiologic Studies

Most patients presenting for emergency intubation will probably have had a recent chest X-ray examination. The chest X-ray is worth reviewing because, in addition to being a useful screening test, it can reveal pathology not evident clinically – pathology that could later be attributed to your intervention. AP and lateral neck films should always be obtained whenever there is encroachment on the airway, regardless of the etiology. Norton et al.[55] recommend dynamic fluoroscopy primarily to assess soft tissue position and motion. If these initial radiologic studies yield insufficient information, it is worthwhile to request a radiology consultation for recommendations on which additional studies will be performed. Appropriate selection is important, since unnecessary studies are time-consuming, costly, and needlessly expose patients to radiation. Modern technological advances in radiology (e.g., computed tomography [CT] and magnetic resonance imaging [MRI]) have greatly improved our ability to diagnose complex airway disorders.

Pulmonary Function Studies

Pulmonary function studies provide additional information about lung function and help distinguish between obstructive and restrictive lung disease. They also allow one to determine the reversibility of airway disease by performing tests before and after various treatments (bronchodilators, steroids, and anticholinergics). Spirometry is the basis of pulmonary function studies and the equipment used for these measurements is called a spirometer, which is a very simple device that measures forced vital capacity (FVC) during exhalation. One of the disadvantages of spirometry is that patient effort is required and repetitive tests are needed (usually three) in order to validate the results. Graphic depiction of a typical

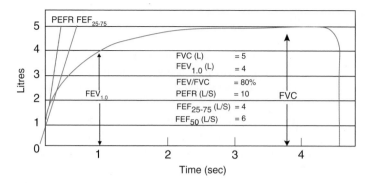

Fig. 2.14 Spirometry

spirogram can be seen in Fig. 2.14. Several useful measurements of lung function can be obtained in this way.[56]

Flow-Volume Loops

Another way of studying pulmonary function is to measure flow and volume in both phases of respiration. The graph generated by this biphasic measurement is called a flow-volume loop. To be more specific, this is a pulmonary function study in which the forced expiratory volume (FEV) and forced inspiratory volume (FIV) are recorded in succession on a spirogram. Flow is plotted on the vertical axis, and volume on the horizontal. Flow-volume loops help distinguish between small and large airway obstructions. They also may help pinpoint the site of a large airway obstruction and whether the obstruction is fixed or variable and whether the obstruction is intrathoracic or extrathoracic.[57] An example of a normal flow-volume loop is depicted in Fig. 2.15a and an abnormal flow-volume loop is depicted in Fig. 2.15b. One of the advantages of flow-volume loops over basic spirometry is that they can distinguish between intrathoracic and extrathoracic obstruction because measurements are made in both phases of respiration. In extrathoracic obstructions, the changes are most noteworthy during the inspiratory phase. Conversely, intrathoracic obstruction is reflected in the expiratory phase of the flow-volume loop.

Difficult Airway Clinic

In 1987, Norton et al.[55] established a "difficult airway" clinic at the University of Michigan. Patients with potential airway difficulties are referred to that clinic by anesthesiologists and surgeons. In that setting, a formal evaluation of the airway is carried out and a plan of action is formulated. One of the important functions of modern preadmission clinics (PAC) is to preemptively detect problem airways

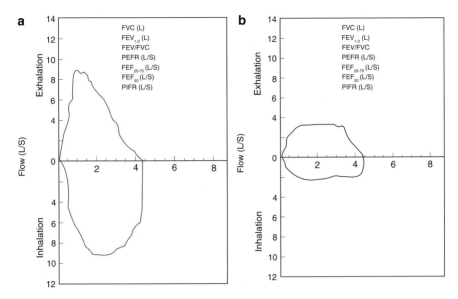

Fig. 2.15 (**a, b**) Showing flow-volume loops. (**a**) Is normal (**b**) is showing airway obstruction

before the scheduled day of surgery. Unfortunately, not all patients are seen in the PAC. Consequently, a number of healthy patients with problem airways present on the day of surgery and, in that setting, the urgency of maintaining "throughput" sometimes takes priority over careful preoperative assessment of patients.

The "Awake Look"

The "awake look" is a procedure used by some anesthesiologists as a final assessment of the airway before making a decision about the safety of inducing anesthesia. We have already discussed in detail the various tests available to determine the status of the airway and the limitations thereof. In a way, the "awake look" is the final test available to us before we make that definitive decision about how to proceed. The procedure is as follows: the patient is prepared as they would be for general anesthesia including preoperative assessment and monitoring. Then the patient is sedated usually using a combination of opiate and benzodiazepine and, when the patient is adequately sedated, topical anesthesia is applied to the supraglottic structures, and direct laryngoscopy is attempted. If the epiglottis can be readily elevated and some part of vocal apparatus seen, we can then assume that it is safe to proceed with general anesthesia. If we cannot see the epiglottis or if the epiglottis is fixed in place, we must then perform an "awake" intubation. This should always be considered before attempting intubation in a patient with suspected airway difficulty if the problem has not been well defined. The "awake look" test has not yet been validated as a useful tool to predict difficult intubation.

Summary

The one very clear message that we have been trying to convey in this chapter is the importance of taking the time to conduct a thorough evaluation of the airway. If you abide by that rule, you will uncover the vast majority of problem airways. We have done a thorough search of the literature to help guide you when performing this task. We have conveyed that there is no single guaranteed test available to predict the problem airway. However, there are now a number of tests that we can perform during our evaluation that will allow us to detect the problem airway in the vast majority of cases. Traditionally, we have focused most of our attention on the task of endotracheal intubation and possible problems with that procedure. We need to ask ourselves a more fundamental question when dealing with airway issues. "Will I be able to oxygenate and ventilate this patient if or when he/she becomes unconscious?" We should be able to answer that question affirmatively in all cases, and if not, we need contingency plans.

References

1. Caplan RA, Posner KL, Ward RJ, Cheney FW. Adverse respiratory events in anesthesia: a closed claims analysis. *Anesthesiology*. 1990;72:828–833.
2. Rose DK, Cohen MM. The airway: problems and predictions in 18,500 patients. *Can J Anaesth*. 1994;41(5):372–383.
3. Combes X, Le Roux B, Suen P, et al. Unanticipated difficult airway in anesthetized patients: prospective validation of a management algorithm. *Anesthesiology*. 2004;100:1146–1150.
4. El-Ganzouri AR, McCarthy RJ, Tuman KJ, Tank EN, Invankovich AD. Preoperative airway assessment: predictive value of a multivariate risk index. *Anesth Analg*. 1996;82:1197–1204.
5. Reissell E, Orko R, Maunuksela EL, Lindgren L. Predictability of difficult laryngoscopy in patients with long term diabetes mellitus. *Anaesthesia*. 1990;45:1024-1027.
6. Salazarulo HH, Taylor LA. Diabetic stiff joint syndrome as a cause of difficult endotracheal intubation. *Anesthesiology*. 1986;64:366–368.
7. Nadal JLY, Fernandez BG, Escobar IC, Black M, Rosenblatt WH. The 'palm print' as a sensitive predictor of difficult laryngoscopy. *Acta Anaesthesiol Scand*. 1998;42:199–203.
8. *Guidelines to the Practice of Anesthesia*. Revised Edition 2010. Supplement the Canadian Journal of Anesthesia 2010;57(1).
9. Lundstrom LH, Moller AM, Rosenstock C, Astrup G, Wetterslev J. High body mass index is a weak predictor for difficult and failed tracheal intubation. *Anesthesiology*. 2008;110:266–274.
10. Stewart DJ, Lerman JL. *Manual of Pediatric Anesthesia*. 5th ed. New York: Churchill Livingston; 2001.
11. Schmitt H, Buchfelder M, Radespiel-Troger F, Fahlbusch R. Difficult intubation in acromegalic patients. *Anesthesiology*. 2000;93:110–114.
12. Aiello G, Metcalf I. Anaesthetic implications of TMJ disease. *Can J Anaesth*. 1992;39:610–616.
13. Block C, Brechner VL. Unusual problems in airway management: the influence of the temporomandibular joint, the mandible and associated structures and endotracheal intubation. *Anesth Analg*. 1971;50:114.
14. Posselt U. *Physiology of Occlusion and Rehabilitation*. 2nd ed. Oxford: Blackwell; 1968.
15. Calder I, Calder J, Crockard HA. Difficult direct laryngoscopy in patients with cervical spine disease. *Anaesthesia*. 1995;50:756–763.

16. Langeron O, Masso E, Huraux C, et al. Prediction of difficult mask ventilation. *Anesthesiology*. 2000;92:1229–1236.
17. Khan ZH, Kashfi A, Ebrahimkhani E. A comparison of the Upper Lip Bite Test (simple new technique) with Modified Mallampati Classification in predicting difficulty in endotracheal intubation: a prospective blinded study. *Anesth Analg*. 2003;96:595–596.
18. Calder I, Picard J, Chapman M, O'Sullivan C, Crockard HA. Mouth opening. A New Angle. *Anesthesiology*. 2003;99:799–801.
19. Finucane BT. Difficult intubation associated with the foetal alcohol syndrome. *Can Anaesth Soc J*. 1980;27(6):574–575.
20. St. Paul Fire and Marine Insurance Co. *Physician and Surgeon Professional Liability Countrywide Summary Report by Allegation;* 1978.
21. Burton JF, Baker AB. Dental damage during anesthesia and surgery. *Anaesth Intensive Care*. 1987;15:262–268.
22. Davies JM, Eagles CJ. Mouths. *Can J Anaesth*. 1991;38:687–688.
23. Conlon N, Sullivan R, Herbison PG, Zacharias M, Buggy DJ. The effect of leaving dentures in place on bag-mask ventilation at induction of anesthesia. *Anesth Analg*. 2007;105:370–373.
24. Mallampati SR. Clinical signs to predict difficult tracheal intubation [hypothesis]. *Can Anaesth Soc J*. 1983;30:316–317.
25. Mallampati SR, Gatt SP, Gugino LD, et al. A clinical sign to predict difficult tracheal intubation: a prospective study. *Can Anaesth Soc J*. 1985;82:429.
26. Samsoon GLT, Young JRB. Difficult tracheal intubation: a retrospective study. *Anaesthesia*. 1987;42:487–490.
27. Oates JD, Oates PD, Pearsall FJ, McLeod AD, Howie JC. Phonation affects Mallampati class. *Anaesthesia*. 1990;45:984.
28. Tham EJ, Gildersleve CD, Sanders LD, Mapelson WW, Vaughan RS. Effects of posture, phonation and observer on Mallampati classification. *Br J Anaesth*. 1992;68:32–38.
29. Lewis M, Keramati S, Benumof JL, Berry CC. What is the best way to determine oropharyngeal classification and mandibular space length to predict difficult laryngoscopy? *Anesthesiology*. 1994;81:69–75.
30. Ezri T, Cohen I, Geva D, et al. The incidence of class zero airway and the impact of Mallampati score, age, sex and body mass on prediction of laryngoscopy grade. *Anesth Analg*. 2001;93:1073–1075.
31. Grover VK, Mahajan R, Tomar M. Class zero airway and laryngoscopy. *Anesth Analg*. 2003;96:911.
32. Cohen SM, Laurito C, Segil LJ. Oral exam to predict difficult intubation: a large prospective study. *Anesthesiology*. 1989;71:A937.
33. Cormack RS, Lehane J. Difficult tracheal intubation in obstetrics. *Anaesthesia*. 1984;39:1105–1111.
34. Pilkington S, Carli F, Dakin MJ, et al. Increase in Mallamapati score during pregnancy. *Br J Anaesth Analg*. 1995;74:638–642.
35. Rocke DA, Murray WB, Rout CC, Gouws E. Relative risk analysis of factors associated with difficult intubation in obstetric anesthesia. *Anesthesiology*. 1992;77:67–73.
36. Jones DH, Cohle SD. Unanticipated difficult airway secondary to lingual tonsillar hyperplasia. *Anesth Analg*. 1993;77:1285–1288.
37. Buckland RW, Pedley J. Lingual thyroid – a threat to the airway. *Anaesthesia*. 2000;55:1103–1105.
38. Rosenberg AD, Young M, Bernstein RL, Albert DB. Tongue rings: just say no. *Anesthesiology*. 1998;89:1279.
39. Brown DC. Anesthetic considerations of a patient with a tongue piercing and a safe solution. *Anesthesiology*. 2000;93:307.
40. Bannister FB, MacBeth RG. Direct laryngoscopy and tracheal intubation. *Lancet*. 1944;1:651.
41. Patil VU, Stehling LC, Zauder HL. *Fiberoptic Endoscopy in Anesthesia*. 1st ed. Chicago: Year Book; 1983.
42. Al Ramadhani S, Mohamed LA, Rocke DA, Gouws E. Sternomental distances a sole predictor of difficult laryngoscopy in obstetric anesthesia. *Br J Anaesth*. 1996;77:312–316.

43. Brodsky J, Lemmens HJM, Brock-Utne JG, Vierra M, Saidman LJ. Morbid obesity and tracheal intubation. *Anesth Analg.* 2002;94:732–736.
44. Gonzalez H, Minville V, Delanue K, et al. The importance of increased neck circumference intubation difficulties in obese patients. *Anesth Analg.* 2008;106:1132–1136.
45. Chou HC, Wu TL. Mandibulohyoid distance in difficult laryngoscopy. *Br J Anaesth.* 1993;71:335–339.
46. Walls RD, Timmis DP, Finucane BT. Difficult intubation associated with calcified stylohyoid ligament. *Anaesth Intensive Care.* 1990;18:110–126.
47. Sherwood-Smith GH. Difficulty in intubation: calcified stylohyoid ligament. *Anaesthesia.* 1976;31:508–510.
48. Akinyemi OO, Elegbe EO. Difficult laryngoscopy and tracheal intubation due to calcified stylohyoid ligaments. *Can Anaesth Soc J.* 1981;28:80–81.
49. Keenan MA, Stiles CM, Kaulman RL. Acquired laryngeal deviation associated with cervical spine disease in erosive polyarticular arthritis. *Anesthesiology.* 1983;58:441.
50. Bellhouse CP, Doré C. Criteria for estimating likelihood of endotracheal intubation with the Macintosh laryngoscope. *Anaesth Intensive Care.* 1988;16:329–337.
51. Kheterpal S, Han R, Tremper KK, et al. Incidence and predictors of difficult and impossible mask ventilation. *Anesthesiology.* 2006;105:885–891.
52. Han R, Tremper KK, Kheterpal S, O'Reilly M. Grading scale for mask ventilation (letter). *Anesthesiology.* 2004;101:267.
53. Kheterpal S, Martin L, Shanks AM, Tremper KK. Prediction and outcomes of impossible mask ventilation. A review of 50, 000 cases. *Anesthesiology.* 2009;110:891–897.
54. Yamamoto K, Tsubokawa T, Shibita K, Ohmura S, Nitta S, Kobayashi T. Predicting difficult intubation with indirect laryngoscopy. *Anesthesiology.* 1997;86:316–321.
55. Norton ML, Wilton N, Brown ACD. The difficult airway. *Anesthesiol Rev.* 1988;15:25–28.
56. Crapo RO. Pulmonary function testing. *N Engl J Med.* 1994;331:25.
57. Ruppel G. *Manual of Pulmonary Function Testing.* 6th ed. St Louis: Mosby; 1994.

Suggested Reading

Hagberg CA. *Benumof's Airway Management.* 2nd ed. St. Louis: Mosby; 2007.
Hagberg CA. *Handbook of Difficult Airway Management.* 1st ed. Philadelphia: Churchill Livingston; 2000.
Hung O, Murphy M. *Management of the Difficult and Failed Airway.* 1st ed. New York: McGraw-Hill; 2008.
Bainton CR. Difficult intubation – what's the best test? *Can J Anaesth.* 1996;43:541–543.
Jacobsen J, Jensen E, Waldau T, Poulsen TD. Preoperative evaluation conditions in patients scheduled for elective surgery. *Acta Anaesthesiol Scand.* 1996;40:421–424.
Tse JC, Rimm EB, Hussain A. Predicting difficult endotracheal intubation in surgical patients scheduled for general anesthesia: a prospective blind study. *Anesth Analg.* 1995;81:254–258.
Kanaya N, Kawana S, Watanabe H, et al. The utility of three-dimensional computed tomography in unanticipated difficult endotracheal intubation. *Anesth Analg.* 2000;91:752–754.
Karkouti K, Rose DK, Wigglesworth D, et al. Predicting difficult intubation: a multivariable analysis. *Can J Anesth.* 2000;47:730–739.
Naguib M, Malabarey T, AlSatli RA, Al Damegh S, Samarkandi AH. Predictive models for difficult laryngoscopy and intubation: a clinical, radiologic and three-dimensional computer imaging study. *Can J Anesth.* 1999;46:748–759.
Nath G, Sekar M. Predicting difficult intubation – a comprehensive scoring system. *Anaesth Intensive Care.* 1997;25:482–486.
Sawwa D. Prediction of difficult tracheal intubation. *Br J Anesth.* 1994;73:149–153.

Chapter 3
Basic Emergency Airway Management and Cardiopulmonary Resuscitation (CPR)

Contents

B.T. Finucane et al., *Principles of Airway Management*,
DOI 10.1007/978-0-387-09558-5_3, © Springer Science+Business Media, LLC 2011

Emergency Airway Management

In an emergency, all basic life support (BLS), advanced cardiac life support (ACLS), and advanced trauma life support (ATLS) techniques focus on the ABCs – *airway, breathing, and circulation* (currently ABCD with *defibrillation* is also used).[1-3] The airway is the most important element of BLS and is correctly allocated as the "A" in the ABCD of resuscitation. Assessment, establishment, and maintenance of a patent airway, with adequate oxygenation and ventilation, form the foundation upon which other resuscitative measures are built. Without this foundation, all other resuscitative measures are doomed to failure, as an inadequate airway leads rapidly to hypoxemia and uncorrected hypoxemia will result in brain damage and ultimately death.

BLS skills form an important foundation for other advanced resuscitation measures such as ACLS and ATLS. BLS primarily consists of cardiopulmonary resuscitation (CPR) and basic airway management. This chapter contains information about BLS and airway management techniques for resuscitating the airway of a victim with cardiopulmonary arrest as well as complete and partial airway obstruction. A detailed review of cardiac arrest, ACLS, or ATLS are beyond the scope of this chapter, although there will be some introduction to the etiology of upper airway obstruction. The comparative table and algorithm included in this chapter provide a synopsis of the various techniques used and highlight essential assessments and interventions required to treat cardiac arrest and other life-threatening conditions. These guidelines and recommendations are updated on a regular basis as new information becomes available and the reader is urged to check the most up-to-date official guidelines and recommendations.

Importance of Basic Life Support

Cardiovascular disease (CVD) is the leading cause of death worldwide. In 2005, CVD was the underlying cause in 35.3% of deaths in the United States, and coronary artery disease caused about one in five deaths (with a total of 445,687 deaths from CHD).[4] The picture in Canada is very similar with 36% of deaths due to CVD.[5] Many victims of cardiac arrest do not receive effective CPR. Of nearly 300,000 out-of-hospital cardiac arrests which are treated annually in the United States by emergency medical services (EMS),[4] many do not survive (60% of unexpected cardiac deaths are treated by EMS).[6] Clearly, treatment does not translate into survival. Worldwide, the survival rate for out-of-hospital sudden cardiac arrests (SCA) remains low (6% or below), despite continual efforts to promote CPR science and education.[7] While asphyxia is the most common mechanism of cardiac arrest in children, SCA and ventricular fibrillation (VF) are not the only causes of death in adults. An unknown number of adult deaths have an asphyxial mechanism, as in drowning or drug overdose. Moreover, a significant number of fatalities due to motor vehicle accidents and other traumatic events are precipitated by upper airway obstruction, secondary to central nervous system (CNS) depression. Together, these facts support the focus on both identification and control of risk factors (for CVD) and improvement in resuscitation science, including recommendations for appropriate and timely emergency intervention (e.g., CPR).

Since many preventable deaths occur outside the hospital, all health professionals should become competent in basic airway management and CPR.[3] (It has also been suggested that operators of facilities where large crowds gather (e.g., factories, schools, office buildings, stadiums) should provide training for security and other personnel in the techniques of CPR and the use of an automated external defibrillator).[8] Even in a hospital setting, the ancillary equipment and experienced personnel may not be immediately available in an emergency situation, and time should not be lost waiting for their arrival. Except in cases of hypothermia (in which the brain's decreased rate of oxygen consumption can prolong survival), patients will suffer irreversible hypoxic encephalopathy if CPR is delayed for more than 4–6 min after cardiopulmonary arrest. Therefore, timing is critical; clinicians, and indeed the population at large, must be prepared to deliver BLS.

Adult Basic Life Support (BLS)

Originally published in 1974, the American Heart Association (AHA) developed training guidelines for CPR and emergency cardiac care (ECC). After reissuing guidelines several times (1980, 1986, and 1992), the AHA became a member of the International Liaison Committee on Resuscitation (ILCOR) and hosted the first two ILCOR conferences in 1999 and 2005 to evaluate resuscitation science and develop common resuscitation recommendations.[3, 9] The AHA now bases its guidelines upon the recommendations reached at the ILCOR conferences, and the 2005 AHA guidelines are based on the most extensive evidence review of CPR ever published.[10]

Over the years, emphasis has always been placed on the need to identify risk factors and focus on primary prevention of CVD in order to prevent incidences of SCA. The concept of the *chain of survival* stresses that survival is contingent upon prioritizing certain variables. Further, the most recent guidelines have been streamlined and clarified with respect to reducing the amount of information required to learn and focusing on those interventions that should be performed frequently and well. Increased emphasis on ensuring that rescuers deliver high-quality CPR includes: providing an adequate number and depth of compressions, allowing for complete chest recoil after compressions, and minimizing interruptions in chest compressions. Beyond knowledge of guidelines, good survival rates (from witnessed VF SCA) have been reported in lay rescuer programs that train rescuers in a planned and practiced response and teach rapid recognition of SCA. As well, prompt provision of bystander CPR and defibrillation within 5 min of collapse improve outcomes.[7] Continuous quality improvement efforts should also be implemented.[11]

The etiology of cardiopulmonary arrest is often a guide to the most effective CPR response. While cardiac arrest with VF is best treated using compressions and defibrillation (especially if initiated immediately after collapse), the best results for asphyxial arrest are obtained with a combination of compressions and ventilation. This is the reason for "Calling First" in adults with sudden collapse and "Calling Fast" (after two cycles of CPR) if there is suspected asphyxial arrest.

Chain of Survival

The chain of survival for victims of SCA VF includes:

1. Early recognition of the emergency and activation of the EMS or local emergency response system ("phone 911" in North America).
2. Early bystander CPR (immediate CPR can double or triple the victim's chance for survival).
3. Early delivery of a shock with a defibrillator.
4. Early ACLS followed by postresuscitation care delivered by health care providers.

Changes in the 2005 and 2010 AHA Recommendations

The main changes in the 2005 AHA Recommendations that were reached by the 2005 ILCOR Consensus Conference include the following:[7]

• The lay rescuer is no longer trained to assess signs of circulation before beginning compressions. They begin compressions after delivering two rescue breaths in the unresponsive victim who is not breathing.
• All breaths should be given over 1 s using sufficient volume to achieve visible chest rise.
• Health care (HC) providers now apply the pediatric BLS guidelines to all *prepubescent* victims.
• Compressions should be fast (100 per minute) and hard (to allow visible chest rise), and there should be full recoil and minimal interruptions in compressions.
• Compression-ventilation ratio of *30:2* is recommended for all *lone rescuers* of victims from infancy (excluding newborns) through adulthood. This ratio is deemed suitable to restore adequate coronary and cerebral blood flow without too many interruptions in compressions and without excessive ventilation, while being appropriate for different causes of cardiac arrest (e.g., asphyxial arrest and VF SCA). This ratio will simplify training in one-rescuer and two-rescuer CPR and all lay rescuer resuscitation. A ratio of *15:2* is recommended for *two-rescuer CPR* [generally only health care providers (HC)] for infant and children (to the

onset of puberty), due to the higher ventilation requirement of asphyxial arrest (more commonly seen in this age category).

- Lay rescuers involved in a public defibrillation program (thus trained to analyze the victim's rhythm) and HC providers who treat cardiac arrest with automated external defibrillators (AED) on-site should always use the AED as soon as it is available. EMS rescuers may provide about five cycles of CPR before attempting defibrillation in victims with VF or pulseless ventricular tachycardia (VT) in the event of greater than 4–5 min of response or when the responders did not witness the arrest. Immediately after shock delivery, it is important to deliver CPR.
- Defibrillation should proceed with one shock followed immediately by CPR, starting with compressions. Checking for circulation should not commence until after about five cycles (2 min) of CPR. Defibrillators with biphasic waveforms require between 120 (rectilinear waveform) and 200 J (150–200 J for truncated exponential waveforms), while doses of 360 J should be administered with those having monophasic waveforms.

In the 2010 AHA guidelines, the order of CPR steps has been rearranged for all ages beyond the newborn. Instead of A -B-C, which stands for airway and breathing first followed by chest compressions, the AHA now recommends the sequence of CPR should change to C-A-B: chest compressions first, then airway and breathing (Fig 3.1). The rationale for these changes is highlighted in following section Compression – only CPR. The pediatric and neonatal guidelines are presented in chap. 10. Table 3.1 is a comparison of health care provider CPR maneuvers for all ages."

The AHA Algorithm and Recommendations for Rescue Breaths, a Universal Compression-Ventilation Ratio, and Defibrillation

The 2005 and 2010 AHA Adult BLS Healthcare Provider Algorithm is found in Fig. 3.1. In addition to detailing the sequence and main recommendations for rescue breathing and the compression-ventilation ratio, there is a discussion relating to the recommended techniques to be used when performing CPR, as well as some theoretical background and additional strategies.

General Sequence for Lay Rescuer and HC Provider

Lone Lay Rescuer

1. Telephone emergency response and retrieve an AED (if available). Return to victim and use CPR and AED when appropriate.
2. Open the airway and check for *normal* breathing; in the absence of normal breathing, give two rescue breaths.
3. Immediately, begin cycles of compressions and ventilations at a ratio of 30:2 and use the AED as soon as possible.

Table 3.1 Comparison of health care provider CPR maneuvers in adults, children, infants, and newborns

	Pulse check (≤10 s)	Airway access	Depth of compressions an hand/finger position	Compression rate (per minute) and technique	Compression-to-ventilation ratio	Ventilation rate (breaths per min) in victim with pulse	Foreign body airway obstruction
Adult	Carotid	Head tilt, chin lift (if trauma suspected, jaw thrust)	At least 2 in. 2 finger-breadths above xiphoid Place heel of 1 hand and other hand on top	At least 100 Push hard and fast, allow complete recoil	30:2	10–12	Heimlich maneuver/abdominal thrusts
Child (1–adolescent[a])	Carotid	Head tilt, chin lift (if trauma suspected, jaw thrust)	1/3–1/2 anteroposterior diameter of chest Place 1 or 2 hands 2 fingers-breadths above xiphoid	At least 100 Push hard and fast, allow complete recoil	30:2 or 15:2 (2 HCP rescuers)	12–20	Heimlich maneuver/abdominal thrusts
Infant (under 1 year)	Brachial or femoral	Head tilt, chin lift (if trauma suspected, jaw thrust)	1/3–1/2 anteroposterior diameter of chest Use 2 fingers just below the intermammary line	At least 100 Push hard and fast, allow complete recoil	30:2 or 15:2 (2 HCP rescuers)	12–20	Back slaps and chest thrusts
Newborn[b]	Brachial or femoral	"Sniffing position" Clear with bulb syringe or suction catheter	1/3–1/2 anteroposterior diameter of chest on the lvower 1/3 of the sternum (2 thumb-encircling hands or two fingers with second hand supporting back)	90 Push hard and fast, allow complete recoil, maintain thumb contact with chest	3:1	40–60 (average initial peak inflating pressures of 30–40 cm H_2O)	Back slaps and chest thrusts

[a] Health care providers now apply the pediatric (child) BLS guidelines to all *prepubescent* victims (1 to about 12–14 years)
[b] Newborn CPR applies to infants from their first hours after birth until leaving the hospital
Compiled from American Heart Association[10]

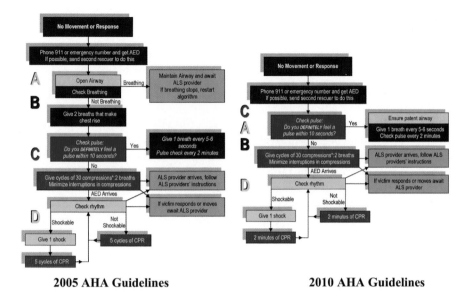

2005 AHA Guidelines   **2010 AHA Guidelines**

Fig. 3.1 Algorithm for basic adult life support. Flow charts based on (*left*) 2005 and (*right*) 2010 AHA guidelines[10a,b]

Lone HC Provider

1. If there was sudden collapse and the victim is unresponsive, phone 911 and get an AED if available. Begin CPR and use the AED as appropriate.
2. If the victim likely has an asphyxial cause of arrest, provide five cycles of CPR (compressions-ventilations ratio of 30:2) before leaving the victim to phone the emergency response number.

If more than one person is present, the actions of providing CPR and calling for the AED will occur simultaneously.

Rescue Breaths

Each rescue breath should be delivered over 1 s and should produce visible chest rise. This recommendation is for all forms of ventilation during CPR. Avoid rapid or forceful breaths. When rescue breaths are provided to victims with a pulse (no compressions provided), the HC provider should provide 10–12 breaths per minute. Once an advanced airway (Combitube, LMA, endotracheal tube) is in place during two-rescuer CPR, the compressor should provide 100 compressions per minute without pausing and the breather should deliver 8–10 breaths per minute. If ventilation is delivered using a bag and mask, use an adult ventilating bag (volume 1–2 L) and a tidal volume of 500–600 mL (as long as there is chest rise).

Chest Compressions

The compression-ventilation ratio is 30:2 for all adult victims. Push hard and fast – compressions should be performed at a rate of 100 per minute, with complete chest recoil between each compression. Allow minimal interruptions between compressions (see previous comment on rescue breaths during two-rescuer CPR), since interruptions in chest compressions for rescue breathing decrease coronary perfusion pressure, myocardial blood flow, and 24-h survival.[12, 13] See the Sect. on "Compression Only CPR" later in this chapter for more information. Compress the chest using the heel of both hands, in the center of the chest at the nipple line. Depress the chest 1.5–2 in.

Defibrillation

In victims with SCA, early defibrillation is critical for survival. Each minute prior to defibrillation decreases the SCA victim's chance of survival by 7–10%.[14] Defibrillation is the treatment for VF, the most common initial rhythm in SCA, and the VF will deteriorate to asystole within a few minutes. CPR prolongs VF and provides a small amount of blood flow that may maintain some oxygen and substrate delivery to the heart and brain. If defibrillation is delayed, bystander CPR can double or triple survival from witnessed SCA at most intervals to defibrillation.[15]

Lay rescuers involved in a public defibrillation program (thus trained to analyze the victim's rhythm) and HC providers who treat cardiac arrest with AEDs on-site should always use the AED as soon as it is available. Defibrillation before CPR may not always be beneficial for victims with VF if the delay between collapse and rescuer intervention is greater than 4–5 min. EMS rescuers may provide five cycles of CPR before checking the ECG rhythm and attempting defibrillation in victims with VF or pulseless VT when more than 4 min has elapsed since the initial call, or when the responders did not witness the arrest. Immediately after shock delivery, it is important to deliver CPR since most victims demonstrate asystole or pulseless electrical activity for several minutes after defibrillation.[10] For in-hospital cardiac arrest, there is insufficient evidence to support or refute providing CPR before defibrillation.[15] There are some safety factors for consideration when performing defibrillation (Box 3.1).[16]

While manual defibrillators will be used in monitored inpatient hospital settings, AEDs may be beneficial in areas where there are no monitored beds as well as in outpatient and diagnostic facilities. The goal with defibrillation is to deliver the first

Box 3.1 Safety Considerations Before Performing Defibrillation

- Check the environment for pools of water or metal surfaces that connect the patient to the operator. Volatile atmospheres, such as gasoline or aviation fumes, can ignite with a spark.
- A bare frontal chest area is required, so clothing should be open or cut to allow access.
- If possible, remove all metal objects such as chains and medallions from the front of the chest (pathway of shock). Do not delay defibrillation to attempt removal of those pieces (e.g., body jewelry) that cannot be removed – the potential benefit of avoiding minor burns from these does not override the risk of delay.
- The patient's chest should be checked for the presence of self-medication patches which may deflect energy away from the heart.
- Oxygen that is being used (e.g., pocket mask) should be directed away from the patient or turned off during defibrillation

Source: data from Colquhoun et al.[16]

shock in less than 3 min from collapse. Recommendations for electrode placement and size, synchronized cardioversion, supraventricular tachycardia, ventricular tachycardia, and pacing are included in the 2005 guidelines.[15]

Defibrillation should proceed with one shock followed immediately by CPR, starting with compressions. Checking for circulation should not commence until after about five cycles (2 min) of CPR. A three-stacked shock sequence is no longer recommended for the treatment of VF/pulseless VT, as in 2000.[9] In contrast to the previous need for multiple defibrillations to overcome the low first-shock efficacy (terminating VF for at least 5 s), modern defibrillators have high first-shock efficacy (greater than 90% reported by current biphasic defibrillators).[17] Moreover, immediate CPR is required for the nonperfusing rhythms displayed after the termination of VF. Implementing the one-shock strategy has modified the energy recommendations required to terminate VF using the lowest effective energy: defibrillators with biphasic waveforms require between 120 (rectilinear waveform) and 200 J (150–200 J for truncated exponential waveforms), while those with a monophasic waveform require doses of 360 J. Nonescalating and escalating energy biphasic waveform shocks can be used safely and effectively. For second and subsequent biphasic shocks, use the same or higher energy.

If multiple biphasic shocks are required when using AEDs, it is important to limit the interruptions in compressions to maintain threshold levels of coronary perfusion pressure. This action is a major determinant of successful cardiac resuscitation.[18] Yu et al.[19] evaluated the effects of compression interruptions during automated defibrillation in a swine model with electrically induced VF and found successful return of spontaneous circulation in all animals when the delay to compression before the delivery of the first and subsequent (up to 3 total) 150-J shocks was preceded by a 3-s interval, but in no animal when the delay was greater than 15 s. The shortest delay (3 min) enabled a sufficient rate of compressions (greater than 80 per min) to provide successful resuscitation. In order to limit interruptions, Yu et al.[19] suggest the aim of perfecting ECG analyses to proceed without loss of sensitivity and specificity, for instance, with the use of advanced signal processing, to remove the artifacts produced by the chest compression.

Techniques of CPR

Establishing Unresponsiveness and Positioning the Victim

Upon encountering a collapsed victim, the rescuer must determine if the environment is safe, then quickly assess any injury and determine unresponsiveness. It should not be assumed that all supine, motionless individuals are in need of CPR. Firstly, it should be *determined if the victim is unconscious* by gentle tapping or shaking and then questioning them with, "Are you all right?" Then, if there is a response, they should be *asked the following questions*:

• Do you have neck pain?
• Do you have numbness in your arms or legs?
• Can you move your arms or legs?

The witness should then call for help and return to the victim to check on their condition frequently.

If there is no response, it is then necessary to make sure the victim is properly positioned. In order to provide effective circulation from chest compressions, the victim must be placed supine on a firm surface. Then, one should kneel beside the victim's shoulders and open the airway. If there is any evidence of trauma to the head or neck, or if cervical spine injury is suspected, the victim should not be moved if at all possible. Otherwise, there is the risk of exacerbating any spinal cord injury that may be present, which could lead to paraplegia or quadriplegia. If such a victim must be moved or rolled, the head, neck, and torso should be controlled as a unit. Spinal motion restriction should be applied manually, rather than with immobilization devices during CPR (devices will be necessary during transport). This method is safer, does not interfere with the airway, and does not increase the intracranial pressure in the head-injured patient.

If cervical trauma is not suspected, the unresponsive victim with spontaneous respirations should be placed in the *recovery position* (Fig. 3.2). This involves rolling the patient onto one or other side and placing the lower arm in front of the body. This position helps to maintain a patent airway and reduces the risk of airway obstruction and aspiration.

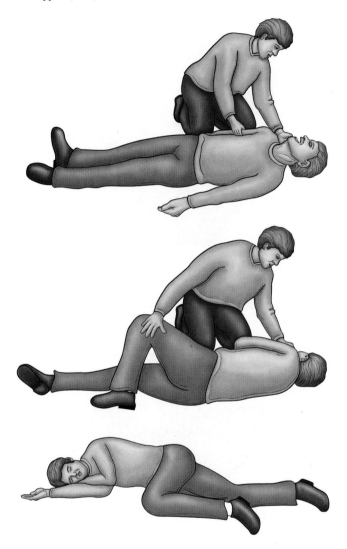

Fig. 3.2 Placing the victim in recovery position

Maneuvers for Opening the Airway

Head Tilt/Chin Lift

The AHA has found that the head tilt/chin lift maneuver (Fig. 3.3) is the most effec-tive technique for opening the airway of an unconscious victim.[10] This is the only maneuver recommended for the lay rescuer and the preferred method for the HC

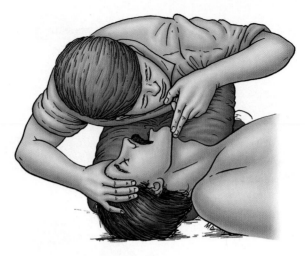

Fig. 3.3 The head tilt/chin lift maneuver

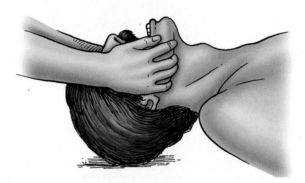

Fig. 3.4 The triple airway maneuver

provider when there is no evidence of head or neck trauma. (The head tilt/neck lift maneuver, although slightly easier to perform, is less effective and *is not* recommended.) The head tilt/chin lift maneuver is achieved with placement of one hand on the victim's forehead and a tilt of the head backward. The fingers of the other hand are placed firmly beneath the bony portion of the victim's chin, lifting it upward.

Vigorous pressure on the soft tissue structures beneath the chin can cause airway obstruction and should be avoided. The chin lift maneuver should be performed with the first two or three fingers and not the thumb. Dentures, if present, should not necessarily be removed, because they help maintain the normal contour of the mouth and facilitate rescue breathing.

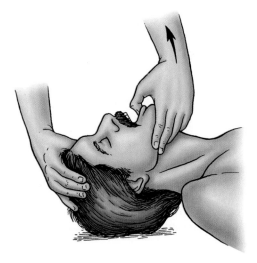

Fig. 3.5 Mandibular displacement

Jaw Thrust

The traditional jaw thrust maneuver is performed by gripping the angles of the mandible with both hands, one on each side, and pulling forward, while at the same time tilting the victim's head backward. However, when cervical spine injury is suspected, the modified jaw thrust maneuver is recommended. Since it does not involve extension of the neck, this maneuver consists of forward traction on the mandible without head tilt.

Triple Airway Maneuver (Not Included in AHA Recommendations)

This technique is a variation or extension of the head tilt/jaw thrust maneuver. In addition to backward tilting of the head and a forward pull on the mandible, the victim's lower lip is retracted using the rescuer's thumb to open the mouth (Fig. 3.4). It is generally used by rescuers with advanced airway management skills.

Mandibular Displacement (Not Included in AHA Recommendations)

The mandible can also be pulled forward by the rescuer placing their thumb in the victim's mouth and their fingers beneath the chin and then lifting upward (Fig. 3.5). This maneuver is very effective in spontaneously breathing edentulous individuals, but it can be dangerous for the rescuer when the victim has teeth.

Determining Breathlessness (Look, Listen, and Feel)

Determine breathlessness while maintaining an open airway. Lay rescuers assess whether the adult victim is breathing *normally*. Agonal gasps or respirations associated with retraction of the substernal region are signs of inadequate respiration and require augmented breathing. HC providers should assess for *adequate* breathing, since some patients will have inadequate breathing which requires assisted ventilation (i.e., treat the victim with occasional breaths as if they are not breathing and provide rescue breaths).

The procedure is as follows:

1. Open the airway
2. Listen for breathing by placing your ear over the victim's mouth
3. Look for the rise and fall of the chest
4. Listen for breath sounds
5. Feel for the exhaled air

If these signs are present, a patent airway should be maintained, although if there is no response, the victim should be moved to the recovery position. However, resuscitation should be initiated if these signs are absent indicating that the victim is not breathing adequately.

Rescue Breathing Technique

The technique of rescue breathing can be difficult to master and is best learned on a mannequin that shows the results on a printout. Effective rescue breathing requires correct head position, an airtight seal, and sufficient force to inflate the victim's lungs (i.e., cause a perceptible rise and fall of the chest). For mouth-to-mouth breathing (Fig. 3.6), the victim's airway is opened, their nose pinched, and an airtight mouth-to-mouth seal is created. The rescuer then provides two breaths, with each given over 1 s and with a pause of one regular breath. If inadequate chest rise results, the airway should be reopened with the head tilt/chin lift. Adequate ventilation is not always possible, especially if a small rescuer is confronted with a large victim. Conversely, a

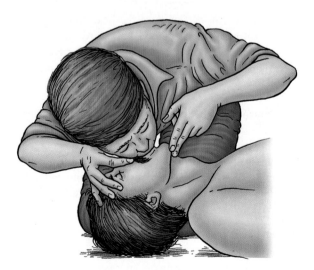

Fig. 3.6 Rescue breathing

large rescuer may use excessive ventilatory volumes in a child, causing barotrauma or gastric distention, leading to regurgitation and aspiration. (This is one of the main reasons that lay rescuers are now required to use a compression ratio of 30:2 which provides more compressions than ventilations). If regurgitation occurs, the victim's head should be turned to one side, their mouth wiped out, and CPR continued.

When mouth-to-mouth ventilation is unsatisfactory or impossible for any reason (e.g., serious injury or inability to open the mouth), mouth-to-nose ventilation may be a viable alternative (Fig. 3.7). For those victims with a tracheostomy, mouth-to-stoma

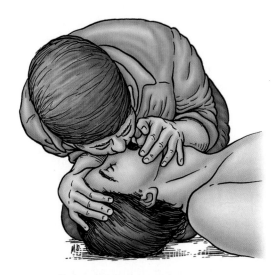

Fig. 3.7 Mouth-to-nose ventilation

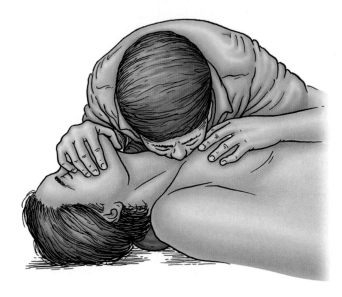

Fig. 3.8 Mouth-to-stoma ventilation

ventilation may be required (Fig. 3.8). If one chooses to use a barrier device when providing rescue breaths (even though they may not reduce the risk of infection and may increase resistance to airflow), breathing should not be delayed. Face masks used for face mask or bag-mask ventilation (BMV) should contain a one-way valve that directs the rescuer's breaths into the patient and diverts the victim's exhaled air away from the rescuer. Ventilating with a bag and mask can use room air or oxygen. Gastric inflation should be avoided with breaths that are provided over 1 s and that provide sufficient volume to cause visible chest rise. See Box 3.2 for requirements of a bag-mask device.[20] An alternative to BMV is the use of an advanced airway, including an endotracheal tube (via tracheal intubation), the esophageal-tracheal Combitube, the King airway or the laryngeal mask airway (LMA). When an advanced airway is in place and functioning appropriately, rescuers should deliver 8–10 breaths per minute, while chest compressions are being delivered continuously at a rate of 100 per minute. These advanced airways are discussed below.

Box 3.2 Requirements of a Bag-Mask Device

- A nonjam inlet valve.
- Either no pressure relief valve or a pressure relief valve which can be bypassed.
- Standard 15-mm/22-mm fittings.
- An oxygen reservoir to allow delivery of high oxygen concentrations.
- A nonbreathing outlet valve that cannot be obstructed by foreign material and will not jam with an oxygen flow of 30 L/min.
- The capability to function satisfactorily under environmental conditions and extremes of temperature.

Source: data from Barnes[20]

Bag-Mask Ventilation

BMV is an extremely important skill and one that all clinicians involved in airway management need to master. One study showed that there was no significant difference in the rate of survival or neurologic outcome in prehospital setting between BMV alone and BMV followed by endotracheal intubation.[21] This result reinforces the importance of proper BMV technique.

BMV is best provided by two rescuers. If performed by a lone rescuer, the rescuer should be experienced enough with the device to simultaneously open the airway, perform ventilation, and observe chest rise. It is important to perform airway clearing maneuvers (see Sect. "Maneuvers for Opening the Airway") and to use airway adjuncts such as oropharyngeal or nasopharyngeal airways when available (see Chap. 4 for description of these devices).

If two operators are present, the mask can be held by two hands of one operator. Conversely, the lone operator will need to hold the mask in one hand (Fig. 3.9).

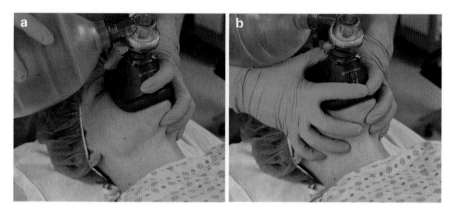

Fig. 3.9 (**a**) One- and (**b**) two-handed technique for holding mask

A step-by-step guide for applying one-operator BMV can be found in Chap. 4. In brief, the techniques are as follows:

1. With the left hand, place the mask over the patient's face seal so that the apex of the mask covers the bridge of patient's nose and the base is between the lower lip and chin.
2. Create and maintain a tight seal by gripping the mask with the thumb and index finger of the left hand.
3. Place the last three fingers of the left hand under the jaw to provide counter pressure to the mask and to keep open the airway by lifting the patient's jaw up.

Two rescue breaths should be delivered during a brief pause between each cycle of 30 chest compressions. The volume required to cause visible chest rise (500–600 mL) should be produced by squeezing a 1-L adult bag about one half to two thirds of its volume or a 2-L bag about one third of its volume. The HC provider should provide supplementary oxygen when available – O_2 >40% with a minimum flow rate of 10–12 L/min. Disadvantages of BMV include gastric inflation, air leak, and failure to protect the airway from aspiration of gastric contents.[22]

Advanced Airway Devices for Airway Control and Ventilation

The use of advanced airway devices such as the LMA, the King airway or Esophageal-Tracheal Combitube should only be used by well-trained and experienced HC providers. The use of devices for airway management during resuscitation aims to provide rapid and reliable restoration and maintenance of the airway, thereby allowing optimal oxygenation and ventilation. Additional aims include the ability to provide positive pressure ventilation, to protect the airway against regurgitation, and to be "fail safe" (thus doing no harm if unsuccessful or inexpertly placed).[22] While there are advantages of using these devices, chest compressions will be interrupted for several seconds and thus the benefits and risks must be considered.

Endotracheal tubes (ETT) can be used to intubate the trachea when adequate ventilation with a bag and mask has been unsuccessful in victims with no protective airway reflexes. Although ETTs are routinely carried by paramedic teams, intubation is a difficult skill to learn and, if infrequently performed (thus generally poorly performed), failure rates (>50%)[23] are unacceptable. Furthermore, unrecognized failure and esophageal intubation are more likely to occur in inexperienced hands.[21] Providers should use some device to confirm the placement of the ETT, such as an exhaled CO_2 detector, at several time points during CPR (without interrupting compressions) and transport. The LMA may be a good option for controlling and ventilating the airway and the AHA states that it is acceptable to use this as an alternative to the ETT in cardiac arrest.[24] The placement of this device may be more frequently successful and faster to perform than the placement of an ETT. It can also be used in cases where it is impossible to position the patient for intubation. Although controversial, the rate of regurgitation is relatively uncommon with use of the classic LMA.[25] There are concerns over the efficacy of ventilation when using a classic LMA. The classic LMA only forms a low-pressure seal; thus if higher pressures are required, there will be some leakage; it is advisable to use low volumes and low pressures. The Proseal LMA may be very suitable for resuscitation, due to its ability to form a higher pressure seal and the incorporation of a gastric tube to lower the chance of aspiration (Fig. 3.10). The Combitube is another alternative to the ETT during resuscitation of cardiac arrest.[24] The Combitube achieves similar ventilation and oxygenation to that of the ETT and is easier to learn. It is critical to identify the location of the distal tube (i.e., whether it is in the esophagus or trachea) to avoid fatal complications. The LMAs and Combitube are covered in more detail in Chaps. 4 and 5.

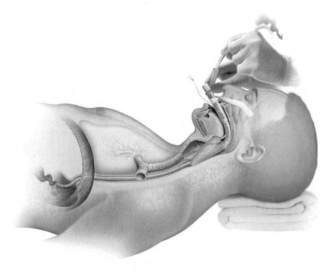

Fig. 3.10 Proseal LMA in situ (Copyright 2009 The Laryngeal Mask Company Limited, with permission)

Determining Pulselessness (HC Providers Only)

Ventilation alone will not sustain an individual who has suffered a cardiac arrest. It is also essential to concurrently reestablish effective circulation for perfusion of the vital organs. Palpation of the carotid or femoral pulse will assess whether the victim has effective circulation. No more than 10 s should be taken when checking for a pulse. If a pulse is present but the patient is apneic, ventilations are initiated at a rate of 10–12 breaths per minute (one every 5–6 s) and the pulse is checked every 2 min. However, if no pulse is detectable (or there is uncertainty), cardiac arrest has occurred and the rescuer must begin external chest compressions.

Layperson rescuers are not expected to assess the circulation by performing the pulse check. Studies have shown that laypeople waste considerable time attempting to feel the pulse and that they fail to recognize the *absence* of a pulse in up to 10% of cases (false negative, or type II error). They also fail to diagnose the *presence* of a pulse in 40% of cases. These errors have serious consequences. In failing to recognize the absence of a pulse, victims are deprived of lifesaving measures (compressions and attachment of the AED). In failing to recognize the *presence* of a pulse (false positive, type I error) in up to 40% of cases, the compressions are needlessly applied and the AED is attached. Therefore, instead of attempting to palpate the pulse, a lay rescuer should look for other signs of circulation:

- Look, listen, and feel for breathing or coughing
- Look for signs of movement
- If the above signs are absent, the rescuer should begin compressions

This assessment should take no longer than 10 s. If there is some doubt about the assessment of the circulation, begin chest compressions.

External Chest Compression Techniques

The mechanism, whereby chest compression results in circulation of blood, is somewhat controversial. There are two main theories. The *cardiac pump theory*[26] postulates that chest compression directly squeezes the heart between the sternum and the vertebral column. In contrast, the *thoracic pump theory*[27] maintains that chest compression increases the intrathoracic pressure, which is transmitted predominantly to the extrathoracic arteries, since they are much less collapsible than the extrathoracic veins. As a result, an arteriovenous pressure gradient is generated outside the thoracic cavity and blood flow occurs. These theories are not mutually exclusive, and it is likely that both may be operative.

Compressions will be most effective if the patient can be positioned supine on a hard surface. To perform external chest compressions, the heel of one hand is placed over the lower half of the victim's sternum and between the nipples and the other hand is placed on top of the first (Fig. 3.11). The rescuer's arms must be straight, with the shoulders directly over the victim's sternum, so they are directing the vector of force vertically. To enhance the effectiveness of chest compressions, each one

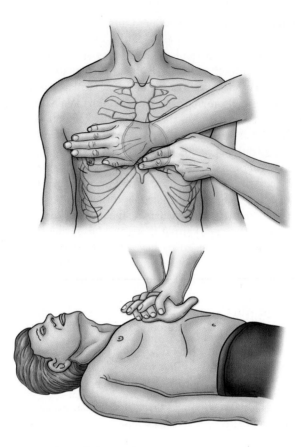

Fig. 3.11 Chest compression technique

should be a smooth motion, equal in duration to the relaxation phase. To minimize the risk of complications (listed below), proper hand position should be maintained at all times. For an adult, the depth of compression is 1.5–2 in. and the rate 100 per minute. The chest should be allowed to recoil after each compression, to allow venous return (incomplete recoil is associated with higher intrathoracic pressures, decreased coronary perfusion, and decreased cerebral perfusion).[28] If two rescuers are present, quickly switch the compressor about every 2 min. Once initiated by lay rescuers, CPR should be continued until an AED arrives, the victim begins to move, or EMS takes over. For HC personnel, CPR should be continued except for specific interruptions such as insertion of an advanced airway or use of a defibrillator.

Compression-Only CPR

Mouth-to-mouth breathing is unquestionably effective in CPR. However, some rescuers are reluctant to use it because of fear of contracting infectious diseases (hepatitis, acquired immunodeficiency syndrome). It is now accepted that the outcome of CPR without ventilations is significantly better than that after no CPR at all for adult cardiac arrest. In fact, survival outcomes have shown to be fairly similar for compression-only CPR to that of conventional CPR in several bystander studies.[29] Assar et al.[30] showed the average time to deliver breaths by a non-HC bystander is 16 s – much longer than the recommended 1 s per breath.[7] Based on that finding, Kern et al.[13] simulated, in pigs, traditional CPR with compressions delivered at a rate of 100 compressions per minute with a 16-s pause in compressions to deliver rescue breaths (simulating bystander CPR) and compared it to continuous cardiac compressions (CCC), delivered also at 100 compressions per minute, but with no pause for delivery of rescue breaths. They found neurological function and 24 h survival to be significantly better in the pigs who received CCC than in those that received the bystander-simulated CPR. There is further evidence to suggest that rescue breathing is not essential during the first 5 min of CPR for VF SCA.[31] Continuity of circulatory support seems to result in more perfusion to the heart and CNS and leads to better outcomes than bystander CPR with longer-than-recommended pauses to deliver rescue breaths.

Special Situations

Drowning

CPR should be given to the victim as soon as they are removed from the water, and the lone rescuer should provide five cycles of CPR prior to leaving the victim to activate the EMS system. Reducing hypoxia is the single most important variable with drowning. Rescue breaths can be performed in the water, although compressions are difficult and may not be effective. Maneuvers to remove foreign body airway obstruction are not recommended.

Hypothermia

Breathing should be assessed by a HC provider for 30–45 s since heart rate and breathing may be very slow. Do not put off CPR until the patient is warmed. Rescue breathing should be performed immediately to those who are not breathing. If the patient does not have a pulse, begin chest compressions.

CPR Devices and Techniques

In the past few years, many new devices and techniques have been investigated to assist ventilation or support circulation during CPR — including automated and mechanical transport ventilators, active compression–decompression CPR, interposed abdominal compression, high-frequency (> 120/min) chest compressions, mechanical piston and impedance threshold devices, load-distributing bands ("Vest CPR"), CPR with medical antishock trousers, and continuous abdominal binding.[9, 32]

Automated transport ventilators are useful for ventilation of adult patients with a pulse who have an advanced airway or an LMA in place. Interposed abdominal compressions have been shown to increase blood flow by about twofold and the rate of return to spontaneous circulation by 25–50%.[33] Impedance threshold devices, when used by trained personnel for intubated cardiac arrest patients, can improve hemodynamic parameters (e.g., increase systolic blood pressure by approximately twofold)[34] and return spontaneous circulation. A mechanical piston device has been shown to improve end-tidal CO_2 and mean arterial pressure in cardiac arrest patients.[35, 36] In McDonald's opinion, "direct measurement of arterial pressure and the use of mechanical chest compression result in a more informed and less frenetic environment during CPR."[35] This device may be considered for patients in cardiac arrest when manual resuscitation is difficult, as long as the device is programmed to deliver the recommended depth and rate of compressions as well as complete chest recoil between compressions.[32]

Limitations and Complications of CPR

Even when performed by experienced personnel, CPR is barely adequate to sustain life. First, exhaled air contains only 15–18% oxygen, which might be adequate if the victim's arterial PO_2 is not lowered substantially by the desaturation of mixed venous blood. Second, gastric distention is common, especially when excessive ventilation is given, and not only interferes with ventilation, but also increases the risk of aspiration. Third, even with adequate chest compressions using standard CPR techniques, cardiac output is only 25% of normal. Luce et al.[27] have shown that in anesthetized dogs with electrically induced VF who received conventional CPR, cerebral blood flow is only approximately 6% of normal and coronary blood flow 3% of normal.

Furthermore, despite proper CPR technique, complications can occur, including rib and sternal fractures, bone marrow emboli to lung, mediastinal bleeding, vegetable material in pulmonary artery, new pericardial bleeding, subcutaneous emphysema, mediastinal emphysema, and bone marrow emboli to heart.[37]

Airway Obstruction

Etiology of Upper Airway Obstruction

When the patency of the airway is compromised, the amount of air entering or leaving the lungs is diminished. There are numerous causes of upper airway obstruction, but for the sake of clarity, they will be classified into two broad groups: central nervous system (CNS) and peripheral.

CNS Causes

CNS depression from any cause leads to diminished tone in the mandibular muscles, resulting in airway obstruction by the tongue. Following are causes of CNS depression:

- Decreased cardiac output (e.g., acute myocardial infarction, cardiac tamponade, congestive heart failure, ventricular tachycardia or fibrillation, hypovolemic shock, septic shock, massive pulmonary embolism)
- Cerebral ischemia
- Head trauma
- Drug overdose (e.g., alcohol, barbiturates, benzodiazepines, opiates, cocaine, or combinations of these and other CNS depressants)
- Hypoxemia/hypercarbia (e.g., chronic obstructive pulmonary disease, adult respiratory distress syndrome, pneumonia, pulmonary embolism)
- Anesthesia
- Metabolic derangements (e.g., hypoglycemia, hyperglycemia, hyponatremia, hypernatremia, hypokalemia, metabolic acidosis, uremia, hepatic encephalopathy)
- Hypothermia
- Hyperthermia

Peripheral Causes

Any disease or condition that allows encroachment on the upper airway is included in this category. Most causes fall under the following headings:

- Congenital anomalies of the airway (e.g., Treacher Collins)
- Infections (e.g., epiglottitis, croup, retropharyngeal abscess)
- Tumors and mass lesions (benign, malignant) (e.g., thymoma; carcinoma of the oropharynx, larynx, and esophagus; aortic aneurysm)
- Trauma
- Drowning
- Foreign body
- Burns
- Gas and smoke inhalation
- Anaphylaxis (secondary to bee stings, pollen, food, drugs)
- Laryngospasm
- Bilateral vocal cord paralysis (secondary to trauma, thyroidectomy, or neoplasm)

The Tongue as a Cause of Airway Obstruction

The tongue is attached firmly to the mandible, hyoid bone, and epiglottis by a number of muscles and ligaments. In the normal conscious state, tone in these muscles prevents the tongue from encroaching upon the airway (Fig. 3.12). However, with

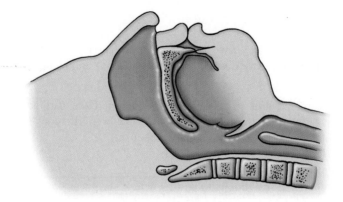

Fig. 3.12 Tongue position in a conscious supine adult

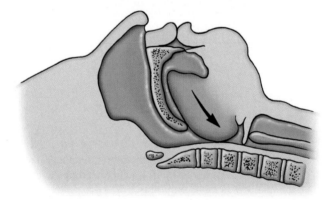

Fig. 3.13 Tongue position in an unconscious supine adult

altered consciousness the tone in these muscles decreases, allowing the tongue to gravitate toward the posterior pharyngeal wall and cause airway obstruction.

Three other factors contribute to airway obstruction by the tongue. First, in the comatose state the cervical spine adopts a semiflexed position, narrowing the distance from the tongue to the pharynx. Second, the epiglottis gravitates toward the glottis. Third, respiratory effort in the presence of airway obstruction pulls the tongue toward the airway (Fig. 3.13). Thus, the most common cause of upper airway obstruction is the tongue.

Foreign Body Airway Obstruction

Complete airway obstruction is a serious emergency that must be addressed as soon as possible. As already noted, the tongue is the most common cause of airway obstruction in unconscious adult patients. The epiglottis may contribute to obstruction caused by the tongue. Blood or solid food contents from the stomach may also obstruct the airway. It has been estimated that there are 1.2 deaths per 100,000 population from choking.[38]

Foreign body airway obstruction has been labeled the "café coronary" because it occurs frequently in restaurants and the signs mimic those of an acute myocardial infarction. Typically, while eating, the individual suddenly stops breathing, becomes cyanotic, and loses consciousness. Factors that predispose to choking include ingestion of food while intoxicated or exercising, and inadequate chewing of meat, especially in elderly people wearing dentures. Most choking deaths occur in individuals who are aged 75 or older, or in children in the 1–4-year range. Meat, particularly steak and hot dogs, is the most common offending agent in adults, whereas children, who often have more eclectic tastes, choke on a variety of organic and inorganic materials, ranging from peanuts to marbles to miniature toy trucks.

The diagnosis of foreign body airway obstruction should be considered in (1) any witnessed acute respiratory arrest and (2) any unwitnessed arrest wherein the rescuer cannot ventilate the victim despite repositioning the head.

The appropriateness of intervention in a conscious choking victim depends upon the adequacy of air exchange, which correlates with the degree of airway obstruction.

Partial Obstruction

In partial obstruction the narrowed portion of the airway still allows some air exchange to occur. Certain characteristic sounds may reveal the site of the obstruction. A crowing sound suggests obstruction at the vocal cords, a wheezing sound obstruction of the trachea or bronchi, and a gurgling sound regurgitation or aspiration. If there is adequate airflow, the victim can generate a powerful cough.

Since spontaneous coughing is more effective than any rescue maneuver in dislodging a foreign body, the victim's attempts to cough should not be impeded. In addition, the victim (who may be panic-stricken) should be prevented from running out of sight (e.g., to the bathroom, where they might collapse and die, unnoticed and unattended), and they should be monitored for signs of deteriorating respiratory status—a feeble cough, stridor, marked chest wall retractions, cyanosis, and ultimately loss of consciousness. The management of partial airway obstruction with poor airflow is the same as for complete airway obstruction.

Complete Obstruction

Complete airway obstruction is present when the victim cannot speak, cough, or breathe. Often the victim grips his throat – the universal distress signal for airway obstruction (Fig. 3.14). No signs of air exchange are detectable upon looking for chest movements, listening for breath sounds, and feeling for airflow. Efforts at inspiration are accompanied by marked chest wall retractions. In an apneic individual, complete obstruction is present when the lungs cannot be inflated by ventilations.

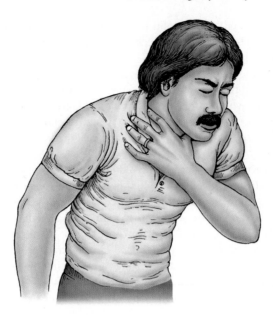

Fig. 3.14 The universal sign of choking

Management of the Obstructed Airway: The Heimlich Maneuver

The Heimlich maneuver, alternatively described as subdiaphragmatic abdominal thrusts, is now considered the standard for relieving foreign body upper airway obstruction in the adult.[13] Theoretically, it causes a sharp increase in intraabdominal pressure, which in turn compresses the lungs. The resulting exhalation should be of sufficient force to expel an obstruction from the airway. The Heimlich maneuver may be performed on a conscious or an unconscious victim, who may stand, sit, or remain supine, and it may even be self-administered.

Conscious Victim

The conscious victim may be either standing or sitting when the Heimlich maneuver is carried out. (For the small rescuer the maneuver may be performed more easily with the conscious victim supine). The victim's waist is encircled from behind. The rescuer makes a fist with one hand, such that the thumb rests firmly on the abdominal wall in the midline slightly above the navel and well below the tip of the xiphoid process (Fig. 3.15a). The fisted hand is gripped with the other hand (Fig. 3.15b) and an inward/upward thrust is applied rapidly. The rescuer's hands must never rest on the xiphoid or lower ribs, otherwise internal organ damage may occur. Repeated thrusts should be delivered until the foreign body is expelled or the victim becomes unconscious.

The Heimlich maneuver may be self-administered by applying a fisted hand to the abdomen as just described and pressing it inward and upward. Alternatively, the victim may lean forcefully over the edge of a firm surface such as a railing or the back of a chair.

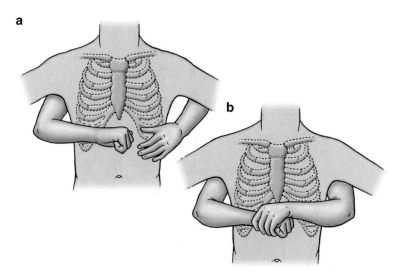

Fig. 3.15 The Heimlich maneuver. (**a**) Thumb facing inward in the midline between the navel and xiphoid process. (**b**) Grip fisted hand and apply a firm inward/upward thrust

Unconscious Victim

The unconscions victim should be lying supine on a firm surface. The rescuer with knees astride or beside the victim, places the heel of one hand in the midline between the xiphoid process and umbilicus (i.e., same hand position as above), and with the other hand covering the first, applies firm inward/upward pressure. Again, contact with the xiphoid process and rib cage is avoided at all times.

Chest Thrusts

In markedly obese individuals, women in advanced pregnancy, and infants, the Heimlich maneuver is contraindicated and the *chest thrust* should be applied instead. (*Note:* In infants, a combination of chest thrusts and back blows is recommended [see Chap. 10]). In adults the hand position for the chest thrust is identical to that for chest compression during CPR (Fig. 3.16).

Finger Sweep

The finger sweep should be used only in an unconscious choking victim. The mouth is opened using the tongue/jaw lift (i.e., gripping the tongue and mandible between the thumb and fingers and lifting upward) and the index finger of the opposite hand is inserted alongside the cheek toward the larynx. A hooking motion can be used in an attempt to dislodge the foreign body into the mouth (Fig. 3.17). In performing this maneuver, it should be remembered that there is a risk of further impacting the object and exacerbating the airway obstruction.

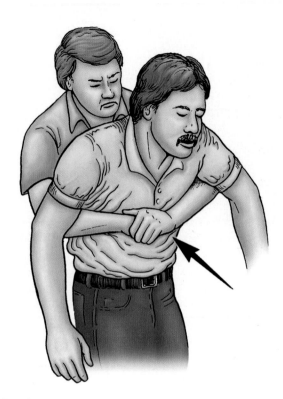

Fig. 3.16 The chest thrust

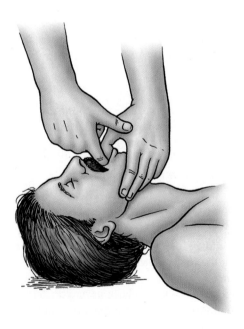

Fig. 3.17 The finger sweep

Recommendations for the Conscious Choking Victim Who Becomes Unconscious (AHA Sequence)

1. Recognize the signs of choking.

   (a) Universal distress
   (b) Inability to speak
   (c) Cyanosis
   (d) Correct scenario

2. Call for help. Activate EMS (call 911 in North America).
3. If victim is conscious and able to speak, cough and breathe, do not interfere with attempts to cough. Otherwise, use the Heimlich maneuver until successful or until the victim loses consciousness.
4. Place the victim in a supine position.
5. Open the mouth (tongue/jaw lift) and perform a "finger sweep."
6. Open the airway (head tilt/chin lift) and attempt to ventilate.
7. If unsuccessful, perform up to five Heimlich maneuvers.
8. Finger sweep.
9. Open the airway and attempt to ventilate.
10. Repeat steps 7 through 9 until successful, or until expert help arrives.

If the proper equipment is available, a qualified person should attempt to visualize the area with a laryngoscope and attempt to remove the foreign body with either a Magill forceps or a Kelly clamp. Failing this, a cricothyrotomy should be performed (see Chap. 12).

CPR and Precautions Against the Transmission of Disease

CPR is predominantly performed by health care workers and public safety personnel, and less so by the lay public. However, laypeople are more likely to perform CPR in the home.

Although the risk of disease transmission during mouth-to-mouth ventilation is miniscule, the perceived risk is quite high. In one survey, 5% of 975 questioned reported a willingness to perform mouth-to-mouth ventilation on a stranger. On the other hand, 68% were willing to perform chest compression alone if it was offered as an alternative. In reality, there have only been 15 reports of CPR-related infections reported in the literature between 1960 and 1998.[39] Organisms identified in these cases of CPR-related transmission include *Helicobacter pylori, Mycobacterium tuberculosis,* meningococcus, herpes simplex, shigella, streptococcus, salmonella, and *Neisseria gonorrhea.* There have been no reports of human immunodeficiency virus (HIV), hepatitis B virus (HBV), hepatitis C, or cytomegalovirus transmission during CPR.[40] Despite these data, both lay personnel and health care workers are reluctant to perform CPR.

Direct mouth-to-mouth ventilation will likely result in exchange of saliva between victim and rescuer. Saliva contaminated with HBV is not infectious to oral

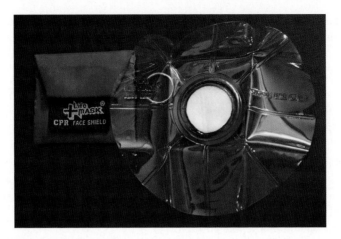

Fig. 3.18 CPR Face Shield

mucous membranes, such as through sharing musical instruments, even among HBV carriers. The risk of infection is far greater with airborne diseases such as tuberculosis. When a health care worker or layperson is exposed to tuberculosis following mouth-to-mouth respiration, the caregiver should have a skin test and should be tested again 12 weeks later. Despite the fact that they may not reduce the risk of infection, some clinicians prefer to use a barrier device such as a pocket face mask or shield. Through such a device it is possible to deliver a breath through a one-way valve while directing the patient's exhaled air away (Fig. 3.18).

Whenever possible, disposable airway equipment should be used, and gloves should be worn when available.[41] Furthermore, known carriers of hepatitis or persons who are HIV positive or have other infections should not teach CPR. In addition, prehospital emergency health care providers — including paramedics, emergency medical technicians (EMTs), police, and firefighters — should become skilled in the technique of BMV.

Health care workers who have a duty to perform CPR on a regular basis should follow guidelines recommended by the Centers for Disease Control and Prevention (CDC) and the Occupational Safety and Health Administration (OSHA) and take precautions to protect themselves (i.e., use latex gloves and bag-mask equipment with one-way valves).

Transmission of Disease from CPR Mannequins

The risk of disease transmission is extremely low during CPR training. Regardless, every effort should be made to avoid the risk of infection by the use of cleansing agents and disinfectants after each use. Both external and internal parts of mannequins must be thoroughly cleaned after each use. There is no evidence that HIV can be transmitted by casual personal contact. The HIV virus is very delicate and is inactivated in less than 10 min at room temperature by a number of disinfectants. If current AHA and mannequin manufacturer recommendations are followed, the risk of HIV, HBV, bacterial, and fungal infection is extremely low.

Summary

Since time is of the essence in the prevention of cerebral hypoxia, the rescuer must always be prepared to perform CPR or relieve airway obstruction at a moment's notice, without using a bag/valve device (Ambu Bag), laryngoscope, or other sophisticated equipment. CPR is best thought of as a series of alternating diagnostic and therapeutic steps. The first step (establishing unresponsiveness) is followed by maneuvers to open the airway (head tilt/chin lift, jaw thrust, triple airway maneuver, mandibular displacement). Subsequently, there is assessment as to whether the victim is breathing and, if necessary, ventilations are initiated (providing 2 breaths). Finally, if no pulse is palpable, cycles of compressions (100/min) and ventilations (30:2 ratio) must begin and occur until a defibrillator arrives, ALS providers take over, or the victim moves. If the patient has a susceptible rhythm, one shock is provided followed immediately by five cycles of CPR.

In managing a choking victim, the rescuer must assess whether the obstruction is partial or complete by evaluating the adequacy of airflow and the victim's ability to speak, cough, and breathe. The Heimlich maneuver (which may have to be repeated several times) proves effective in most cases of foreign body airway obstruction. Only if proper equipment is available and the rescuer is trained, should the airway be viewed and attempts made to remove the foreign body.

Now that the basic elements of the airway have been dealt with, the ensuing chapters will deal with more advanced aspects of airway management.

Acknowledgments The author would like to thank Jennifer Pillay, Nikki Stalker, Jenkin Tsui, and Adam Dryden for their contribution to this chapter.

References

1. American Society of Anesthesiologists Task Force on Management of the Difficult Airway. Practice guidelines for management of the difficult airway. *Anesthesiology*. 1993;78:597–602.
2. Emergency Cardiac Care Committee and Subcommittees AHA. Guidelines for cardiopulmonary resuscitation and emergency cardiac care. Part I. Introduction. *JAMA*. 1992;268:2171–2183.
3. International Liaison Committee on Resuscitation. 2005 International consensus on cardiopulmonary resuscitation and emergency cardiovascular care science with treatment recommendations. *Circulation*. 2005;112:III-1–III-136.
4. American Heart Association Statistics Committee and Stroke Statistics Subcommittee. Heart disease and stroke statistics – 2009 Update. *Circulation*. 2009;199:e21–e181.
5. Heart and Stroke Foundation of Canada. *The Changing Face of Heart Disease and Stroke in Canada 2000*. Ottawa: Statistics Canada, Health Canada; 1999:107p.

6. Chugh SS, Jui J, Gunson K, et al. Current burden of sudden cardiac death: multiple source surveillance versus retrospective death certificate-based review in a large U.S. community. *J Am Coll Cardiol.* 2004;44:1268–1275.

7. Hazinski MF, Nadkarni VM, Hickey RW, O'Connor R, Becker LB, Zaritsky A. Major changes in the 2005 AHA Guidelines for CPR and ECC: reaching the tipping point for change. *Circulation.* 2005;112:IV206–IV211.

8. Lund I, Skulberg A. Cardiopulmonary resuscitation by lay people. *Lancet.* 1976;2:702–704.

9. American Heart Association in Collaboration with the International Liaison Committee on Resuscitation. Guidelines 2000 for cardiopulmonary resuscitation and emergency cardiovascular care science, international consensus on science. *Circulation.* 2000;102:1–384.

10a. American Heart Association. 2005 American heart association guidelines for cardiopulmonary resuscitation (CPR) and emergency cardiovascular care (ECC). *Circulation.* 2005;112:IV1–IV203.

10b. American Heart Association. 2010 American Heart Association Guidelines for Cardiopulmonary Resuscitation and Emergency Cardiovascular Care." *Circulation.* 2010;122(suppl 3):S640–S656. Guidelines for Cardiopulmonary Resuscitation and Emergency Cardiovascular Care." *Circulation.* 2010;122(suppl 3):S639–S946.

11. Hazinski MF, Idris AH, Kerber RE, et al. Lay rescuer automated external defibrillator ("public access defibrillation") programs: lessons learned from an international multicenter trial: advisory statement from the American Heart Association Emergency Cardiovascular Committee; the Council on Cardiopulmonary, Perioperative, and Critical Care; and the Council on Clinical Cardiology. *Circulation.* 2005;111:3336–3340.

12. Berg RA, Sanders AB, Kern KB, et al. Adverse hemodynamic effects of interrupting chest compressions for rescue breathing during cardiopulmonary resuscitation for ventricular fibrillation cardiac arrest. *Circulation.* 2001;104:2465–2470.

13. Kern KB, Hilwig RW, Berg RA, Sanders AB, Ewy GA. Importance of continuous chest compressions during cardiopulmonary resuscitation: improved outcome during a simulated single lay-rescuer scenario. *Circulation.* 2002;105:645–649.

14. American Heart Association [Internet]. Dallas: The Association. c2009 [Updated 2008 May 8, cited 2009 Nov 12]. CPR Facts and Statistics; [about 1 screen]. Available from: http://www.americanheart.org/presenter.jhtml?identifier=3034352.

15. American Heart Association. Part 5: Electrical therapies, 2005 American Heart Association guidelines for cardiopulmonary resuscitation and emergency cardiovascular care. *Circulation.* 2005;112:IV35–IV46.

16. Colquhoun M, Handley AJ, Evans TR. *ABC of Resuscitation.* 5th ed. London: BMJ Books; 2004.

17. Schneider T, Martens PR, Paschen H, et al. Multicenter, randomized, controlled trial of 150-J biphasic shocks compared with 200- to 360-J monophasic shocks in the resuscitation of out-of-hospital cardiac arrest victims. Optimized Response to Cardiac Arrest (ORCA) Investigators. *Circulation.* 2000;102:1780–1787.

18. Sanders AB, Kern KB, Atlas M, Bragg S, Ewy GA. Importance of the duration of inadequate coronary perfusion pressure on resuscitation from cardiac arrest. *J Am Coll Cardiol.* 1985;6:113–118.

19. Yu T, Weil MH, Tang W, et al. Adverse outcomes of interrupted precordial compression during automated defibrillation. *Circulation.* 2002;106:368–372.

20. Barnes TA. Emergency ventilation techniques and related equipment. *Respir Care.* 1992;37:673–690.

21. Gausche M, Lewis RJ, Stratton SJ, et al. Effect of out-of-hospital pediatric endotracheal intubation on survival and neurological outcome: a controlled clinical trial. *JAMA.* 2000;283:783–790.

22. Cook TM, Hommers C. New airways for resuscitation? *Resuscitation.* 2006;69:371–387.

23. Sayre MR, Sakles JC, Mistler AF, Evans JL, Kramer AT, Pancioli AM. Field trial of endotracheal intubation by basic EMTs. *Ann Emerg Med.* 1998;31:228–233.

24. American Heart Association. Part 7.1: Adjuncts for airway control and ventilation. 2005 American Heart Association guidelines for cardiopulmonary resuscitation (CPR) and emergency cardiovascular care (ECC). *Circulation.* 2005;112:IV51–IV57.
25. Stone BJ, Chantler PJ, Baskett PJ. The incidence of regurgitation during cardiopulmonary resuscitation: a comparison between the bag valve mask and laryngeal mask airway. *Resuscitation.* 1998;38:3–6.
26. Rudikoff MT, Maughan WL, Effron M, Freund P, Weisfeldt ML. Mechanisms of blood flow during cardiopulmonary resuscitation. *Circulation.* 1980;61:345–352.
27. Luce JM, Ross BK, O'Quin RJ, et al. Regional blood flow during cardiopulmonary resuscitation in dogs using simultaneous and nonsimultaneous compression and ventilation. *Circulation.* 1983;67:258–265.
28. Yannopoulos D, McKnite S, Aufderheide TP, et al. Effects of incomplete chest wall decompression during cardiopulmonary resuscitation on coronary and cerebral perfusion pressures in a porcine model of cardiac arrest. *Resuscitation.* 2005;64:363–372.
29. Nolan JP, Soar J. Airway techniques and ventilation strategies. *Curr Opin Crit Care.* 2008;14:279–286.
30. Assar D, Chamberlain D, Colquhoun M, et al. Randomised controlled trials of staged teaching for basic life support. 1. Skill acquisition at bronze stage. *Resuscitation.* 2000;45:7–15.
31. Hallstrom AP. Dispatcher-assisted "phone" cardiopulmonary resuscitation by chest compression alone or with mouth-to-mouth ventilation. *Crit Care Med.* 2000;28:N190–N192.
32. American Heart Association. Part 6: CPR Techniques and Devices, 2005 American Heart Association Guidelines for Cardiopulmonary Resuscitation and Emergency Cardiovascular Care. *Circulation.* 2005;112:IV-47–IV-50.
33. Babbs CF. Interposed abdominal compression CPR: a comprehensive evidence based review. *Resuscitation.* 2003;59:71–82.
34. Pirrallo RG, Aufderheide TP, Provo TA, Lurie KG. Effect of an inspiratory impedance threshold device on hemodynamics during conventional manual cardiopulmonary resuscitation. *Resuscitation.* 2005;66:13–20.
35. McDonald JL. Systolic and mean arterial pressures during manual and mechanical CPR in humans. *Ann Emerg Med.* 1982;11:292–295.
36. Ward KR, Menegazzi JJ, Zelenak RR, Sullivan RJ, McSwain NE Jr. A comparison of chest compressions between mechanical and manual CPR by monitoring end-tidal PCO2 during human cardiac arrest. *Ann Emerg Med.* 1993;22:669–674.
37. Powner DJ, Holcombe PA, Mello LA. Cardiopulmonary resuscitation-related injuries. *Crit Care Med.* 1984;12:54–55.
38. National Safety Council [Internet]. Chicago: The Council; c2009 [Updated 209; cited 2009 May 2]. Injury Facts 2009 Edition; [about 2 screens]. Available from: http://www.nsc.org/lrs/injuriesinamerica08.aspx.
39. Liaison committee on Resuscitation. Part 1: Introduction to the International Guidelines 2000 for CPR and ECC: a consensus on science. *Circulation.* 2000;102:I1–I11.
40. Mejicano GC, Maki DG. Infections acquired during cardiopulmonary resuscitation: estimating the risk and defining strategies for prevention. *Ann Intern Med.* 1998;129:813–828.
41. Risk of infection during CPR training and rescue: supplemental guidelines. The Emergency Cardiac Care Committee of the American Heart Association. *JAMA.* 1989;262:2714–2715.

Chapter 4
Basic Equipment for Airway Management

Contents

Introduction

Proper management of a patient's airway during elective and emergency situations is of vital importance for any clinician. Because of this, a multitude of airway aids and devices are available for airway management. These devices include not only face masks, laryngeal masks (e.g., LMA) oral/nasal airways, conventional/video laryngoscopes, and endotracheal tubes, but also oxygen delivery systems for oxygenation and ventilation. The purpose of this chapter is to describe basic oxygen delivery systems and basic equipment for intubation and ventilation. Subsequent

B.T. Finucane et al., *Principles of Airway Management*,
DOI 10.1007/978-0-387-09558-5_4, © Springer Science+Business Media, LLC 2011

chapters will discuss the use of this equipment as well as the use of more advanced equipment and techniques.

Oxygen Sources

The primary goal of airway management is to oxygenate the patient. If oxygenation is inadequate, all other supportive care will fail. An understanding of the equipment and networks used for oxygen storage, delivery, and monitoring will help one to avoid making fundamental mistakes that could interfere with oxygenation.

Wall Oxygen

Commercially available oxygen is obtained from the fractional distillation of air and is at least 99% pure. Wall oxygen is stored either in liquid form or as a gas in large cylinder reservoirs. Oxygen is piped throughout most hospitals to wall outlets. At an outlet, oxygen passes through a reducing valve at a pressure of 50 psi, which is maintained at all flow rates to every outlet.

In addition, piping systems are arranged in defined zones throughout the hospital to allow the termination of oxygen delivery to a specific area while providing normal flow to other areas. This allows manual shutoff of a specified zone of outlets (e.g., in the case of fire in an isolated area). In the event of a central system failure, low-pressure alarms are activated throughout the hospital, alerting responsible individuals to take appropriate action. The standards for oxygen reservoir and piping systems are set forth by the National Fire Protection Association and the Compressed Gas Association.[1]

Each wall station is capped by an outlet, usually the Diameter Index Safety System (DISS) or quick-connect system (Figs. 4.1 and 4.2). To obtain oxygen at a reduced pressure and manageable flow rate, a flowmeter is connected to the outlet (Fig. 4.3). Flowmeters are either back-pressure compensated or nonback-pressure compensated, depending on the location of the needle valve that regulates the flow. In a nonback-pressure compensated system the actual flow may be different from the indicated flow, owing to back pressure within the device. If in doubt as to which type of flowmeter is in use, consult the respiratory therapy department for details concerning the model used in a particular hospital.

From the flowmeter, oxygen tubing may be connected directly to the oxygen-delivery equipment, whether it is a self-inflating bag, a face mask, or nasal prongs.

To ensure proper oxygen delivery from a wall outlet, follow these guidelines:

- Be sure that the flowmeter is properly fitted in the wall outlet.
- Check that the ball in the flowmeter is freely floating. Set the flow in liters per minute.
- Inspect the oxygen tubing from the flowmeter, making sure that all connections are tight and the tube is not kinked or obstructed.
- Listen for or feel oxygen flow at the mask or self-inflating resuscitation bag.
- If there is any doubt about the nature or content of the gas coming from the wall outlet, use an O_2 analyzer for verification.

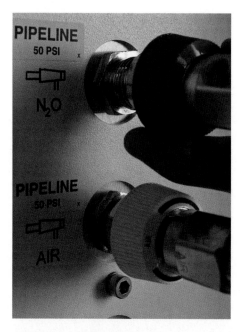

Fig. 4.1 The Diameter Index Safety System (DISS) connector

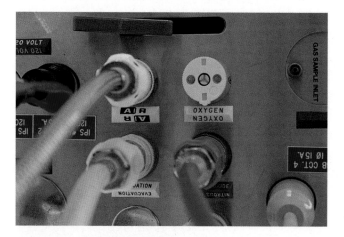

Fig. 4.2 A modern oxygen quick-connect outlet

Tank Oxygen

Another type of oxygen storage system commonly used is the portable oxygen cylinder with an affixed regulator and flowmeter (Figs. 4.4 and 4.5). The regulator reduces the pressure within the system to 50 psi for delivery through the flowmeter. There is still no uniform color coding system for cylinders containing gas under pressure, which is potentially dangerous as physicians move from country to

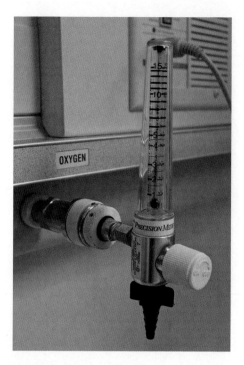

Fig. 4.3 An oxygen flowmeter inserted into the wall outlet

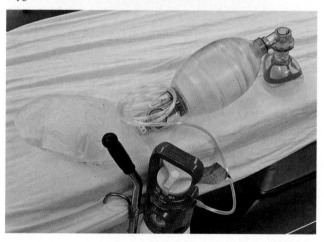

Fig. 4.4 An oxygen E cylinder, showing the regulator and flowmeter

country. Several countries including Canada – but not the United States – have adopted International Standards Organization's color code system for marking gas cylinders for medical use.[2] Oxygen tanks, under this system, are colored white (in some countries only on the shoulder), while in the US, tanks are green and carry various markings that document the manufacturer and inspection dates. The common E cylinder is pressurized to between 1,800 and 2,400 psi at 70°F and 14.7 psi absolute

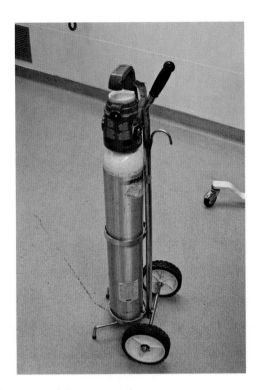

Fig. 4.5 A portable oxygen tank for transportation

(atmospheric pressure) and contains 659 L of oxygen; therefore, the cylinder will last approximately 1 h at a flow rate of 10 L per minute. To calculate tank life in minutes of a partially used cylinder:[3]

Tank life in minutes = (tank pressure in psi × 0.28)/liters per minute flow
or
Tank volume in L/flow rate in L/min.

To ensure proper oxygen flow from a portable tank, follow these guidelines:

- Check that the seal is in place between the cylinder valve and regulator yoke.
- Make sure that all connections are tight between the cylinder valve and regulator yoke.
- Open the cylinder valve with a key or wrench (Fig. 4.6).
- Read the pressure on the regulator pressure gauge.
- Open the flowmeter and check for flow in liters per minute.
- Inspect the oxygen tubing from the flowmeter and make sure that it is unobstructed and connected to the mask or self-inflating resuscitation bag.

As simple as these suggestions seem, in an emergency it is easy to overlook fundamental details that could interfere with oxygen flow.

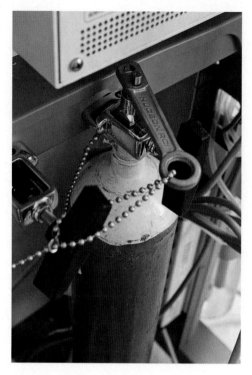

Fig. 4.6 The tank wrench used to open an E cylinder

Pulse Oximetry and Capnography

The pulse oximeter is used to document the level of oxyhemoglobin saturation in capillary tissue and the capnograph is used to measure end-tidal CO_2 as expired from the lungs. These monitors are used routinely in the operating room, recovery room, emergency room, and the intensive care unit. Practitioners of airway management must learn to apply the monitors correctly and to interpret the data properly. These monitors can be used to help diagnose various anatomic abnormalities as well as mechanical problems with oxygenation/ventilation equipment. One may learn about these monitors (and their limitations and problems) in formal anesthesiology and intensive-care medicine textbooks.

Vacuum Suction Apparatus

Occasionally secretions, vomitus, and blood may interfere with gas exchange. For these reasons, a suction apparatus is necessary for airway management. Suction may be obtained from a wall or portable vacuum source (Fig. 4.7).

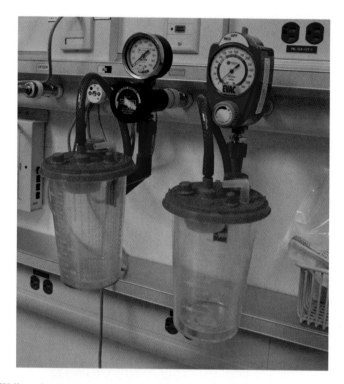

Fig. 4.7 Wall suction apparatus

Prolonged suctioning can lead to deoxygenation. Thus, suctioning should be limited to less than 10 s per application and 100% oxygen should be delivered in the intervals between applications.

Suction tubing may be attached to:

- A flexible catheter (Fig. 4.8a). The flexible catheter is useful for decompressing the stomach and suctioning the esophagus, pharynx, and endotracheal tube (Fig. 4.8b).
- A rigid tonsillar tip (Fig. 4.9a). The tonsillar tip is useful for rapid suctioning of large volumes of fluid from the oropharynx (Fig. 4.9b). However, these tips can damage the teeth, and overzealous suctioning can dislodge an endotracheal tube.

Both types should be immediately available to the person managing the airway. Both types, however, can induce laryngospasm, mucosal damage, or bradycardia, so care must be exercised whenever they are being used.

Some publications warn that traditional suction equipment, even the Yankauer tip suction, is not big enough to clear common particulate material in vomitus.[4] Therefore, larger-diameter suction tubing and tips should be available to the airway manager. Contact the sales representatives of airway equipment manufacturers to review the latest suction system modifications and design improvements.

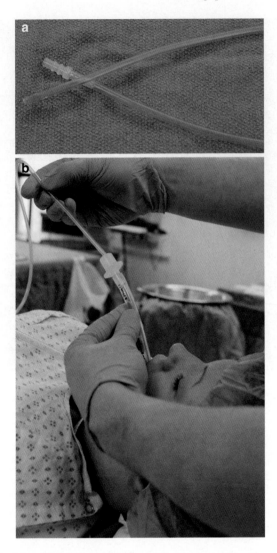

Fig. 4.8 (a) A flexible suction catheter. (b) The catheter can be used to clear secretions from an endotracheal tube or the patient's upper airway

Oxygen Delivery Systems for Spontaneously Breathing Patients

Many patients who do not require ventilatory support need supplemental oxygen, particularly those with pneumonia, postoperative atelectasis, or cardiac disease. In patients with normal hemoglobin concentration and cardiac output, the goal of oxygenation should be to achieve an oxyhemoglobin saturation of at least 90%. Some characteristics of oxygen delivery systems are found in Table 4.1.

In the spontaneously breathing patient, the simplest method to supplement oxygen is with nasal cannulae (prongs) (Fig. 4.10a, b) or a nasopharyngeal catheter. These are lightweight and usually well tolerated, and they do not allow rebreathing of

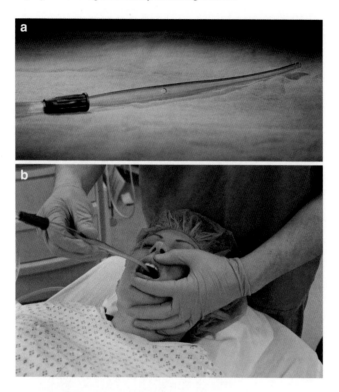

Fig. 4.9 (**a**) A rigid tonsillar suction tip. (**b**) The tip can be used to remove large volumes of fluid from a patient's upper airway

Table 4.1 Characteristics of some oxygen delivery devices

Delivery device	Flow rate (L/min)	Percent O_2[a]	Advantages
Nasal catheter	1–8	30–50	
Nasal prongs/cannula	1–8	22–50	Simple, comfortable; Allows patient to eat or drink
Simple mask	6–12	35–60	Delivers a higher flow rate than nasal prongs
Partial rebreathing	6–12	60–90	
Nonrebreathing	6–8	Up to 100	Higher FiO_2 (Recently disputed[18])
Venturi	(See instructions for partial mask)	24, 28, 35, 40	More precise control of FiO_2
Oxygen reservoir mask	10–16	90	
Blow-by	Varies	Varies	May be used for pediatric patients and the extremely claustrophobic patient

[a]Approximate ranges for adults
Source: Data from Stewart,[3] Hunsinger,[16] McPherson,[17] and Waldau[19]

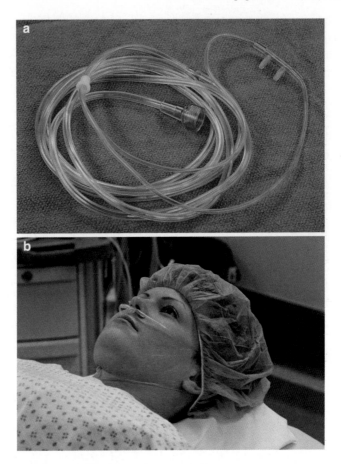

Fig. 4.10 (a) Nasal prongs. (b) In use

expired air. The actual FiO_2 delivered is variable and depends upon the flow rate and the fraction of inspired oxygen.[5] Note, most patients will not tolerate oxygen flow rates exceeding 6 L/min. Some literature suggests that patients with depressed respiratory drives (i.e., chronic obstructive pulmonary disease [COPD]) should not be administered high-flow oxygen as they rely on greater CO_2 levels in the bloodstream to elicit a sufficient stimulus to breath. This is unsubstantiated advice and should be ignored.[6]

The monitoring of $PETCO_2$ with nasal oxygenating systems is becoming more common, especially if the patients are receiving "conscious sedation." Many nasal oxygenation–CO_2 sampling systems are available. Be aware that different systems are tolerated differently by patients and that CO_2 sampling is affected by oxygen flow rates. Woda et al.[7] reported that the Hospitak (HOS) nasal cannula (Lindenhurst, NY) is well tolerated and that CO_2 sampling is not affected by respiratory rate and the oxygen flow rates tested (2–6 L/min). Another nasal cannula–CO_2 sampling system is the Smart CapnoLine Plus™ O_2 (Oridion Medical, Jerusalem, Israel)

(Fig. 4.11). Carbon dioxide monitoring can be performed by operating room analyzers or the portable Microcap™ (Oridion) monitor (Fig. 4.12).

One study reports that nasal cannulae may be modified so that one nasal prong supplies O_2, while CO_2 is sampled via the other. Clamping between the prongs allows for unaffected oxygen delivery and continuous monitoring of end-tidal CO_2

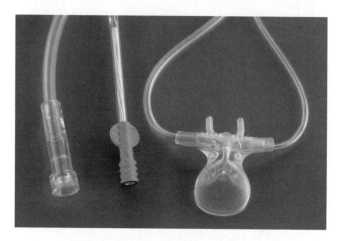

Fig. 4.11 Smart CapnoLine Plus™ (copyright 2009 Oridion Medical 1987 Ltd., with permission)

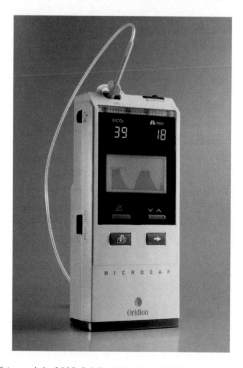

Fig. 4.12 Microcap™ (copyright 2009 Oridion Medical 1987 Ltd., with permission)

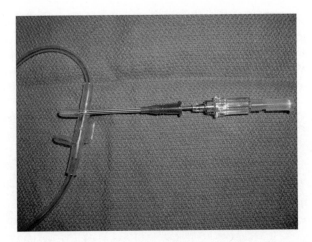

Fig. 4.13 Modified nasal cannula

in the spontaneously breathing, sedated patient.[8] Future studies will carefully document how accurately various nasal sampling systems reflect true PETCO$_2$ and how well nasal PCO$_2$ correlates with PaCO$_2$. For example, an angiocatheter or any clean, unused syringe cap can be cut at a 45° angle for this use (Fig. 4.13).[9]

Nasal cannulae and modified oxygen masks (with the top cut off just above the insufflation holes and other "custom" designs) are sometimes used to supply oxygen to patients whose lower face (including the nose) is covered by surgical drapes, such as for eye surgery. There is debate in the literature as to the best oxygen delivery system. Adding a system to suction CO$_2$ from under the drapes, to decrease FiCO$_2$ and increase patient comfort, should be considered along with oxygenation systems.[10–15]

A plastic mask may also be used. Commonly used masks are called: simple, Venturi (air entrainment), partial rebreathing, and nonrebreathing (Fig. 4.14). The Venturi is designed to deliver specified percentages of oxygen (Table 4.1),[3, 16–19] depending upon the size of the entrainment ports and/or the jet of oxygen. All of these masks can be used on spontaneously breathing patients who are alert enough to protect their airway from the aspiration of secretions or vomitus. If a patient cannot protect his airway (e.g., because he is obtunded or does not manifest a gag, cough, or swallow reflex), an endotracheal tube must be inserted. All the masks illustrated are made of plastic and equipped with a head strap for support. The type of mask used depends on the desired FiO$_2$.

Oxygenation and Ventilation Systems

The remainder of this chapter describes different types of equipment used to support the patient who has lost control of his airway. Patients in this category may be obtunded, perhaps from drugs, hypoxia, or anesthesia or are, for some reason, unable to maintain adequate gas exchange and oxygenation. This section reviews the use of airways, masks, resuscitation bags, and intubation equipment.

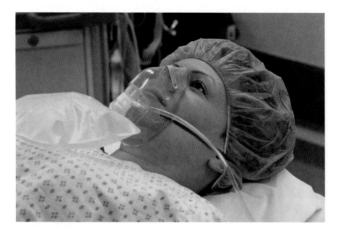

Fig. 4.14 A partial rebreathing oxygen mask in use

Airways

A patient's oropharynx can become occluded when the tongue falls posteriorly. This obstruction is often relieved by repositioning the head or anteriorly displacing the mandible. If these maneuvers are unsuccessful, an artificial airway may be inserted either orally or nasally and will usually provide a route through and around which ventilation can be maintained. However, the jaw lift maneuver is usually required even with a nasal or oral airway in place.

Oral Airway

The first oral airway was described by Hewitt in 1908.[20] Oral airways come in different lengths and designs (Fig. 4.15). They may be inserted easily behind the tongue that has been anteriorly displaced by a wooden tongue blade or a finger (Fig. 4.16). Alternatively, they may be inserted into the mouth by pointing them initially toward the hard palate (Fig. 4.17a) and then advancing the airway and simultaneously rotating it 180° so that the tip slides behind the tongue into the hypopharynx (Fig. 4.17b). This maneuver can cause trauma to the lips, teeth, or oropharyngeal mucosal surfaces. In short, an oral airway is primarily used for two purposes: to help establish a patent, unobstructed airway when a face mask is used, and often as a bite block to prevent the patient from biting on the ET tube during emergencies.

It must be stressed that the insertion of an oral airway may not relieve soft tissue obstruction. Often, atlantooccipital joint dorsiflexion is necessary, even after the airway is in place.[21] Oral airways can stimulate the gag and vomit reflexes and it is usually recommended that it only be used in patients whose protective reflexes have been obtunded, or who have been anesthetized.

This gag reflex is a normal defense mechanism whose afferent impulses are carried by the glossopharyngeal nerve, activation of which results in distinctive spasmodic

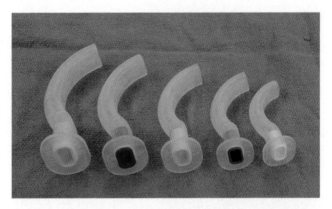

Fig. 4.15 Oral airways (commonly made of plastic)

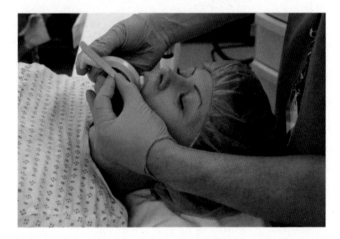

Fig. 4.16 An oral airway can be inserted over the tongue that has been displaced by a wooden tongue blade

and uncoordinated muscle movements. Both physical and psychological stimuli may induce gagging. Methods to reduce gagging include relaxation, hypnotherapy, acupuncture, and "hypnopuncture," among others.[22–24] These methods stem from the concept that neural pathways from the gagging center to the cerebral cortex permit the gag reflex to be modified at higher centers (i.e., psychologically controlled). The novel concept of "patient-controlled airway insertion," in contrast to clinician-assisted insertion, has been suggested.[25] By letting patients insert the oral airway (Fig. 4.18), they are in control of the rate of entry and can pause when they feel themselves gagging.

As with patient-controlled analgesia, this empowered role might increase patient satisfaction and confidence in the procedure. Furthermore, the lidocaine coating of the intubating airway provides additional topicalization as the airway directly

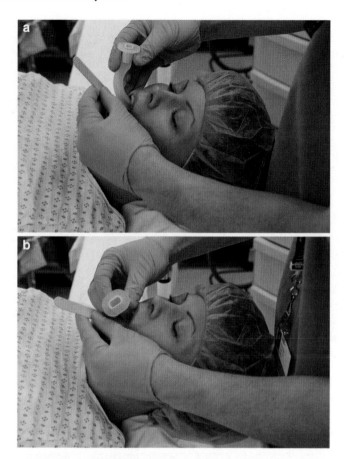

Fig. 4.17 The oral airway can also be inserted using a two-step method. (**a**) Step one: the tongue is depressed and the airway tip angled toward the roof of the mouth. (**b**) Step two: the airway is rotated 180° so its tip slides into the hypopharynx

contacts the oropharynx tissue during the procedure. This technique does not add risk as long as therapeutic guidelines for topical anesthesia dosage are followed, and the procedure is explained carefully and performed slowly by the cooperative awake patient. Although this author found this technique very useful for placing the oral intubating airway in preparation for fiberoptic intubation (Fig. 4.19), future studies will be needed to assess the true merit of this technique.

Nasal Airway

Nasal airways are manufactured in various diameters and lengths (Fig. 4.20). Care must be taken to ensure that airway has a ring, cone, or pin through its proximal

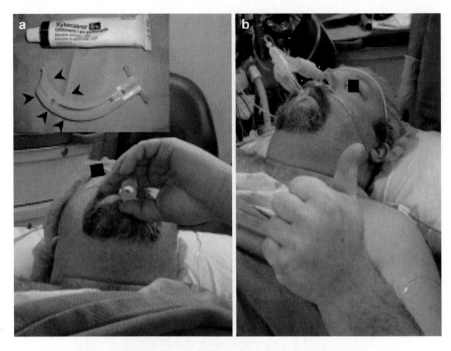

Fig. 4.18 (**a**) Patient-controlled airway insertion. (**b**) Successful outcome (from Tsui,[25] reprinted with permission from Springer Science + Business Media)

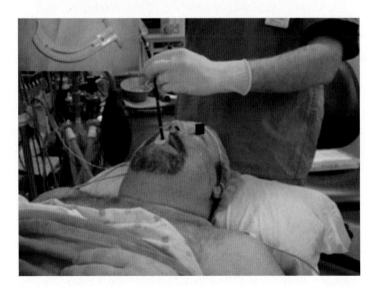

Fig. 4.19 Oral intubation airway for awake fiberoptic intubations

end so that it does not slip into the esophagus or trachea (Fig. 4.21). It should be inserted gently through a passage that has been lubricated with viscous lidocaine or K-Y Jelly and should be advanced parallel (not superiorly) against the turbinates (Fig. 4.22). If resistance to insertion is encountered, the other nostril or a smaller-sized airway should be tried. Remember that nasal airways can induce laryngospasm, epistaxis, or vomiting, and if left in place for a prolonged period, they can cause tissue necrosis. One should seriously consider using another type of airway if the patient has a basilar skull fracture.[26] If the airway is too long, its tip can enter the esophagus or trachea.

Stoneham[27] commented that "the ideal position for the distal tip of the nasopharyngeal airway is within 1 cm. of the epiglottis tip" and that a 150-mm airway is appropriate for most male patients, while a 130-mm airway is suitable for most female patients. Stoneham also studied the position of the nasopharyngeal airway tip fiberoptically and noted that the tip's position did not change very much

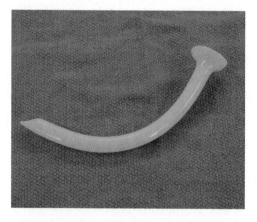

Fig. 4.20 Nasal airways (trumpets). The most commonly used are made of soft plastic or rubber

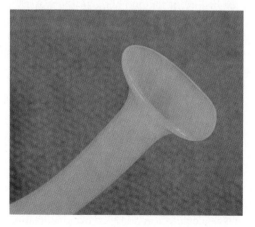

Fig. 4.21 The distal end of the nasal airway should have a cone or ring on it so that it does not slip into the pharynx, esophagus, or trachea

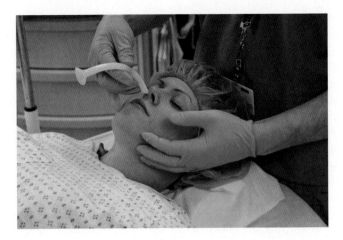

Fig. 4.22 The nasal airway, well lubricated, is inserted parallel to the turbinates

with flexion or extension of the head. Beattie[28] described the "modified nasal trumpet" maneuver. He prepared an airway by inserting a 15-mm adapter from a 7.5 or 8.0 endotracheal tube into the proximal end of a nasal airway that had been modified by cutting a "Murphy eye" into its distal end (Fig. 4.23). He then inserted the modified nasal airway and attached the distal end to an anesthesia machine circuit and attempted to ventilate the patient. If ventilation was unsuccessful, he pulled the nasal airway back 1–2 cm and attempted to ventilate again. He was able to provide ventilation easily to most patients. He described performing fiberoptically guided nasotracheal intubation through the other nostril with the modified airway in place used to ventilate and oxygenate the patient during the intubation. Those interested in the history of the oral and nasal airway should read the scholarly article by John McIntyre[29] that succinctly reviews the subject. He writes, "Currently for supraglottic airway management during general anesthesia, four types of airway should be available: a Guedel (oral) airway, a nasopharyngeal airway, a laryngeal mask airway [LMA], and an airway specifically designed to facilitate blind tracheal intubation." (see Chap. 5)

Anesthesia Masks and Resuscitation Bags

Adequate ventilation and oxygenation can be maintained with a bag and mask system that is connected to an oxygen source (Fig. 4.24). Do not abandon the mask for intubation unless the added protection of a cuffed endotracheal tube is indicated. All too often, bag/mask ventilation is neglected or underutilized and intubation becomes the main priority of the individual managing the airway, occasionally to the detriment of the patient. Mask ventilation should be maintained until all intubation equipment is on hand and checked out.

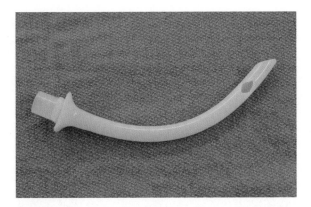

Fig. 4.23 The modified nasal trumpet (MNT). Ordinary nasal airway with an endotracheal tube (ETT) connector wedged into the flared end. Also shown is an optional "Murphy eye," a fenestration cut (with scissors) into the distal end opposite and slightly proximal to the bevel

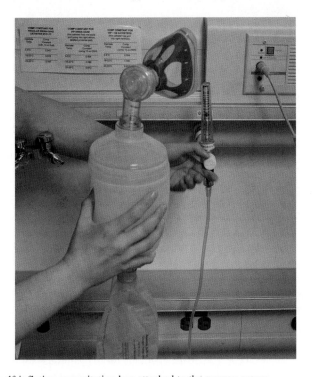

Fig. 4.24 A self-inflating resuscitation bag attached to the oxygen source

Masks

There are many shapes and sizes of anesthesia/resuscitation masks (Fig. 4.25). A mask should fit over the bridge of the nose, cheeks, and chin to produce an airtight seal. This seal should allow maintenance of at least 20–30 cm H_2O pressure with a minimal leak. However, the operator should avoid airway pressure greater than 25 cm

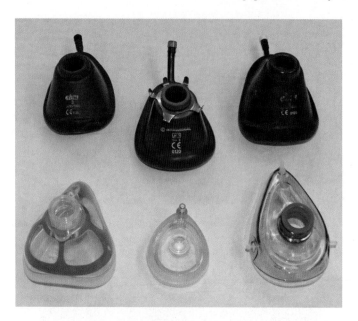

Fig. 4.25 Anesthesia resuscitation masks. These come in a variety of sizes, shapes, and materials

H_2O in order to minimize the risk inflating the patient's stomach. If a seal is difficult to establish, reshaping the mask's malleable perimeter or selecting a different-sized mask may be helpful. The mask should be pressed against the nasal bridge with the thumb while the index finger exerts downward pressure on the base of the mask over the chin. The little finger should engage the angle of the mandible. With the hand thus positioned, one can lift the mandible upward to open the airway (Fig. 4.26). Although the grip must be tight, intermittent relaxation of one or two fingers at a time will prevent the hand and arm from tiring. Anesthetists often maintain mask airways for 1–2 h after they have mastered the technique. New more ergonomic masks, which make one-hand face mask ventilation easier, are beginning to emerge and are meeting with positive reception.[30]

All masks increase dead space, so larger tidal volumes are required. Note also that opaque masks may conceal vomit or secretions within the mouth; thus, clear masks are preferable. Perhaps the masks of the future will be designed with more attention to anatomical considerations.

A variety of devices have been used to assist with mask fit and the maintenance of a patent airway. Most have been used in the operating room by anesthesiologists. Some are of simple design, such as the head strap, others more complex (Fig. 4.27). Be aware that the use of a mask with or without supporting devices can cause nerve or eye injury.

Manual Resuscitation Bags

The self-inflating manual resuscitation bag/valve/mask is the primary system utilized by clinicians involved in airway management. Ventilation and oxygenation can be

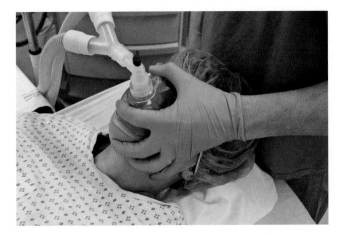

Fig. 4.26 Proper mask fit. Note the position of the hand, with two fingers holding the mask, and three lifting the mandible

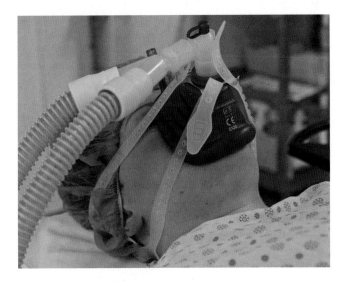

Fig. 4.27 To improve the fit, a mask may be supported by a head strap

maintained for long periods while other supportive therapy is initiated. It may also be preferable to use a bag/valve/mask device so that in the event of oxygen system failure, at least room air can be delivered. The bag/valve/mask device should have standard fittings for connection to an endotracheal tube or face mask (15 mm inside, 22 mm outside, diameter delivery port) (Fig. 4.28). A self-inflating system can deliver enriched oxygen mixtures when connected to an oxygen storage tank or wall outlet. The valves of the system should be designed to function during either spontaneous or controlled positive-pressure ventilation. To avoid the development of high airway pressures, pediatric bag/valve devices should be fitted with a 25–30 cm H_2O release valve. All systems should also be able to accept a positive

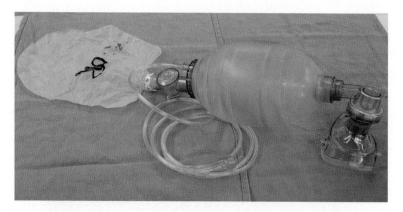

Fig. 4.28 A complete mask/resuscitation bag/oxygen reservoir/tubing system

end-expiratory pressure (PEEP) valve and should be designed so that either a tube-type reservoir or a reservoir bag can be fitted to deliver high FiO_2. Before use, check the valves for proper operation and gas flow and make sure that the plastic connections are properly secured.

Despite the advantages of bag mask ventilation (BMV) in emergency situations, there are some disadvantages. To be fully prepared while using a bag/valve/mask:

- Ensure thorough training in the correct use of the BMV.
- Create a tight seal prior to ventilating the patient and monitor the seal periodically during patient transport and CPR procedures.
- Beware of the danger of gastric distention caused by the device.
- Watch for blood, fluid, and vomitus, which can be forced up into the airway.

How to use a BMV:

1. Place the body of the mask in the left hand and grip the mask with the thumb and index finger of the left hand.
2. Place the narrow end of the mask over the bridge of the nose.
3. Place the chin end of the mask on the alveolar ridge.
4. Provide jaw lift with the remaining three fingers of the left hand to create counter pressure on the mask. These three fingers will ensure that the mask is properly sealed by pulling the jaw into the mask (avoid placing pressure on the soft tissue under the chin).
5. Using the right hand, fully compress the bag firmly, but not too forcefully. Time the squeezing of the bag to deliver breaths with the patient's inhalations where evident. Note, squeezing the bag too rapidly or forcefully can cause gastric distention. If tachypnea is present, alternate assisted breaths with the patient's own breaths.
6. Insert an airway (oral or nasal) if obstruction occurs despite jaw lift, and reposition the patient's head.

Even without other mitigating factors, it can be difficult to maintain a perfect seal using the one-person method noted above. Many authors describe *two-person* or *two- or three-handed*[31–33] mask ventilation when one operator has trouble maintaining a mask fit with one hand and providing positive-pressure ventilation with the other. These maneuvers are performed with one person applying the mask with two hands and providing jaw lift while the other ventilates the patient. The person ventilating the patient can also help to position the mask on the patient's face with a free hand. Two-person mask ventilation is often effective when one-person ventilation is not. BMV operator stress should not be discounted as a complicating factor in successful outcomes and understanding variables such as inspiratory flow rates and peak airway pressure are crucial.[34]

Some of the difficulties encountered during BMV are:

- Lack of a proper seal. This could be caused by a thick beard (applying surgical lubricant and carefully monitoring the seal may be beneficial), or in the edentulous patient whose facial muscles may be collapsed.
- Facial trauma such as mandibular fractures and open wounds may interfere with the operator's ability to properly place the mask.
- Limited chest excursion due to bronchospasm.
- Ineffective chest excursion due to a large chest wall or distended abdomen.
- Poor neck stability.
- Obesity or bull neck.
- Other causes of airway obstruction.

In summary, the basic equipment required to oxygenate and ventilate a patient includes an oxygen source, an oral or nasal airway, a face mask, a resuscitation bag, and a reliable suction apparatus. One must master the technique of manual airway support using these relatively simple and inexpensive pieces of equipment, before advancing to more sophisticated airway management techniques.

Equipment for Endotracheal Intubation

This section describes basic laryngoscopes and various types of basic laryngoscope blades, endotracheal light sources, the endotracheal tube, and stylets used for intubation.

Laryngoscope

Although intubation can be accomplished without a laryngoscope ("blind" intubation), one of the best ways to ensure proper tube placement is to see the tube pass between the vocal cords.

This chapter provides a basic understanding of laryngoscopes and a selection of the standard options. There are many types of blades (Fig. 4.29). Some are of ingenious design to facilitate difficult intubation, such as the Siker mirror blade, the Huffman prism, and the Bellhouse blade. Many of these specialty blades are

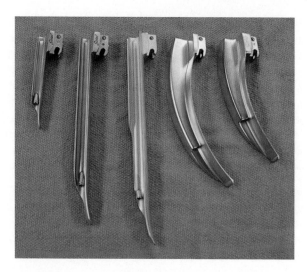

Fig. 4.29 Laryngoscopes blades

described in Chap. 6. One should become familiar with one or two simple designs of blades before graduating to the more sophisticated varieties.

In an article addressing laryngoscope blade design and function, John McIntyre[35] evaluates many types of laryngoscope blades and suggests anatomic findings that should trigger the intubationist to consider a particular blade design. Dr. McIntyre writes, "Selection of the laryngoscope for the task must be based on problems identified at clinical examination, the patient's history, and an intuitive matching of a laryngoscope that appears to have characteristics that will offset these factors. ... Thus, an axiom for anesthesiologists is: 'Examine your patient, understand laryngoscopes, and learn how to use them.' " This is sound advice reflecting years of study and experience. One needs to become familiar with only two basic designs – the straight blade (Miller) and the curved blade (Macintosh). In one analysis of laryngoscope blade shape and design, the authors state[36]: "Since the advent of tracheal intubation in anesthesia, at least 50 descriptions of laryngoscope blade designs have been published, and many more designs exist unpublished."

Conventional laryngoscope blades are fitted with a small light that screws into an outlet on the blade. Newer blades are fitted with a fiberoptic light-delivery channel; the light source may be housed in the handle of the laryngoscope. The laryngoscope consists of a handle and a blade (Fig. 4.30). The handle houses the batteries that power the light. The surface of the handle is usually machined to afford a rough surface for improved grip. The top of the handle has a fitting into which the blade is secured and through which electricity is supplied to the bulb. To ensure good electrical or fiberoptic contact, the blade end that mates with the handle should be clean (Fig. 4.31) and batteries should always be fresh.

Laryngoscope blades are designed to enter the mouth, displace the soft tissues, elevate the epiglottis (either directly [straight blade] or indirectly [curved blade with the tip in the vallecula]), and expose the vocal cords. All resuscitation trays should contain at least two laryngoscope handles with a variety of straight and curved blades.

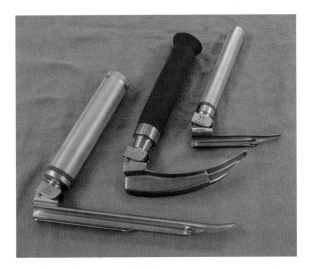

Fig. 4.30 Laryngoscopes

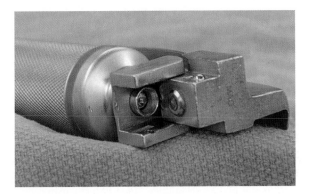

Fig. 4.31 To ensure good contact and bright illumination, the electrical connections of the laryngoscope handle and blade must be clean

The laryngoscope blade has four main features:

- A light source or fiberoptic channel (the light source should be tightly secured so that the bulb produces constant illumination and is not dislodged in the oropharynx).
- A spatula for compression or manipulation of soft tissue.
- A flange to help guide the tube.
- A tip to contact and support the epiglottis or vallecula for exposure of the vocal cords.

Fiberoptic laryngoscopes are made by many manufacturers such as Anesthesia Associates (SanMarcos, CA), Heine (Herrsching, Germany), Medicon (Tuttlingen, Germany), Penlon (Abingdon, UK), Riester (Jungingen, Germany), and Upsher (Foster City, CA).[37] One needs to keep in mind the observations of Bucx et al.,[38] Tousignant and Tessler,[39] and Fletcher[40] when using fiberoptic laryngoscopes. These scopes are designed with the light source in the handle of the scope. The light is transmitted towards the tip of the blade with a fiberoptic channel. When new and functioning optimally, the light intensity directed toward the airway is bright and focused. However, these authors report that sterilization and handling of the blades can compromise the quality and intensity of the light directed into the airway. The quality of the light produced with traditional scopes can also be altered with cleaning and handling, and the bulbs and batteries need to be checked on a regular basis.

Laryngoscopes with a "levering" tip have been introduced into practice. These scopes employ a Macintosh blade with a hinged tip that can be "levered" upward, causing the tip to exert more force to the vallecula, a maneuver that purportedly will more efficiently elevate the epiglottis. It is postulated that less lifting needs be applied to the scope and that neck movement can be minimized. Avoiding neck movement might make laryngoscopy safer for patients with cervical spine pathology.[41] Two such scopes are the McCoy Levering Laryngoscope (Penlon Ltd., Abingdon, UK) and the Heine CL (Corazzelli-London) Flexible Tip Laryngoscope Blade (Heine USA Ltd., Dover, NH) (see Chap. 6 for more on these laryngoscopes).

The "ultimate" blade has not been designed, but more study of the shape, size, and classification of laryngoscope blades is under way, and in the future, selection of the best blade for intubation in the widest variety of clinical scenarios should be more predictable, based upon scientific data rather than traditional clinical bias and anecdote.[36, 37, 42–44] Recent research shows that, despite the variety of laryngoscope designs, proficiency is quickly attained with new devices.[45] In concluding this section on laryngoscopes and blade design, one is encouraged to become familiar with the use of standard Macintosh and Miller blades before experimenting with blades of more sophisticated design (described in detail in Chap. 6).

Alternative Light Source

The more sophisticated airway tray might contain an alternative light source – a headlight,[46] pen light,[47] a pocket flashlight,[48] or a high-intensity external fiberoptic light source.[49] These devices have been used to illuminate the airway when the primary light source (on the laryngoscope blade) has failed because of loose connections, weak batteries, blood covering the bulb, or poor illumination.

Endotracheal Tube

The endotracheal tube is one of the most essential tools for airway management. Despite the fact that tracheal intubation is often lifesaving, both the technique and instruments used can be hazardous to the patient. An understanding of tube design and function is essential for safe application.

Compared to the normal airway, an endotracheal tube increases the resistance to gas flow. In certain cases it may also increase dead space. Tubes are calibrated in external and internal diameters (mm) and in length (cm). To prevent excessive airway resistance, a tube should not become kinked or sharply bent. Also, whenever possible, straight or large-bore connectors should be used in the circuit from the tube to the resuscitation bag. Modern tracheal tubes are usually made of polyvinyl chloride or medical-grade silicone rubber. Since many chemicals are involved in the manufacture of plastic tubes, tissue toxicity from the tubes themselves has long been a concern. Most manufacturers now tissue-test their tubes and document the lack of tissue toxicity by printing "IT" (implant tested) or Z-79 (Z-79 Committee of the American National Standards Institute) on the tubes. Only tubes with these safety designations should be used. Endotracheal tubes should not be reused.

This section will describe some of the common types of tracheal tubes available and special types of tubes are discussed in Chap. 6. Most tubes incorporate a high-volume, low-pressure cuff (Fig. 4.32). Cuff pressure should not exceed 25 torr (capillary pressure) lest mucosal ischemia or tracheal necrosis occur. Standard endotracheal tubes may be used for nasal and oral intubation. The tip of the tube is beveled and should include a side port or Murphy eye (Fig. 4.33). The side port may allow ventilation even if the main port becomes occluded by the tracheal wall, blood clot, or secretions. The other end of the tube is fitted with a standard 15-mm adapter for connection to a resuscitation bag or ventilator. The cuff of the tube may be inflated by injecting air into the valve, which is attached to a side port. *Uncuffed*

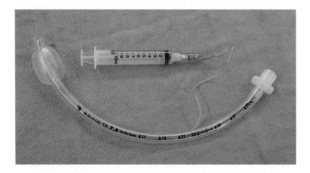

Fig. 4.32 Standard endotracheal tube with inflated cuff

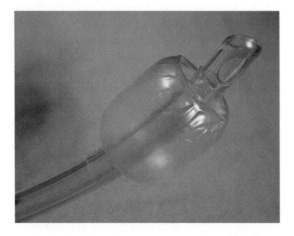

Fig. 4.33 Tip of a standard endotracheal tube, demonstrating the Murphy eye or side port

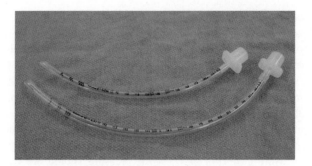

Fig. 4.34 Uncuffed pediatric endotracheal tubes

tubes are generally inserted in pediatric patients (Fig. 4.34). Cuffs are not necessary in most children under 8 years of age because the narrowest portion of a small child's airway is at the cricoid cartilage and an uncuffed tube of appropriate size should afford a reasonable seal at this level. Recent articles document that cuffed endotracheal tubes are safe to use in pediatric patients. The old dogma of using only uncuffed tubes in children is no longer accepted by many practitioners.[50–52]

Newly designed tubes and cuffs have been introduced that will hopefully make ventilation easier (less airway resistance) and decrease the likelihood of pressure-related trauma and injury to the mouth, larynx, or trachea.

One should consider the *orientation and shape of the tip* of the endotracheal tube, especially if one has difficulty passing a standard tube through the vocal cords over a fiberoptic scope or a gum bougie. West et al.[53] described an experimental tube that had the bevel reversed and found that it was very easy to pass over a bougie under "simulated" difficult airway conditions. A tube manufactured by Parker Medical (Highlands Ranch, CO) is called the Parker Flex-Tip. This tube has its bevel pointing toward the back of the tube. It also has a smooth, "hooded" tip that could facilitate passage of the tube through the glottic opening.

Much is written concerning the pressures exerted against the mucosal surfaces by the tube and its cuff. An article by Brimacombe et al.[54] warns that indirect methods to measure mucosal pressure, such as cuff pressure, are of "moderate predictive value" and may not accurately reflect true mucosal pressure. These investigators also remind us that mucosal pressures vary at different anatomic levels and with different head movements. When evaluating manufacturer's claims with respect to the mucosal pressure exerted by various designs of airway equipment, it is important to verify that the methods used to measure mucosal pressure are accurate and precise. Sridermaa et al.[55] recently recommended that endotracheal cuff inflation should be guided by a manometer to achieve appropriate cuff pressure (30 cm H_2O) every 8 h.

Stylet

A stylet is a malleable metal or plastic stent over which an endotracheal tube is passed (Fig. 4.35). It allows the curvature of the tube to be altered to facilitate a difficult

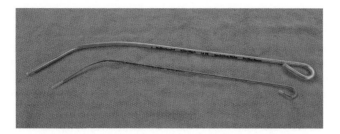

Fig. 4.35 Stylets

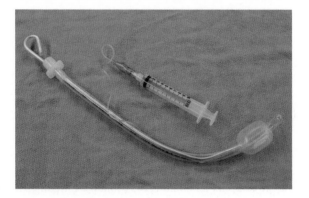

Fig. 4.36 When used in an endotracheal tube, the stylet will hold its hockey-stick configuration to assist in directing the tube toward the airway when the larynx is not readily visible

intubation (Fig. 4.36). Withdrawal of the stylet may cause the tip of the endotracheal tube to move anteriorly, a maneuver documented by Stix and Mancini.[56] This anterior movement could help direct the tube through an anteriorly positioned glottis.

Other Useful Airway Tools

One's arsenal of basic airway equipment should include a gum elastic bougie, various intubating catheters such as the Aintree catheter,[57, 58] Magill forceps,[59] and possibly mouth gags or other mouth-opening devices used by ear, nose, and throat (ENT) surgeons.[60] Consult an experienced instructor when learning to use this equipment.

Cleaning, Disinfecting, and Sterilizing Equipment

There have been documented cases in the literature of respiratory infection transmissions and concern over Variant Creutzfeld-Jakob Disease (vCJD) transmission via reusable airway management devices, underscoring the need for ongoing research into best practices for eliminating cross-infections.[61–64]

Understanding the process of cleaning, disinfecting, and sterilizing airway devices is important to understanding the risks of cross-contamination and infection. Cleaning involves the physical removal of particles from an instrument, disinfection refers to the removal of microorganisms to varying degrees, and sterilization involves the complete removal of microorganisms. The varying degrees of disinfection are divided into three categories: low-level (kills some viruses and bacteria with an FDA-approved and -registered chemical germicide), intermediate (kills mycobacteria, and the majority of viruses and bacteria with a tuberculocide-registered germicide), and high-level (kills all organisms except high levels of bacterial spores with a chemical germicide, FDA approved as a sterilant). Sterilization kills or denatures all organisms, including bacterial endospores.

Spaulding's Classification Scheme is a tool for evaluating the necessary level of disinfection required to eliminate disease-transmitting pathogens by classifying devices according to their risk of disease transmission and the nosocomial infections associated with their use.[65] According to this system, devices that come into direct contact with mucous membranes are classified as semicritical and require high-level disinfection. This includes laryngoscope blades and handles, airways, breathing circuits, connectors, fiberoptic endoscopes, forceps, masks, self-inflating bags, some LMAs, transducer tubing, and transesophageal probes. It should be noted that the Association of Perioperative Registered Nurses suggests that because handles only come into contact with skin, they may undergo a low-level of disinfection.[66] This guideline does not take into consideration the findings in the literature about nosocomial contamination of laryngoscope handles.[67]

Most common methods of disinfection involve steam heat (autoclaving) and cold chemicals. Heat disinfection is only appropriate for materials that can withstand high temperatures without damage. One study placed a clean, unused LMA in an autoclave with other, previously used and contaminated LMAs and found that protein staining occurred on all LMAs that had been batch cleaned, suggesting that instruments should be autoclaved in isolation.[68] Prion proteins responsible for CJD seem to accumulate and replicate within the lymphoreticular system of the individual prior to neuroinvasion.[69] Because LMAs and other airway devices can come into contact with the lymphoreticular tissue of the tonsil bed, they may be at risk of prion transmission.[70] Supplementary cleaning with potassium permanganate 8 mg L^{-1} has shown to eliminate protein deposits from reusable metallic and synthetic rubber airway equipment.[71]

While the maximum level of decontamination might seem desirable, the degree of wear on the instrument with each cleaning must also be taken into consideration. For example, fiberoptic laryngoscopes may be affected by thermal disinfection. Bucx et al.[38] showed that machine washing and disinfection at 90°C achieved a high level of disinfection, but not the highest level of sterilization associated with the widest margin of safety. To achieve this, the instruments were exposed to 134°C, resulting in decreased light intensity, and in some cases, fractures, changes, and discoloration in the instruments.

Concerns over chemical sterilants include compromised tensile strength of endotracheal tubes soaked in 2% activated glutaraldehyde or sterilized with ethylene oxide gas.[72] Glutaraldehyde is toxic, irritant, and allergenic, and ethylene oxide gas is carcinogenic, so proper handling instructions must be followed.

Every airway device manufacturer provides a manual for the disinfection or sterilization of its devices (and which methods and materials are contraindicated) and these guidelines, in conjunction with institutional guidelines, should be followed to achieve maximum disinfection/sterilization, and subsequent patient safety. Whenever possible, disposable airway devices should be considered.

Equipment Problems

Rule No. 1: Any piece of equipment can break or fail
Rule No. 2: Have backup equipment immediately available

The literature is replete with articles and letters describing examples of equipment failure. It is important to check equipment before use and to have backup equipment immediately available if an instrument fails or breaks. Any piece of equipment can fail. The following table summarizes problems the airway manager may encounter (Table 4.2).

Table 4.2 Potential problems with basic airway devices

Device	Potential problems
Oxygen source	Failure of the central oxygen piping system
	Plumbing and piping errors that allow gases other than oxygen to be delivered from the oxygen outlet
	A broken flowmeter[73]
	A contaminated oxygen tank[74]
	Occluded or obstructed oxygen tubing
	Scavenging system failures[75,76]
	Gas sensing line malfunction[77]
Endotracheal tube	Obstruction by a wall defect, membranes, or other manufacturing flaw[78–81]
	Leaks[82–84]
	Cuff herniation or rupture[85]
	Cracks, leaks, or obstruction of the cuff-inflation valve[86]
	A malfunction that makes it difficult to deflate the cuff[87,88]
	Kinking or dislodgment by another device (e.g., a suction catheter)[89]
	Fire (with laser surgery)
	A broken or slipped 15-mm adapter
	Tube connector defect[90]
Laryngoscope	A broken handle or blade[91–95]
	Short-circuiting that leads to excessive heating of the handle[96,97]
	Dead batteries
	A dead or loose lightbulb[98]
	Flexi-tip breakage[99]
Stylet	Direct tissue damage
	Fracture if the plastic coating with pieces is left in the airway[100]
	Broken in the airway[101,102]
	Bent so as to obstruct the cuff side-port
Oral airways	Irritation of salivary duct, causing transient sialadenopathy[103]
	Manufacturing defects[104]
Nasal airways	Cannula displaced submucosally[105]

"The Dedicated Airway" and the "Ideal Airway Device"

Charters and O'Sullivan[106] define the "dedicated airway" to be "an upper airway device dedicated to the maintenance of airway patency while other major airway interventions are anticipated or in progress." Charters[107] lists the features one may expect from the "ideal airway device." These authors remind us that the development of equipment traditionally used in airway management has evolved empirically. The designs are not necessarily based on observations derived from anatomic or physiologic scientific study. They recommend that future design considerations should reflect new knowledge obtained from controlled research designed to define upper airway anatomy and physiologic function.

Summary

A visit to the anesthesiology or respiratory therapy department in *advance* of an emergency will allow you to become familiar with all the equipment available. In an emergency, such a visit can save time, minimize anxiety, and ultimately benefit patients. Important rules to follow are:

- Learn to examine the airway quickly.
- Know the various equipment options available for airway support and instrumentation.
- Choose the correct piece of equipment for the job. Consider backup equipment and techniques.
- Ensure oxygen and suction are always available.
- Never leave the patient with an airway problem unattended.
- Do not forget the basics in the case of equipment failure.
- Get immediate help when doubt or unanticipated difficulty is encountered with a patient's airway. Waste no time in preventing the irreversible sequelae of hypoxia!

Acknowledgments The author would like to thank Jennifer Pillay, Nikki Stalker, and Adam Dryden for their contribution to this chapter.

References

1. Dorsch JA, Dorsch SE. *Understanding Anesthesia Equipment*. 3rd ed. Baltimore: Williams & Wilkins; 1994.
2. Dorsch JA, Dorsch SE. *Understanding Anesthesia Equipment*. 5th ed. Philadelphia: Lippincott Williams & Wilkins; 2008.
3. Stewart C. Oxygenation and ventilation aids. In: Beacom K, Kashickey K, eds. *Advanced Airway Management*. Upper Saddle River, New Jersey: Prentice Hall; 2002:60.
4. Vandenberg JT, Vinson DR. The inadequacies of contemporary oropharyngeal suction. *Am J Emerg Med*. 1999;17:611–613.

5. Ooi R, Joshi P, Soni N. An evaluation of oxygen delivery using nasal prongs. *Anaesthesia.* 1992;47:591–593.
6. Aubier M, Murciano D, Milic-Emili J, et al. Effects of the administration of O_2 on ventilation and blood gases in patients with chronic obstructive pulmonary disease during acute respiratory failure. *Am Rev Respir Dis.* 1980;122:747–754.
7. Woda RP, Dzwonczyk R, Beckmeyer W, Fuhrman T. Cost-benefit analysis of nasal cannulae in non-tracheally intubated subjects. *Anesth Analg.* 1996;82:506–510.
8. Yanagidate F, Dohi S. Modified nasal cannula for simultaneous oxygen delivery and end-tidal CO2 monitoring during spontaneous breathing. *Eur J Anaesthesiol.* 2006;23:257–260.
9. Tsui BC. A simple method with no additional cost for monitoring $ETCO_2$ using a standard nasal cannulae. *Can J Anesth.* 1997;44:787–788.
10. Guzeldemir ME. A mask for operations on and above the eye. *Can J Anesth.* 1998;45:709.
11. Kurt I, Kurt NM, Erel VK, Gursoy F, Gurel A. A simple and inexpensive nasal cannula to prevent rebreathing for spontaneously breathing patients under surgical drapes. *Anesth Analg.* 2001;93:667–668.
12. Langer RA. Simple modification of a medium concentration (Hudson type) oxygen mask improves patient comfort and respiratory monitoring with capnography. *Anesth Analg.* 1996;83:202.
13. Livingston M. Questions use of nasal cannula for oxygen supplementation during cataract surgery. *Anesthesiology.* 1999;91:1176.
14. Schlager A, Luger TJ. Oxygen application by a nasal probe prevents hypoxia but not rebreathing of carbon dioxide in patients undergoing eye surgery under local anaesthesia. *Br J Ophthalmol.* 2000;84:399–402.
15. Williams AR, Tomlin K. The modified bitegard: a method for administering supplemental oxygen and measuring carbon dioxide. *Anesthesiology.* 1999;90:338–339.
16. Hunsinger DL. *Respiratory Technology Procedure and Equipment Manual.* Reston: Reston Publishing; 1980.
17. McPherson SP. *Respiratory Therapy Equipment.* 2nd ed. St. Louis: Mosby; 1981.
18. Sim MA, Dean P, Kinsella J, Black R, Carter R, Hughes M. Performance of oxygen delivery devices when the breathing pattern of respiratory failure is simulated. *Anaesthesia.* 2008;63:938–940.
19. Waldau T, Larsen VH, Bonde J. Evaluation of five oxygen delivery devices in spontaneously breathing subjects by oxygraphy. *Anaesthesia.* 1998;53:256–263.
20. Ball C, Westhorpe R. Clearing the airway–the development of the pharyngeal airway. *Anaesth Intensive Care.* 1997;25:451.
21. Marsh AM, Nunn JF, Taylor SJ, Charlesworth CH. Airway obstruction associated with the use of the Guedel airway. *Br J Anaesth.* 1991;67:517–523.
22. Bassi GS, Humphris GM, Longman LP. The etiology and management of gagging: a review of the literature. *J Prosthet Dent.* 2004;91:459–467.
23. Eitner S, Wichmann M, Holst S. "Hypnopuncture"–a dental-emergency treatment concept for patients with a distinctive gag reflex. *Int J Clin Exp Hypn.* 2005;53:60–73.
24. Fiske J, Dickinson C. The role of acupuncture in controlling the gagging reflex using a review of ten cases. *Br Dent J.* 2001;190:611–613.
25. Tsui BC, Dillane D, Yee MS. Patient-controlled oral airway insertion to facilitate awake fibreoptic intubation. *Can J Anesth.* 2008;55:194–195.
26. Muzzi DA, Losasso TJ, Cucchiara RF. Complication from a nasopharyngeal airway in a patient with a basilar skull fracture. *Anesthesiology.* 1991;74:366–368.
27. Stoneham MD. The nasopharyngeal airway. Assessment of position by fibreoptic laryngoscopy. *Anaesthesia.* 1993;48:575–580.
28. Beattie C. The modified nasal trumpet maneuver. *Anesth Analg.* 2002;94:467–469, table.
29. McIntyre JW. Oropharyngeal and nasopharyngeal airways: I (1880-1995). *Can J Anesth.* 1996;43:629–635.
30. Matioc AA. The adult ergonomic face mask concept: historical and theoretical perspectives. *J Clin Anesth.* 2009;21:300–304.
31. Benumof JL. *Airway Management and Principles and Practice.* St Louis: Mosby; 1996.

32. Ward ME. A new look at the breath of life. *Br J Anaesth.* 1992;69:339–340.
33. Wheeler M. The difficult pediatric airway. In: Hagberg CA, ed. *Handbook of Difficult Airway Management.* Philadelphia: Churchill Livingstone; 2000:268.
34. von Goedecke A, Wenzel V, Hormann C, et al. Effects of face mask ventilation in apneic patients with a resuscitation ventilator in comparison with a bag-valve-mask. *J Emerg Med.* 2006;30:63–67.
35. McIntyre JWR. Airway equipment. *Anesthesiol Clin North America.* 1995;13:309.
36. Marks RR, Hancock R, Charters P. An analysis of laryngoscope blade shape and design: a new criteria for laryngoscope evaluation. *Can J Anesth.* 1993;40:262–270.
37. McIntyre JW. Laryngoscope design and the difficult adult tracheal intubation. *Can J Anesth.* 1989;36:94–98.
38. Bucx MJ, Veldman DJ, Beenhakker MM, Koster R. The effect of steam sterilisation at 134 degrees C on light intensity provided by fibrelight Macintosh laryngoscopes. *Anaesthesia.* 1999;54:875–878.
39. Tousignant G, Tessler MJ. Light intensity and area of illumination provided by various laryngoscope blades. *Can J Anesth.* 1994;41:865–869.
40. Fletcher J. Laryngoscope light intensity. *Can J Anesth.* 1995;42:259-260.
41. Uchida T, Hikawa Y, Saito Y, Yasuda K. The McCoy levering laryngoscope in patients with limited neck extension. *Can J Anesth.* 1997;44:674–676.
42. McIntyre JW. Tracheal intubation and laryngoscope design. *Can J Anesth.* 1993;40: 193–196.
43. Norton ML. Laryngoscope blade shape. *Can J Anesth.* 1994;41:263–265.
44. Relle A. Laryngoscope design. *Can J Anesth.* 1994;41:162–163.
45. Savoldelli GL, Schiffer E, Abegg C, Baeriswyl V, Clergue F, Waeber JL. Learning curves of the Glidescope, the McGrath and the Airtraq laryngoscopes: a manikin study. *Eur J Anaesthesiol.* 2009;26:554–558.
46. Stowell DE. An alternative light source for laryngoscopy. *Anesthesiology.* 1994;80:487.
47. Kubota Y, Toyoda Y, Kubota H. Endotracheal intubation assisted with a pencil torch. *Anesthesiology.* 1988;68:167.
48. Przemeck M, Vangerow B, Panning B. Mini flashlight as a spare light source for a failing fiberoptic laryngoscope. *Anesthesiology.* 1997;86:1217.
49. Arthurs GJ. Fibre-optically lit laryngoscope. *Anaesthesia.* 1999;54:873–874.
50. Deakers TW, Reynolds G, Stretton M, Newth CJ. Cuffed endotracheal tubes in pediatric intensive care. *J Pediatr.* 1994;125:57–62.
51. Khine HH, Corddry DH, Kettrick RG, et al. Comparison of cuffed and uncuffed endotracheal tubes in young children during general anesthesia. *Anesthesiology.* 1997;86:627-631.
52. Weber T, Salvi N, Orliaguet G, Wolf A. Cuffed vs non-cuffed endotracheal tubes for pediatric anesthesia. *Pediatr Anesth.* 2009;19(Suppl 1):46–54.
53. West MR, Jonas MM, Adams AP, Carli F. A new tracheal tube for difficult intubation. *Br J Anaesth.* 1996;76:673–679.
54. Brimacombe J, Keller C, Giampalmo M, Sparr HJ, Berry A. Direct measurement of mucosal pressures exerted by cuff and non-cuff portions of tracheal tubes with different cuff volumes and head and neck positions. *Br J Anaesth.* 1999;82:708–711.
55. Sridermma S, Limtangturakool S, Wongsurakiat P, Thamlikitkul V. Development of appropriate procedures for inflation of endotracheal tube cuff in intubated patients. *J Med Assoc Thai.* 2007;90(suppl 2):74–78.
56. Stix MS, Mancini E. How a rigid stylet can make an endotracheal tube move. *Anesth Analg.* 2000;90:1008.
57. Avitsian R, Doyle DJ, Helfand R, Zura A, Farag E. Successful reintubation after cervical spine exposure using an Aintree intubation catheter and a Laryngeal Mask Airway. *J Clin Anesth.* 2006;18:224–225.
58. Zura A, Doyle DJ, Orlandi M. Use of the Aintree intubation catheter in a patient with an unexpected difficult airway. *Can J Anesth.* 2005;52:646–649.
59. Ehrensperger C, Gross J, Hempel V, Henn-Beilharz A, Rau A. The modified Magill forceps. *Anaesthesist.* 1992;41:218–220. Abstract in English.

60. Ball C, Westhorpe R. Clearing the airway–mouth gags, wedges and openers. *Anaesth Intensive Care*. 1997;25:335.

61. Kressel AB, Kidd F. Pseudo-outbreak of Mycobacterium chelonae and Methylobacterium mesophilicum caused by contamination of an automated endoscopy washer. *Infect Control Hosp Epidemiol*. 2001;22:414–418.

62. Ramasamy I. The risk of accidental transmission of transmissible spongiform encephalopathy: identification of emerging issues. *Public Health*. 2004;118:409–420.

63. Murdoch H, Taylor D, Dickinson J, et al. Surface decontamination of surgical instruments: an ongoing dilemma. *J Hosp Infect*. 2006;63:432–438.

64. Will RG, Ironside JW, Zeidler M, et al. A new variant of Creutzfeldt-Jakob disease in the UK. *Lancet*. 1996;347:921–925.

65. Muscarella LF. Recommendations to resolve inconsistent guidelines for the reprocessing of sheathed and unsheathed rigid laryngoscopes. *Infect Control Hosp Epidemiol*. 2007;28: 504–507.

66. Recommended practices for cleaning. handling and processing anesthesia equipment. *AORN J*. 2005;81:856–870.

67. Call TR, Auerbach FJ, Riddell SW, et al. Nosocomial contamination of laryngoscope handles: challenging current guidelines. *Anesth Analg*. 2009;109:479–483.

68. Richards E, Brimacombe J, Laupau W, Keller C. Protein cross-contamination during batch cleaning and autoclaving of the ProSeal laryngeal mask airway. *Anaesthesia*. 2006;61:431–433.

69. Hill AF, Butterworth RJ, Joiner S, et al. Investigation of variant Creutzfeldt-Jakob disease and other human prion diseases with tonsil biopsy samples. *Lancet*. 1999;353:183–189.

70. Greenwood J, Green N, Power G. Protein contamination of the Laryngeal Mask Airway and its relationship to re-use. *Anaesth Intensive Care*. 2006;34:343–346.

71. Laupu W, Brimacombe J. The effect of high concentration potassium permanganate on protein contamination from metallic and synthetic rubber airway equipment. *Anaesthesia*. 2007;62: 824–826.

72. Yoon SZ, Jeon YS, Kim YC, et al. The safety of reused endotracheal tubes sterilized according to Centers for Disease Control and Prevention guidelines. *J Clin Anesth*. 2007;19:360–364.

73. Szocik JF. Preoperative hypoxemia. *Anesth Analg*. 1993;76:681–682.

74. Coveler LA, Lester RC. Contaminated oxygen cylinder. *Anesth Analg*. 1989;69:674–676.

75. Hwang NC. Hidden hazards of scavenging. *Br J Anaesth*. 2000;84:827.

76. Khorasani A, Saatee S, Khader RD, Nasr NF. Inadvertent misconnection of the scavenger hose: A cause for increased pressure in the breathing circuit. *Anesthesiology*. 2000;92:1501–1502.

77. Eggemann I, Bottiger BW, Spohr F. Accidentally opened adjustable pressure-limiting valve. Failure of manual ventilation. *Anaesthesist*. 2009;58:301–302. Abstract in English.

78. Barst S, Yossefy Y, Lebowitz P. An unusual cause of airway obstruction. *Anesth Analg*. 1994;78:195.

79. Campbell C, Viswanathan S, Riopelle JM, Naraghi M. Manufacturing defect in a double-lumen tube. *Anesth Analg*. 1991;73:825–826.

80. McCoy E, Barnes S. A defect in a tracheal tube. *Anaesthesia*. 1989;44:525.

81. McLean RF, McLean J, McKee D. Another cause of tracheal tube failure. *Can J Anesth*. 1989;36:733–734.

82. Gettelman TA, Morris GN. Endotracheal tube failure: undetected by routine testing. *Anesth Analg*. 1995;81:1313.

83. Lewer BM, Karim Z, Henderson RS. Large air leak from an endotracheal tube due to a manufacturing defect. *Anesth Analg*. 1997;85:944–945.

84. Saini S, Chhabra B. A tracheal tube defect. *Anesth Analg*. 1996;83:1129–1130.

85. Patterson KW, Keane P. Missed diagnosis of cuff herniation in a modern nasal endotracheal tube. *Anesth Analg*. 1990;71:563–564.

86. Basagoitia JN, LaMastro M. Another complication of tracheal intubation. *Anesth Analg*. 1990;70:460–461.

87. McCaskill KR. Polamedco endotracheal tubes. *Can J Anesth*. 1993;40:577–578.

88. Oystan J, Holtby H. Fracture of a RAE endotracheal tube connector. *Can J Anesth*. 1988;35:438–439.

89. Saade E. Unusual cause of endotracheal tube obstruction. *Anesth Analg*. 1991;72:841–842.
90. Yapici D, Atici S, Birbicer H, Oral U. Manufacturing defect in an endotracheal tube connector: risk of foreign body aspiration. *J Anesth*. 2008;22:333–334.
91. Desmeules H, Tremblay PR. Laryngoscope blade breakage during intubation. *Can J Anesth*. 1988;35:202–203.
92. Jolly DT, Hawthorn G, Wan T. Fibreoptic laryngoscope blade. *Can J Anesth*. 1998;45:382.
93. Norman PH, Coveler LA, Daley MD, Dugas MJ. Failure of a laryngoscope blade. *Anesth Analg*. 1998;86:448.
94. Paterson JG. Laryngoscope breakage. *Can J Anesth*. 2000;47:927.
95. Smith MB, Camp P. Broken laryngoscope. *Anaesthesia*. 1989;44:179.
96. Alexander PD, Meurer-Laban M. Rechargeable optima laryngoscopes. *Br J Anaesth*. 1995;74:724–725.
97. Siegel LC, Garman JK. Too hot to handle–a laryngoscope malfunction. *Anesthesiology*. 1990;72:1088–1089.
98. Hall DB. Takes a lickin' and keeps on tickin'. *Anesth Analg*. 1999;88:1424.
99. Porter JM, Osborn KD. Flexi-tip laryngoscope breakage with airway trainer. *Anesth Intensive Care*. 2003;31:592.
100. Larson CE, Gonzalez RM. A problem with metal endotracheal tubes and plastic-coated stylets. *Anesthesiology*. 1989;70:883–884.
101. Fishman RL. Reuse of a disposable stylet with life-threatening complications. *Anesth Analg*. 1991;72:266–267.
102. Sharma A, Jain V, Mitra JK, Prabhakar H. A rare cause of endotracheal tube obstruction: a broken stylet going unnoticed–a case report. *Middle East J Anesthesiol*. 2008;19:909–911.
103. Gupta R. Unilateral transient sialadenopathy: another complication of oropharyngeal airway. *Anesthesiology*. 1998;88:551–552.
104. Michelsen LG, Valdes-Murua H. An intubating airway with teeth. *Anesthesiology*. 2001;94:938–939.
105. Ickx BE, Lamesch F. Life-threatening upper airway obstruction caused by oxygen administration with a nasal catheter. *Anesthesiology*. 2000;92:266–268.
106. Charters P, O'Sullivan E. The 'dedicated airway': a review of the concept and an update of current practice. *Anaesthesia*. 1999;54:778–786.
107. Charters P. Airway devices: where now and where to? *Br J Anaesth*. 2000;85:504–505.

Chapter 5
The Laryngeal Mask Airway (LMA™) and Other Extraglottic (Supraglottic) Airway Devices

Contents

B.T. Finucane et al., *Principles of Airway Management*,
DOI 10.1007/978-0-387-09558-5_5, © Springer Science+Business Media, LLC 2011

Introduction

The LMA™ was invented by Dr. Archie Brain in 1981.[1] Commercial products were introduced in England in 1988 and approved for use in the United States in 1991.[2] Over the past 21 years, the LMA™ (Laryngeal Mask Airway) has been modified to offer more clinical options as well as to enhance patient safety. As of 2009, LMA™

products had been used in over 200 million surgical procedures.[3] Articles on the LMA™ peaked in the mid-1990s[2]; however, research interest in the LMA™ remains keen. An analysis of the literature documented that the LMA ProSeal™ had the highest "immediacy index" in 2003.[4] The index was designed to reflect the topic's rank as a nidus for scientific inquiry. The LMA™ has established itself as a revolutionary airway management device that is a mainstay in the armamentarium of airway managers.

The LMA™ in all of its clinical variations is the most popular extraglottic airway device and will be presented as the prototype. Many other extraglottic devices will be described in this chapter. Finally, a recurrent controversy will be addressed, i.e., *Is the extraglottic airway device interchangeable with the endotracheal tube in the practice of anesthesia?*

The definitive textbook on the LMA™ was written by Joseph R. Brimacombe, MB ChB, FRCA, MD. His book entitled Laryngeal Mask Anesthesia: Principles and Practice, 2nd Edition[2] was published in 2005 and is a complete thesis on the subject. Readers are referred to this book if they require more thorough consideration of the material presented in this chapter.

The "Ideal" Extraglottic Airway

Although the design of extraglottic airway devices has been "somewhat empirical,"[5] many features of an "ideal" airway were taken into account by their inventors. Table 5.1 lists some of these features.

The question of which extraglottic device has proven to be most "ideal" was examined by Miller[6] who devised a scoring system to compare supraglottic sealing airways. Although he admitted that his scoring system might be considered

Table 5.1 Features of the "ideal" extraglottic airway

Efficient conduit for pulmonary ventilation bypassing the upper airway
Easy, appropriate insertion even by a nonspecialist
Good first-time insertion success rate
Efficacy not drastically impaired by suboptimal placement
Stable airway once positioned (capable of "hands free" anesthesia)
Works equally well in abnormal as well as normal airways
Sufficient sealing quality to apply positive pressure ventilation
Easily converted to tracheal tube placement
Good acceptance by patient (through various phases of anesthesia)
Minimal/no risk of aspiration
Minimal risk of cross-infection (single use device vs. effective sterilization)
Sealing should be with minimal pharyngeal distortion and/or distension
Cricoid pressure friendly
Negligible or minimal risk of side effects

Source: Adapted from Charters[5] and Miller[6]

"premature," "subjective," and would "likely be controversial" he reported that the LMA Classic™ and LMA Fastrach™ (Intubating LMA™) incorporated the most "ideal" properties. The COPA® (Mallinckrodt Medical, Athlone, Ireland) and the GO$_2$ (Glottic Aperture Seal Airway, Augustine Medical, Inc.) airways had the next best scores. An editorial by Cook[7] commented on many medical, environmental, and financial aspects of the LMA Classic™ (reusable airway) compared to newer single use LMA Classic™ "look alike" airways. He concluded that the LMA Classic™ had become the "standard supraglottic airway (SGA)" in many countries. He warned that many arguments used to persuade practitioners to switch to single use airways were based on advertisement and not supported by comparative scientific studies. Each practitioner must decide which extraglottic device is his "ideal" airway. One should examine the literature when comparing his choice to the gold standard, the LMA Classic™, especially when evaluating issues of utility and patient safety.

Classification of Extraglottic (Supraglottic) Airway Devices

The literature often describes the airway devices to be discussed in this chapter as supraglottic. However, Brimacombe[8] challenged the appropriateness of the term supraglottic when he noted that some devices are designed to be inserted with a distal tip below the level of the glottis (infraglottically). Thus, a more precise term to describe this class of airways is extraglottic. The classification of extraglottic airway devices can be based on anatomic, functional, design, and clinical criteria. One such classification scheme was proposed by Brimacombe[8] in which extraglottic devices were categorized by the presence or absence of a cuff, the oral or nasal route of insertion, and the anatomic location of the airway's distal tip. Miller[6] proposed another classification system based on an airway's sealing mechanism, or lack thereof.

Sinha and Misra[9] present another system classifying airways by presence or absence of a cuff, route of insertion, and anatomic level of the device's seated distal end. In practice, each clinician can develop his own classification scheme with respect to extraglottic airways to remind him of the device's design features, function, and clinical applications.

The following topics will be presented in this chapter:

1. Description of extraglottic airways: design, function, clinical use
2. Insertion techniques including use of the gum-elastic bougie (GEB)
3. Removing the extraglottic airway
4. Size selection
5. Consideration of cuff sealing pressure
6. Ventilation
7. Pediatric use
8. Innovative uses of the extraglottic airway
9. Patient positioning considerations

10. Use of adjunctive airway equipment with the extraglottic airway
11. Difficult airway management
12. Use outside the operating room
13. Problems and complications
14. Food and Drug Administration (FDA) regulations concerning medical devices including extraglottic airways
15. Is the extraglottic airway interchangeable with the endotracheal tube in the practice of anesthesia?

Description of Extraglottic Airways

Every manufacturer provides literature explaining the following concerning their extraglottic airway devices:

1. Description of the airway
2. Indications and contraindications for use
3. Insertion directions
4. Instructions for proper use
5. Care of the airway (sterilization of reusable airways, storage, etc.)
6. Potential problems, complications, risks, and adverse effects
7. Disclaimers

Basic Extraglottic Airway Design and Function

Since the literature of every manufacturer cannot be presented in this chapter, two companies have been chosen as representatives of the industry: LMA™ North America, Inc., San Diego, CA and Ambu® Inc., Glen Burnie, MD. Product information from these companies will be presented as examples of that provided by a typical manufacturer. The information addresses concepts of extraglottic airway design and function that are applicable to similar products. Unique claims may be made by each manufacturer. Support for unique claims can be researched in the literature, as most manufacturers can provide an extensive bibliography of articles that relate to their products. *Before using a specific airway, consult the product information supplied by the manufacture to assure safe and proper use of the device.* Check the company's website for more information, i.e.: *LMA™ North America, Inc. Extraglottic Airway Products.*

In 1992 the inventor of the LMA™, Dr. Archie Brain, wrote: "The aim [of developing the LMA] was to form a direct connection with the patient's airway which might afford greater security and convenience than the face mask."[1] When the LMA™ is inserted correctly, the tip rests against the upper esophageal sphincter, the sides face into the pyriform fossae, and the upper border faces the base of the tongue. Proper positioning of the LMA™ brings the glottic and airway apertures into alignment. The LMA™ "forms a seal around the laryngeal, not the pharyngeal, perimeter."[1] Two practical features of the LMA™ are that it provides a "much more reliable airway than the face mask,"[1] and when the LMA™ is secured, the practitioner can use both hands to perform other tasks. The LMA™ was designed to be used on patients breathing spontaneously and those whose ventilation was controlled. Dr. Brain has cautioned that the LMA™ is not a substitute for an endotracheal tube when the latter device is clearly indicated. The LMA™ does not necessarily protect the patient from aspiration of regurgitated gastric contents. The glottic sphincter may still close with the LMA™ in place, especially if the patient is inadequately anesthetized or the airway is used by "less experienced"[1] clinicians.

The LMA™ Instruction Manual[10] as well as other useful information is available on the Internet at www.lmana.com.[3] The current manual contains information the manufacturer deems important and covers all aspects of LMA™ use.

Indications for LMA use (Verbatim from LMA™ Instruction Manual[3] [numbers added]).

1. The LMA™ is indicated for use as an alternative to the face mask for achieving and maintaining control of the airway during routine and emergency anesthetic procedures.
2. The LMA™ airway is not indicated for use as a replacement for the endotracheal tube, and is best suited for use in elective surgical procedures where tracheal intubation is not necessary.
3. The LMA™ airway is also indicated in a known or unexpected difficult airway situation.
4. The LMA™ airway is also indicated as a method of establishing a clear airway during resuscitation in the profoundly unconscious patient with absent glossopharyngeal and laryngeal reflexes who may need artificial ventilation. In these cases, the LMA™ airway should be used only when tracheal intubation is not possible.

Contraindications to LMA™ use (Verbatim from LMA™ Instruction Manual[10] [numbers added])

1. Due to the potential risk of regurgitation and aspiration, do not use the LMA™ airway as a substitute for an endotracheal tube in the following elective or difficult airway patients on a nonemergency pathway:

   (a) Patients who have not fasted, including patients whose fasting cannot be confirmed.
   (b) Patients who are grossly or morbidly obese, more than 14 weeks pregnant or those with multiple or massive injury, acute abdominal or thoracic injury, any conditions associated with delayed gastric emptying, or using opiate medication prior to fasting.

2. The LMA™ airway is also contraindicated in:

   (a) Patients with fixed decreased pulmonary compliance, such as patients with pulmonary fibrosis, because the LMA™ airway forms a low-pressure seal around the larynx.

   (b) Patients where the peak airway inspiratory pressures are anticipated to exceed:

      (i) 20 cm H_2O with LMA Classic™, LMA Unique™, or LMA Flexible™/ single use LMA Flexible™.

      (ii) 30 cm H_2O with LMA ProSeal™.

3. Adult patients who are unable to understand instructions or cannot adequately answer questions regarding their medical history, since such patients may be contraindicated for LMA™ airway use.

4. When used in the profoundly unresponsive patient in need of resuscitation or in a difficult airway patient on an emergency pathway (i.e., "cannot intubate/cannot ventilate"), the risk of regurgitation and aspiration must be weighed against the potential benefit of establishing an airway.

The LMA™ Instruction Manual offers many guidelines concerning the device's safe use including mandates concerning cleaning and sterilization of reusable airways, airway preparation, insertion instructions, performance testing, and use with adjunctive equipment. Some of these topics will be presented in this chapter. The reader is encouraged to read the instruction manual for an excellent general overview of all LMA™ products.

Cleaning and Sterilization of Reusable LMA™ Products

"Steam autoclaving is the only recommended method for sterilization" of reusable LMA™ products (LMA Classic™ and LMA ProSeal™)[10] [Note: The LMA Fastrach™, LMA Flexible™, and LMA Excel™ are also reusable]. It is essential to follow all of the cleaning and sterilization instructions in the LMA™ Instruction Manual to protect the patient from contamination and to prolong the life of the LMA™. The manufacturer recommends that reusable LMA™'s should be recycled a maximum of 40 times. It is necessary to keep a log documenting each airway's cleaning, sterilization, and usage. Even with the added cost of caring for a reusable airway, it may be less expensive to use than its disposable counterpart. Consult the LMA™ Instruction Manual for further details concerning cleaning and sterilization.

Basic LMA™ Design Features

All LMA™ devices have three main components:

1. An airway tube with a standard 15 mm connector
2. A mask that conforms to the contours of the hypopharynx with its lumen facing the glottis
3. An inflation channel

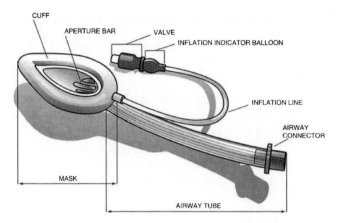

Fig. 5.1 The components of the LMA Classic (courtesy of LMA™ North America, Inc.) (*LMA Manual* 2000: Fig. 5.1, p. 1)

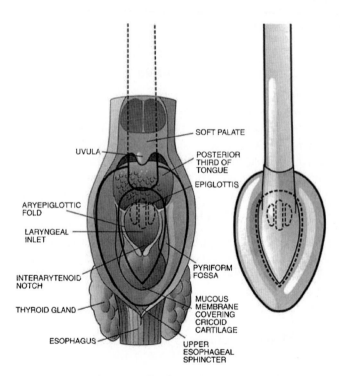

Fig. 5.2 Dorsal view of the LMA Classic showing position in relation to the pharyngeal anatomy. Note that the aperture of the airway and the glottic opening are aligned when the LMA is properly positioned (courtesy of LMA™ North America, Inc.) (*LMA Manual* 2000: Fig. 5.2, p. 2)

These features are the same for all similar extraglottic airway devices (see Figs. 5.1 and 5.2).

LMA™ Models

There are nine LMA™ airway models and two LMA™ endotracheal tubes on the market. Reusable models are made of medical grade silicone while single use models are made of medical grade polyvinylchloride (PVC).

Reusable LMA Models

1. LMA Classic™
2. LMA ProSeal™
3. LMA Fastrach™
4. LMA Flexible™
5. LMA Excel™
6. LMA™ Endotracheal Tube

Single Use LMA™ Models

1. LMA Unique™
2. LMA Supreme™
3. LMA Fastrach™
4. LMA Flexible™
5. LMA™ Endotracheal Tube

Ambu® Line of Extraglottic Airway Products

Ambu®, Inc. (Glen Burnie, MD) markets five models of extraglottic airways. Each model has the word Aura™ in its name and is referred to as a "laryngeal mask airway." The airways come in a variety of sizes for use on patients from infant to adult.

Information concerning the Ambu® airways can be obtained on the company's website www.ambuusa.com.[11] General information concerning the airways is presented in the following sections. The features of each model will be presented later in the chapter with those of other manufacturers' airways.

General Information Concerning Ambu® LMAs

The company's product information describing Ambu® airways appropriately begins with warnings and cautions concerning their safe use. Each model's manual presents information specifically referring to that model. The lists of indications and contraindications that follow summarize, quote, and paraphrase comments from the manuals of the various models.

Indications for Ambu® LMAs

1. The Ambu® airway is intended for use as an alternative to a facemask for achieving and maintaining control of the airway during routine and emergency anesthetic procedures in fasted patients.
2. The Ambu® airway may also be used where unexpected difficulties arise in connection with airway management.
3. The mask may also be preferred in some critical airway situations.
4. The Ambu® may also be used to establish a clear airway during resuscitation in profoundly unconscious patients with absent glossopharyngeal and laryngeal reflexes who may need artificial ventilation.
5. The device is not intended for use as a replacement of the endotracheal tube, and is best suited for use in surgical procedures where tracheal intubation is not deemed necessary.

Contraindications

The Ambu® airway does not protect the patient from the consequences of regurgitation and aspiration. The following contraindications apply in the case of routine use in elective surgical procedures or in difficult airway patients.

1. Patients who have not fasted (including those cases where fasting cannot be confirmed).
2. Patients who are pathologically obese or more than 14 weeks pregnant.
3. Patients with massive or acute injury to the abdomen or thorax.
4. Patients with any condition associated with delayed gastric emptying, or using opiate medication prior to fasting.
5. Patients where peak airway inspiratory pressures are anticipated to exceed 20 cm H_2O (because the Ambu® forms a low-pressure seal around the larynx).

Use of Ambu® LMAs for Resuscitation

The company's instruction manuals also address use of the airways for resuscitation. Following is a quote from the manual:

> When the Ambu® [airway] is used in profoundly unconscious patients in need of resuscitation or in an emergency patient with a difficult airway situation (i.e., "cannot intubate, cannot ventilate"), there is a risk of regurgitation and aspiration. This risk must be carefully balanced against the potential benefit of establishing an airway (see the guidelines established by your own local protocol). The Ambu® [airway] should not be used for resuscitation or emergency treatment of patients who are not profoundly unconscious and who may resist insertion.[11]

Each model's instruction manual addresses the device's principles of operation, adverse effects associated with its use, preparation and inspection advice, and detailed directions for proper insertion, placement, and removal. Ambu® extraglottic airways are designed to be used with anesthetized patients who are breathing spontaneously as well as those who are receiving positive pressure ventilation with

"…peak airway pressures less than 20 cm H_2O and tidal volumes less than 8 ml/kg while capnography is closely monitored."[11]

The basic designs and uses of two companies' extraglottic airways have been presented. There are many manufacturers of similar devices. Consult their instruction manuals and the scientific literature to obtain information concerning a specific airway.

Sizing of Extraglottic Airways

The sizes of extraglottic airways are usually referenced to the patient's weight. Summarizing the recommendations of several popular manufacturers, Table 5.2 is a general reference to airway sizing.

Descriptions of Extraglottic Airway Design and Features

Table 5.3 summarizes data on a multitude of extraglottic airway devices from many manufacturers. The information is adapted from excellent articles by Hagberg[12] and Osborn and Reinhard[13] and contains additional information taken from manufacturers' published materials. (The author of this chapter does not imply that all manufacturer claims are supported by conclusive scientific investigation just because they are included in the table. Some claims may be promotional and speculative). This table is presented as a "summary table" to make it easier for the reader to reference a single source to get the names of and basic information concerning many extraglottic airway devices.

Illustrations of Extraglottic Airway Devices

Illustrations of extraglottic airway devices are grouped by manufacturer. The most common design has a laryngeal mask. This design is that of the prototypical LMA Classic™. The second most common design has a distal tip that is positioned in the esophagus. A third type of airway does not have an inflatable cuff: I-gel, and Slipa™ airways. Each

Table 5.2 General suggestions for extraglottic airway size

Size of airway	Patient size
1	<5 kg: Neonates and infants
1½	5–10 kg: Infants
2	10–20 kg: Infants and children
2½	20–30 kg: Children
3	30–50 kg: Children
4	50–70 kg: Small adults
5	70–100 kg: Adults
6	>100 kg: Adults

Table 5.3 Descriptions and features of extraglottic airway devices

Name of airway and manufacturer	Description	Reusable or single use	Sizes	Features
LMA™ Airways LMA North America, Inc.				LMA™ products other than Fastrach™ are MRI compatible but may distort image if not used properly. See Instruction Manual for each product
LMA Classic™	Soft silicone rubber cuff. Attaches to standard 15 mm airway equipment	Reusable (40 times)	8 Sizes (1–6)	First LMA™ device. Part of the ASA difficult airway algorithm. has epiglottic and aperture bars. Accommodates ETT 3.5–7.0 mm ID
LMA Unique™	Packaged for single use. Made of soft, flexible material	Single use	7 Sizes (1–5)	First disposable LMA™ Same as LMA Classic™
LMA ProSeal™	Silicone rubber cuff. Built-in bite block. Two channels to isolate respiratory and GI tracts	Reusable	6 Sizes (1.5–5)	50% higher cuff pressure (up to 30 cm H$_2$O) providing tighter seal. Provides more airway security if PPV used. Optimal insertion tool available
LMA Supreme™	Larger precurved cuff for improved fit. Molded fins protect airway form epiglottic obstruction. Bite block built-in. Two channels to isolate respiratory and GI tracts	Single use	3 Sizes (3–5)	Easier gastric tube insertion than with ProSeal™. Other features same as ProSeal™ First and only disposable LMA™ with built-in drain tube

LMA Fastrach™	Designed to facilitate tracheal intubation. Set comes with wire-reinforced endotracheal tube and stabilizer rod. Reusable Fastrach™ made with silicone rubber. Single use Fastrach™ made of PVC Contraindicated for MRI use	Reusable and single use models	3 Sizes (3–5)	Accommodate 6.0–8.0 ETT. (Special wire-reinforced tubes included with set). Can be used for blind or fiberoptic-guided intubation. Movable epiglottic elevating bar. Fastrach™ can be left in place or removed after intubation
LMA Flexible™	Reinforced airway tube may be positioned away from the surgical field	Reusable and single use models	6 Sizes (2–6)	ID 5.1–8.7 mm. Wire-reinforced tube resists kinking
LMA Excel™	Armored airway connector increases tube strength. Removable connector to facilitate intubation. Soft silicone rubber cuff. Epiglottic elevating bar	Reusable (60 times)	3 Sizes (3–5)	Accommodates ETT's from 6.0 to 7.5 mm ID. May be left in place or removed after intubation. Designed to facilitate fiberoptic intubation through the LMA
Ambu® Extraglottic Airways Ambu®, Inc.				
Ambu® Aura40 Straight	Clearly marked guidelines for easy insertion, cuff inflation volume, and patient weight printed on the airway tube. Silicone rubber construction	Reusable (40 times)	8 Sizes (1–6)	No epiglottic bars
Ambu® Aura40 Curved	Special curve replicates human anatomy. Convenient depth marks. Color-coded pilot balloon identifies mask size and provides precise tactile indication of degree of inflation. Extra soft cuff	Reusable (40 times)	8 Sizes (1–6)	Cuff and airway tube molded as single unit. Flexible airway tube adapts to individual anatomical variances and a wide range of head positions

(continued)

Table 5.3 (continued)

Name of airway and manufacturer	Description	Reusable or single use	Sizes	Features
Ambu® AuraOnce	Curved to replicate human anatomy. D-shaped airway tube to offer better grip during positioning. Soft cuff. Pilot balloon identifies mask size and provides precise tactile indication of degree of inflation. Depth marks imprinted on airway	Single use	8 Sizes (1–6)	Curve ensures that the patient's head remains in a natural supine position without stressing the upper jaw. Easy access for fiberoptic scope. Accommodates ETT's 3.5–7.0 mm ID. Recommended to use Aintree airway exchange catheter as an intubation guide
Ambu® AuraFlex	Long flexible wire-reinforced airway tube. Integrated (protected) pilot tube. Depth marks printed on tube. Color-coded packaging	Single use	6 Sizes (2–6)	May be positioned for surgical field avoidance. Kink resistant
Ambu® AuraStraight	Similar in shape to LMA Unique™. Color-coded packaging. Depth marks printed on airway. Soft cuff	Single use	8 Sizes (1–6)	No epiglottic bars
King Systems Extraglottic Airways				
King Systems Corporation (manufactured by VBM Medizintechnik GmbH)				
King LAD™ Silicone	Silicone rubber Similar to LMA Classic™ in design	Single use	7 Sizes (1–5)	MRI compatible
King LAD™ Flexible	Silicone rubber cuff. Similar to LMA Classic™ in design	Single use	5 Sizes (2–5)	Reinforced flexible tubing (PVC)
King ClearSeal™	PVC	Single use	7 Sizes (1–5)	
King LT™	Single lumen double-cuffed tube (oropharyngeal and esophageal cuffs). Two ventilation outlets. Insertion marks. Color-coded connectors	Reusable (50 times)	Sizes 3–5 worldwide 0–2 outside of North America	No epiglottic bars. Possible aspiration protection. May be used for fiberoptic or AEC (airway exchange catheter) guided intubation

Device	Description	Reusability	Sizes	Comments
King LT-D™	Same as LT®	Single use	Adult: 3–5 Peds: 2–2.5	
King LTS-D™	Similar to LT™ but has a second lumen at the distal tip. Distal tip is specially designed to assist the airway's passable into the esophagus	Single use	Adult sizes 3–5	Second lumen provides a vent for gastric pressure and regurgitated material. A gastric tube up to 18 Fr can be passed through the second lumen
AES Laryngeal Mask Airways AES, Inc.				
Cuff Pilot™ Valve (CPV)	The CPV on certain AES laryngeal masks is a color-coded bellows built into the inflation cuff			The CPV shows the airway operator if the cuff pressure increases or decreases
AES Ultra™ and AES Ultra CPV™	Silicone rubber tube and cuff. Anatomically correct tip. No bars. Color-coded packaging	Single use	Ulta™ 4 sizes: 3–6 Ultra CPV™: 8 sizes: 1–6	MRI compatible
AES Ultra Clear™ and AES Ultra Clear CPV™	Silicone rubber cuff and PVC tube. Otherwise same as Ultra™	Single use	Same as Ultra™	MRI compatible
AES Ultra EX™ and Flex EX™	100% silicone. Soft cuff. Flexible body. Reusable airways in Ultra™ and Flex™ models	Reusable	8 Sizes (1–6)	Absence of bars makes cleaning and instrumentation through the tube easier
Flexicare, Inc. USA LarySeal™ Multiple	Silicone, autoclavable LMA. Color-coded pilot balloon indicates size of airway. Info printed on tube provides guidance for air volume and size. Designed to give a clear view of the glottis using an endoscope	Reusable (40 times)	7 Sizes (1–5)	Crush resistant airway tube. Universal connector (15 mm). Thin walled pilot balloon. Highly elastic cuff that forms itself to the contour of the oropharyngeal area thus providing a seal
LarySeal™ Blue	Same as LarySeal™	Single use	Same as LarySeal Multiple™	Single use protects against patient cross contamination. "Cost effective" according to manufacturer

(continued)

Table 5.3 (continued)

Name of airway and manufacturer	Description	Reusable or single use	Sizes	Features
LarySeal™ Clear	PVC. Soft construction material	Single use	7 Sizes (1–5)	Cost effective
LarySeal™ MRI	PVC. No metal in construction	Single use	7 Sizes (1–5)	For use in MRI suite. Contains no metal that could cause image distortion
LarySeal™ Flexi	PVC. Wire-reinforced main tube. Satin cuff texture similar to silicome	Single use	5 sizes (2–5)	Flexible tube for surgical field avoidance
LarySeal™ Cuff Inflator Syringe	Syringe has color-coded markings to deliver a specific volume of air to the LMA. The color-code is matched to the color of the pilot balloon on the mask size. The colors vary with LMA size. The volume of air delivered will produce a cuff pressure of 60 cm H_2O			
Cookgas® (Distributed by Mercury Medical®)				
Air-Q Laryngeal Mask (formerly known as Intubating Laryngeal Airway [ILA])	Color-coded removable airway connector. Tip designed to resist folding. Larger diameter tube to facilitate standard ETT tube passage for endotracheal intubation. Integrated bite block. Accompanying air-Q Removal Stylet to hold ETT in place during LMA removal	Single use and Reusable models (40 times)	4 sizes (1.5–4.5)	May be used as standard LMA devices. Designed to facilitate tracheal intubation with standard ETT sizes 5.5–8.5

Intersurgical, Inc.				
I-gel	Made from a medical grade thermoplastic elastomer. Noninflatable seal designed to encompass pharyngeal, laryngeal, and perilaryngeal structures while avoiding compression trauma. Integrated bite block and gastric channel. Buccal cavity stabilizer designed to maintain airway position	Single use	3 sizes (3–5) Supplied in color-coded protective cradle	For use during routine and emergency anesthetics of fasted patients. Can be used with spontaneously ventilating patients or to deliver intermittent positive pressure ventilation
Solus™ Standard LMA	Standard LMA design	Single use	7 Sizes (1–5)	
Solus™ MRI compatible LMA	Standard LMA design	Single use	7 Sizes (1–5)	
Solus™ Flexible Wire-Reinforced LMA	Standard LMA design	Single use	5 Sizes (2–5)	
Smiths Medical				
Portex® Silicone Laryngeal Mask	Silicone construction. Low atrium with epiglottic bars. One piece design to minimize insertion trauma	Single use	5 Sizes (2–5)	
Portex® Soft Seal® Laryngeal Mask	Cuff is less permeable to nitrous oxide than that of reusable LMAs thus reducing pressure while minimizing potential trauma. Clear tubing. Higher atrium contributing to better seal. Atraumatic tip. No epiglottic bars. Nonreturn valve. Printed pilot balloon. Integrated pilot line and radio opaque Blue Line®	Single use	7 Sizes (1–5)	Lack of epiglottic bars may make fiberoptic intubation easier

(continued)

Table 5.3 (continued)

Name of airway and manufacturer	Description	Reusable or single use	Sizes	Features
Slipa Medical, Ltd. Slipa™ Airway	Preformed shape lines the pharynx. No inflatable cuff or epiglottic bars	Single use	6 adult sizes (47–57) Refer to Slipa™ Size Chart	Seal provides for "excellent quality positive pressure ventilation." Hollow structure allows for storage of regurgitated liquids. Rescue intubation possible with fiberoptic scope and airway exchange catheter
Teleflex Medical Rusch Easytube®	Designed for use in managing difficult or emergency airway. Blind insertion. Distal tip placed in esophagus. Double-lumen design. Pharyngeal and distal cuffs. Single lumen at distal tip. Can be used to ventilate with distal tip in trachea or esophagus. Set supplied with prefilled syringes and suction catheter	Single use	2 sizes (Large 41 French, Small 28 French)	When placed with distal tip in esophagus the tube allows the use of fiberoptic devices or passage of suction catheter or tube exchanger
Covidien Combitube® Esophageal/Tracheal Double-Lumen Airway	Designed for difficult or emergency blind airway intubation. Designed to provide patent airway with either esophageal or tracheal placement. Oropharyngeal balloon is *latex*. Distal cuff designed to be low-pressure. Kit includes syringes and suction catheters. ventilatory holes between cuffs. Packaged nonsterile	Single use	2 sizes (37 and 41 French)	Reduced risk of gastric contents claimed by manufacturer. May be used during surgical procedures Contains latex

Engineered Medical Systems

Device	Description	Use	Sizes	Comments
CobraPLA™ (Perilaryngeal Airway)	PVC/polycarbonate. Tapered head centers grill in front of the glottis. Ultra thin cuff is positioned in the upper hypopharynx creating a high-volume, low-pressure seal allowing for "moderate controlled ventilation with a peak airway pressure limited to 20 cm H_2O"	Single use	Adult and Pediatric	"Ramping" in head design helps direct ETT towards glottis. Secretions can be suctioned. Allows passage of NG tube, if indicated
CobraPLUS™	Similar to CobraPLA™. All sizes include temperature monitor. Ped sizes ½, 1, and 1½ have distal CO_2 gas sampling ports	Single use	8 Sizes (0.5–6)	
Elisha Medical Technologies, Ltd.				
Elisha Airway Device[182]	Silicone. Three separate channels for ventilation, intubation, gastric tube insertion. Proximal balloon seals the oro and nasopharynx. Distal cuff seals the esophagus. Balloons are inflated through single pilot port with 50 ml air resulting in intraballoon pressure of approximately 70 cm H_2O	Reusable		Intubating channel accommodates 8.0 mm ID ETT for blind or fiberoptic tracheal intubation

Note: All airways are latex-free except for the Combitube® (Covidien)
MRI use: Check each airway's instruction manual prior to use to assure that it is MRI compatible

manufacturer has a website if the reader desires to learn more about a specific airway. (Some airways are not shown because their manufacturers did not give permission to publish images of their products.)

LMA™ Airways (Figs. 5.3–5.11)
Ambu® Extraglottic Airways (Figs. 5.12–5.16)
King Systems Extraglottic Airways (Figs. 5.17–5.20)

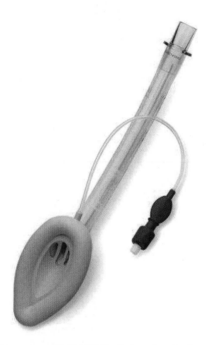

Fig. 5.3 LMA Classic™ (courtesy of LMA™ North America, Inc.)

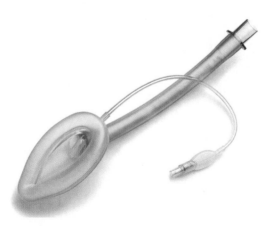

Fig. 5.4 LMA Unique™ (courtesy of LMA™ North America, Inc.)

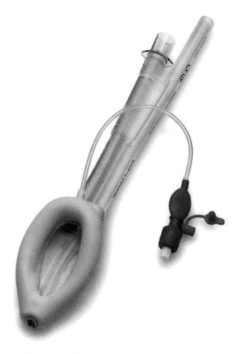

Fig. 5.5 LMA ProSeal™ (Courtesy of LMA™ North America, Inc.)

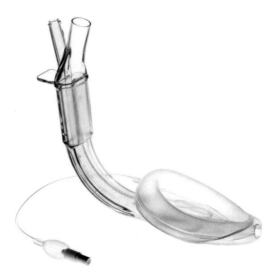

Fig. 5.6 LMA Supreme™ (Courtesy of LMA™ North America, Inc.)

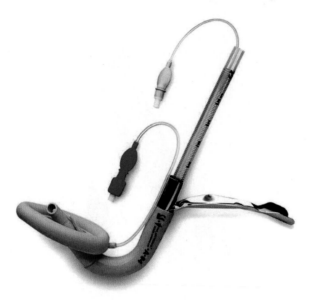

Fig. 5.7 LMA Fastrach™ Multiple Use (courtesy of LMA™ North America, Inc.)

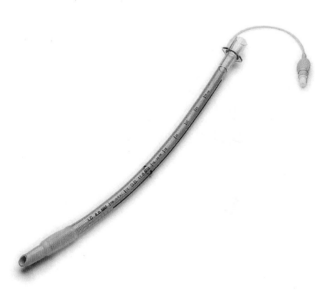

Fig. 5.8 LMA™ Endotracheal Tube for use with LMA Factrach™ (courtesy of LMA™ North America, Inc.)

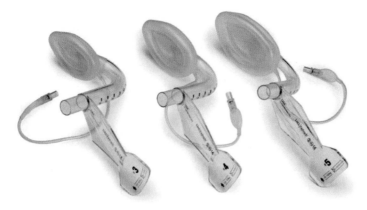

Fig. 5.9 LMA Fastrach™ Single Use (courtesy of LMA™ North America, Inc.)

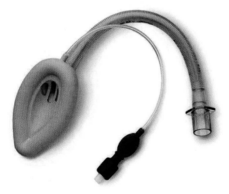

Fig. 5.10 LMA Flexible™ Multiple Use and Single Use (courtesy of LMA™ North America, Inc.)

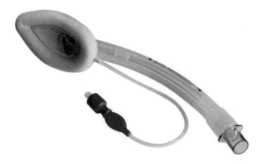

Fig. 5.11 LMA Excel™ Single Use (courtesy of LMA™ North America, Inc.)

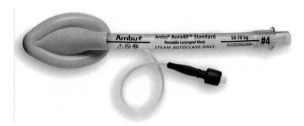

Fig. 5.12 Ambu® Aura40 Straight

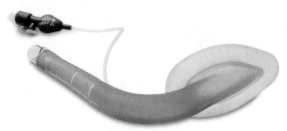

Fig. 5.13 Ambu® Aura40 Curved

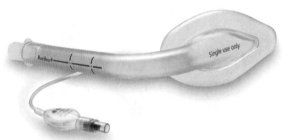

Fig. 5.14 Ambu® AuraOnce

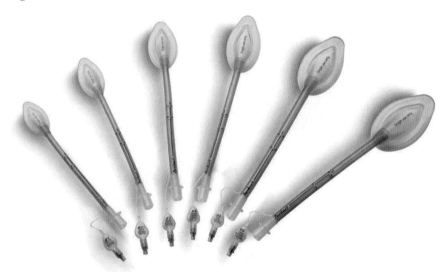

Fig. 5.15 Ambu® AuraFlex Family

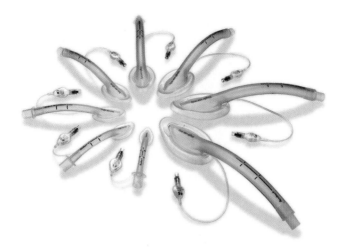

Fig. 5.16 Ambu® AuraStraight Family

AES LMAs (Figs. 5.21–5.27)
Flexicare, Inc. USA Airways (Figs. 5.28–5.33)
Cookgas® (Distributed by Mercury Medical®) (Fig. 5.34)
Intersurgical, Inc. (Figs. 5.35–5.37)

Insertion Techniques

A detailed description of the insertion techniques recommended by the manufacturers
of each extraglottic airway is available on the Internet. The insertion techniques of
selected airways will exemplify principles of insertion applicable to airways of
similar design. Insertion techniques for the following airways are presented: most
LMA™ devices with special consideration of the LMA ProSeal™ and LMA
Fastrach™, Ambu® AuraStraight™, SLIPA™, and the King LTS-D™.

Preinsertion Recommendations

All manufacturers make preinsertion recommendations. Tables 5.4 and 5.5 show
recommendations that apply to all extraglottic airways.

LMA™ Insertion Recommendations

Before inserting any LMA™ airway, it is recommended to deflate and preshape the
cuff. Manually, or using a deflation device sold by the manufacturer, form the

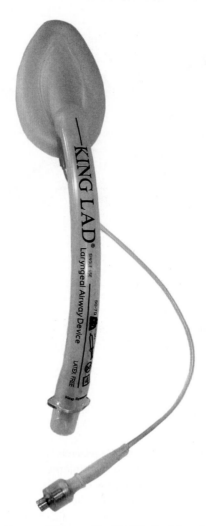

Fig. 5.17 King LAD™ Airways: (Silicone, ClearSeal™, flexible options)

deflated cuff into a "wedge shape" with the cuff having a smooth leading edge. Make sure the red plug has been inserted into the inflation tube and pull back on the tube to assist shaping. Lubricate the posterior surface of the airway cuff with a water-soluble jelly (Fig. 5.38).

LMA™ Insertion

Four techniques for inserting LMA™ airways are recommended. The "Index Finger Insertion Technique" and the "Thumb Insertion Technique" are applicable to the LMA Classic™, Flexible™, Unique™, Excel™, and the ProSeal™ airways.

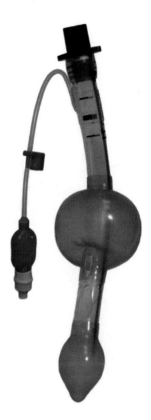

Fig. 5.18 King LT™

The ProSeal™ can also be inserted with a specially designed introducer that will be described in the next section. Finally, the LMA Supreme™ and Fastrach™ manuals have instructions for insertion of these airways.

Concerning basic LMA™ insertion techniques, the LMA™ Instruction Manual states[10]:

> To position the LMA™ airway correctly, the cuff tip must avoid entering the valleculae or the glottic opening and must not become caught up against the epiglottis or the arytenoids. The cuff must be deflated in the correct wedge shape and should be kept pressed against the patient's posterior pharyngeal wall. To avoid contact with anterior structures during insertion, the inserting finger must press the tube upwards (cranially) throughout the insertion maneuver.

Index Finger Insertion Technique

The following figures illustrate the "Index Finger Insertion Technique." Depending on the size of the patient, the index finger may have to be inserted to its fullest extent before resistance is felt upon seating of the cuff. This is especially true for the LMA Flexible™ and the single use LMA Flexible™ airways (Figs. 5.39–5.43).

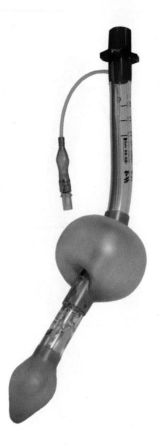

Fig. 5.19 King LT-D™

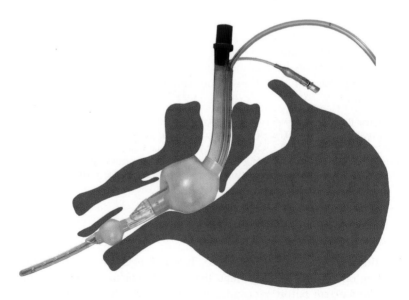

Fig. 5.20 King LTS-D™ in position showing relationship of balloon cuffs to the glottis and esophagus

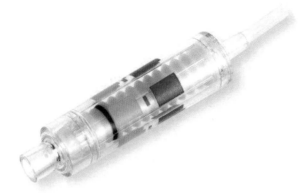

Fig. 5.21 AES Cuff Pilot™ Valve (CPV)

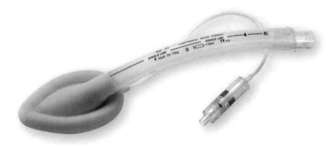

Fig. 5.22 AES Ultra™ with CPV™

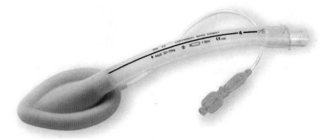

Fig. 5.23 AES Ultra™

Thumb Insertion Technique

The "Thumb Insertion Technique" may be used if the airway is not managed from behind. The thumb is advanced to its fullest extent. The pushing action of the thumb against the hard palate extends the head facilitating airway insertion. Figures 5.44–5.48 illustrate this technique.

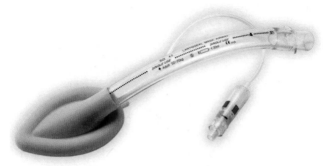

Fig. 5.24 AES Ultra Clear™ with CPV™

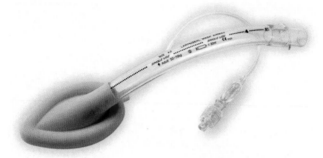

Fig. 5.25 AES Ultra Clear™

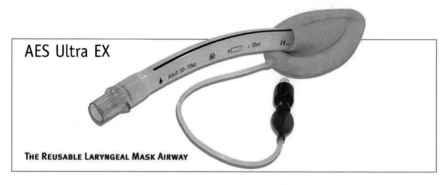

Fig. 5.26 AES Ultra EX™ with CPV™

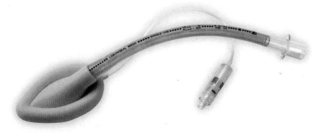

Fig. 5.27 AES Ultra Flex™ with CPV™

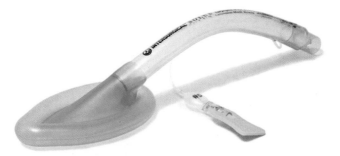

Fig. 5.37 Solus™ MRI compatible LMA

Table 5.4 Preinsertion recommendations concerning extraglottic airways

Make sure the airway is the proper size based on age and weight of the patient. See Table 5.4
    or follow manufacturer recommendations for airways of unique design: e.g., SLIPA™,
    Combitube™, etc.

Make sure the airway has been properly sterilized if a multiple use device is utilized

Visually inspect the airway to make sure it is not damaged and none of its components is loose
    or missing

Insure that all of the tubes and openings of the airway are clean and unobstructed

Examine the 15 mm connector

Performance test the airway by deflating the cuff and inspecting for manufacturing defects.
    While deflated, remove the syringe and observe whether the valve functions properly
    (deflation maintained). Overinflate the cuff and remove the syringe. Insure valve integrity
    and observe all surfaces of the cuff. Make sure all tubes and openings remain patent. Make
    sure the valve balloon retains pressure

Have backup airways of different sizes available

Use nonanesthetic lubricants. Anesthetic lubricants might blunt or ablate protective airway
    reflexes

Table 5.5 Preinsertion recommendations concerning the patient

Make sure the airway is the proper size for the patient

Make sure the patient is anesthetized and will not struggle or fight against airway insertion

Place the patient's head in the "sniff position" and hold it in place with the nondominant hand,
    that which is not directing the airway device. A pillow may help support the head

Avoid excessive force at all times while inserting any airway device

Testing the LMA ProSeal™ for Proper Positioning: "Malpositioning Test"

Pass a suction catheter through the drainage channel of the airway to make sure it is patent. Perform a "malpositioning test" by placing a small bolus of lubricant gel at the proximal end of the drainage tube then deliver a positive pressure breath through the airway. If the gel is ejected, the mask is not positioned properly.

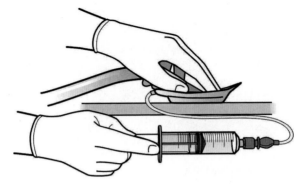

Fig. 5.38 LMA™ cuff properly deflated for insertion: "wedge shape" (courtesy of LMA™ North America, Inc.)

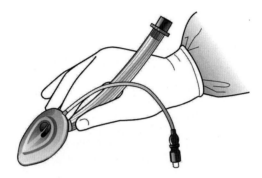

Fig. 5.39 Hold the LMA™ airway with the index finger at the cuff/tube junction or in the LMA ProSeal™ introducer strap (courtesy of LMA™ North America, Inc.)

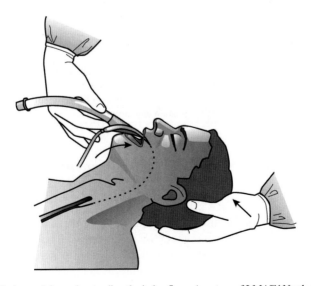

Fig. 5.40 Slide the mask inward, extending the index finger (courtesy of LMA™ North America, Inc.)

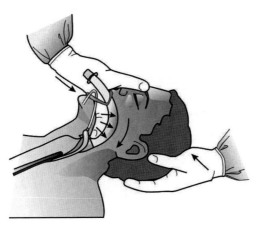

Fig. 5.41 Press the mask up against the hard palate. Note the flexed wrist (courtesy of LMA™ North America, Inc.)

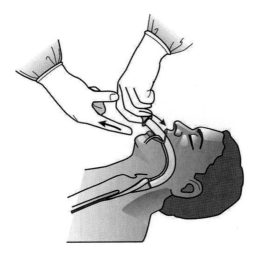

Fig. 5.42 Remove the index finger while holding the LMA™ in place with the other hand (courtesy of LMA™ North Amereica, Inc.)

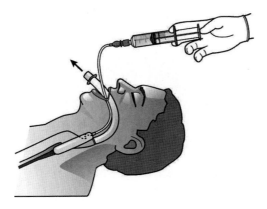

Fig. 5.43 Inflate the cuff (courtesy of LMA™ North America, Inc.)

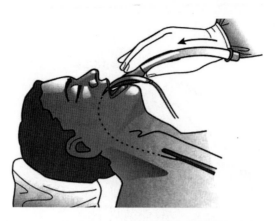

Fig. 5.44 Method for holding the LMA for thumb insertion (courtesy of LMA™ North America, Inc.) (*LMA Manual* 2000: Fig. 5.14, p. 29)

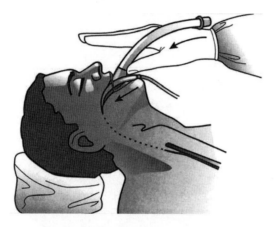

Fig. 5.45 With the fingers extended, press the thumb along the posterior pharynx (courtesy of LMA™ North America, Inc.) (*LMA Manual* 2000: Fig. 5.15, p. 29)

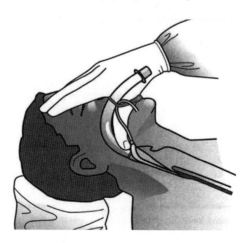

Fig. 5.46 Advance the thumb to its fullest extent (courtesy of LMA™ North America, Inc.) (*LMA Manual* 2000: Fig. 5.16, p. 30)

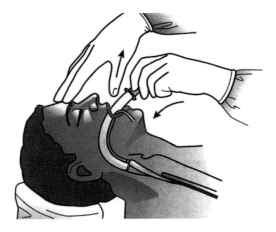

Fig. 5.47 Press gently in the place with the nondominant hand while removing the thumb (courtesy of LMA™ North America, Inc.) (*LMA Manual* 2000: Fig. 5.17, p. 30)

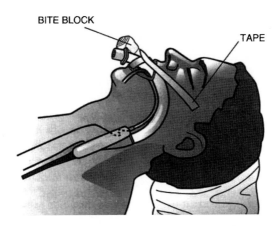

Fig. 5.48 Tape the bite block and airway tube together with the tube taped downward against the chin (courtesy of LMA™ North America, Inc.) (*LMA Manual* 2000: Fig. 5.18, p. 31)

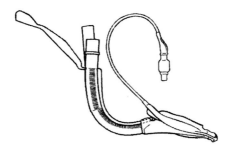

Fig. 5.49 LMA ProSeal with introducer in place (courtesy of LMA™ North America, Inc.) (*LMA-ProSeal Manual* 2000: Fig. 5.6, p. 23)

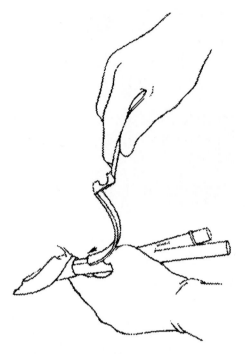

Fig. 5.50 Place the tip of the introducer into the flap of the ProSeal (courtesy of LMA™ North America, Inc.) (*LMA-ProSeal Manual* 2000: Fig. 5.5a, p. 21)

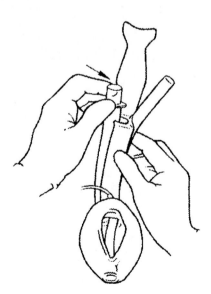

Fig. 5.51 Fold the tubes around the introducer and fit the proximal end of the airway tube into the matching slot (courtesy of LMA™ North America, Inc.) (*LMA-ProSeal Manual* 2000: Fig. 5.5b, p. 21)

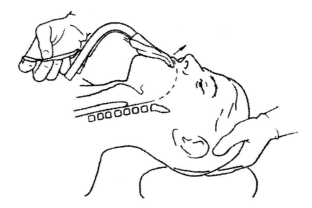

Fig. 5.52 Press the tip of the cuff against the hard palate (courtesy of LMA™ North America, Inc.) (*LMA-ProSeal Manual* 2000: Fig. 5.7, p. 23)

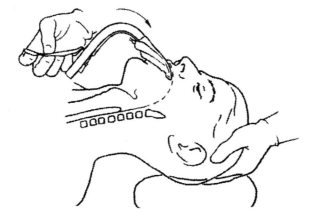

Fig. 5.53 Press the cuff further into the mouth, maintaining pressure against the palate (courtesy of LMA™ North America, Inc.) (*LMA-ProSeal Manual* 2000: Fig. 5.8, p. 23)

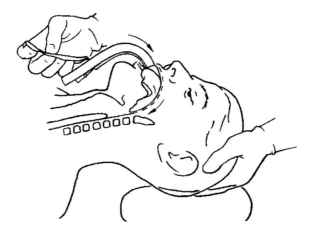

Fig. 5.54 Swing the device inward with a circular motion, pressing against the contours of the hard and soft palate (courtesy of LMA™ North America, Inc.) (*LMA-ProSeal Manual* 2000: Fig. 5.9, p. 24)

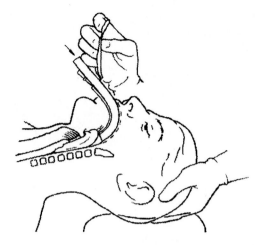

Fig. 5.55 Advance the LMA ProSeal in the hypopharynx until resistance is felt (courtesy of LMA™ North America, Inc.) (*LMA-ProSeal Manual* 2000: Fig. 5.10, p. 24)

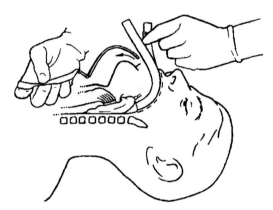

Fig. 5.56 Hold the ProSeal tube in place while removing the introducer (courtesy of LMA™ North America, Inc.) (*LMA-ProSeal Manual* 2000: Fig. 5.11, p. 24)

LMA Fastrach™ Insertion and Intubation Through the Airway[14]

The LMA Fastrach™ Instruction Manual (2006) describes the use of the airway in detail. This manual serves as the reference for this section of the chapter and should be studied before using the LMA Fastrach™. All of the recommendations for cleaning, sterilizing, inspecting, and handling the airway should be followed at all times. Perhaps the most important cautionary note, a principle that should be applied to all airway devices is: "Do not use force under any circumstances" when using the airway.

The LMA Fastrach™ is a reusable extraglottic airway that is designed to function as a primary airway or as a guide to facilitate blind or fiberoptic endotracheal intubation. (Recent publications question use as a primary airway because of high mucosal pressures exerted by the cuff and possible cervical spine displacement in patients with neck injuries. See subsequent section in this chapter that deal with these issues.) The airway should be used with an LMA Fastrach™ Endotracheal Tube. The tube is sold in five sizes: 6.0, 6.5, 7.0, 7.5, and 8.0 mmID, and two models: Reusable or Disposable. In addition to the contraindications for other LMA™ airways, additional contraindications specific to the Fastrach™ include:

1. Patients whose heads need to be turned during a case
2. Patients placed in the prone position
3. Patients in the MRI suite since it has metal parts
4. Patients who are undergoing procedures involving use of a laser or electrocautery in the vicinity of the device

Table 5.6 is a selection guide referring to LMA Fastrach™ size selection. Figures 5.57–5.64 illustrate insertion and intubation techniques applicable to the LMA Fastrach™ (see also Table 5.7).

Intubation Through the LMA Fastrach™

LMA™ recommends that the LMA Fastrach™ Endotracheal Tube be used to intubate through their airway. The tube is straight, wire-reinforced and specially designed for use with the Fastrach™. The following figures illustrate intubation using the Fastrach™ Endotracheal Tube (Figs. 5.65–5.67).

Removal of the LMA Fastrach™ While Leaving the Endotracheal
Tube in Position

The manufacturer recommends removal of the LMA Fastrach™ after intubation because of reports of pharyngeal edema and increased mucosal pressure attributed

Table 5.6 LMA Fastrach™ selection guidelines

LMA Factrach™	Patient size (kg)
Size 3	Children 30–50
Size 4	Adults 50–70
Size 5	Adults 70–100

(Laryngeal depth is not directly related to patient size or weight)
Source: LMA Fastrach™ Instruction Manual. 2005: www.lmana.com[14] (courtesy of LMA™ North America, Inc.)

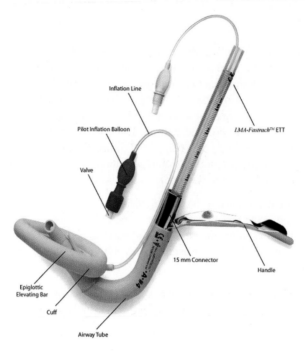

Fig. 5.57 LMA Fastrach™ Extraglottic Airway (courtesy of LMA™ North America, Inc.)

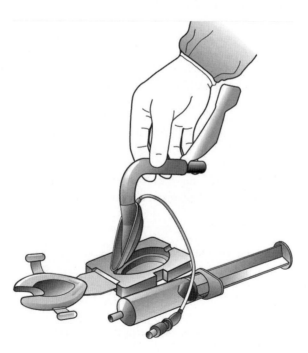

Fig. 5.58 Preshape the LMA Fastrach™ by deflating the cuff completely then folding it into the "wedge" shape with a sharp leading edge. This can be done by hand or with the LMA™ Cuff Deflator (courtesy of LMA™ North America, Inc.)

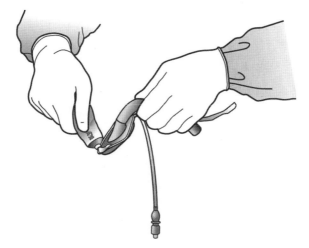

Fig. 5.59 Lubricate the posterior surface of the airway with a water-soluble lubricant. "Lubricants containing lidocaine are not recommended for use as lidocaine may delay the return of protective reflexes, provoke an allergic reaction, or affect surrounding structures, including the vocal cords" (courtesy of LMA™ North America, Inc.)

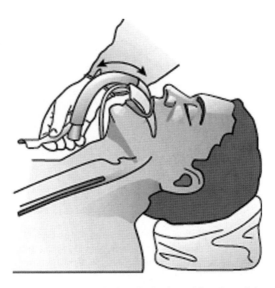

Fig. 5.60 Hold the LMA Fastrach™ by the handle that is positioned parallel to the patient's chest. Position the tip of the airway so it is flat against the hard palate just inside the mouth immediately posterior to the upper incisors. Slide the mask tip back and forth to distribute lubricant holding the cuff against the palate to prevent folding of the tip. Slide the mask backwards following the curve of the rigid airway tube. It may be necessary to draw the mouth open momentarily to permit the widest part of the mask to enter the oral cavity (courtesy of LMA™ North America, Inc.)

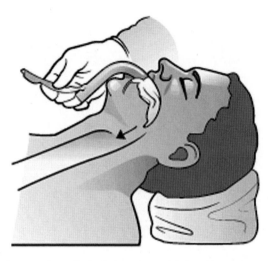

Fig. 5.61 Ensure the curved metal tube is in contact with the chin prior to rotation (courtesy of LMA™ North America, Inc.)

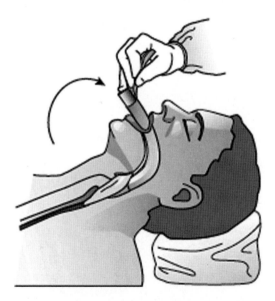

Fig. 5.62 Swing the mask into place in a circular movement maintaining pressure against the palate and posterior pharynx. After insertion, the tube should emerge from the mouth directed somewhat caudally, lying approximately parallel to the plane of the inner surface of the upper incisors (courtesy of LMA™ North America, Inc.)

to the rigidity inherent in the airway's design. *Note: Removal of the extraglottic device may cause inadvertent extubation. Be prepared to secure the airway should this happen.* Figures 5.68–5.70 illustrate the LMA Fastrach™ removal maneuver leaving the endotracheal tube in place.

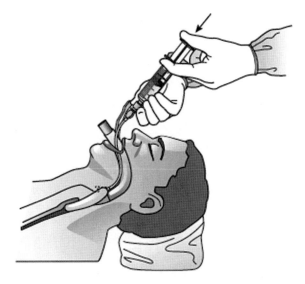

Fig. 5.63 Inflate the cuff just enough to obtain a seal. Do not overinflate the cuff

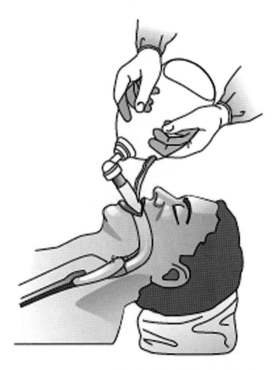

Fig. 5.64 Ventilate the patient (courtesy of LMA™ North America, Inc.)

Table 5.7 Maximum cuff inflation volumes

LMA Fastrach™ size	Maximum air volume (ml)
3	20
4	30
5	40

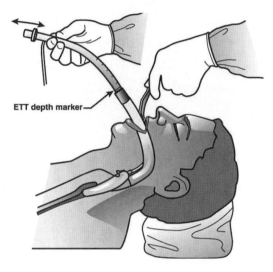

Fig. 5.65 After lubricating the endotracheal tube, insert it into the LMA Fastrach™ with the tube's black line rotated towards the handle. Insert the tube no further than the 15 cm transverse line that is printed into the wall of the tube (courtesy of LMA™ North America, Inc.)

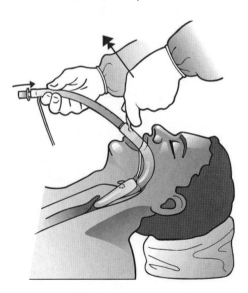

Fig. 5.66 Grip the handle and lift gently to draw the larynx forwards a few millimeters. This "Chandy maneuver" seals the cuff and aligns the axes of the trachea and endotracheal tube to facilitate intubation (courtesy of LMA™ North America, Inc.)

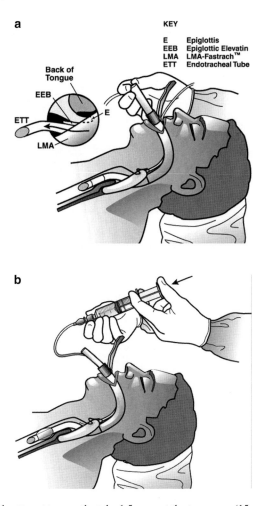

KEY

E	Epiglottis
EEB	Epiglottic Elevatin
LMA	LMA-Fastrach™
ETT	Endotracheal Tube

Fig. 5.67 (**a**) Gently attempt to pass the tube 1.5 cm past the transverse (15 cm) line. Do not press the handle downwards. If no resistance is felt, it is likely the epiglottic elevating bar is lifting the epiglottis upwards as designed, allowing the endotracheal tube to pass easily into the trachea. Continue to advance the tube using clinical judgment to determine when intubation has been accomplished. (**b**) Inflate the endotracheal tube cuff and confirm tube position by standard methods (courtesy of LMA™ North America, Inc.)

Intubation with a Fiberoptic Scope

The fiberoptic scope can be passed through a seated LMA Fastrach™ to confirm proper positioning. Alternatively, the fiberoptic scope can be used to pass the endotracheal tube into the trachea. Make sure the tip of the fiberoptic scope does not pass the epiglottic elevating bar as the scope may be damaged (Fig. 5.71).

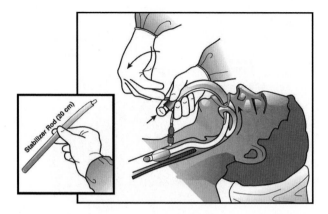

Fig. 5.68 Take the connector off of the endotracheal tube. Deflate the cuff of the LMA Fastrach™. Swing the mask out of the pharynx into the oral cavity, applying counterpressure to the endotracheal tube with a finger prior to insertion of a stabilizer rod (courtesy of LMA™ North America, Inc.)

Troubleshooting Problems Associated with LMA Fastrach™ Intubation

The LMA™ Instruction Manual addresses many of the problems encountered when using the Fastrach™ to guide blind intubation. Some of these problems include the following:

1. Downfolded epiglottis or tube impaction
2. Fastrach™ too small or too large
3. Inadequate anesthesia or muscle relaxation

Figure 5.72 summarizes an approach to deal with problems associated with blind LMA Fastrach™ intubation.

Insertion of Ambu® Mask Airways

Insertion instructions for the Ambu® AuraStraight™ Single Use LMA are presented as representative of Ambu's® line of products.[15] An instruction manual can be obtained for any Ambu® airway at the AMBU.com website.

Preparation

When preparing to use an Ambu® product, first make a visual inspection of the airway looking for cracks, loose parts, blockages, or other damage. Next, test the cuff's integrity by overinflating and totally deflating inspecting the cuff at each extreme for defects and/or leaks. Do not use an airway that is defective in any manner.

Before inserting the airway, deflate the cuff completely so it is flat and non-wrinkled. One can flatten the cuff on a sterile surface as shown in Fig. 5.73. When

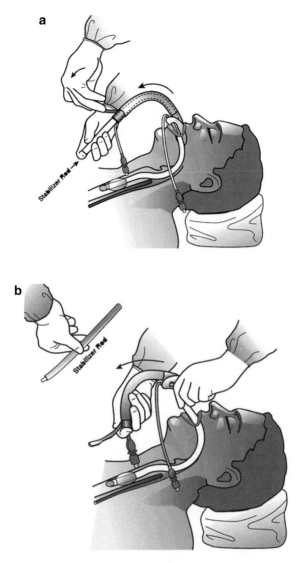

Fig. 5.69 (**a**) When the proximal end of the endotracheal tube is level with the proximal end of the metal tube, insert the LMA™ Stabilizer Rod to keep the endotracheal tube in place. Using the stabilizer rod, slide the LMA Fastrach™ out over the rod until it is clear of the mouth. (**b**) Remove the stabilizer rod and steady the endotracheal tube at the level of the incisors (courtesy of LMA™ North America, Inc.)

the cuff is flattened properly, it will take on a saucer shape. (Some practitioners prefer to use an airway with a mask shape other than the recommended saucer with equal success of insertion.)

To facilitate insertion, a nonanesthetic sterile water-based lubricant should be applied to the distal posterior surface of the cuff.

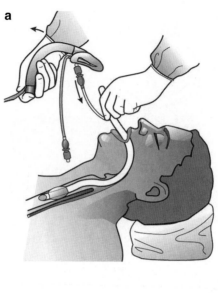

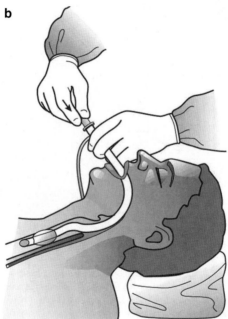

Fig. 5.70 (**a**) Remove the LMA Fastrach™ completely, gently unthreading the inflation line and pilot balloon of the endotracheal tube. (**b**) Replace the endotracheal tube connector. Verify proper endotracheal tube position and ventilate the patient (courtesy of LMA™ North America, Inc.)

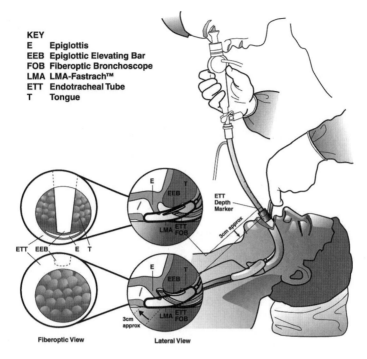

Fig. 5.71 Intubation with fiberoptic endoscope (courtesy of LMA™ North America, Inc.)

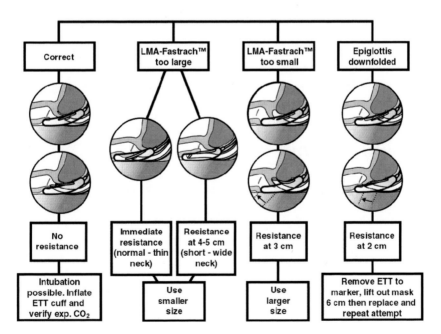

Fig. 5.72 Summary of approach to deal with problems associated with blind LMA Fastrach™ intubation (courtesy of LMA™ North America, Inc.)

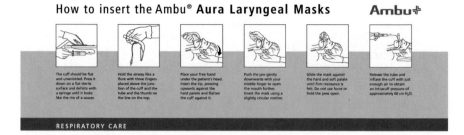

Fig. 5.73 Ambu Insertion Card (courtesy of Ambu)

The Ambu® AuraStraight™ manual[15] states:

The following points are extremely important:

1. Check for correct deflation and lubrication as described.
2. The size of the Ambu® AuraStraight™ must fit the patient. Use the sizing guidelines combined with clinical judgment to select the correct size.
3. Always have a spare Ambu® AuraStraight™ ready for use.
4. Preoxygenate and use standard monitoring procedures.
5. Check that the level of anesthesia (or unconsciousness) is adequate before attempting insertion.
6. The head of the patient should be positioned in an extended, flexed position normally used for intubation ("sniffing position").
7. Never use excessive force (from the Ambu® AuraStraight™ Product Information Manual, with modification[15]).

Consult the product information manual[15] for complete details of Ambu® mask insertion including problems and troubleshooting.

Insertion of the SLIPA™ SGA[16]

The SLIPA™ SGA is anatomically preformed to line the pharynx. The heel of the airway seats in the nasopharynx providing stability. "A unique feature of the SLIPA™ is a hollow chamber which provides a large capacity reservoir for storing regurgitated liquids from the stomach"[16] (Fig. 5.74).

Indications for Use

The SLIPA™ User Guide[16] lists the indications for use of the airway as follow:

1. For use in the unconscious patient

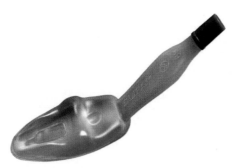

Fig. 5.74 Slipa Airway (courtesy Slipa Medical, Ltd.)

2. For routine and emergency anesthesia in fasted patients for spontaneous breathing and for intermittent positive pressure ventilation
3. For use in fasted patients with esophageal reflux
4. As a routine rescue airway when other SGAs fail
5. For limited mouth opening abilities
6. For fast airway management in cardio-respiratory arrest patients
7. For prehospital airway management when expertise for placement of tracheal tubes is lacking or has failed
8. For use by ambulance personnel and paramedics in prehospital care

Contraindications for Use

The User Manual lists the following contraindications for use of the SLIPA™ airway:

1. Nonfasted patients
2. Infection or anatomical distortion in the pharynx
3. When there is a suspected full stomach
4. When high airway pressures are anticipated above 35 cm H_2O
5. For procedures longer than 3–4 h

Sizes of SLIPA™ Airway

The airway is marketed in six adult sizes from 47 to 57 depending on the patient's height:

1. Size 47: 5′ 0″
2. Size 49: 5′ 3″
3. Size 51: 5′ 6″
4. Size 53: 5′ 8″
5. Size 55: 6′ 0″
6. Size 57: 6′ 3″ (Fig. 5.75)

SLIPA Size (Thyroid Cartilage)	Equivalent LMA Size	Patient Size	Median Height	Height Range
47	3.0	Very Small Female	152cm	145-160cm
49	3.0 – 3.5	Small Female	160cm	152-168 cm
51	3.5 – 4.0	Medium Female	168cm	160-175 cm
53	4.0 – 4.5	Large Female to Small Male	173cm	163-182 cm
55	4.5 – 5.0	Medium Male	182cm	173-193 cm
57	5.0 – 5.5	Large Male	190cm	180-200 cm

- Size number indicates in millimetre the width across the bridge of the particular SLIPA which corresponds to the size of thyroid cartilage.
- Choose size of SLIPA by the patient's height, and/or by the size of their thyroid cartilage.
- Elderly may need one size larger than usual because the tissues are lax.
- Size ranges actually overlap quite significantly.

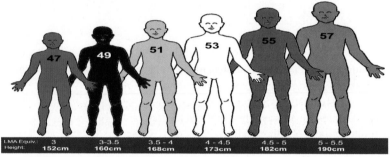

NOTE: If unsure between sizes choose the larger size!

Fig. 5.75 Slipa airway size table (courtesy Slipa Medical, Ltd.)

Preuse Checks

1. Ensure the packaging is not damaged. If so, discard the airway.
2. Examine the SLIPA™ for obvious defects and sharp edges.
3. Ensure a suitable selection of alternative sizes is available.

Preinsertion Preparation

1. Always wear gloves
2. Remove SLIPA™ from the sterile package
3. Apply lubricant to the concave SLIPA™ chamber

Insertion of SLIPA™ Airway

The product's user manual states that the insertion technique of the SLIPA™ airway is not the same as that used for the LMA™. The steps recommended by the manufacturer follow:

1. Induce anesthesia.
2. Place the patient in the "sniff position" (head extended, neck flexed).
3. Have an assistant open the patient's mouth and lift his jaw. The assistant should work from below opening the mouth with his thumbs and lifting the jaw with his index fingers.
4. While the SLIPA is cold and fairly rigid, direct the toe of the airway to the back of the throat at an acute angle with the toe pointing towards the esophagus following the natural curve of the SLIPA™. The tongue may be lifted with the airway using a laryngoscope blade to facilitate insertion.
5. Once the airway slides off the back of the throat and past the teeth, push the device down until the heel lodges in the nasopharynx following the natural curve of the SLIPA™. At this point, the axis of the stem is approximately perpendicular with the axis of the chamber.
6. It is easily felt when the chamber is firmly up against the back of the throat. Push the stem towards the back until firm resistance is felt. The heel in the nasopharynx creates stability that requires no need to tie the device in position (Fig. 5.76).

Consult the SLIPA™ User Guide for a complete description of the airway including troubleshooting recommendations.

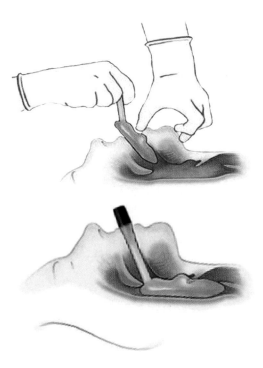

Fig. 5.76 Insertion of Slipa Airway (courtesy Slipa Medical, Ltd.)

Insertion of the King LT(S)-D® Airway[17]

The King LT(S)-D® airway has been selected as representative of extraglottic airways that are seated with their distal tip in the esophagus. (Consult the specific user manual pertaining to airways of similar design for safe and proper insertion instructions. The user manual can be found on the Internet for every manufacturer of extraglottic airway devices.)

The King LT(S)-D® airway offers the following design features:

1. Soft and conforming cuffs that disperse pressure over the largest surface area possible, which stabilizes the airway device at the base of the tongue
2. When properly inserted there is a low incidence of gastric insufflation
3. Ease of insertion, with minimal movement of the head
4. Latex-free
5. Disposable
6. Allows passage of an 18 Fr gastric tube through a separate channel

Sizes

The King LT(S)-D® airway is marketed in five sizes. The appropriate airway size is determined by the patient's height and/or weight (see Table 5.8).

Insertion Technique

The steps for inserting the King LT(S)-D® Airway follow:

1. Hold the airway at the connector with the dominant hand. With the nondominant hand, hold the mouth open and apply chin lift, unless contraindicated by C-spine precautions or patient position. Using a lateral approach, introduce the tip into the corner of the mouth.
2. Advance the tip behind the base of the tongue while rotating the tube back to midline so that the blue orientation line faces the chin of the patient.
3. Without exerting excessive force, advance the tube until the base of the connector is aligned with the teeth or gums.

Table 5.8 King LT(S)-D® airway sizing information[17]

Size	Patient height	Patient weight (kg)
2	35–45 in.	12–25
2.5	41–51 in.	25–35
3	4–5 ft.	
4	5–6 ft.	
5	6-ft.	

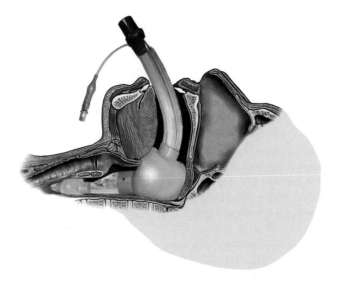

Fig. 5.77 King LT(S)-D® Airway: properly seated position (with permission, King Systems, Noblesville, IN)

4. Inflate the cuffs to 60 cm H_2O or to "just seal" volume (see user manual for suggested volumes).
5. Attach the breathing circuit or resuscitator bag to the airway. While gently bagging the patient to assess ventilation, withdraw the airway until ventilation is easy and free flowing (large tidal volume with minimal airway pressure).
6. If necessary, add additional volume to the cuffs to maximize the seal of the airway (Fig. 5.77).

Modified Insertion Techniques

Even though an early study of 12,000 patients reported a successful insertion rate of 99.8%[18] using the manufacturer's recommended insertion technique, clinicians have suggested modifications to facilitate LMA™ placement. One such modification is to partially inflate the cuff with air before insertion.[19] Another is to start LMA™ insertion with a partially inflated cuff with its breathing grille pointed towards the hard palate. The LMA™ is advanced into the hypopharynx, then twisted 180°[20] (the "Charlottetown twist"). A distinct "pop" is felt when the LMA™ seats itself. Brimacombe offered negative comments on the efficacy and safety of these modifications.[21,22] In a recent study, rotation of the LMA ProSeal™[23] was found to facilitate insertion. Once the cuff was placed in the mouth, the airway was rotated 90° counterclockwise, advanced until resistance was felt, then rotated back into the normal position. Other authors have suggested that the cuff could be molded into shapes at variance with the manufacturer's recommended saucer shape to ease insertion.[24,25] Another popular modification is to displace the tongue with a wooden blade when inserting the LMA™. Aoyama et al. [26] reported that the triple airway maneuver, a combination of head extension, mouth opening, and jaw thrust used on anesthetized/paralyzed patients, resulted in less epiglottic downfolding by the LMA™. These same authors reported that the application of cricoid pressure to anesthetized/paralyzed patients impeded the positioning of and ventilation through the LMA™.[27] Once the practitioner has mastered the manufacturer's suggested insertion technique for any extraglottic airway, modifications may be tried. Modifications must not add a risk to the patient such as trauma to the teeth or other airway structures. Remember, *the manufacturer of the LMA™ has developed and tested insertion techniques that have been used on millions of patients. These techniques have proven to be safe and effective for over 20 years.* The manufacturers of other airways have developed instructions that they too believe are safe and effective for their extraglottic devices.

Use of the GEB (Gum Elastic Bougie) for LMA ProSeal™ Insertion

Howarth et al.[28] first described using a GEB to guide placement of an LMA ProSeal™ in 2002. Subsequent studies primarily by Joseph Brimacombe and colleagues standardized and popularized the technique. His book discusses the topic in detail. The technique "…involves railroading the drain tube along a GEB placed in the proximal esophagus under direct vision"[2] (p. 521). The technique purportedly has six advantages over the standard ProSeal™ insertion techniques[2] (p. 251):

1. It allows the distal cuff to be guided into its correct position in the hypopharynx
2. It minimizes impaction at the back of the mouth
3. Folding over off the cuff cannot occur
4. It is compatible with finger-free insertion
5. It allows unexpected oropharyngeal pathology to be identified
6. It provides information about ease of laryngoscope-guided tracheal intubation (LG-TI)
7. Tests for the position and patency of the drain tube are not necessary

The main disadvantage is the potential for causing trauma with the rigid GEB such as pharyngeal wall perforation.[29] From 2002 to 2005, Brimacombe and others admitted that the potential for trauma by the GEB needed more study and that it be used as a backup technique. Similar techniques using a softer gastric tube,[30] a fiberoptic scope,[31] or a suction catheter,[32] were described documenting successful placement of the LMA ProSeal™ with these adjuncts. A 2004 study by Brimacombe et al.[33] generated comments both supportive and critical. The authors compared the digital insertion technique, the ProSeal™ introducer tool technique, and a two-operator GEB assisted technique and concluded that the "…GEB-guided insertion technique is more frequently successful than the digital or IT [introducer tool] techniques. The authors suggested that the GEB-guided technique may be a useful backup technique for when the digital and IT techniques fail." Matioc and Arndt[34] suggested a modification involving handling of the ProSeal™ preloaded with the GEB to make it a one-operator technique vs. the two-operator technique of Brimacombe. Reier[35] responded negatively to the study and cited concerns with pathologic definitions, interpretation of morbidity statistics, perceived lack of follow-up by the researchers, as well as assertions concerning use of the technique in the "difficult airway" management scenario. Brimacombe et al.[36] responded to all of Reier's comments offering peer-reviewed studies rebutting much of Reier's criticism. None-the-less, all concerned agreed in 2004 that further research was needed to establish the safety of the GEB-guided ProSeal™ insertion technique. In support of the technique, Brimacombe et al.[36] reported use of the GEB-guided technique in more than 6,000 patients "...with a first-time insertion failure rate of 0.07%" and a "...first-time ventilation failure rate of 0.5%." Ventilation failure was treated with more anesthesia/muscle relaxants (patients with laryngospasm), repositioning the airway or adjusting the amount of air in the cuff (by jaw thrust maneuvers, reinsertion of the airway, taking air out of the cuff, or using a smaller airway) and the overall ventilation failure rate was reduced to 0.08%. They reported no cases of esophageal or pharyngeal injury.[36]

Since 2004, many authors have studied the GEB-guided insertion technique applied to LMA ProSeal™. Following is a list of studies and reports documenting a wide variety of variables and observations that have been associated with the technique:

1. Brimacombe et al.[37] case report of the technique used to establish an airway in an adult patient with occult tonsillar hypertrophy.
2. Brimacombe and Keller.[38] GEB-guided insertion compared to the ProSeal™ Introducer Tool guided insertion in 100 adult patients who had failed digital placement of the ProSeal™. Researchers reported a higher success rate and faster insertion time with the GEB-guided group compared to the Introducer Tool guided group.
3. Brimacombe and Keller.[39] GEB-guided rapid sequence induction. The ProSeal™ was left in for the case. The stomach was suctioned and the cuff pressure and seal were deemed sufficient to protect the trachea.
4. Lopez-Gil et al.[40] In a study of 120 children aged 1–16 years weighing between 10 and 50 kg, the authors concluded that the group who had an LMA ProSeal™ inserted with GEB-guidance had a higher first attempt success rate when compared to a group who had the ProSeal™ inserted with the standard digital technique. The insertion time for the ProSeal™ group was slightly longer (37. vs. 32 s). There was no difference in the efficacy of the seal, the ease of gastric tube placement, hemodynamic responses, blood staining ,or postoperative airway morbidity.
5. Hohlrieder et al.[41] Laryngoscope-guided GEB-guided ProSeal™ insertion was compared to laryngoscope-guided tracheal intubation in a group of first-month anesthesia residents after brief manikin-only training. The authors concluded "...that laryngoscope-guided, GEB-guided insertion of the ProSeal LMA is

superior to conventional laryngoscope-guided tracheal intubation for airway management in terms of insertion after brief manikin-only training. The guided ProSeal technique has potential for cardiopulmonary resuscitation by novices when conventional intubation fails."

6. Eschertzhuber et al.[42] In a simulated "difficult airway" scenario, the authors concluded that GEB-guided ProSeal™ insertion was more frequently successful than either digital or introducer tool-assisted insertion in adult female patients. Another study reported that GEB-guided ProSeal™ insertion was the "best" backup technique if either the digital or IT techniques failed.[43]

7. El Beheiry et al.[44] Fiberoptic examination revealed that a group of adult patients in whom a ProSeal™ was inserted with a GEB-guided technique had better esophageal and laryngeal alignment of the airway's ports compared to a group in which an introducer tool was used to guide insertion. Insertion time was longer for the GEB-guided group (47.8s vs. 29.7s).

8. Taneja et al.[45] The authors concluded that ProSeal™ insertion was more successful, faster, more accurately positioned, and associated with less airway trauma when the GEB-guided technique was used compared to insertion with an introducer tool or digitally-guided.

Laryngoscope-Guided, GEB-Guided LMA ProSeal™ Insertion Technique[2] (p. 521)

The insertion technique described in Brimacombe's textbook[2] is summarized as follows:

1. The ProSeal™ drain tube is primed with a lubricated GEB otherwise known as an Eschmann™ (Smiths Medical, Keene, NH) Tracheal Tube Introducer. [El-Orbany et al.[46] point out that the Eschmann™ Introducer is neither a true bougie, nor is it made of gum elastic material. In fact, the introducer is now marketed as the Portex® Venn Tracheal Tube Introducer (Smiths Medical, Keene, NH). In spite of their scholarly admonition, virtually every writer and researcher refers to the Eschmann™ Introducer as a GEB. The author of this chapter offers his apology to El-Orbany et al. and has chosen to follow the popular vernacular.] The angled end of the bougie protrudes out of the proximal port of the airway and should be of adequate length for an assistant to grip. The straight end of the bougie protrudes from the distal end of the drain tube. It is this straight end of the bougie that is guided into the esophagus. Before beginning the insertion sequence make sure the cuff is deflated and lubricated (Fig. 5.78).

2. Perform "gentle" laryngoscopy (the vocal cords do not have to be exposed). Perform a visual inspection of the upper airway to assess ease of laryngotracheal intubation if necessary.

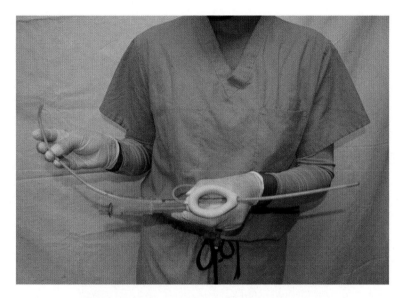

Fig. 5.78 The LMA ProSeal™ Primed with an Eschmann™ Gum Elastic Bougie (GEB) (the bougie is marketed by Smiths Medical, Keene, NH. The current name of the device is the Portex® Venn Tracheal Tube Introducer)

3. Place the straight distal end of the Eschmann™ bougie 5–10 cm into the esophagus while the assistant holds the angled proximal end and the ProSeal™.
4. The laryngoscope is carefully removed.
5. The operator railroads the ProSeal™ into place. The airway is passed in the midline of the tongue. An assistant holds the proximal end of the Eschmann™ bougie to insure that it is not pushed into the esophagus.
6. Inflate the cuff.
7. Secure the ProSeal™ to the patients face.
8. Remove the GEB. Hold the airway in place to prevent dislodgement.
9. Ventilate the patient. Verify correct placement using clinical observations. A fiberoptic endoscope may be used to check both mask and distal drain tube placement.

Two variations to the technique are offered by Brimacombe.[2] First, the laryngoscope can be kept in place during insertion of the ProSeal™. One might detect epiglottic downfolding with the scope in place. Secondly, if a GEB has been placed in the esophagus in a failed intubation attempt, leave it there and pass a lubricated ProSeal™ over the GEB (Figs. 5.79–5.82).

Critics have commented that the GEB-guided LMA ProSeal™ insertion technique may be too hazardous to oral, tracheal, and esophageal tissue because of the rigid nature of the Eschmann™ bougie. Others have commented that it adds an

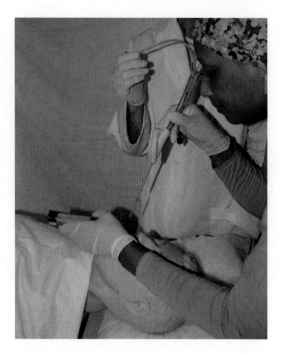

Fig. 5.79 After gentle laryngoscopy, pass the straight distal end of the Eschmann™ bougie 5–10 cm into the esophagus. An assistant stabilizes the airway and holds the proximal end of the bougie. Gently remove the laryngoscope

unnecessary intermediate step to establishing a secure airway. They opine that if one is performing laryngoscopy as the first step to guide the GEB into the esophagus, why not intubate the trachea at that point? Why bother with the GEB and the LMA™? However, the investigators who have studied the technique and authors who have reported anecdotal cases where it has proven successful in difficult airway situations assert that GEB-guided LMA ProSeal™ insertion has proven itself to be an acceptable option available to the airway management practitioner trained in its safe use. It has applications in routine as well as difficult airway scenarios. All techniques have problems and complications associated with their application in clinical practice. All airway management techniques should be learned under the guidance of a skilled and experienced teacher. Never use excessive force when inserting an instrument or manipulating the structures of the airway. Brimacombe states in his papers that the Eschmann™ bougie may not prove to be the best designed stenting device for the technique. However, at this time, no other bougie or exchange catheter has been studied as thoroughly as the Eschmann™. In a letter to the editor, Micaglio et al.[47] suggested using a gastric tube instead of the rigid bougie and a Glidescope™ video laryngoscope instead of a standard laryngoscope, equipment they suggested might cause less mouth (airway) trauma. Future research may define a more optimal stent and other modifications to the technique to enhance safety.

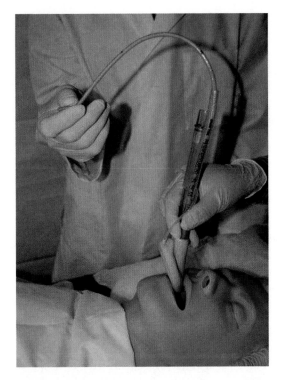

Fig. 5.80 Place the mask of the ProSeal™ into the midline of the mouth

Removing the Extraglottic Airway

Extraglottic airways of the LMA™ configuration are well-tolerated by patients emerging from anesthesia. Keep the intracuff pressure 60 cm H_2O or less. Allow the patients to breath spontaneously. Keep all monitors on the patient to assure that the vital signs are stable, the oxyhemoglobin saturation is optimal (usually above 98%), and the end-tidal CO_2 is normal. Document that all neuromuscular drugs are reversed and that the patient's strength has returned to baseline. Leave the cuff inflated, avoid pharyngeal or tracheal suctioning, and do not disturb the patient by moving him. Observe for the return of airway reflexes. Allow the patient to wake-up and observe his ability to follow commands. Suction the pharynx if necessary. Deflate the cuff and remove the airway when the patient opens his mouth on command. Nunez[48] reported that removal of the LMA™ in accordance with the manufacturer's recommendations resulted in fewer complications than when the device was removed with the patient still anesthetized. Whatever removal strategy one employs, be ready to intervene immediately if the patient experiences any postremoval problems.

For airways designed with a subglottic esophageal tip, one should follow the manufacturer's recommendations when removing the device.

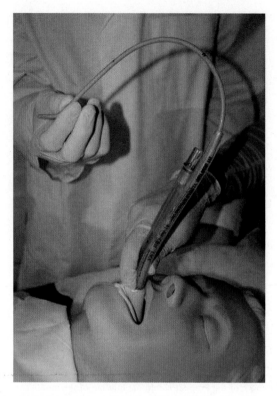

Fig. 5.81 Insert the ProSeal™ using the digital insertion technique. An assistant holds the proximal end of the Eschmann™ bougie so it is not passed further into the esophagus

Further Comments on LMA™ Size

Three strategies can be used to select an appropriately sized LMA™. First is to use the manufacturers' recommendation based on the patient's weight (see Table 5.2). Second, a formula such as the one suggested by Kagawa and Obara[49] can be used: LMA size = Square root of (patient weight (kg)/5).

Finally, for adult patients, gender-based strategies recommend a size 3 airway for females and a size 4 for males[50] or size 4 for females and size 5 for males[51,52] without regard to the patient's weight.

Ease of LMA™ Insertion and Airway Grading Systems

In 1995 McCrory and Moriarty[53] reported "…that the Mallampati classification indicates difficulty not only in tracheal intubation but also in achieving an adequate airway with the LMA." By contrast, a more recent metaanalysis of the literature

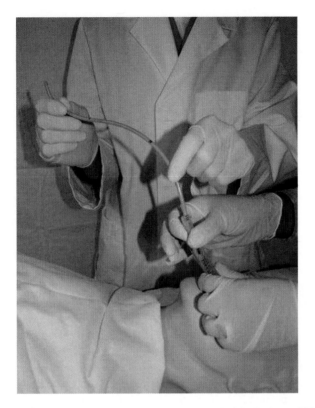

Fig. 5.82 Seat the ProSeal™. An assistant holds the distal end of the Eschmann™ bougie so it is not passed further into the esophagus

conducted by Brimacombe[2] (p. 314) and reported in 2005 found that there is no correlation between the Mallampati score or the Cormack and Lehane score and ease of LMA™ insertion.

Comparison of Methods to Assess LMA™ Airway Sealing Pressures

The maximum amount of air that should be inflated into the cuff of an LMA™ airway depends on the size of the airway. The manufacturer's recommendations are reported in Table 5.9.

One should inject enough air to produce a cuff seal of 20 cm H_2O. At this cuff pressure, the mucosal pressure exerted by the airway on surrounding tissues ranges between 2 and 20 cm H_2O for all LMA airways except for the LMA Fastrach™.[54–57] The mucosal pressure exerted by the Fastrach™ "…exceeded [the] capillary perfusion pressure" and the authors recommended removing the Fastrach™ after intubation.[58]

Table 5.9 Airway size vs. maximal volume of air inflated
into cuff to achieve a 60 cm H_2O intracuff pressure

Airway size	Maximum cuff inflation volume (ml)
1	4
1½	7
2	10
2½	14
3	20
4	30
5	40
6	50

Source: Courtesy of LMA™ North America, San Diego, CA

The Fastrach™ airway should not be used as a primary extraglottic device. The same authors reported that in anesthetized patients, the use of muscle relaxants or the modality of ventilation did not affect pharyngeal mucosal pressure,[59] nor did head flexion, extension, or rotation.[60] Finally, they reported that the most efficient cuff seal and the best fiberoptic view through the LMA™ were achieved with the cuff inflated with volumes below the maximum recommended volume.[61, 62]

Many clinical tests are used to assess the efficiency of the airway seal when an LMA™ is positioned. One should choose an appropriately sized airway and fill the cuff with enough air to achieve a seal at around 20 cm H_2O. Keller et al.[63] compared four tests to assess the airway seal as follows: (1) detection of audible noise by listening over the mouth; (2) capnography: detection of CO_2 by placing a sampling tube 5 cm inside the mouth alongside the LMA™; (3) manometric stability: observing the "…aneroid manometer dial as the pressure from the breathing system [is] increased and noting the airway pressure at which the dial reached stability"; (4) auscultation: "…detection of an audible noise using a stethoscope placed just lateral to the thyroid cartilage." They reported a mean airway sealing pressure ranging between 19.5 and 21.3 cm H_2O. All of the tests were deemed to be excellent for clinical purposes. These tests should be used to verify that the LMA™ is inflated to a safe and effective volume. In conclusion, the LMA™ cuff should be inflated with a volume below the maximum recommended volume to achieve a seal at 20 cm H_2O. Other manufacturers of extraglottic devices make recommendations concerning maximum cuff inflation volumes and cuff pressures. For example, Ambu® recommends inflation volumes the same as those recommended by LMA™ to achieve a cuff pressure of 60 cm H_2O.[15] Consult the insertion instructions of each manufacturer's airway before use.

LMA™ and Modalities of Ventilation

Large clinical studies from 1993 onward reported the successful and safe use of the LMA™ to manage the airways of anesthetized patients who received positive pressure ventilation. For example, the classic study of Verghese and Brimacombe[18] reported on 11,910 patients who were managed with an LMA™. Intraabdominal surgical procedures were undertaken on 2,222 of these patients and 5,240 received positive pressure ventilation (PPV). The incidence of experiencing a critical airway event was 0.21% for patients receiving PPV vs. 0.11% for those breathing spontaneously (not statistically different). Only one case of aspiration was reported. Brimacombe[2] (p. 246) reported that analysis of a metapopulation composed of 30,041 patients from nine large studies suggested that PPV with the LMA was safe and effective. Besides positive pressure ventilation, other modalities of ventilation have been demonstrated to be safe. These include: spontaneous[2] (pp. 244–245), PEEP,[64] pressure support ventilation,[65,66] and high-frequency ventilation.[67,68] Pediatric patients have been successfully ventilated with positive pressure.[69,70] The authors of these studies warned to keep the peak positive pressure from 10 to 18 cm H_2O and to watch for signs of abdominal distension.

   In summary, the literature supports the claim that positive pressure ventilation can be used safely when the patient's airway is maintained with an extraglottic airway device such as the LMA™. This contention applies whether or not neuro-muscular blocking drugs are administered. In practice, *the LMA™ can be used when it would be appropriate to use a face mask.* The manufacturers of extraglottic airways recommend that the level of positive pressure should not exceed 20 cm H_2O, with the exception of the ProSeal™ for which a peak inspiratory pressure of 30 cm H_2O is endorsed. This pressure should not be exceeded no matter which modality of ventilation is utilized.

Use of the LMA™ with Pediatric Patients

Extraglottic airway devices have been used successfully to manage patients of all ages including neonates. The airways are most frequently used by anesthetists caring for surgical patients. The airways have found utility managing children with difficult airways as well as those undergoing resuscitation. All adult applications apply to children.

Insertion Techniques for Pediatric Patients

The standard insertion techniques recommended for adults are also applicable to children including the midline and lateral approaches and the thumb insertion technique[2] (p. 365) Dr. Brain[71] reconfirmed that the standard technique described for adults is applicable to children. He stressed the need to maintain "…firm flexion of the neck with head extension by the nondominant hand," a maneuver that opens the space behind the larynx. He also wrote that "…the inserting finger must imitate the action of the tongue, which requires the person doing the insertion to point his or her finger toward his or her own umbilicus during the whole insertion maneuver.

This means the direction of the applied pressure is different from the direction in which the mask moves, a point rarely appreciated."

Clinicians have presented alternative insertion strategies including using a Mac #2 laryngoscope blade and inserting the LMA™ under direct vision,[72] applying a "rotary method" if blind insertion was difficult,[73] or using a straight laryngoscope blade to assist insertion.[74]

Removal of the LMA™ in Pediatric Patients

Controversy exists as to when the LMA™ should be removed from children emerging from general anesthesia. Some have reported fewer complications when the airway was removed with the children in a deeper plane of anesthesia[75] while others have advised allowing the airway to remain in place until spontaneously ejected by the patient.[76] Samarkand[77] concluded that "...there was no difference in the incidence of airway complications whether the LMA was removed in the anesthetized or the awake child."

Whether one removes the LMA™ with the child awake or at a deeper level of anesthesia, depends on many variables such as the type of surgery undertaken, whether or not regional anesthetics were used to control postoperative pain, the patient's risk of regurgitation and aspiration after airway removal, the experience of the airway manager, and the preexisting anatomy of the child's airway to name a few. Brimacombe[2] (p. 370) offered thoughtful advice in this regard. He suggested keeping the cuff inflated during removal to allow for the "...maintenance of an effective seal up until the instant of removal." He claimed more secretions could be swept from the mouth if the cuff remained inflated. Finally, he wrote: "The end point for awake removal in older children is mouth opening to command, but in small children is spontaneous mouth opening (usually the first cry or yawn). Deep removal should be in the lateral position. Postremoval management is similar to adults."

Use of the LMA™ to Manage Patients with Congenital Airway Anomalies

Many congenital syndromes are associated with abnormal airway anatomy. While no device or technique is guaranteed to be effective, the LMA™ has been used to manage the airways of children with many different types of congenital anomalies. These include the following: Freeman–Sheldon syndrome,[78] Pierre–Robin syndrome,[79,80] Schwartz–Jampel syndrome,[81] Beckwith–Wiedemann syndrome,[82] and laryngo-tracheo-esophageal clefts[83] to name a few. Muraika et al.[84] reported a case of airway rescue involving the fiberoptically-guided tracheal intubation via an LMA™ in a 3-year-old with Treacher–Collins syndrome. For a complete list of

LMA™ use in pediatric patients with coexisting diseases, including congenital syndromes, see Brimacombe[2] (pp. 372–373).

LMA™ and Neonatal Resuscitation

Paterson et al.[85] evaluated the use of the LMA™ in a prospective study of 21 neonates who underwent resuscitation in the delivery room. The LMA™ was inserted successfully in every newborn and PPV was quickly established. A size 1 LMA™ was used for all patients. All of the LMA's™ were successfully inserted on the first attempt in an average of 8.6 s. The investigators recommended that further investigation was needed to more clearly define the role of the LMA™ in neonatal resuscitation. Other studies have supported the use of the LMA™ to secure the airway during neonatal resuscitation. Brimacombe and Berry[86] recommended that the LMA™ should receive serious consideration for inclusion in neonatal resuscitation protocols. This recommendation was seconded by Arkoosh[87] in a 2001 American Society of Anesthesiologists Refresher Course Lecture. The recommendation should be considered seriously by clinicians who are tasked with the responsibility of neonatal resuscitation.

Diagnostic Fiberoptic Bronchoscopy with LMA™ Assistance

Diagnostic fiberoptic bronchoscopic examination to evaluate conditions such as stridor or pulmonary infiltrate is common in pediatric hospitals. Traditionally, airway management included: (1) fiberoptic examination with no supportive airway intervention, (2) examination through a modified facemask that allowed passage of the bronchoscope, or (3) examination through an endotracheal tube. Many clinicians now use the LMA™ to facilitate diagnostic fiberoptic examinations in pediatric patients.[88–92]

Use of the LMA™ in Pediatric Surgical Patients with Upper Respiratory Tract Infections (URI's) and Mild Bronchopulmonary Dysplasia (BPD)

Tait et al.[93] compared the LMA™ to the endotracheal tube as the method of airway management in 82 patients ranging from age 3 months to 16 years. All children had active URI's at the time of surgery. No airway surgeries were performed. No statistically significant differences were found between groups with respect to the incidence of coughing, laryngospasm, breath holding, arrhythmias, excitement, or excessive secretions. There was a significantly greater incidence of mild broncho-spasm and oxyhemoglobin desaturation below 90% during placement of an endo-tracheal tube. At least one laryngospasm was noted in each group. All airway complications were easily managed. The authors concluded that if surgery had to be performed on patients with a URI, the LMA™ "...provides a suitable alterna-tive to the endotracheal tube."

Von Ungern–Sternberg et al.[94] studied the use of the LMA™ in two groups of pediatric patients who underwent different types of surgical procedures including ENT. The two groups were defined as one consisting of children who had experi-enced a recent URI (within 2 weeks preceding surgery) and the other consisting of children who had not had a recent URI (not within the 2 weeks preceding surgery) based on a questionnaire completed by parents. They concluded that the incidence of laryngospasm, coughing, and oxygen desaturation was higher in the group who had experienced a URI within the 2 weeks preceding surgery. The incidence was also higher in younger children and those undergoing ENT surgery. No severe sequelae resulted from the complications. In their discussion section, the authors stated that a subgroup (those who had not had a URI within 2–4 weeks of surgery) had a similar outcome to the group whose surgery was undertaken at the 2 week mark. They concluded that waiting 2 weeks after URI to have surgery would decrease the risk of adverse respiratory events. Critics of the study stated in a letter: "The specific question that remains unanswered is: does postponing anesthesia by 2 weeks after a URI result in fewer airway-related complications?"[95] The critics were unconvinced that the recommended 2 week waiting period had been established as the "optimum" waiting period. They did concede that: "From a clinical standpoint, we support the authors' view that children who have not had a URI within the past few weeks may be safely anesthetized despite the perhaps unavoidably increased risk." The waiting period controversy remains but the literature supports the use of the LMA™ in children who have had a recent URI, especially when comparing it to the endotracheal tube to secure the airway. *No matter which airway technique or device is used, children who have had a recent URI do have an increased incidence of respiratory problems in the perioperative period compared to healthy children. Expect complications and be prepared to treat them.*

With respect to children with mild bronchopulmonary dysplasia, Ferrari and Goudsouzain[96] compared the use of LMA™ to the endotracheal tube in a study of 27 premature patients undergoing eye surgery. They found no statistically significant differences with respect to airway complications in the intraoperative period. Patients in the LMA™ group opened their eyes and were discharged from the recovery room sooner than those in the endotracheal tube group. Three children in the endotracheal tube group had transient postoperative respiratory complica-tions. They concluded that children with mild BPD could be managed with an LMA™ during minor surgical procedures. Mayhew and Dalmeida[97] in a letter questioned the safety of using an LMA™ to manage patients with BPD. In reply, Ferrari and Goudsouzain[98] maintained that their study had presented their unique experience of using the LMA™ to manage children with BPD who had undergone minor surgical procedures. They had not claimed to have established conclusively the superiority of the LMA™ over other airway management techniques when dealing with children with BPD. Future comparisons will be undertaken.

The Learning Curve for Use of the LMA™ on Pediatric Patients

Lopez-Gil et al.[99] studied 8 third year anesthesiology residents who had no prior experience using the LMA™. Each resident was observed performing 75 LMA™ insertions on pediatric patients using the standard insertion technique. The overall rate of experiencing problems with insertion declined from 62 to 2% comparing the first 15-case epoch to the last. The residents with the highest insertion problem rates after 60 insertions all recorded rates less than 10%. The authors concluded: "Pediatric anesthesiologists with problem rates greater than 10% should determine if they are using the device suboptimally."

Long-Term Use of the LMA™ on Pediatric Patients

The LMA™ has been reported to have been used for long-term airway management in a few case reports. For example, Ames et al.[100] reported managing the airway of a 3-week-old infant for 8 days following surgery. Examination of the patient's oropharynx after removal found no apparent injury associated with the long-term use of the LMA™. Others reported LMA™ use from 4 to 6 days. Obviously, further study into the long-term use of the LMA™ to manage pediatric patients' airways is necessary to establish efficacy and safety of the practice.

The Use of the LMA ProSeal™ on Pediatric Patients

Much of the literature dealing with pediatric patients up to 2005 examined use of the LMA Classic™. Now, manufactures offer a wide variety of extraglottic devices in sizes down to 1. The LMA ProSeal™ is offered in sizes 1.5–5. This range of sizes covers patients of just about every weight category from the neonate to the obese adult. Since the ProSeal™ has been so extensively studied in recent years a comment on its use in pediatric patients is in order.

Noting that the ProSeal™ in sizes 1.5, 2, and 2.5 does not have a rear cuff, Shimbori et al.[101] compared the ease of insertion and the sealing pressures in pediatric ProSeal™ airways to LMA Classic™ airways. They concluded that in children ranging from 12 to 72 months (average age about 40 months), the two airways had similar success with respect to ease of insertion and airway sealing pressures (18–19 cm H_2O). Another study of 240 patients ranging in age from 1 to

16 years found that the ease of insertion, the frequency of mucosal trauma, and the fiberoptically confirmed that the position of the ProSeal™ and Classic™ were similar.[102] The cuff leak pressure was higher and gastric insufflation was lower in the ProSeal™ group. The investigators found that a gastric tube could be passed easily if the ProSeal™ was seated properly. Goldman et al.[103] studied two groups of pediatric patients without lung disease whose airways were managed with a ProSeal™. Both groups received pressure controlled ventilation. PEEP was applied to one of the groups. After 60 min of ventilation, the PEEP group had a significantly higher PaO_2. They concluded that the application of PEEP improved gas exchange. Goldman and Jakob[104] conducted a randomized crossover comparison of the size 2.5 LMA ProSeal™ with the LMA Classic™ on a group of pediatric patients (age 7.7 ± 2 year). They attempted to pass a gastric tube when the ProSeal™ was in place. Ease of insertion of both devices was similar. They concluded that the quality of the initial airway and the fiberoptically verified position were better for the ProSeal™. They also found that the airway leak pressure with various head positions was higher for the ProSeal™. Air entry into the stomach occurred with the Classic™ but not the ProSeal™. Finally, maximum airway volumes were higher for the ProSeal™. They concluded that the ProSeal™ showed some advantages compared to the Classic™ in their crossover study. They warned that the ProSeal™ could cause airway obstruction and its users had to be ready to substitute that model with a Classic™ or an endotracheal tube. The same investigators reported similar favorable results for the 1½ LMA ProSeal™ in another study comparing it to the Classic™ of similar size.[105] Finally, Micaglio and Parotto[106] reported using a 1 LMA ProSeal™ (size not available in USA) to establish the airway in 7 neonates who required PPV in the delivery room. The babies' weight averaged 3,455 g. Insertion was easy and successful on the first attempt. Insertion required use of the introducer tool because the patient's mouths were too small to allow for digital insertion.

In summary, the literature supports the efficacy of using the LMA ProSeal™ in pediatric patients. Safety issues such as complications and airway trauma will be addressed when the ProSeal™ is compared with other airway devices in future studies.

Innovative Uses of the LMA™

When the LMA™ was first marketed, the manufacturer's recommendation was that it be used as an alternate to the face mask, not as a replacement for the endotracheal tube. From the beginning, it was recognized that the LMA™ might have other applications. For example, it proved to be an effective rescue device when tracheal intubation failed. Now the LMA™ and airways of other manufacturers are available in many models with features that allow them to be used in a variety of cases that were formally managed with an endotracheal tube. Table 5.10 lists a few of the innovative uses that have been reported using the LMA™.

Table 5.10 Innovative and special uses of the LMA™

Oral and maxillofacial surgery[107]
Neurosurgery[108–110]
Tonsillectomy
Ventilation through a tracheotomy stoma[111]
Route for tracheal drug administration[112]
Dental surgery
Management of laryngeal polyposis[113]
Gastroscopy[114,115]
Transesophageal echocardiography examination[116]
Obstetrics (Elective Caesarian Section)[117]

Each application has associated complications and failures. For example, during tonsillectomy, Kanniah[118] noted that in addition to laryngeal spasm and airway obstruction from the throat gag, in one case, the surgeon severed the LMA™'s pilot tube with the snare used to remove the tonsil, leading to cuff failure. Parenthetically, a 2007 national survey of British anesthesiologists[119] disclosed that for patients undergoing tonsillectomy, the tracheal tube was the most frequently used airway across all age groups: 87% less than 3 year olds; 79% for 3–16 year; 73% for adults. An LMA™ was used to manage the remainder of patients, ranging from 13 to 27% depending on the patient's age. The incidence of LMA™ use to manage tonsillectomy patients in the United States is not known. Many other innovative uses of the LMA™ are reported by Brimacombe.[2] When evaluating a new application for the LMA™, carefully research the most recent literature and know the complications and problems associated with that application.

Patient Position

The LMA™ has been used with patients in the sitting, lateral, lithotomy, head-down Trendelenburg, reverse Trendelenburg, jack-knife, and prone positions.

Prone Position

The LMA™ has been used to establish an emergency airway with patients in the prone position. Brimacombe and Keller[120] reported a GEB-guided LMA ProSeal™ insertion in a 58-year-old man positioned prone. Dingeman et al.[121] reported placement of a #3-LMA™ in a 5-year-old girl undergoing a neurosurgical procedure in the prone position. In the nonemergent scenario, two studies presented case series of patients' whose anesthesia was induced in the prone position. After induction, an LMA ProSeal™ was inserted to secure the airway. The first[122] was an audit of 73 patients undergoing ambulatory surgery in the prone position. The patients were positioned in the prone position with a soft ring placed under the head. They faced either left or right. A description of the insertion technique follows: "After loss of consciousness, the head ring was removed and the face mask was applied firmly, allowing manual ventilation of the lungs with 100% oxygen. Then, with the anesthesiologist's nondominant hand placed on the patient's forehead that was turned slightly to the side and the assistant opening the mouth by holding the tip of the patient's chin, the LMA was inserted. As the LMA passed the incisors, the patient's chin was released, allowing the tongue to fall forwards, thereby opening up the posterior oropharyngeal space for the LMA. After inflation of the cuff of the LMA, the patient's head was carefully laid to the left or right onto the head ring." During surgery the patients breathed spontaneously. The investigators reported one case of laryngospasm treated with the intravenous administration of more anesthetic drug and four cases of LMA™ malpositioning, three of which were corrected with simple adjustments, with one requiring the anesthesiologist to hold the LMA™ during the procedure. No serious complications were reported. In the other study, Brimacombe et al.[123] reported findings after a retrospective audit of 245 patients who had undergone LMA ProSeal™ insertion in the prone position after induction of anesthesia. The patients were ventilated with volume controlled ventilation. ProSeal™ insertion was accomplished with digital insertion in 237 patients and the GEB was used to guide insertion in 8 patients. Three patients experienced partial obstruction which was easily corrected. None of the patients experienced "… hypoxia, hypercapnia, displacement, regurgitation, gastric insufflation, or airway reflex activation." The investigators concluded that insertion of an LMA ProSeal™ in an anesthetized patient in the prone position was a feasible option.

Lateral Position

Brimacombe[2] (p. 249) reported that 2–4% of LMA™ cases are in patients in the lateral position. Many of these patients were induced in the supine position then turned. Three studies support various airway management techniques with the anesthetized patient already positioned laterally. McCaul et al.[124] demonstrated that the success of LMA™ (unspecified model) placement was higher than success of laryngoscopic endotracheal intubation (96 vs. 79%). Insertion time of the LMA™ was shorter than endotracheal intubation time. Dimitriou et al.[125] demonstrated that flexible lightwand-guided endotracheal intubation through an LMA Fastrach™ (Intubating LMA™) was equally successful for patients in the left lateral, right lateral, and supine positions. On the first attempt, between 90 and 96% of patients were intubated. All were intubated by the third attempt after adjustments were made, most consisting of maneuvering of the ILMA handle. Finally, Komatsu et al.[126] reported a 96% success rate of blind intubation through the Intubating LMA™ in patients placed in either the left or right lateral positions, the same as for patients in the supine position. All of these reports support the contention that the LMA™ can be used in anesthetized patients in the lateral position as well as a rescue device should mask ventilation or endotracheal intubation prove unsuccessful.

LMA™ Oropharyngeal Leak Pressure (OLP) and Head Position

Brimacombe[2] (p. 141) summarized the data available up to 2005 and reported that LMA ProSeal™ oropharyngeal leak pressure was increased with neck flexion and decreased with neck extension. He reported that the OLP increased slightly with rotation. Two more recent studies[127,128] supported the flexion and extension findings but one[128] showed a slight decrease in OLP with rotation. The same study showed that OLP was lower for the LMA ProSeal™ than for the CobraPLA (Engineered Medical Systems) or the LTS (laryngeal tube suction, VBM, Medizintechnid, Germany) with the patient's neck extended.

Adjunctive Equipment to Aid Endotracheal Intubation Through the Extraglottic Airway

The most common adjunct to assist endotracheal intubation through an extraglottic airway is the fiberoptic endoscope. Any extraglottic airway can be used as a guide to fiberoptic directed intubation. Many studies have demonstrated the use of the fiberoptic scope with LMA™ products. The most dedicated LMA™ product is the LMA Fastrach™. However, other airways such as the air-Q Laryngeal Mask (Cookgas®) are specifically designed to facilitate endotracheal intubation. When selecting which extraglottic airway one plans to use to facilitate intubation, consider its design. Does it have epiglottic bars or an epiglottic elevator? What rescue equipment needs to be on hand? What size endotracheal tube will fit through the airway? Is the tube long enough to remove the airway after intubation? Does intubation require special equipment such as endotracheal tubes or a stabilizer bar? (Both are available with the LMA Fastrach™). If intubation requires a longer tube, consider using a Mallinckrodt MLT® tube (Covidien-Nellcor, Boulder, CO). These microlaryngeal tubes are longer than normal endotracheal tubes. The extraglottic airway can be withdrawn over the longer tube then the tube can be cut to proper length.

Extraglottic Airways and the "Difficult Airway"

The "difficult airway" has many definitions. It is not simply an anatomic description. Usually a "difficult airway" involves trouble with one or both of two standard airway management maneuvers: facemask ventilation and/or endotracheal intubation guided with the rigid laryngoscope. Definitions of the "difficult airway" address cause, degree, and clinical endpoint. Dealing with the "difficult airway" is the paramount demand made on the airway manager. The "difficult airway" is further defined by applying one of two classifications: anticipated or unanticipated. The "difficult airway" can present at one extreme described as: "cannot ventilate/ cannot intubate." More commonly it presents with lesser degrees of acuity. For clinical purposes, the "difficult airway" can be described as one in which two man mask ventilation is troublesome and/or endotracheal intubation guided by the rigid laryngoscope has failed in 2–3 attempts by a skilled airway manager. The "difficult airway" is addressed in detail in Chap. 9. The remainder of this section will consider the specific role(s) of extraglottic airway devices in the management of the "difficult airway."

In order to offer its members guidance in dealing with the "difficult airway," the American Society of Anesthesiologists published its first Difficult Airway Algorithm in 1991. Updates were made in 1993 and 2003.[129] In 1996 Benumof[130] suggested five places where the LMA could be added to the Algorithm. Other publications had documented how the LMA had been used to manage many different types of airway emergencies and difficulties.[131] Also, successful LMA Fastrach™ guided endotracheal intubation in anticipated and unanticipated difficult airway scenarios had been documented in the literature.[132–135] In the 2003 edition of the Algorithm, the Combitube®(Covidien) received mention along with the LMA (Fig. 5.83). ASA Refresher Course Lectures in 2003[136] and 2006[137] highlighted the LMA's place on the Algorithm. Many other extraglottic airway devices have been used successfully to manage the "difficult airway." These include the LMA ProSeal,[138–140] LMA Supreme™,[141] Combitube® (Covidien),[142] the Laryngeal Tube (Marketed in USA as the King LT™ (King Medical Systems),[143] and the Intubating Laryngeal Airway™ now known as the air-Q Laryngeal Mask (Cookgas®).[144] Hagberg included just about every type of extraglottic airway in her article on difficult airway management implying that the airway manager could reasonably incorporate any device with which he had clinical competence into his personal difficult airway algorithm.[12] The LMA and other extraglottic devices have been incorporated into other difficult airway algorithms including the following:

1. Canadian Focus Group Algorithm: 1998[145]
2. Airway Approach Algorithm (AAA): 2003 (Rosenblatt and Whipple)[146]
3. Critical Airway Algorithm: 2005 (Matioc and Arndt)[147]
4. K.O.O.T Algorithm (Keep Out of Trouble): 2005 (Lee)[148]

Studies have shown that following a progressive, escalating algorithm when dealing with the management of the difficult airway can lead to beneficial results.[138] However, many authors comment that the dissemination of Difficult Airway Algorithms has not lead to widespread changes in practice.[149–151] Old habits die hard. Many surveys reveal that anesthesiologists the world over often are not prepared to respond to a critical airway scenario in the fashion recommended by algorithms such as that of the ASA. For those who believe that the algorithms have merit, there is some evidence that training programs are doing a better job of teaching new residents to deal with the "difficult airway" in an organized progressive manner. Extraglottic airway devices are important components on all airway algorithms. One should select and master the use of one or two extraglottic airway devices. One such device should be a device like the LMA Fastrach™ or the air-Q Laryngeal Mask™ that are designed to facilitate intubation. Future research will define which extraglottic device is most useful in the management of the "difficult airway."

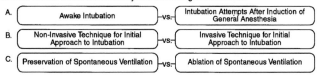

DIFFICULT AIRWAY ALGORITHM

1. Assess the likelihood and clinical impact of basic management problems:
   - A. Difficult Ventilation
   - B. Difficult Intubation
   - C. Difficulty with Patient Cooperation or Consent
   - D. Difficult Tracheostomy

2. Actively pursue opportunities to deliver supplemental oxygen throughout the process of difficult airway management

3. Consider the relative merits and feasibility of basic management choices:

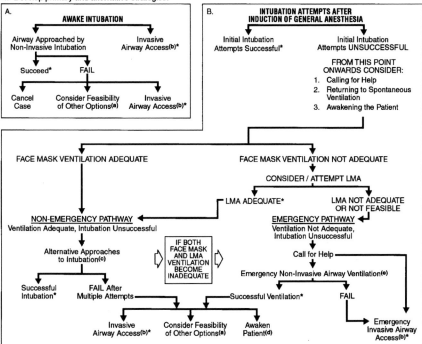

4. Develop primary and alternative strategies:

* Confirm ventilation, tracheal intubation, or LMA placement with exhaled CO_2

a. Other options include (but are not limited to): surgery utilizing face mask or LMA anesthesia, local anesthesia infiltration or regional nerve blockade. Pursuit of these options usually implies that mask ventilation will not be problematic. Therefore, these options may be of limited value if this step in the algorithm has been reached via the Emergency Pathway.

b. Invasive airway access includes surgical or percutaneous tracheostomy or cricothyrotomy.

c. Alternative non-invasive approaches to difficult intubation include (but are not limited to): use of different laryngoscope blades, LMA as an intubation conduit (with or without fiberoptic guidance), fiberoptic intubation, intubating stylet or tube changer, light wand, retrograde intubation, and blind oral or nasal intubation.

d. Consider re-preparation of the patient for awake intubation or canceling surgery.

e. Options for emergency non-invasive airway ventilation include (but are not limited to): rigid bronchoscope, esophageal-tracheal combitube ventilation, or transtracheal jet ventilation.

Fig. 5.83 ASA difficult airway algorithm. Use of the LMA™ is cited at multiple points of the algorithm. The Combitube is cited in footnote (e) (reprinted with permission from American Society of Anesthesiologists Task Force on Management of the Difficult Airway,[118] courtesy of the American Society of Anesthesiologists)

For now, the device should be one that the airway manager uses in daily practice and with which he is comfortable and proficient.

The author of this chapter disagrees with Dr. Brimacombe on one point concerning the role of awake fiberoptic-guided intubation in managing the difficult airway. Brimacombe states that "...awake intubation is so unpleasant (and without guaranteed success) that the induction-LMA insertion sequence would seem a reasonable option for many patients with predicted difficult airways"[2] (p. 331). On the contrary, a fiberoptically-guided endotracheal intubation can be performed safely, expeditiously, and comfortably on an awake patient. Those who practice the technique believe that it is frequently safer for the patient to maintain his own airway and to retain the ability to breath spontaneously during the intubation process. This is especially true if it is likely that the airway would become tenuous or altogether lost due to anatomic abnormalities, pathology, or trauma following the administration of a general anesthetic. While directed LMA™ insertion is an option for those as proficient as Dr. Brimacome in its application, for others, awake fiberoptic-guided intubation may be the technique of choice.

Use of the LMA™ to Manage the Difficult Airway in Obstetric Patients

Case reports and surveys dealing with extraglottic airway devices and the management of the difficult airway in obstetric patients predominantly involve the use of LMA™ products. Keller et al.[152] reviewed 44 cases in which LMA™ products 58including the LMA ProSeal™ were used to manage difficult airway cases in obstetric patients. Another report documented use of the Fastrach™ to manage the airway of an obstetric patient with Treacher–Collins Syndrome.[153] Gataure and Hughes[154] reported that of 209 anesthesiologists who responded to a survey sent to 250 obstetric centers, 72% "were in favor of using the LMA to maintain oxygenation when tracheal intubation had failed and ventilation using a face mask was inadequate." Many of the case reports stated that cricoid pressure had been maintained after insertion of the LMA. One should keep in mind that the application of cricoid pressure might make inserting of the LMA ProSeal™ more difficult and it might alter the oropharyngeal seal off the cuff. Furthermore, it might make the passage of an endotracheal tube more difficult.

In the obstetric difficult airway scenario, after inserting an LMA™, a critical decision the airway manager must make is whether or not to proceed with surgery (C-section) with the LMA™ in place or to choose another airway management option. A few of these options would be to try to intubate the trachea through the LMA™, wake-up the patient and administer a regional anesthetic, or to perform an awake endotracheal intubation. This is a difficult decision to make and is based on the condition of the mother and the baby. The literature supports using the LMA™ in the management of the difficult airway in obstetric patients as the primary airway device. Where it is incorporated into the management algorithm is up to each practitioner. The LMA™ or another extraglottic airway device should be in every obstetric operating room immediately available for use.

Use of the LMA™ and the Difficult Pediatric Airway

Brimacombe[2] (p. 338) analyzed the data of multiple reports where the LMA™ was used to manage the airways of children with a wide variety of congenital diseases. The LMA™ was used as a successful ventilating device in 98% of these patients, as a guide for blind endotracheal intubations in 94% of cases where attempted, and as a guide for fiberoptic-guided intubation in 98% of cases where attempted. Three strategies for intubation using the LMA™ are presented. First, the fiberoptic scope can be used in the customary fashion as a stent placed through the LMA™ into the trachea over which a preloaded endotracheal tube is passed (see Chap. 11). Secondly, if the child is smaller, the method reported by Osses et al.[155] can be tried. The authors described 6 cases of endotracheal intubation in pediatric patients (3 neonates, 3 infants). Under anesthesia, they examined the airway with a laryngoscope and could not see the epiglottis in any patient. After removing the laryngoscope, they inserted an LMA™ and verified correct position with capnography. Then they blindly passed an oral RAE tube (Mallinckrodt Medical) through the unmodified LMA™ into the trachea and confirmed its position. They removed the 15-mm adapter from the tube, attached an adult intubating stylet onto the endotracheal tube, and used the stylet to hold the tube in place as the LMA™ was withdrawn. The 15-mm adapter was reinserted and the patient ventilated. They reported 100% success with the technique. Another method reported by Walker[156] described using the LMA™ to facilitate fiberoptic-guided intubation in children ranging in age from 5 months to 18 years who had a variety of airway abnormalities. Under general anesthesia an LMA™ was placed. A fiberoptic endoscope was passed through the LMA™ into the trachea. A guidewire was passed through the scope until the wire's tip reached the right mainstem bronchus. The scope was removed and a "stiffening" catheter was passed over the wire. The wire was removed and the "stiffening" catheter was left in the trachea. An attempt was made to monitor CO_2 through the catheter to verify position. The LMA™ was removed and an endotracheal tube was passed over the catheter into the trachea. The catheter was removed and the tube's position verified. The author reported 100% success rate for his technique. All of these methods require special equipment and training. Before one uses any of these methods, get all of the equipment together and practice ahead of time on an airway manikin or model. *It is highly advisable to attend an advanced airway management workshop where these and other techniques are taught by experienced, competent instructors before practicing the techniques alone.* Nothing constructive can be said of the *Jack-of-all-trades, master-of-none* in the difficult airway business.

These and other reports support the use of the LMA™ in the management of the difficult pediatric airway, both anticipated and unanticipated.

The LMA™ and the Morbidly Obese Patient

Traditionally, the LMA™ had not been recommended for use in morbidly obese patients. Recognizing that the morbidly obese often posed challenges to the airway manager, Keller et al.[157] published a study in 2002 which investigated the utility of the LMA ProSeal™ to manage the airways of morbidly obese patients. They inserted an LMA ProSeal™ into 60 morbidly obese patients at induction of anesthesia for elective surgical cases. All insertions were with the aid of the "introducer tool." All insertions were performed within 15 s with a 90% success rate on the first try and the remaining 10% on the second. The patients were ventilated for 3 min with PPV, tidal volume 8 ml/kg, and a rate of 12 breaths per minute. I:E ratio was set at 1:1.5. At the end of 3 min, the LMA™ was replaced with an endotracheal tube. The oropharyngeal leak pressure averaged 32 cm H_2O and ventilation was successful in over 95% of patients. No gastric or drainage tube air leaks were detected. After this study, others reported that nearly 1,000 obese patients had been managed successfully either with the LMA Classic™, ProSeal™, or Fastrach™2 (p. 299). Furthermore, studies by Frappier et al.[158] and Coumbes[159] documented the utility of the LMA Fastrach™ as a guide to endotracheal intubation in obese patients. In a study that compared the effectiveness of the LMA Classic™ to the ProSeal™, Natalini et al.[160] concluded that either could be used to deliver mechanical ventilation to moderately obese patients with no problems except for postoperative sore throat. They noted that the cuff seal pressure was higher and that the drainage tube of the ProSeal™ sometimes kinked. The literature has clearly documented that the LMA™ can be used to manage the airways of obese and morbidly obese patients undergoing surgical procedures and receiving PPV. Clearly, clinical judgment reinforced with experience must be exercised when choosing to manage the airway of an obese patient with an extraglottic device.

Use of the LMA™ in Patients with Cervical Spine Pathology

The LMA™ has been used to manage the airways and to facilitate fiberoptic-guided intubation in patients with many types of cervical spine pathology including trauma, contracture,[161] previous cervical radiotherapy,[162] and patients with fixed flexion of the neck.[163]

The recommended position of the head and neck for insertion of the LMA™ is the standard "sniff" position. This position differs from the neutral position maintained with in-line traction. (Consult the neurosurgeon before manipulating the neck prior to LMA™ insertion.) Maintenance of in-line traction or the application of supportive neck devices may affect ease of LMA™ insertion.

Asai et al.[164] compared the time and ease of insertion of the LMA Classic™ in anesthetized, paralyzed patients who were placed either in the "sniff" or neutral position with manual in-line stabilization. LMA insertion was faster and easier when the patients were placed in the "sniff" position (11.7 vs. 20.1 s).

The same investigators[165] reported that the LMA Fastrach™ was easier and faster to insert than the Classic™ in anesthetized patients whose necks and heads were placed in neutral position with in-line stabilization.

Nakazawa et al.[166] reported that 36 of 40 patients with cervical spine disease (24 of whom had limited or prohibited neck extension and 10 of whom presented in stabilization devices) were blindly intubated through an LMA Fastrach™. The others were intubated with fiberoptic guidance through the Fastrach™. They attributed failed blind intubation to improper LMA™ size.

Wakeling and Nightingale[167] reported finding LMA Fastrach™ insertion and blind passage of an endotracheal tube to be difficult, if not impossible, in patients whose necks were stabilized with a rigid collar. By comparison, Moller et al.[168] reported that the stiff neck collar "…produced no serious obstacle to insertion, ventilation, and blind intubation through the ILMA [Proseal™]" in their case series. Obviously, more controlled studies need to be undertaken to address the effects of stiff collar neck immobilization on extraglottic airway insertion and function.

Ferson et al.[135] reported using the Fastrach™ to ventilate and intubate 12 of 12 patients whose necks were immobilized with stereotactic frames. They found that the Fastrach™ proved to be a "…particularly valuable" tool and that its use should be considered "…in the treatment of patients with immobilized cervical spines."

International Anesthesia Clinics[169] has compiled an excellent collection of articles concerning all aspects of LMA™ use including its application to manage the airways of patients with cervical spine pathology.

Cervical Pressure and Movement Associated with LMA™ Use

Brimacombe et al.[170] studied the pressure exerted on the second and third cervical vertebrae during standard LMA insertion. Twenty fresh cadavers were studied and the investigators reported that pressure exerted on the vertebrae during insertion rose transiently to 224 cm H_2O and decreased rapidly to less than 20 cm H_2O after seating of the LMA. The pressure was caused by the index finger used to exert posterior pressure on the mask to hold it against the palate and posterior pharynx during insertion. They suggested that further research was needed to determine the clinical implications of their findings. They recommended "that clinicians be careful to avoid excessive posterior force when using the LMA in [patients with an] unstable cervical spine." They also did not recommend using an LMA Fastrach™ as an alternative to the standard LMA™ because a recent study had shown that the Fastrach™ had "…been shown to exert substantial static pressures (approximately 160 cm H_2O) against the mucosa overlying the cervical vertebrae, and the implications of this have not been evaluated." In a later study, Keller et al.[171] reported their findings after study of 20 fresh cadavers. High cervical pressures were found with insertion of both the Fastrach™ and the Classic™. Highest pressures were found when the Fastrach™ handle was depressed or moved up and down. In another cadaver study [10 subjects with posteriorly destabilized third cervical vertebra],

Brimacombe et al.[172] "...found that significant displacement of the injured segment occurred during airway management with the face mask, laryngoscope-guided oral intubation, the esophageal tracheal combitube, the intubating and classic LMA, but not with fiberoptic-guided nasal intubation." They concluded that the safest maneuver, with respect to cervical vertebral displacement was with the nasal fiberoptic-guided intubation. Brimacombe[2] (p. 474) commented that the Intubating LMA had been used in 106 patients with unstable cervical spines and only one case of neurological deterioration was related to airway management maneuvers.

Kirara et al.[173] recorded cervical movement in 20 anesthetized patients whose necks were stabilized with in-line traction. They studied the effects of LMA Fastrach™ insertion and removal. Insertion of an endotracheal tube was guided with a lightwand. They reported that Fastrach™ insertion was successful on the first try in all patients. During insertion, intubation, and LMA removal, various cervical segments were flexed between 1 and 4°. Posterior movement ranged between 0.5 and 1.0 mm on insertion and intubation. No posterior movement was observed with removal of the LMA. All airway maneuvers were associated with some degree of cervical movement in spite of in-line traction.

Before initiating any type of airway maneuver involving patients with cervical spine pathology, consult the attending surgeon. Determine which maneuvers are safe and which could exasperate neurological injury. Remember that in-line traction does not assure that the cervical vertebrae will not move during airway management operations. If using an LMA Fastrach™, keep the handle as immobile as possible. Minimize handle depression. Do not leave the LMA Fastrach™ in place after intubation. If using the LMA Classic™, minimize posterior pressure applied with the index finger. Clinical judgment and experience are absolute prerequisites when dealing with patients who have cervical spine pathology. Extraglottic airways, especially the LMA™, based on history and clinical study, have a place in the management of these challenging patients.

Role of the LMA Outside of the Operating Room (PreHospital and Emergency Room)

When first marketed, the LMA™ was intended for use by anesthesia personnel. In 1994, Brimacombe[174] noted that two national authorities, one in Japan the other in the UK, had approved programs to train "paramedical staff" in the use of the LMA™. A review by Pollack[175] written for emergency physicians stated that it was appropriate to use the LMA™ in the emergency setting. He wrote that a pilot study conducted in his emergency department to train emergency medicine residents had proven successful. More recent studies document successful use of extraglottic airway devices in the prehospital setting or by nonanesthesia personnel. Kurola et al.[176] reported that inexperienced firefighter-EMT students could successfully insert a King Systems LT™ in timely fashion in anesthetized patients after receiving a 2-h training course. Timmermann and Russo[178] wrote that "Extraglottic airway devices are increasingly used for airway management not only in patients for elective surgery, but also in out-of-hospital settings, when less experienced personnel have to secure the airway." Timmermann et al.[184] reported that 11 of 11 patients were ventilated and intubated in the field by emergency physicians using the Intubating LMA™. Previous oral intubations were unsuccessful for 8 of the patients while in 3, the ILMA™ was the first intervention employed to secure the airway. McCall et al.[179] reported that Tasmanian paramedics intubated 106 patients in the field during the study period. They reported equal success of intubation when comparing the ILMA™ to the standard laryngoscopic directed technique. The success rate for intubation on the first attempt was higher for the ILMA™. Finally, guidelines from a task force from the Scandinavian Society for Anaesthesiology and Intensive Care Medicine[180] recommend that when nonanesthesiologists perform advanced cardiopulmonary resuscitation a SGA device should be used. Furthermore, they suggested that a "… supraglottic device such as the laryngeal tube or the [intubating] laryngeal mask should also be available as a backup device for anesthesiologists in failed ETI [endotracheal intubation]."

In conclusion, the literature supports incorporating an extraglottic airway device into one's prehospital airway management algorithm. Trained but inexperienced nonanesthesiologists have been shown to have a high success rate securing the airway using these devices in the prehospital setting. If emergency personnel are expected to retain proficiency with extraglottic airways they must receive periodic retraining and be observed by experienced teachers in a controlled setting (operating room).

Problems Associated with the Use of Extraglottic Airway Devices

Because of its long clinical history, use in over 200 million anesthetics, and its subjugation to vigorous scientific scrutiny at every step of its evolution, most of the literature concerning problems associated with the use of extraglottic airways has to do with devices manufactured by LMA™. At the start, the company openly addressed problems associated with the LMA™ in its manuals. On its website (lmana.com), the company has directions on how to report problems and how to contact an expert should a problem arise. If one searches the "Bibliography" at the bottom of the website's page, a link to PubMed.com is made. A search of LMA™ related problems can be undertaken immediately. As will be reported, some of the problems associated with the LMA™ are serious in nature. Other manufacturers address problems associated with their products. For example, the Ambu® AuraStraight™ product information manual[15] states in Sect. 5. Adverse effects: "Use of the Ambu AuraStraight may cause minor adverse effects (e.g., sore throat) and major adverse effects (e.g., aspiration)." All of the Ambu® product manuals address adverse effects in an honest effort to caution users to beware of potential problems. As products of manufacturers other then LMA™ gain larger market share, future studies will analyze problems associated with their use.

Table 5.11 Adverse events reported with LMA use

Aspiration	Regurgitation	Vomiting	
		Pharyngolaryngeal reflexes	
Bronchospasm	Hiccup	Coughing	Laryngeal spasm
Gagging	Transient glottic closure	Retching	Breath holding
		Trauma	
Arytenoid dislocation	Larynx	Minor abrasions	Tonsils
Epiglottis	Posterior pharyngeal wall	Uvula	
		Neurovascular	
Tongue cyanosis	Vocal cord paralysis	Hypoglossal nerve paralysis	Parotid gland swelling
Lingual nerve paralysis	Tongue macroglossia		
		Postoperative	
Dry mouth	Sore throat	Dysphonia	Pharyngeal ulcer
Dysphagia	Mouth ulcer	Hoarseness	
Feeling of fullness	Dysarthria	Stridor	
		Coincidental	
Pulmonary edema	Stridor edema	Laryngeal hematoma	Head and neck
		Nonairway	
Myocardial ischemia	Dysrhythmias		

Source: Brain et al. [181]

Table 5.11 summarizes information taken from an instruction manual that LMA™ North America, Inc. previously included with its products. This table is presented because of its historic value and as evidence that LMA™ has always been forthcoming in dealing with problems associated with the use of its products.

Since 2000, a myriad of articles has been published concerning the problems associated with using LMA™ and other extraglottic airway devices. Table 5.12 lists a few of these.

Many problems are associated with the use of the LMA™ and other extraglottic airway devices. Fortunately, serious problems are extremely rare. For a thorough examination of the topic refer to Brimacombe's textbook,[2] Chap. 21. In conclusion, the following points from his textbook constitute a practical take-home summary of the vast literature dealing with the common problems associated with the use of the LMA™.

1. Incidence of clinically detectable pharyngeal regurgitation using LMA: 0.07%
2. Incidence of aspiration in fasted patients using LMA: 0.012%
3. Sore throat using LMA: 17% (39% LG-TI and 4% with face mask)
4. Dysarthria using LMA: 15% (21% with LG-TI)
5. Dysphagia using LMA: 20% (10% with LG-TI)
6. The incidence of sore throat and dysphagia increase with cuff volume

Table 5.12 Additional problems associated with (or during) use of the LMA™

Pharyngolaryngeal problems
Airway obstruction caused by vagal nerve stimulator[182]
Trauma or infection
Dental damage with LMA Fastrach™[183]
Frenular injury[184]
Acute transient submandibular sialadenopathy[185–187]
Acute unilateral macroglossia[188]
Esophageal rupture[189]
Retropharyngeal abscess (LMA™ and Bosworth Introducer)[190]
Pulmonary problems
Negative pressure pulmonary edema[191]
Nerve damage
Review Article: Lingual, Hypoglossal, Recurrent Laryngeal Nerve Involvement[192]
Equipment problems
LMA™ obstruction: nematode,[193] piece of cleaning machine,[194] cuff herniation[195]
Damaged equipment: fractured mask,[196] Fastrach™ tube damage,[197] hole in pilot tube,[198] detached cuff weld[199]
LMA ProSeal™ Cuff Folding[200–202]
MRI Interference[203]
Cleaning Problems with Reusable LMA™ Devices: Protein Residue[204–208]
Venous congestion associated with high cuff pressure[209]
Distorted anatomy
Mechanical closure of vocal cords with Airway Management Device [AMD™][210] ("…airway device(s) with a large and/or inflatable hypopharyngeal component can cause mechanical airway obstruction by vocal cord closure secondary to glottic compression")[211]

What to Do if the Patient Regurgitates with an Extraglottic Airway in Place

Regurgitation and/or vomiting usually occur if the patient's plane of anesthesia is too light. To prevent complications from this phenomenon be sure to select patients prudently, make sure the airway is properly seated and the cuff pressure is appropriate, and assure that the patient is properly anesthetized.

One's response to witnessed regurgitation of stomach contents in a patient with an extraglottic airway in place should be based on a preconsidered plan of action to save time and eliminate unnecessary actions. Following is one suggested plan to deal with witnessed regurgitation or vomiting. For practical purposes, assume that the patient has a normal airway and that endotracheal intubation would not be difficult.

Management of witnessed regurgitation

1. LMA Classic™ or ProSeal™ is in place.
2. Witnessed regurgitation.
3. Increase FiO_2 to 1.0.
4. Apply no PPV. Apply cricoid pressure if no active vomiting observed.

5. Place patient in head-down position. Consider turning patient laterally.
6. Suction above LMA™ cuff.
7. Suction stomach. This can be done through the ProSeal™ vent channel or by inserting an NG tube.
8. Auscultate chest, look for clinical signs of pulmonary aspiration.
9. Consider deepening anesthetic.
10. Consider whether to continue with surgery if the patient is stable and no signs of aspiration are observed. Consider exchanging the LMA™ with an endotracheal tube.
11. If changing to an endotracheal tube, apply cricoid pressure during maneuver.
12. If one suspects pulmonary aspiration, consider fiberoptic examination of lungs.
13. Collect sample of regurgitated stomach contents and check for pH. This step may not change immediate management but if the pH is high one could reasonably predict that the pulmonary sequelae would be less severe.
14. If patient suffers signs of significant pulmonary aspiration and injury, intubate, and initiate treatment for aspiration pneumonitis.

If the patient has a known or suspected difficult airway, one should have a more detailed plan to respond to regurgitation as well as to the loss of the airway for any reason. Make plans and preparations before starting any case.

U.S. FDA Regulations Concerning the Introduction of Extraglottic Airway Devices to the Market: "510(k) Exempt" Classification

Medical devices that are classified as 510(k) exempt do not require FDA review before marketing. To quote the FDA, "These medical devices are mostly low-risk, Class I devices and some Class II devices that have been determined not to require a 510(k)…to provide a reasonable assurance of safety and effectiveness."[212] These devices are exempt from complying with premarket notification requirements. However, they must meet certain general controls such as:

1. Be suitable for their intended use
2. Be adequately packaged and properly labeled
3. Have establishment registration and device listing forms on file with the FDA
4. Be manufactured under a quality system (with the exception of a small number of Class I devices that are subject only to complaint files and general recordkeeping requirements)

Examples of Class I devices that are exempt from 510(k) regulation include "Anesthesiology Devices" under Part 868. All LMA™ devices including reusable and disposable Fastrach™ endotracheal tubes are Class I, 510(k) exempt devices (Communication from LMA North America, Inc.). Furthermore, the FDA apparently classifies all oropharyngeal airways as Class I, 510(k) exempt under Regulation

Number 868.5110. One should be aware that FDA regulations concerning these devices require no review of premarket testing or notification. It is up to the manufacturers to assure that the devices are safe and of "suitable" design to function as intended.

Is the Extraglottic Airway Device Interchangeable with the Endotracheal Tube in the Practice of Anesthesia?

Six points to consider on the question of "interchangeability" of the EGA with the endotracheal tube are the following:

1. Cost: What are the comparative costs of each device to the patient and the healthcare system?
2. Efficacy: Considerations of oxygenation and ventilation; use with adjunctive airway devices; ease of use.
3. Educational Considerations: How hard is it to learn to use each device safely and proficiently?
4. Safety: What are the risks to the patient? (Not including the risk of aspiration)
5. Security: Which airway is less likely to become displaced, fall out, kink, or obstruct?
6. Aspiration Risk: The facts and the consensus of opinion.

The points are ordered from the easiest to answer to most difficult. Each will be addressed in turn. Finally, an attempt will be made to answer the question presented above.

1. Cost:

The cost of an airway device depends on many things such as a hospital's contract with suppliers and the pressure of competition. The LMA™ will face stiffer competition in the future due to the introduction of so many new extraglottic devices. The cost of endotracheal tubes also varies depending on a facility's purchasing contracts and competition. The more sophisticated reusable extraglottic airways are often cheaper to use than their disposable counterparts (LMA ProSeal™ can be used 40 times and is cheaper to use per application than the LMA Supreme™). In reality, the cost of a disposable extraglottic airway such as the LMA Unique™ and a standard PVC endotracheal tube is not too different ($10 vs. $1.50). However, when one considers the other costs of endotracheal intubation such as that for laryngoscope handles and blades (that always seem to disappear), the routine use of neuromuscular drugs to facilitate intubation, a deeper level of anesthesia required to tolerate the endotracheal tube, and cleaning costs for airway equipment, the actual cost to purchase and use an LMA™ could be less than the actual cost of using an endotracheal tube. Should newly trained anesthesiologists move to standardize the use of video laryngoscopes, the cost to provide instant access to a videoscope in every operating room would run into the hundreds of millions of dollars.

(By comparison, the net sales of LMA™ International in 2009 was \$107,634,000).[3] Furthermore, cost to the healthcare provider is not the same as cost to the patient. Who knows what a hospital charges the patient for an endotracheal tube vs. an LMA™? The patient's cost is paid for by insurance premiums, cash, or taxpayers' money and must be added to the total cost of using the device. For now it appears that the cost between the extraglottic device and the endotracheal tube is about the same. This could change in the future.

2. Efficacy:

Both the extraglottic airway and the endotracheal tube are effective and reliable devices used to channel oxygen to the patient as well as to permit the application of every useful mode of ventilation. This includes spontaneous and controlled ventilation and the application of moderate levels of CPAP, PEEP, and pressure support ventilation. If the peak inspiratory pressure is in excess of 20 cm H_2O (30 cm H_2O for the LMA ProSeal™) or if the distending airway pressure needs to be above 10 cm H_2O, an endotracheal tube would be indicated to support ventilation. These limits are based on manufacturers' recommendations. Concerning the efficacy of using adjunctive equipment with either airway, consider the fiberoptic scope: The skilled manager can use the scope with either device equally as well depending on the clinical situation and demands of the airway management task. In fact, the LMA™ may be the airway of choice if the fiberoptic scope is being used to observe laryngeal function and anatomy. Special intubating extraglottic airways are available to enhance efficacy. Other adjunctive equipment such as an NG tube can be inserted easily with either device in place. Finally, with respect to ease of insertion, both devices can be used safely and with facility by the trained airway manager. In summary, both devices are about equal with respect to efficacy in the majority of cases.

3. Educational considerations:

The learning curves for using of the LMA™ and intubating the trachea using a laryngoscope are multiphasic. The first plateau of the curve can be defined as that of "marginal competency." To reach this endpoint with the LMA™, a student must perform between 15 and 75 insertions under the guidance of a skilled teacher.[213,214] With respect to endotracheal intubation, it has been suggested that after 70 oral and nasal intubations most students will have been exposed to the majority of intubation related problems. During training, a resident is expected to become proficient (at least safe) to perform many more sophisticated airway management techniques. After successfully completing a 3-year anesthesiology residency and having managed thousands of airways, the new anesthesiologist is deemed to be clinically competent to manage the airway at the consultant level. In reality it will take many years for one to appreciate nuances of every airway device and technique. For a specific group of professionals, though, learning to use the LMA™ for one specific task has been shown to be easier than learning to use the laryngoscope to guide intubation. That group is nonanesthesiologist technicians and physicians who must secure the airway in an emergency situation either in the field or in the ER. For this group, studies confirm and difficult airway management algorithms recommend using an extraglottic device as the first-line airway management tool. This group of healthcare providers can use the extraglottic airway very effectively after a relatively short training period. In summary, concerning educational considerations, learning curves for either device are similar. This applies to the formal training of an anesthesiologist and on a very limited basis, to nonanesthesiologist first responders.

4. Safety:

The risks associated with using an extraglottic airway or performing an endotracheal intubation, although rare, can be catastrophic. The ASA Closed Claims Project[215] lists respiratory events as the leading cause of death and brain damage in anesthesia related Law suits. Many of the respiratory event claims are associated with endotracheal intubation. An analysis of the respiratory event claims associated with the LMA™ has not been published. Miller[216] reviewed Closed Claims difficult airway data in 2000 and stated that the Project "…cannot yet evaluate the effect of new airway management tools such as the LMA on anesthesia liability arising from airway management problems." Cheney[217] made a similar claim in a paper reviewing aspiration data. In March 2010, the Closed Claims Project (Posner. ASA Closed Claims Project. Personal email: 1 March 2010) provided this chapter's author with the following quote concerning the association of the LMA™ with database claims: "The ASA Closed Claims Project database, a national collection of anesthesia malpractice claims, contains 10 claims for aspiration during LMA use. Five of these aspirations occurred during induction of general anesthesia (with conversion to endotracheal intubation), four intraanesthesia, and one at emergence. Most of these claims resulted in temporary injury to the patient. There was one claim for permanent severe brain damage and three for death of the patient. All of these severe injuries resulted in payment to the patient. Most patients who aspirated with LMA use had risk factors for aspiration such as GERD, diabetes, hiatal hernia, trauma, or an ongoing intraabdominal process. In addition to claims for aspiration, there were seven claims for airway injuries with LMA. Four patients complained of sore throat, with two of these having retropharyngeal air or abscess. Another sore throat resulted from improper LMA preparation and sterilization causing chemical irritation. Other injuries included hypoglossal nerve compression and displaced arytenoids cartilage. One patient sustained airway obstruction after biting down on the LMA at emergence, requiring tracheotomy to secure the airway. All of these injuries resolved. Only two of these claims resulted in payment to the patient." Since the device has been incorporated into the ASA Difficult Airway Algorithm it will be used to manage patients already at risk for developing injury resulting from respiratory system mishaps. As a result, more claims will surface in the future associated with the LMA™ and other extraglottic airway devices.

At this time, it is accurate to say that both devices can cause significant trauma and have been associated with many types of respiratory complications. The incidence of severe outcome is rare, though it can be as catastrophic as brain injury or death.

The literature does offer data with respect to more common problems associated with the extraglottic airway compared to endotracheal intubation.

(a) Endotracheal intubation[218]

    i. Difficult laryngoscopic view: 1.5–8.5%
    ii. Difficult/failed ventilation: 0.01–0.07%
    iii. Failed intubation: 0.13–0.3%
    iv. "Cannot ventilate/cannot intubate": 0.01–2/10,000

(b) LMA™: (Classic™, ProSeal™, Flexible™, Fastrach™)[2] (p. 570)

    i. Failure: 1–2% (failed insertion/seal/obstruction)

(c) Comparisons of common problems[2] (p. 570):

    i. *Sore throat*: Lower for LMA™ than LG-TI
    ii. *Dysphagia*: Higher for LMA™ than LG-TI
    iii. *Dysarthria*: Similar for both devices

Concerning the problem of contamination, the incidence is very low for both devices. Certainly, if one is worried about this problem, disposable equipment should be used. In summary with respect to the safety issue, both devices have a low incidence of significant problems associated with their use. However, experience and training will guide the practitioner to apply clinical judgment when choosing the airway tool and technique most appropriate to do the job safely.

5. Security:

Both the LMA™ and endotracheal tube have been used in patients positioned every imaginable way. This includes supine, lateral, prone, lithotomy, head-up or down, jackknife, and sitting. With respect to security of the airway, one cannot argue one technique is better than the other based on scientific evidence. Any airway can dislodge or fallout making it ineffective. One way to look at the security issue is the following: Apply then Plus 2 Rule When Dealing with Airway Security

> When deciding issues of airway security, be prepared to intervene immediately with at least 2 options to reestablish or salvage a displaced airway device. These options must be those for which the manager is fully trained and proficient to carry out. Consider whether or not the patient's position eliminates any rescue option.

Remember, turning the patient supine to reestablish the airway is always an option, but it might not be the best in the opinion of the surgeon and it might increase risk to the patient.

Another important consideration concerning the patient's position is:

> Does the position predispose the patient to regurgitation and possibly tracheal aspiration of stomach contents?

If so, one must choose the airway he feels is both secure and protects the patient most effectively against aspiration.

In summary, with respect to airway security, it is a judgment call by the airway manager. His decision must be based on training, experience, and ability to salvage a dislodged airway. He must select the airway, secure it in place, have a backup plan, and consider the effects of position on security, emergency management, and the risk of aspiration.

6. Aspiration risk:

Experts agree that the overall risk of aspiration in patients managed with an LMA™ is about the same as for those who are endotracheally intubated. The estimated risk varies from 0.003 to 0.047% of cases (p. 118)[2,219] (perioperative aspiration carries a 5% mortality rate.) If the risk of aspiration is the same, why does the question persist?

Is the extraglottic airway device interchangeable with the endotracheal tube in the practice of anesthesia?

There is no consensus of opinion or definitive study to answer the question. However, in the past decade, more anesthesiologists have used extraglottic airway devices, mostly LMA™ products, in applications that were not endorsed by the manufacturer when the LMA™ was introduced. Now, the company's website lists many "Advanced use(s) of an LMA™."[3] These include using an appropriate LMA™ airway to manage patients undergoing intraabdominal, laparoscopic, intraoral plastic surgery, and other ENT procedures. A Forum was published in the 2008 *Gazette* of the Society for Airway Management.[220] Anesthesiologists were asked to comment on the use of a SGA in patients with a history of reflux (GERD). A few pertinent comments are quoted from the publication expressing anesthesiologists' points of view on the subject (The names of the commentators have been deleted at the discretion of this chapter's author):

Commentator #1: The risk of aspiration in using the LMA is approximately 1 in 10,000 (similar to the incidence of an ETT). No clinical study of this magnitude is likely to be performed. (To determine which airway is safer with respect to aspiration during use.)

Commentator #2: I use only the Proseal (PLMA) or Supreme in patients with suspected GERD, especially if it is not well-controlled.

Commentator #3: My personal approach for the "full stomach" in second trimester patients has changed over the years. I might manage a short procedure in an asymptomatic patient with an SGA. The problem is that we taught "full stomach" in OB patients so effectively for 20–30 years that it would be difficult to justify if a patient aspirated. As always, there's some plaintiff's authority/expert who would cite chapter and verse and destroy the individual who gave anesthesia.

Commentator #4: (Commenting on using the LMA Supreme™ to manage the airways of two pregnant patients of 17-week and 23-week gestation for dilatation and extraction, both of whom were fasted, not obese, and had small amounts of gastric contents suctioned from the gastric port) I verified that the device was properly positioned before proceeding and provided adequate anesthetic depth. This may be the beginning of a new era in managing these patients.

Commentator #5: The rationale for deviating from community standards of care may be defendable in some situations (and also supported by the literature). The use of the ProSeal™ (and little data exist for the Supreme) for elective surgery where definite conditions for increasing the risk of aspiration exist, has certainly not become a standard of care in the U.S.

An excellent review of the ProSeal™ in 2005[221] cited many improvements attributed to the airway's design. The authors concluded that the risk of aspiration may be less with the ProSeal™ compared to other devices but at the time of publication this contention had not been proven. Finally, as a reminder that severe problems can arise with ProSeal™ use, Keller et al.[222] reported three serious aspiration related complications including the first case of brain injury and death.

To answer the question posed at the beginning of this section, the first five considerations of cost, efficacy, educational considerations, security, and safety with respect to nonaspiration related problems do not favor either the extraglottic airway device or the endotracheal tube. However, with the additional consideration of aspiration related morbidity, the author of this chapter answers the question as follows:

> At this time, for patients who are not fasted or who have a definite risk of aspiration, or who may develop an increased risk of aspiration due to positioning, the endotracheal tube is the airway of choice when compared to an extraglottic airway device.

More importantly, the world's expert on the LMA™, Dr. Joseph Brimacombe (Personal email communication) provided the following quotation concerning his thoughts on the question:

> The ProSeal LMA, with its high seal for ventilation and gastric access for prevention of aspiration and gastric insufflation, can be used in most elective situations where a tracheal tube is considered standard practice, particularly when inserted using a guided technique.

> Joseph Brimacombe, MD: 1 May 2008

"Most elective situations" does not include nonfasted patients. Dr. Brimacombe leaves a lot of choice open to each practitioner. One thing he does not leave open is that the anesthesiologist must know how to insert an LMA ProSeal™ properly and to use some form of "guided technique." This may include a GEB. In addition to knowing the proper insertion technique, the airway manager must know how to verify proper airway position (with a fiberoptic scope). He must also be able to diagnose and correct problems associated with the LMA ProSeal™.

Dr. Brimacombe's quotation is the best answer to the question: *Is the extraglottic airway device interchangeable with the endotracheal tube in the practice of anesthesia?* Keep in mind that his answer applies to one specific airway, the LMA ProSeal™, and to no others.

A quote from an editorial by Cooper[223] offers thoughtful advice to those wishing that there was a clear-cut answer the question at hand. He states:

> It is important that our clinical practice be guided by the best evidence we can marshal; such evidence might ultimately come from well-designed, sufficiently powered randomized trials. Until that evidence exists, it is important that we make use of surveys, metaanalyses, case

94. Von Ungern-Sternberg BS, Boda K, Schwab C, et al. Laryngeal mask airway is associated with an increased incidence of adverse respiratory events in children with recent upper respiratory tract infections. *Anesthesiology.* 2007;107:714–719.

95. Eikermann M, Cote CJ. Laryngeal mask airwayand children's risk of perioperative respiratory complications: randomized controlled studies are required to discriminate cause and effect. *Anesthesiology.* 2008;108(6):1154.

96. Ferrari LR, Goudsouzian NG. The use of the laryngeal mask airway in children with bronchopulmonary dysplasia. *Anesth Analg.* 1995;81:310.

97. Mayhew JF, Dalmeida RE. Letter. *Anesth Analg.* 1996;82(4):886.

98. Ferrari LR, Goudsouzian N. Response to Ref. 82. *Anesth Analg.* 1996;82(4):886–897.

99. Lopez-Gil M et al. Laryngeal mask airway in pediatric practice: a prospective study of skill acquisition by anesthesiology residents. *Anesthesiology.* 1996;84(4):807.

100. Ames WA, Fischer SF, Dear GD. Long-term use of the laryngeal mask airway in a neonate. *Anesth Analg.* 2006;103:792.

101. Shimbori H, Ono K, Miwa T, et al. Comparison of the LMA-Proseal™ and LMA-Classic™ in children. *Br J Anaesth.* 2004;93(4):528–531.

102. Lopez-Gil M, Brimacombe J, Garcia G. A randomized non-crossover study comparing the Proseal™ and Classic™ laryngeal mask airway in anaesthetized children. *Br J Anaesth.* 2005;95(6):827–830.

103. Goldmann K, Roettger C, Wulf H. Use of the Proseal™ laryngeal mask airway for pressure-controlled ventilation with and without positive end-expiratory pressure in paediatric patients: a randomized, controlled study. *Br J Anaesth.* 2005;95(6):831–834.

104. Goldmann K, Jakob C. A randomized crossover comparison of the size 2½ laryngeal mask airway Proseal™ versus laryngeal mask airway-Classic™ in pediatric patients. *Anesth Analg.* 2005;100:1605–1610.

105. Goldmann K, Roettger C, Wulf H. The size 1½ Proseal™ laryngeal mask airway in infants: a randomized, crossover investigation with the Classic™ laryngeal mask airway. *Anesth Analg.* 2006;102:405–410.

106. Micaglio M, Parotto M. Size 1 Proseal™ laryngeal mask airway in neonates. *Anesth Analg.* 2006;103(4):1044–1045.

107. Bennett J et al. Use of the laryngeal mask airway in oral and maxillofacial surgery. *J Oral Maxillofac Surg.* 1996;54:1346.

108. Agarwal A, Shobhana N. Letter. *Can J Anaesth.* 1995;42(8):750.

109. Agarwal A, Shabhana R. Letter. *Can J Anaesth.* 1995;42(12):1176.

110. Silva LC, Brimacombe JR. Letter. *Anesth Analg.* 1996;82(2):430.

111. Morita Y, Takenoshita M. Laryngeal mask airway fitted over a tracheostomy office: a mean to ventilate a tracheotomized patient during induction of anesthesia. *Anesthesiology.* 1998;89(5):1295.

112. Alexander R et al. The laryngeal mask airway and the tracheal route for drug administration. *Br J Anaesth.* 1997;78(2):220.

113. Pennant JH et al. The laryngeal mask airway and laryngeal polyposis. *Anesth Analg.* 1994;78:1206.

114. Brimacombe J et al. The laryngeal mask for percutaneous endoscopic gastrostomy. *Anesth Analg.* 2000;91:635.

115. Brimacombe J. Laryngeal mask airway for access to the upper gastrointestinal tract. *Anesthesiology.* 1996;84(4):1009.

116. Salvi L, Pepi M. Pressure-assisted breathing through a laryngeal mask airway during transesophageal echocardiography. *Anesth Analg.* 1999;89:1585.

117. Han T, Brimacombe J, Lee E, Yang H. The laryngeal mask airway is effective (and probably safe) in selected healthy parturients for elective cesarean section: a prospective study of 1067 cases. *Can J Anesth.* 2001;48(11):1117.

118. Kanniah SK. Laryngeal mask airway and tonsillectomy. *Anesth Analg.* 2006;103(4):1051.

119. Clarke MB, Forster P, Cook TM. Airway management for tonsillectomy: a national survey of UK practice. *Br J Anaesth.* 2007;99(3):425.

120. Brimacombe J, Keller C. An unusual case of airway rescue in the prone position with the proseal laryngeal mask airway. *Can J Anesth*. 2005;52(8):884.
121. Dingeman RS, Goumnerova LC, Goobie SM. The use of a laryngeal mask airway for emergent airway management in a prone child. *Anesth Analg*. 2005;100:670–671.
122. Ng A, Raitt DG, Smith G. Induction of anesthesia and insertion of a laryngeal mask airway in the prone position for minor surgery. *Anesth Analg*. 2002;94(5):1194–1198.
123. Brimacombe JR, Wenzel V, Keller C. The proseal laryngeal mask airway in prone patients: a retrospective audit of 245 patients. *Anaesth Intensive Care*. 2007;35(2):222–225.
124. McCaul CL, Harney D, Ryan M, et al. Airway management in the lateral position: a randomized controlled trial. *Anesth Analg*. 2005;101:1221–1225.
125. Dimitriou V, Voyagis GS, Iatrou C, Brimacombe J. Flexible lightwand–guided intubation using the intubating Laryngeal Mask Airway™ in the supine, right, and left lateral positions in healthy patients by experienced users. *Anesth Analg*. 2003;96:896–898.
126. Komatsu R, Nagata O, Sessler DI, Ozaki M. The intubating laryngeal mask airway facilitates tracheal intubation in the lateral position. *Anesth Analg*. 2004;98(3):858–861.
127. Xue FS, Mao P, Liu HP, et al. The effects of head flexion on airway seal, quality of ventilation and orogastric tube placement using the proseal laryngeal mask airway. *Anaesthesia*. 2008;63(9):079–085.
128. Park SH, Han SH, Do SH, Kim JW, Kim JH. The influence of head and neck position on the oropharyngeal leak pressure and cuff position of three supraglottic airway devices. *Anesth Analg*. 2008;108(1):112–7.
129. American Society of Anesthesiologists Task Force on Management of the Difficult Airway. Practice guidelines for management of the difficult airway: an updated report by the American Society of Anesthesiologists Task Force on Management of the Difficult Airway. *Anesthesiology*. 2003;98(5):1269–1277.
130. Benumof JL. Laryngeal mask airway and the ASA difficult airway algorithm. *Anesthesiology*. 1996;84(3):686.
131. Parmet JL et al. The laryngeal mask airway reliably provides rescue ventilation in cases of unanticipated difficult tracheal intubation along with difficult mask airway. *Anesth Analg*. 1998;87:661.
132. Joo HS et al. The intubating laryngeal mask airway after induction of general anesthesia versus awake fiberoptic intubation in patients with difficult airways. *Anesth Analg*. 2001;92:1342.
133. Shung J et al. Awake intubation of the difficult airway with the intubating laryngeal mask airway. *Anaesthesia*. 1998;53:645.
134. Fukutome T et al. Tracheal intubation through the intubating laryngeal mask airway (LMA-Fastrach™) in patients with difficult airways. *Anaesth Intensive Care*. 1998;26:387.
135. Ferson DZ et al. Use of the intubating LMA-Fastrach™ in 254 patients with difficult-to-manage airways. *Anesthesiology*. 2001;95:1175.
136. Ferson DF. LMA: what's old-what's new, patients with difficult airways. *ASA Refresher Course;* 2003:236.
137. Ovassapian A. The role of LMA, combitube and fiberoptics in the difficult airway. *ASA Refresher Course;* 2006:120.
138. Rosenblatt WH. The use of the LMA-Proseal™ in airway resuscitation. *Anesth Analg*. 2003;97:1773–1775.
139. Dunn SM, Robbins L, Connelly NR. The LMA Proseal™ may not be the best option for difficult to intubate/ventilate patients. *Anesth Analg*. 2004;99:310.
140. Rosenblatt WH. Response to Ref. 139. *Anesth Analg*. 2004;99:311.
141. Pearson DM, Young PJ. Use of the LMA-Supreme™ for airway rescue. *Anesthesiology*. 2008;109:356.
142. Mort TC. Laryngeal mask airway and bougie intubation failures: the combitube as a secondary rescue device for in-hospital emergency airway management. *Anesth Analg*. 2006;103:1264–1266.

143. Matioc AA, Olson J. Use of the Laryngeal Tube™ in two unexpected difficult airway situations: lingular tonsillar hyperplasia and morbid obesity. *Can J Aneath*. 2004;51(10):1018–1021.
144. Wong DT, McGuire GP. Endotracheal intubation through a laryngeal mask/supraglottic airway. *Can J Anesth*. 2007;54(6):489–490.
145. Crosby ET, Cooper RM, Douglas MJ, et al. The unanticipated difficult airway with recommendations for management. *Can J Anesth*. 1998;45:759–776.
146. Rosenblatt WH, Whipple J. The difficult airway algorithm of the American society of anesthesiologists. *Anesth Analg*. 2003;96:1230–1242.
147. Matioc AA, Arndt G. The critical airway. *Can J Anesth*. 2005;52(9):993–995.
148. Lee LW. "Keep out of trouble" airway algorithm. *Can J Anesth*. 2005;52(9):995–996.
149. Crosby E. The unanticipated difficult airway-evolving strategies for successful salvage. *Can J Anesth*. 2005;52(6):562–567.
150. Hung O. Airway management: the good, the bad, and the ugly. *Can J Anesth*. 2002;49(8):767–771.
151. Hung O, Murphy M. Changing practice in airway management: are we there yet? *Can J Anesth*. 2004;51(10):963–968.
152. Keller D, Brimacombe J, Lirk P, Puhringer F. Failed obstetric tracheal intubation and post-operative respiratory support with the Proseal™ laryngeal mask airway. *Anesth Analg*. 2004;98:1467–1470.
153. Morillas P, Fornet I, de Miguel I, et al. Airway management in a patient with treacher collins syndrome requiring emergent cesarean section. *Anesth Analg*. 2007;105(1):294.
154. Gataure PS, Hughes JA. The laryngeal mask airway in obstetrical anaesthesia. *Can J Anaesth*. 1995;42(2):130.
155. Osses H et al. Laryngeal mask for difficult intubation in children. *Paediatr Anaesth*. 1999;9:339.
156. Walker RWM. The laryngeal mask airway in the difficult paediatric airway: an assessment of positioning and use in fibreoptic intubation. *Paediatr Anaesth*. 2000;10:53.
157. Keller C et al. The laryngeal mask airway Proseal™ as a temporary ventilatory device in grossly and morbidly obese patients before laryngoscope-guided tracheal intubation. *Anesth Analg*. 2002;94:737.
158. Frappier J, Guenoun T, Journois D, et al. Airway management using intubating laryngeal mask airway for the morbidly obese patient. *Anesth Analg*. 2003;96:1510–1515.
159. Coumbes X, Sauvat S, Leroux B, et al. Intubating laryngeal mask airway in morbidly obese and lean patients. *Anesthesiology*. 2005;102(6):1106–1109.
160. Natalini G, Franceschetti M, Pantelidi M, et al. Comparison of the standard laryngeal mask and the proseal laryngeal mask airway in obese patients. *Br J Anaesth*. 2003;90(3):323–326.
161. Dimitriou V et al. Letter. *Anesthesiology*. 1997;86(4):1011.
162. Giraud O et al. Limits of laryngeal mask airway in patients after cervical or oral radiotherapy. *Can J Anaesth*. 1997;44(2):1237.
163. Asai T, Shingu K. Tracheal intubation through the intubating laryngeal mask in a patient with a fixed flexed neck and deviated larynx. *Anaesthesia*. 1998;53:1199.
164. Asai T et al. Ease of placement of the laryngeal mask during manual in-line neck stabilization. *Br J Anaesth*. 1998;80(5):617.
165. Asai T et al. Placement of the intubating laryngeal mask is easier than the laryngeal mask during manual in-line neck stabilization. *Br J Anaesth*. 1999;82(5):712.
166. Nakazawa K et al. Using the intubating laryngeal mask airway (LMA-Fastrach™) for blind endotracheal intubation in patients undergoing cervical spine operations. *Anesth Analg*. 1999;89:1319.
167. Wakeling HG, Nightingale J. The intubating laryngeal mask airway does not facilitate tracheal intubation in the presence of a neck collar in simulated trauma. *Br J Anaesth*. 2000;84(2):254.
168. Moller F et al. Intubating laryngeal mask airway (iLMA) seems to be an ideal device for blind intubation in cases of immobile spine. *Br J Anaesth*. 2000;85(3):493.
169. International Anesthesia Clinics 1998;36(2): Spring Edition.

170. Brimacombe J et al. Laryngeal mask usage in the unstable neck. *Anesth Analg*. 1999;89(2):536.
171. Keller C, Brimacombe J, Keller K. Pressures exerted against the cervical vertebrae by the standard and intubating laryngeal mask airway. A randomized, controlled crossover study in fresh cadavers. *Anesth Analg*. 1999;89:1296–1300.
172. Brimacombe J, Keller C, Kunzel KH, et al. Cercical spine motion during airway management. A cinefluoroscopic study of the posteriorly destabilized third cervical veterbrae in human cadavers. *Anesth Analg*. 2000;91:1274–1278.
173. Kihara S et al. Segmental cervical spine movement with the intubating laryngeal mask during manual in-line stabilization in patients with cervical pathology undergoing cervical spine surgery. *Anesth Analg*. 2000;91:195.
174. Brimacombe J. Does the laryngeal mask have a role outside the operating theatre? *Can J Anaesth*. 1995;42(3):258.
175. Pollack CV. The laryngeal mask airway: a comprehensive review for the emergency physician. *J Emerg Med*. 2000;20(1):53.
176. Kurla JO, Turnen MJ, Laakso JP, et al. A comparison of the laryngeal tube and bag-valve-mask ventilation by emergency medical technicians: a feasibility study in anesthetized patients. *Anesth Analg*. 2005;101:1477–1481.
177. Timmermann A, Russo SG. Which airway should I use? *Curr Opin Anaesthesiol*. 2007;20(6):595–599.
178. Timmermann A, Russo SG, Rosenblatt WH, et al. Intubating laryngeal mask airway for difficult out-of-hospital airway management: a prospective evaluation. *Br J Anaesth*. 2007;99(2):286–291.
179. McCall MJ, Reeves M, Skinner M, et al. Paramedic tracheal intubation using the intubating laryngeal mask airway. *Prehosp Emerg Care*. 2008;12(1):30–34.
180. Berlac P, Hyldmo PK, Kongstad P, et al. Pre-hospital airway management: guidelines from a task force from the Scandinavian society for anaesthesiology and intensive care medicine. *Acta Anaesth Scand*. 2008;52(7):897–907.
181. Brain AIJ, Denman WT, Goudsouzian NG. *LMA-Classic and LMA-Flexible Instruction Manual*. San Diego: LMA North America, Inc.; 2000.
182. Bernards CM. An unusual cause of airway obstruction during general anesthesia with a laryngeal mask airway. *Anesthesiology*. 2004;100:1017–1018.
183. Asai T. Dental damage caused by the intubating laryngeal mask airway. *Anesth Analg*. 2006;103(3):785.
184. Haris ZM, Loo WT, Brimacombe J. Frenular injury during insertion of the proseal laryngeal mask airway using the introducer tool technique. *Anesth Analg*. 2006;102:1906–1907.
185. Hooda S et al. Acute transient sialadenopathy associated with laryngeal mask airway. *Anesth Analg*. 1998;87(6):1438.
186. Brimacombe J, Keller C. Sialadenopathy with the laryngeal mask airway. *Anesth Analg*. 1999;89:261.
187. Ogata J et al. The influence of the laryngeal mask airway on the shape of the submandibular glands. *Anesth Analg*. 2001;93:1069.
188. Maltby J et al. Acute transient unilateral macroglossia following use of a LMA. *Can J Anaesth*. 1996;43(1):94.
189. Branthwaite MA. An unexpected complication of the intubating laryngeal mask. *Anaesthesia*. 1999;54:166.
190. Casey ED, Donelly M, McCaul CL. Severe retropharyngeal abscess after the use of a reinforced laryngeal mask with a Bosworth introducer. *Anesthesiology*. 2009;110(4):943–945.
191. Devys JM et al. Biting the laryngeal mask: an unusual case of negative pressure pulmonary edema. *Can J Anesth*. 2000;47(2):176.
192. Brimacombe J, Clarke G, Keller C. Lingual nerve injury associated with the proseal laryngeal mask airway: a case report and review of the literature. *Br J Anaesth*. 2005;95:420–435.
193. Roy K, Kundra P, Ravishankar M. Unusual foreign body airway obstruction after laryngeal mask airway insertion. *Anesth Analg*. 2005;101:294–295.
194. Hardy D. An unusual case of laryngeal mask airway obstruction. *Can J Anesth*. 2003;50(9):969.

195. Wrobel M, Ziegeler S, Grundmann U. Airway obstruction due to cuff herniation of a classic reusable laryngeal mask airway. *Anesthesiology.* 2007;106(6):1255–1256.
196. Wong DT et al. Fractured laryngeal mask airway (LMA). *Can J Anesth.* 2000;47(7):716.
197. Mesa A, Miguel R. Hidden damage to a reinforced LMA-Fastrach™ endotracheal tube. *Anesth Analg.* 2000;90(1):1250.
198. Nagi H, Brown PC. Undetected hole in a laryngeal mask. *Anesth Analg.* 1999;88:232.
199. Asai T. Airway obstruction due to a damaged to the laryngeal mask. *Anesth Analg.* 2005;100:1549.
200. Christodoulou D. Proseal laryngeal mask airway foldover detection. *Anesth Analg.* 2004;99(3):312.
201. Brimacombe J, Keller C. Reply to 201. *Anesth Analg.* 2004;99(3):312.
202. Brimacombe J, Keller C. A proposed algorithm for the management of airway obstruction with the proseal laryngeal mask airway. *Anesth Analg.* 2005;100:289–299.
203. Anez C, Fuentes A, Jubera P. The proseal laryngeal mask airway interferes with magnetic resonance imaging. *Can J Anesth.* 2005;52(1):116–117.
204. Clery G, Brimacombe J, Stone T, et al. Routine cleaning and autoclaving does not remove protein deposits from reusable laryngeal mask devices. *Anesth Analg.* 2003;97:1189–1191.
205. Brimacombe J, Stone T, Keller C. Supplementary cleaning does not remove protein deposits from re-usable laryngeal mask devices. *Can J Anesth.* 2004;51(3):254–257.
206. Laupu W, Brimacombe J. Potassium permanganate reduces protein contamination of reusable laryngeal mask airways. *Anesth Analg.* 2004;99(2):614–616.
207. Coetzee GJ. Proteinaceous material on routinely cleaned laryngeal mask airways. *Anesth Analg.* 2004;98:1817–1818.
208. Walsh EM. Time to dispose of nondisposable LMAs. *Anesth Analg.* 2005;100:896.
209. Lenoir RJ. Venous congestion of the neck; its relation to laryngeal mask cuff pressures. *Br J Anaesth.* 2004;93:476–477.
210. Stacy MR, Sivasankar R, Bahlmann UB, et al. Mechanical closure of the vocal cords with the airway management device. *Br J Anaesth.* 2003;91(2):299.
211. Brimacombe J, Keller C. Response to Ref. 211. *Br J Anaesth.* 2003;91(2):299.
212. http://www.fda.gov/AboutFDA/Basics/ucm194468.htm. Accessed 20.02.10.
213. McCrirrick A, Ramage DT, Pracillo JA, et al. Experience with the laryngeal mask airway in two hundred patients. *Anaesth Intensive Care.* 1991;19:256–60.
214. Lopez-Gil M, Brimacombe J, Cebrain J, et al. Laryngeal mask airway in pediatric practice-a prospective study of skill acquisition by anesthesia residents. *Anesthesiology.* 1996;84:807–811.
215. www.asaclosedclaims.org. Accessed 22.02.10.
216. Miller CG. Management of the difficult intubation in closed malpractice claims. *ASA Newsl.* 2000;64(6):13–16.
217. Cheney FW. Aspiration: a liability hazard for the anesthesiologist? *ASA Newsl.* 2000;64(6):5–6; 26.
218. Crosby ET, Cooper R, Douglas MJ, et al. The unanticipated difficult airway with recommendations for management. *Can J Anaesth.* 1998;45:757–776.
219. Tasch MD, Stoelting RK. Aspiration prevention and prophylaxis: preoperative considerations. In: Hagberg CA, ed. *Benumof's Airway Management.* 2nd ed. Philadelphia: Mosby Elsevier; 2007:281–302.
220. Goldman AJ. E-lights of the SAM forum. *The Airway Gazette: Official Publication of the Society for Airway Management.* 2008;13(3):12–14.
221. Cook TM, Lee G, Nolan JP. The proseal laryngeal mask airway: a review of the literature. *Can J Anesth.* 2005;52(7):739–760.
222. Keller C, Brimacombe J, Bittersohl J, et al. Aspiration and the laryngeal mask airway: three cases and a review of the literature. *Br J Anaesth.* 2004;93(4):579–582.
223. Cooper RM. The LMA, laparoscopic surgery and the obese patient-can vs. should. *Can J Anesth.* 2003;50(1):5–10.

Chapter 6
Advanced Airway Devices

Contents

B.T. Finucane et al., *Principles of Airway Management*,
DOI 10.1007/978-0-387-09558-5_6, © Springer Science+Business Media, LLC 2011

Introduction

As anesthesia and technology advance, more powerful techniques and more complicated equipment are utilized for airway management. Although early equipment
was quite rudimentary, tremendous advances have been made during the past 50
years, and now modern-day equipment provides clinicians with sophisticated and
versatile methods of ventilation and intubation. The aim of this chapter is to provide
a brief description and information about a wide variety of commonly available
advanced airway devices beyond the basic oxygen supplies, standard mask, conventional laryngoscope, and endotracheal tubes discussed in Chap. 4.

Supra and Infraglottic Devices

Supraglottic Devices

Supraglottic devices are alternative devices to ensure airway patency by bridging the oral/pharyngeal space and to allow both positive pressure as well as spontaneous ventilation. Ideally, they produce low resistance to respiratory gas flow and protect the respiratory tract from gastric and nasal secretions. The ability of a foreign body to be accepted by the oropharynx largely depends upon its shape, cuff position, cuff volume, and material.[1] Supraglottic devices may be classified according to their sealing mechanism, and generally whether they are cuffed or anatomically preshaped.[2] Some can be considered cuffed perilaryngeal sealers (e.g., LMAs), some cuffed pharyngeal sealers (e.g., Combitube and Laryngeal Tube), and others uncuffed anatomically preshaped sealers (e.g., I-Gel Airway, Streamlined Liner of the Pharynx Airway). Within each group there may be preference for their use (reusable vs. single-use) and for their ability to protect the airway from aspiration of gastric contents. Several devices will be introduced below, although more discussion of these devices (particularly the LMA) can be found in Chap. 5.

Laryngeal Masks

The laryngeal mask airway (LMA), developed and described by AIJ Brain in 1983, seals the laryngeal inlet through an inflatable cuff that surrounds the entrance to the larynx.[3] Originally developed for routine cases of airway management with spontaneous ventilation, the LMA is now incorporated into the ASA Difficult Airway Algorithm and is described as useful in the AHA resuscitation guidelines. It is very safe and can be used as an airway, a conduit for endotracheal intubation, a mode of stress-reduced extubation, or as pressure support or positive pressure ventilation. It has also been described as part of a management strategy for accidental extubation of patients in the prone position.[4-6] The impact of this device on routine anesthetic practice is evident in view of the fact that 30–60% of all general anesthetic procedures are performed with an LMA.[1] Once newly manufactured devices hit the market (e.g., Softseal by Portex), these devices are collectively considered Laryngeal Masks rather than LMAs.

LMA Classic

The original LMA Classic (The Laryngeal Mask Company Ltd., St. Helier, UK or LMA North America, San Diego, CA) is composed of a curved tube attached to the lumen of a small ellipsoid bowl containing an inflatable cuff. The device has many advantages over the facemask, largely due to the "hands free" anesthesia that is offered. The device has excellent success for first time insertion and achieves an effective airway in approximately 30 s. The intracuff pressure should be limited to

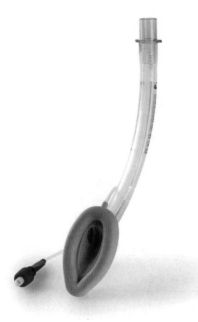

Fig. 6.1 LMA Classic (Copyright 2009 The Laryngeal Mask Company Limited, with permission)

≤60 cm H_2O, in order to avoid oropharyngeal mucosal damage. So rather than increasing pressure to compensate for low airway leak pressures, it is suggested to adjust the device position or reinsert the device.[1] While this classic device (Fig. 6.1) is still widely used today, modified versions may replace its use due to their ability to either protect against aspiration, or serve as a conduit for intubation, or both. Because one of the main disadvantages of the LMA Classic is the production of seal pressures below those adequate for positive pressure ventilation, newer versions have been developed with improved structure for providing higher seal pressures.

LMA Unique and Portex Softseal (Single-Use Variants of LMA Classic)

There are several single-use products on the market, including:

- LMA-Unique (The Laryngeal Mask Company Ltd., St. Helier, UK or LMA North America, San Diego, CA) (Fig. 6.2).
- Portex Softseal LM (Smiths Medical International Limited, Hythe, UK).
- Ambu AuraOnce LM (Ambu Inc., Glen Burnie, MD).

These were generally introduced since it was found that protein deposits remain on reusable LMAs and thus may contribute to disease transmission.[7] This, as well as the desire to reduce time spent on cleaning and preparing the LMAs, has led to the production of several single-use variants. These devices have been shown to perform similarly to reusable LMAs with respect to ease of insertion and incidences of bleeding and postoperative sore throat.[8] The lack of increased cuff pressure during

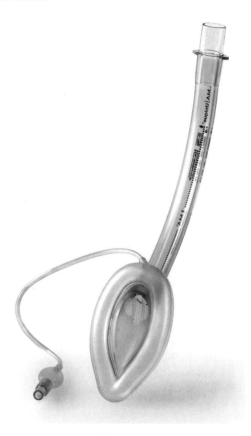

Fig. 6.2 LMA Unique (Copyright 2009 The Laryngeal Mask Company Limited, with permission)

anesthesia with nitrous oxide, as seen with the Classic LMA, offers additional
evidence of their clinical feasibility.

LMA ProSeal

The ProSeal (The Laryngeal Mask Company Ltd., St. Helier, UK or LMA North
America, San Diego, CA) variant of the LMA Classic provides higher seal pressures and protection against aspiration (it can be considered the "gastric LMA").
It features a dorsal cuff (in sizes 3.0 and up), which pushes the ventral cuff into the
periglottic tissue, effectively directing the pressure against the glottis off the posterior
pharyngeal wall (Fig. 6.3). For detailed description of the forces produced by various
supraglottic airways, the reader is referred to Miller's[2] work, which proposes a classification and scoring system for these devices. The airway tube has been wire-
reinforced to allow for the double-lumen structure, whereby an incorporated
drainage tube allows passage of a gastric tube. The protection of aspiration will be
highly dependent upon the position of the device on the laryngeal inlet.[9] This device

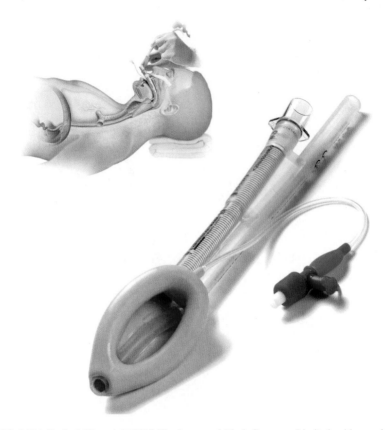

Fig. 6.3 LMA ProSeal (Copyright 2009 The Laryngeal Mask Company Limited, with permission)

is also available in pediatric sizes 1.5 and 2. Cook, Lee, and Nolan[10] have written a highly comprehensive review of this device.

LMA Flexible (Wire-Reinforced Flexible LMA)

This LMA (The Laryngeal Mask Company Ltd., St. Helier, UK or LMA North America, San Diego, CA) has a wire-reinforced flexible airway intended for use in ENT procedures where the device allows access to the surgical field without loss of seal (Fig. 6.4). The airway tube, which is smaller than that of other LMAs, is of similar internal diameter to endotracheal tubes. These tubes are available in reusable and single-use versions and in sizes suitable for adults and children.

LMA Supreme

The LMA Supreme (The Laryngeal Mask Company Ltd., St. Helier, UK or LMA North America, San Diego, CA) is a single-use LMA (as is the LMA Unique) which features a gastric drain tube located within its airway tube, a strengthened

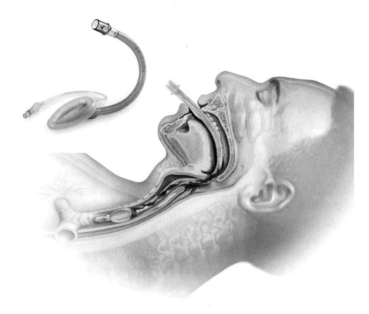

Fig. 6.4 LMA Flexible (Copyright 2009 The Laryngeal Mask Company Limited, with permission)

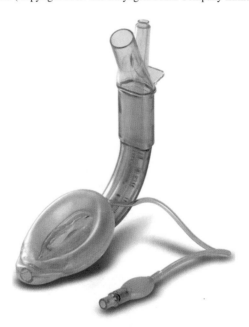

Fig. 6.5 LMA Supreme (Copyright 2009 The Laryngeal Mask Company Limited, with permission)

inner cuff to prevent airway obstruction from infolding, and epiglottic fins to prevent epiglottic downfolding (wedging of the epiglottis in the airway) (Fig. 6.5).[11]
In comparison to the reusable LMA ProSeal (both enabling gastric access and
providing high seal pressures), the LMA Supreme provided similar insertion

success (35/36), glottic seal pressure (28 cm H_2O), and gastric access in 36 female paralyzed and anesthetized patients.[12]

LMA Fastrach (Intubating LMA)

The LMA Fastrach (The Laryngeal Mask Company Ltd., St. Helier, UK or LMA North America, San Diego, CA) is intended for use in the management of both anticipated and unanticipated difficult tracheal intubation situations, as well as for rapid oxygenation and ventilation in failed intubation scenarios (Fig. 6.6). It may be particularly useful for rescuers who are inexperienced with tracheal intubation, since it allows for continuous ventilation during intubation. It may also prove beneficial for intubation in the presence of in-line neck stabilization.[13] Intubation is accomplished by the passage of an 8.00 mm cuffed endotracheal tube and is facilitated by elevation of the epiglottis (with its elevating bar) and a ramp that directs the tube centrally and anteriorly. Baskett et al.[14] showed the device to have a success rate for blind tracheal intubation of over 96% within three attempts and to have excellent rates of providing satisfactory ventilation.

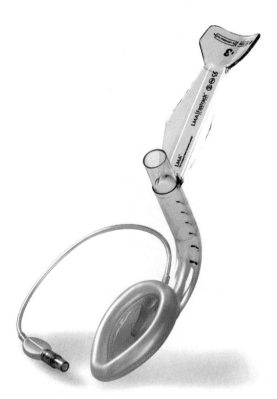

Fig. 6.6 LMA Fastrach (Copyright 2009 The Laryngeal Mask Company Limited, with permission)

LMA CTrach

The LMA CTrach (The Laryngeal Mask Company Ltd., St. Helier, UK or LMA North America, San Diego, CA) is an intubating LMA (as is the LMA Fastrach), which contains fiberoptics to enable viewing on a liquid crystal display (the Viewer) (Fig. 6.7). Once the airway is secured and ventilation initiated, the wireless and portable Viewer (<200 g) is attached to the airway via a magnetic connector and a clear image of the larynx can be displayed on the screen, thus allowing real-time visualization of the intubation. At the distal end of the airway tube, fiberoptic bundles emerge under the modified Epiglottic Elevating Bar, the latter facilitating endotracheal tube passage. After insertion of the LMA CTrach (as with the LMA Fastrach), maneuvers may be required for optimizing ventilation ("up and down" including withdrawal for 6 cm and reinsertion) and enabling the smooth passage of the endotracheal tube during intubation (part of the Chandy maneuver including lifting of the LMA CTrach away from the posterior laryngeal wall to avoid collision with arytenoids).[15] Even though the LMA CTrach can be sterilized, the fiberoptics deteriorate with use and the image quality will not match that offered by video laryngoscopes or fiberoptic bronchoscopes.[16]

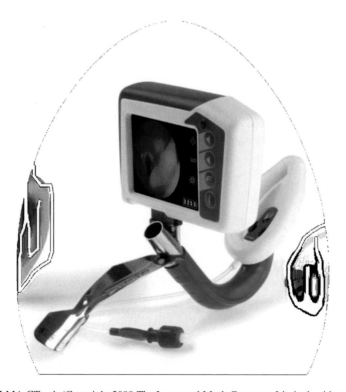

Fig. 6.7   LMA CTrach (Copyright 2009 The Laryngeal Mask Company Limited, with permission)

Initial evaluation of the LMA CTrach in surgical patients with normal airways found that this device offered high success with insertion and ventilation (100%), as well as intubation on first attempt (≥96%), but variable views of the larynx (84% laryngeal view or 40% grade III and IV).[17, 18] Further evaluation of the initial laryngeal views (as assessed with fiberoptic laryngoscopy) and the effectiveness of subsequent corrective measures in 100 patients found that downfolding of the epiglottis was the most common cause of poor views (57 of 69 patients) and simple corrective measures were effective in most patients. Overall, this study recorded high rates of ventilation (100%), glottic viewing (94%), and intubation (97%).[19] The high intubation rates, despite common initial grade III and IV views, of these studies suggest that the LMA CTrach can successfully enable intubation in the difficult airway.

Intubation through an intubating LMA (ILMA) such as LMA Fastrach can be performed blindly, but the first-attempt success rate can be improved with fiberoptic tracheal intubation through the ILMA. Tracheal intubation using the LMA CTrach has been compared to both blind and fiberoptically assisted intubation using an ILMA. The LMA CTrach enabled higher first- attempt and overall success with intubation compared to blind intubation through the LMA. Yet, Fastrach (93.3% vs. 67.9% and 100% vs. 96.4%) required more time due to optimizing maneuvers to view the larynx. Again, the lack of correlation between Cormack and Lehane grade and intubation parameters indicates that these devices are useful for difficult airway management.[16] Compared to the fiberoptically assisted intubation through the ILMA, the LMA CTrach requires less time (31 s less) for intubation and does not require the operator to have skills with endoscopy. The use of the LMA CTrach was preferred to that of the fiberoptically assisted ILMA technique.[20]

Quantitatively reviewing the performance of nonstandard laryngoscopes (bladed laryngoscopes, optical bougies, and conduits) and rigid fiberoptic intubation (FOI) aids in adult patients. Mihai et al.[21] found that the LMA CTrach and the Bonfils were the only devices that were studied in homogeneous studies (via chi-square test for heterogenicity) and had >90% first-attempt and overall success rates in both normal and difficult airways.

Laryngeal Tube and Laryngeal Tube S

The laryngeal tube (LT) was designed as an alternative to intubation or mask ventilation and for use during positive pressure ventilation or spontaneous breathing. It has a single-lumen, two low-pressure cuffs (pharyngeal and esophageal) in order to seal the pharyngeal airway and esophageal inlet, and an intermediary ventilation outlet which is placed in front of the vocal cords. The newer LTS (LT & LTS: VBM Medizintechnik GmbH, Sulz, Germany, or King Systems, Indianapolis, MN) has a suction port allowing the passage of an (up to) 18 French gastric tube in order to improve the device's ability to protect the airway from aspiration of gastric contents. Dorges and colleagues[22, 23] have shown that the devices are easy to use (100% first-attempt rate) and provide seals adequate for peak airway pressures.

Further studies have shown that the LT provides similar ease of insertion with a higher peak pressure than the Classic LMA, although may be less effective than the LMA ProSeal during controlled ventilation under general anesthesia.[24, 25] One main disadvantage with the device as shown in these studies is that it may require adjustments in position to obtain a clear airway. Adjustments to obtain ventilation include lifting the angle of the mandible vertically, further extension of the patient's head, turning the patient's head to the side, and a gentle push or pull of the device.[26] This readjustment may be most applicable to its use in children.[26] While the LT is available in sizes from newborn to adult, the LTS is only available for small to large adults. The use of the LT in children has not been studied with any sufficiency. Both the LT and LTS are available in reusable or disposable versions.

I-Gel Airway

In contrast to LMAs, which are supraglottic airway devices that involve inflation of the mask to provide a perilaryngeal seal, the I-Gel (Intersurgical Ltd., Wokingham, Berkshire, UK) is composed of a gel-like thermoplastic elastomer which fits anatomically within the perilaryngeal and hypopharyngeal structures (Fig. 6.8). There is a gastric channel for gastric tube exchange, a bite guard to improve the device's patency (prevent occlusion), and a widened buccal cavity to reduce axial rotation and, thus, maintain its position. It can be used suitably for perioperative airway management, positive pressure ventilation, and weaning from ventilation. It may also be used as an intubation aid as well as during resuscitation. Easy insertion of a gastric tube will help confirm the device's proper placement in front of the larynx.[27] In a cadaver study, the I-Gel consistently achieved proper positioning for supraglottic ventilation.[28] The mean percentage of glottic opening (as seen through the lumen) for 73 insertions in 65 nonembalmed cadavers was 82%, with all insertions producing at least 50% glottic opening. Experience in adult surgical patients has

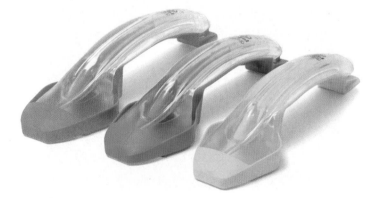

Fig. 6.8 I-Gel Airway (Copyright 2009 Intersurgical Incorporated, with permission)

thus far shown the device to be easy to insert, remove, and use, without causing trauma or impeding access during nasal or eye surgery.

The I-Gel was successfully applied within 10 s in all but 3 of 300 patients.[29] Studying the ease and efficacy of I-Gel insertion for use as a resuscitation aid in 50 manikins and 40 anesthetized patients, Wharton et al.[30] found that the I-Gel was successfully (82.5% at first and 97.5% at second attempt) and rapidly (17.5 s, range 7–197) inserted by novice users and compared favorably with other supraglottic devices. A neck extension maneuver was used for insertion in 57.5% of patients. In children, the I-Gel has shown to be very easy to insert and carry a high success rate (100% first attempt). Moreover, a positive pressure was easy to achieve without gastric inflation or pharyngeal leak.[27]

Cobra Perilaryngeal Airway (PLA)

The CobraPLA (Engineered Medical Systems, Indianapolis, IN) is a cuffed, pharyngeal sealer, supraglottic airway which is disposable, sterile, and latex-free (Fig. 6.9). The construction of it consists of: a head containing slotted openings to hold both the soft tissue and epiglottis away and permit air exchange, a circumferential pharyngeal large-volume, low-pressure cuff, and a breathing tube which can

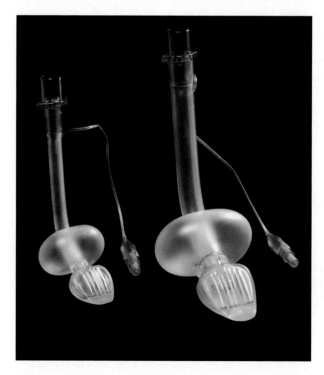

Fig. 6.9 Cobra Perilaryngeal Airway (Copyright 2009 Engineered Medical Systems, with permission)

be attached to a standard 15 mm ID connector. There is a distal curve in the breathing tube to avoid kinking. A recently introduced model, The Cobra Plus, contains both a distal thermistor probe (for core temperature) and a gas sampling line for the three smallest pediatric sizes. Its use does not prevent gastric regurgitation and pulmonary aspiration, thus it should not be used in aspiration-risk patients. A review of the clinical experience with the CobraPLA between 1996 and 2006 summarized this device as one which had been used primarily to maintain the airway during spontaneous and controlled ventilation for short surgical procedures.[31] It was shown to have similar insertion times and first-pass success as the LMA Classic, but has higher airway sealing pressures. Its use may be preferable to the LMA Classic for patients with limited mouth opening or if the use of a Classic LMA results in a poor seal. Findings from a recent comparison of the Classic LMA with the CobraPLA agreed that the PLA provides a superior seal to the LMA, and also found it did this at a lower intracuff pressure.

Streamlined Liner of Pharyngeal Airway (SLIPA)

The noncuffed, single-use SLIPA (Medical Ltd, London, UK) is designed like the LMA Unique and is intended for use in an emergency or as a primary airway device for short surgical procedures.[32] The primary aim of its development by Miller was for reducing the chance of aspiration as compared to conventional LMAs. Its preformed shape, the hollow blow-molded chamber with a toe, a bridge that seals at the base of the tongue, and a heel for anchoring the device between the esophagus and nasopharynx, lines the larynx, so positive pressure ventilation can be achieved without cuff inflation[33] Clinically, the SLIPA has similar efficacy to the ProSeal[33] and Classic LMA.[34] Although its large chamber (capacity of up to 50 mL) may hold the volume of most fasted patient's gastric contents, its efficacy in prevention of aspiration requires further study. The insertion technique differs from that for the LMAs; therefore, there may be a learning curve.[35]

Infraglottic Devices

Combitube

The Combitube (Tyco-Kendall-Sheridan, Mansfield, MA) or ETC (esophagotracheal Combitube) is a variation of the esophageal obturator airway that may be useful in the event of a difficult intubation or the "can't intubate, can't ventilate" situation.[36, 37] It is also increasingly used in clinical anesthesiology where endotracheal intubation is contraindicated. The Combitube (Fig. 6.10) is a double-lumen tube with an open distal end on the longer lumen and eight small perforations at the supraglottic level of the second lumen, which has a blind end.[38] No preparations are required for intubation, although a laryngoscope is recommended for experienced

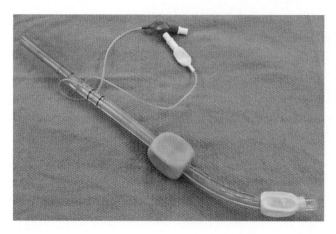

Fig. 6.10 Combitube

users during insertion. If it enters the esophagus, which is the most likely destination following a blind insertion, the esophageal cuff is inflated to prevent regurgitation around the tube. The proximal cuff occupies the pharynx above the airway and prevents leakage externally through the mouth and nose. The perforations in the esophageal lumen allow ventilation of the airway. If the ETC enters the trachea, ventilation may take place via the tracheal lumen.

This device is a major advance over the esophageal obturator airway, which proved to be quite dangerous if accidentally inserted into the airway. The major disadvantage of the ETC is that it does not allow suctioning of the trachea if it enters the esophagus.

The efficacy of the Combitube has been tested in field management of the airway by Rumball et al.[39] They compared successful insertion of the Combitube, the pharyngotracheal lumen airway (PTLA), the LMA, and an oral airway by EMTs in 470 cardiac arrest victims. The Combitube was inserted successfully and ventilation achieved in 86% of patients, compared with 82% with the PTLA and 73% with the LMA. The Combitube may be more advantageous in the field and the emergency room, where those performing airway management are more familiar with it and where patients are more likely to regurgitate. The LMA may be more advantageous in an operating room setting, where anesthesiologists are more familiar with its use and where passive regurgitation is less likely to occur. There is a greater risk of damage to the airway, the pharynx, or the esophagus when the Combitube is used by inexperienced personnel.[40]

Easy Tube

The Easy Tube (EzT) (Teleflex Medical, Rusch, Kernen, Germany) was developed for airway management in emergencies and difficult airways.[41] This disposable device combines the essential features of an endotracheal tube with those of a

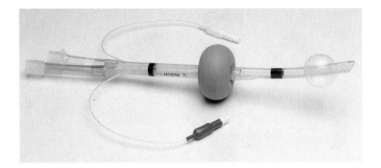

Fig. 6.11 Easy tube (Copyright 2009 Teleflex Incorporated, with permission)

supraglottic device (Fig. 6.11). It is a sterile, single-use double-lumen tube with a pharyngeal proximal cuff and a distal cuff and is positioned either blindly or using a laryngoscope. Blind insertion likely positions the tip within the esophagus in 95% of cases.[38] It provides sufficient ventilation whether it is placed in the esophagus or trachea. One of the lumen opens as if it were a tracheal tube and the other lumen serves as a supraglottic ventilation outlet between the two cuffs. The pharyngeal aperture allows for a flexible fiberoptic bronchoscope, bougie, or suction catheter. The initial experience with this device in patients with unanticipated difficult airways is encouraging.[42]

Laryngoscope Handles and Blades

Handles

Both conventional and fiberoptic laryngoscopes come with a variety of handles in several profiles, from pediatric, penlight/slender, standard, and large, to bantam (shorter and lighter than standard) and adjustable. Adjustable handles, such as the Penlon and Patil-Syracuse designs (Anesthesia Associates Inc. San Marcos, CA) (Fig. 6.12), allow the blade to be positioned at varying angles for special purposes, including the 45° angle achieved by the Howland adapter/lock. Early fiberoptic laryngoscope handles and blades were not compatible between manufacturers, but with standardization, the green system of laryngoscopes allows interchangeability between different manufacturer's handles and blades.

There has been much discussion in the literature about the lack of clear protocols for cleaning laryngoscope handles between uses and about subsequent cases of cross-infection.[43-46] The ASA also does not provide specific guidelines on disinfection. Some groups advocate for thorough low-level sterilization, at minimum, while others suggest high-level sterilization is prudent.[44,47]

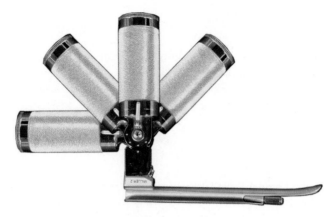

Fig. 6.12 Patil-Syracuse adjustable laryngoscope handle (Copyright 2009 Anesthesia Associates Inc. [AincA], San Marcos, CA, with permission)

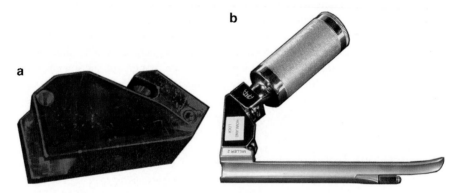

Fig. 6.13 (a) Howland lock (Copyright 2009 Anesthesia Associates Inc. [AincA], San Marcos, CA, with permission) (**b**) with Bantam handle and Miller-2 blade (Copyright 2009 Anesthesia Associates Inc. [AincA], San Marcos, CA, with permission)

Howland Adapter/Lock

The Howland adapter (Anesthesia Associates Inc. San Marcos, CA) (Fig. 6.13a, b) is an example of how the laryngoscope handle may be modified to aid exposure of the larynx, even in the presence of a receding chin, anterior larynx, protruding teeth, "bull neck," facial confractures, and decreased jaw mobility. This modification decreases the angle that the blade makes with the horizontal axis of the patient, providing a definite mechanical advantage. However, because of the design of the handle, it may be difficult to insert the blade into the mouth, especially in patients with an increased anteroposterior chest diameter. Ideally, the Howland adapter should have a shorter handle.

Blades

The "ultimate" blade has not yet been designed, but more study of the shape, size, and classification of laryngoscope blades is under way. In the future, selection of the best blade for intubation in the widest variety of clinical scenarios should be more predictable, based upon scientific data rather than traditional clinical bias and anecdote.[48-51]

Left-Handed Macintosh Blade

Left-handed Macintosh blades (Anesthesia Associates Inc. San Marcos, CA) may have originally been designed for left-handed anesthesiologists, but since both hands must be dextrous when using the laryngoscope, its application is most notable in facilitating intubation by using the left side of the mouth when anatomical abnormalities exist on the right side of the face and mouth[52,53] (Fig. 6.14). This reverse Macintosh laryngoscope is held in the right hand while the left hand places the endotracheal tube.[54]

Polio Blade

The polio blade (Anesthesia Associates Inc. San Marcos, CA) is also a modification of the Macintosh and was made by altering the angle between the blade and the handle (Fig. 6.15).[55] It was originally designed for use in patients confined to the Drinker respirator (iron lung). It may now be used when the anteroposterior diameter of the chest is such that insertion of a laryngoscope into the mouth is impossible. Its main disadvantage is that all mechanical advantages of the conventional blade are lost.[56] Alternatively, a regular Macintosh blade with a "stunted" handle may be used.

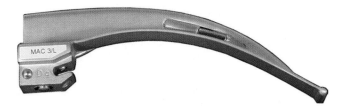

Fig. 6.14 Left-handed Macintosh blade (Copyright 2009 Anesthesia Associates Inc. [AincA], San Marcos, CA, with permission)

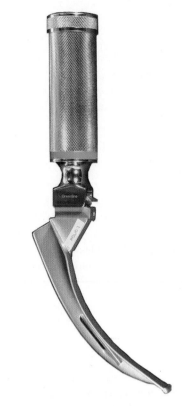

Fig. 6.15 Polio blade (Copyright 2009 Anesthesia Associates Inc. [AincA], San Marcos, CA, with permission)

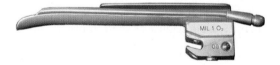

Fig. 6.16 Miller-Port blade (Copyright 2009 Anesthesia Associates Inc. [AincA], San Marcos, CA, with permission)

Oxiport Blades

Both Macintosh and Miller blades (Anesthesia Associates Inc. San Marcos, CA) have been modified to include an oxygen port (Fig. 6.16), allowing the oxygenation (and other gas mixtures) of patients during intubation attempts.

Siker Blade (Mirror Laryngoscope)

The Siker blade (Anesthesia Associates Inc. San Marcos, CA) is curved and contains a mirror located 3 cm proximal from the tip (Fig. 6.17).[57] This blade may help see the anterior larynx and may enable laryngoscopy with less neck hyperextension

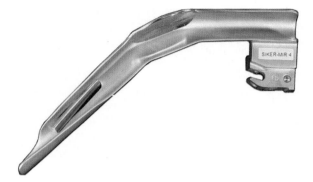

Fig. 6.17 Siker blade size 4 (Copyright 2009 Anesthesia Associates Inc. [AincA], San Marcos, CA, with permission)

than when using the Macintosh blade. This laryngoscope is awkward to use, however, since practice is required to interpret the inverted image.

Belscope

The Belscope (Avulunga Pty. Ltd., Murwillumbah, Australia) is an angulated laryngoscope blade. The straight blade has been modified to form a wide V-shaped angle.[58, 59] It was designed to improve the view of the larynx in cases of difficult intubation where the curved Macintosh blade may obscure vision. Further, the distance between the upper teeth and the vertical portion of the blade is greater than with the Miller blade, such that the mandible will not need to be forcibly drawn anteroinferiorly, risking dental damage.[60] The view beyond the blade may, though, be obscured when the blade angle cannot be pulled forward sufficiently during insertion for the larynx to be seen directly. This blade has been designed to fit a prism for obtaining an indirect view around the corner.

Levering Laryngoscope Blades

Laryngoscopes with a "levering" tip have been introduced into practice. These scopes generally employ a Macintosh blade with a hinged tip that can be "levered" upward, causing the tip to exert more force to the vallecula, a maneuver that purportedly will more efficiently elevate the epiglottis. It is postulated that less lifting needs be applied to the scope and that neck movement can be minimized. Avoiding neck movement might make laryngoscopy safer for patients with cervical spine pathology.

McCoy Levering Laryngoscope

The McCoy Levering Laryngoscope (InterMed Penlon Ltd., Abingdon, UK) is one of the first levering laryngoscopes designed.[61] This is another modification

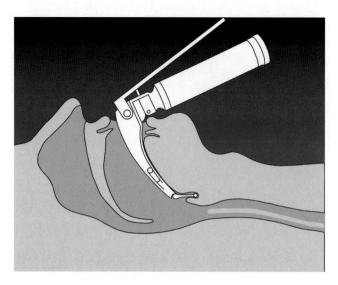

Fig. 6.18 McCoy levering laryngoscope (Copyright 2009 Penlon Ltd., Abingdon, UK, with permission)

(originally of the standard Macintosh blade) that enables you to have a good view of the vocal apparatus without the force often required when using the Macintosh blade in difficult situations.[62, 63] The blade is designed to eliminate contact with the upper teeth and to have its fulcrum at a lower point within the pharynx. Its tip is hinged, and the angle of the hinged portion can be altered by a lever attached to the handle (Fig. 6.18).

The main advantage of this modification is improved visualization without altering the axis of the handle. In a small clinical trial involving about 50 patients with simulated difficult airways via neck immobilization in the neutral position, laryngoscopic views improved by one grade in 70% of patients with a grade 2 Cormack and Lehane view and 83% of patients with a grade 3 view, compared with the view obtained with the standard Macintosh blade. However, no improvement occurred with a grade 4 view.[64] These results have been corroborated by other investigators.[65-67]

The utility of this design of laryngoscope blade is still under investigation. Some authors report that it is useful when neck extension is limited or undesirable.[64, 68] The stress responses to laryngoscopy may be reduced when using the McCoy in comparison to the Macintosh blade, and pretreatment with opioids is not required when using this blade.[62, 69] Others report that the McCoy blade can be used to facilitate FOI even if the laryngoscopic view is not significantly improved.[70, 71] The reports of Randell et al.[72] and Ochroch and Levitan[73] suggest that laryngoscopic visualization is more improved by external tracheal manipulations ("B.U.R.P." maneuver) than by utilization of the McCoy scope placed in the "sniff" position for elective intubation of patients. One case report by Usui et al.[74] documents arytenoid dislocation in a patient intubated with a McCoy scope (this injury is also reported with standard blade designs). A disadvantage of using a lever to operate the blade tip is that the grip on the handle must be relaxed (at a time necessary for maximal stability and control) in order to use the thumb to depress the lever.[75] Benham and Gale[75] describe how the lever can be operated by a button mechanism attached to a secondary handle attached to the standard handle. Currently, this blade is manufactured with Macintosh designs for sizes 3 and 4 and Seward designs for sizes 1 and 2.

Pediatric McCoy

The pediatric version of the McCoy blade comes in a straight Seward style. A study comparing the pediatric McCoy (#1) with the conventional Miller (#1) blade for laryngoscopy and intubation of 40 normal infants found that the McCoy blade had no advantages over the Miller in laryngoscopy and may in fact delay intubation.[76]

Dorges Universal

The Dorges blade (Karl Storz GmbH, Tuttlingen, Germany) was designed to be universal with several features designed to facilitate tracheal intubation. The blade has a lower profile (height 15 mm vs. 22 mm) which requires less mouth opening than a Macintosh laryngoscope blade size 3 or 4. The space requirements and costs required would be reduced if using this blade as compared to the Macintosh, since only one or two blades would be required. A preliminary comparison with the Macintosh blades sizes 2–4 found that orotracheal intubation in an adult airway management trainer took significantly less time when using the Dorges blade.[77] In a high-fidelity simulator in both normal and difficult airway settings, the McCoy, Macintosh, and Dorges blades performed similarly, suggesting that the use of an alternative blade in unsuccessful difficult intubation may be unsupported.[78]

Viewmax

Designed to improve the view of the vocal cords during intubation, the Viewmax laryngoscope (Rusch, Deluth, GA) is a curved blade alongside which is a view tube containing a patented lens system (Fig. 6.19). The use of this blade requires an unconventional technique and the learning curve for this technique, as performed in manikins with normal airways, seems steep. A manikin study showed that the Viewmax provided a better laryngeal view than the McCoy and Macintosh laryngoscopes, but provided no advantage in the success of intubation and in fact took longer to use than the other blades.[79]

While it is commonly reported that intubation times may be longer with the optical laryngoscopes (and therefore they may not be useful during rapid sequence intubation), the failure to improve success is also noteworthy. Furthermore, the

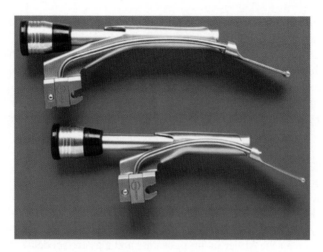

Fig. 6.19 Viewmax laryngoscope (Copyright 2009 Teleflex Incorporated, with permission)

view tube provides a narrower and smaller field of vision and its angulated view of
the larynx necessitates a gum elastic bougie to direct the endotracheal tube.
The view tube requires separate disinfection process to prevent damage to the lens
and an antifog wipe should be at hand to avoid fogging.[79]

Fiberoptic Laryngoscopes

Fiberoptically assisted intubation is one of the most important advances in airway
management since the introduction of the laryngoscope. It allows endotracheal
intubation to be performed even in the most difficult circumstances.

Truview EVO2

The Truview blade (Truphatek Holdings Ltd., Netanya, Isreal), designed with an
optical system and a specially profiled slim steel blade, is indicated especially for
cases where neck extension is limited. The view field is enlarged via a 46° refrac-
tion angle and an oxygen port provides flow at 10 L/min to oxygenate while also
keeping the lens clear of secretions and fogging. The Truview eyepiece can be connected to an endoscopic camera head with a monitor to enable training. A comparison of laryngoscopy and intubation using the Truview blade and the Macintosh
blade in 170 patients found that the Truview blade offered a better laryngoscopic
view, produced less force during intubation, and resulted in less bleeding and soft
tissue damage following intubation.[80] The duration of intubation was longer,

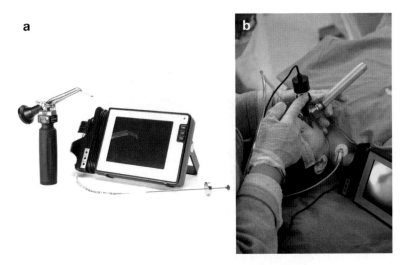

Fig. 6.20 (**a**) Truview pediatric set. (**b**) In use (Copyright 2009 Truphatek International Ltd., with permission)

though, which would limit its use in some cases. A study in manikins with normal and difficult airways found similar results, concluding that the Truview did not facilitate endotracheal intubation in any of the difficult scenarios created.[81] The time taken for intubation in this study was significantly, statistically but not clinically, longer for the Truview blade. The Truview has recently become available in an infant size and has shown to compare favorably to the Miller blade (size 0) for glottic view (Figs. 6.20a, b).[82]

Heine FlexTip+

This is a MacIntosh blade with a tip which is adjustable through 70°. The handle contains a lever to control the movement at the tip (Fig. 6.21). There are integrated fiber optics in this blade. Heine (Heine USA Ltd., Dover, NH) also produces Mac Modular+ and Miller Modular Fiberoptic Laryngoscopic blades.

Flipper

This fiberoptic laryngoscope blade (Rusch, Teleflex Medical, Durham, NC) is designed to provide more anterior exposure during difficult intubation (Fig. 6.22). It has an articulating tip which can be raised via a lever attached to the handle. Rusch produces several other fiberoptic laryngoscopes (Emerald and Snaplight and FOCS).

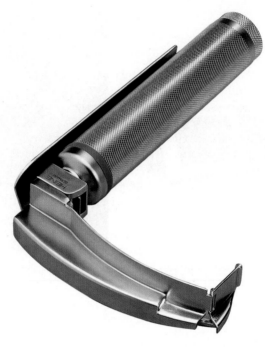

Fig. 6.21 Heine Flexible tip laryngoscope blade (Copyright 2009 Heine Ltd., with permission)

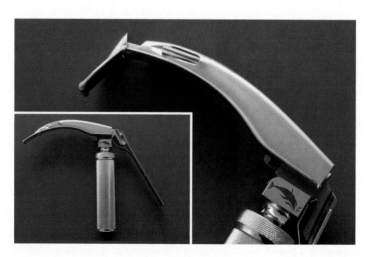

Fig. 6.22 Flipper fiberoptic laryngoscope (Copyright 2009 Teleflex Incorporated, with permission)

Bullard

The Bullard laryngoscope (Circon Corp., Santa Barbara, CA) was designed for difficult intubations.[83,84] Consisting of a rigid curved blade with a fiberoptic bundle posteriorly, it may be used in both adults and children. It is battery operated or may be connected to a light source. It comes with an eyepiece attached to the main body of the scope at a 45° angle, and a teaching head is also available. The Elite version comes with the suction channel which can be used to deliver oxygen to patients. The Bullard device is not immediately user-friendly, however, and practice on normal airways is recommended first.

Some studies have shown that the learning curve for the Bullard laryngoscope is similar to that required to learn fiberoptic-assisted intubation.[83,85] The Bullard laryngoscope functions well with the head and neck in the neutral position and when there is limited mouth opening. It has two ports, one for oxygen, suction, or injection, and the other to house a malleable, intubating stylet. A number of studies have reported high success rates when the Bullard is used in difficult airway situations by experienced personnel.[86]

WuScope

Described in 1994, the WuScope (Achi Corp., Freemont, CA) was designed to facilitate endotracheal intubation for the routine or difficult airway in the awake or anesthetized patient, and via the oral or nasal route. Intubation is performed with the patient in the neutral head position. The WuScope is a combination of a rigid laryngoscope blade (tubular, curved, and bivalved) and a flexible fiberscope (Fig. 6.23).[87] The handle receives the fiberscope body, and the main blade and bivalve element form passageways for the endotracheal tube and the fiberscope insertion cord, with an oxygen channel located alongside the latter passageway.

While the endotracheal tube passageway should remove the need for a stylet, O'Neill et al.[88] reported that they found the use of an intubation guide (Flexiguide) helpful in some patients. This intubating device has applicability in a large range of situations, including emergency awake intubation and tube exchange in critical care, and for numerous difficult scenarios (e.g., obesity, pharyngeal obstruction, cervical spinal lesions).[87,89] The use of the device is limited technically in cases where blood and secretions, or anatomic derangements such as tumors, are in the airway. As with other flexible fiberscopes, care should be taken when handling and assembling.[90]

One needs to keep in mind the observations of Bucx et al.,[91] Tousignant and Tessler,[92] and Fletcher[93] when using fiberoptic laryngoscopes that are designed with the light source in the handle of the scope. The light is transmitted toward the tip of the blade with a fiberoptic channel. When new and functioning optimally, the light intensity directed toward the airway is bright and focused. However, sterilization

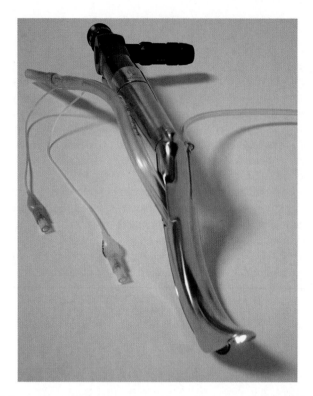

Fig. 6.23 WuScope fiberoptic laryngoscope with double-lumen tube (Copyright 2009 Achi Corp., with permission)

and handling of the blades can compromise the quality and intensity of the light directed into the airway.[91] The quality of the light produced with traditional scopes can also be altered with cleaning and handling, and the bulbs and batteries need to be checked on a regular basis. Some newer blades have an incorporated, but removable, light source that will remove the bulb from the oral cavity and allow standard handles to be used.

Video Laryngoscopes

Video laryngoscopes may aid in laryngoscopy and intubation due to a variety of factors. The magnified view enables easier identification of anatomy and anomalies, and the ability for the operator to have valuable assistance (e.g., for external laryngeal manipulation) when required. Effective coordination of efforts between operator and assistant is possible as both can see the exact same image. Chapter 11 discusses in greater detail the variety of fiberoptic endoscopes such as bronchoscopes, laryngoscopes, rhinoscopes, intubating laryngoscopes, and portable scopes, while this chapter focuses on video laryngoscopes. The video laryngoscope will also be very valuable for teaching purposes to help avoid unnecessary intubation attempts.[94] No attempt was made to include every available system, and new systems will without doubt be marketed while this chapter goes to press. One example of a new system not discussed is the C-MAC video laryngoscope system by Karl Storz Endoscopy. A discussion of results found from comparisons of indirect laryngoscopy devices follows after the descriptions below.

Storz DCI Video Intubating System

Berci, Kaplan, and Ward[94] designed a video laryngoscope system (Karl Storz Endoscopy, Mississauga, Canada), incorporating a TV camera into a standard Macintosh laryngoscope handle, with a short image-light bundle threaded into a small metal guide in the blade to reach two thirds of the length of the blade (Fig. 6.24). The cart that is required to carry the video equipment (and comes as part of the Universal Intubating System) contains an 8-in. monitor positioned on a swivel arm to enable the intubator to position the screen above the patient's chest and work in one axis. The developers of this system believe that there is a very

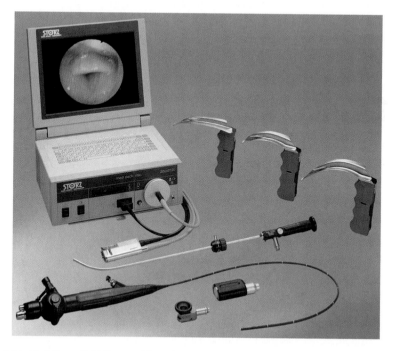

Fig. 6.24 Karl Storz DCI System (Copyright 2010 Karl Storz Endoscopy-America, Inc., with permission)

small learning curve for its use. Despite that, there is a requirement for learning eye-hand coordination and becoming comfortable with the handling requirements of the system. Part of the reason for this is the standard blade design which is familiar to anesthesiologists. The Macintosh video laryngoscope is now available as part of the Storz DCI Video Laryngoscopy System.

A multicenter trial compared direct and video-assisted laryngoscopy for their views of the glottic opening.[95] In 865 patients, after obtaining the best possible view using direct, naked-eye vision (using the Macintosh video laryngoscope and allowing for the use of external laryngeal pressure or backward, upward, and rightward pressure), the view was improved where necessary with maneuvers using the video monitor. The monitor improved the view from difficult to easy in 100 patients, while it hindered the view in 7 patients. Most of the patients in this study were considered to have easy laryngoscopy, although difficult laryngoscopy occurred in 21 (2.4%) patients. Comparison of direct and video laryngoscopy, using this device, in 200 patients with a Mallampati score of III or IV found that video laryngoscopy produced better glottic views, enabled higher intubation success in less time, and required fewer optimizing maneuvers.[96]

The Storz DCI Video Intubating System may also be used in pediatrics. The pediatric video laryngoscope integrates a fiberoptic lens (60°) into the light source of a standard Miller type blade with the handle coupling the camera and blade. This device has been used successfully as a rescue technique after two failed attempts at direct laryngoscopy in a neonate with Desbuquois syndrome.[97] Recently, the Miller 1 video laryngoscope was compared to a standard Miller 1 laryngoscope during simulated difficult intubations by 32 anesthesiologists.[98] The video laryngoscope provided a better laryngeal view and improved the view by at least 1 grade for 78% of the anesthesiologists. There was no difference between the techniques in terms of intubation times.

Karl Storz has recently manufactured a new, portable video laryngoscope called the C-MAC. This system was designed for routine use in the operating room and intensive care in the emergency room, in addition to prehospital use in road and air ambulances. It weighs less than 1.5 kg and has a battery life of more than 2 h. There will likely soon be data published about this system in anesthesia journals.

GlideScope

The GlideScope video laryngoscope (Verathon Inc., Bothell, WA) was developed to provide an alternative to direct laryngoscopy (when obtaining a direct view of the glottis fails) while enabling a view of the endotracheal tube as it passes through the glottis (Fig. 6.25). It is designed for difficult and unpredictable airways.

The specialized laryngoscope contains a charged-coupled device (digital) camera with a wide angle lens at the inferior aspect of its blade, which provides miniature video clips. Illumination is provided by two light emitting diodes and a cable attached to an LCD monitor that emerges from the handle. It is similar to a standard

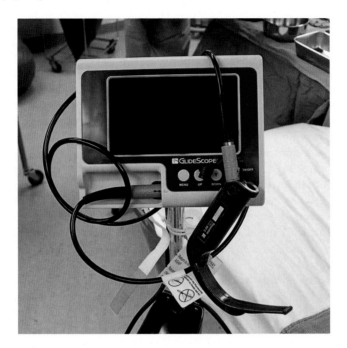

Fig. 6.25 Glidescope

Macintosh blade, but it is nondetachable, is made from medical grade plastic, and there is a sharp upward 60° angulation.[99] This angulation was designed to view the anterior glottis without the need for a direct line of sight.

The GlideScope is inserted along the midline of the tongue and advanced until the glottis is visible on the monitor. The manufacturer's guidelines suggest that when preshaping the tracheal tube over the stylet, it will be helpful to match the 60° angle of the blade. While a standard malleable stylet may be used, there is also a dedicated GlideScope rigid stylet available. There is some controversy as to whether the dedicated stylet is beneficial or not.[100]

The original GlideScope system included a black and white monitor, while the second generation, produced by Verathon, has a color monitor. The GlideScope is available in four sizes, to enable its use in neonates, infants and children, adolescents and adults, and large or obese adults. Newer versions are also available: the GlideScope Ranger is a portable and compact system, and the GlideScope Cobalt (in adults and infants sizes) is single-use.

The initial clinical assessment of the device demonstrated its use for laryngoscopy and intubation in routine orotracheal intubation.[99,101,102] It provided at least a good (Cormack and Lehane grade 1 or 2) view in 99% of 722 patients, improved the view in several patients with poor grades, and enabled successful intubation in 96.3% of patients. Cooper et al.[99] recommend strict adherence to the manufacturer's directions and the use of a malleable stylet. This is echoed by Rai et al.[101] who mention that there may be some resistance when advancing the tracheal tube. In a randomized controlled trial comparing the laryngoscopic views and times to intubate using the GlideScope and direct laryngoscopy (Macintosh size 3), the time to intubate using this device was similar to direct laryngoscopy for patients with Cormack and Lehane grade 3 laryngoscopic views, but was prolonged in patients with better views (Cormack and Lehane grades 1 or 2). Obtaining these results, Sun et al. conclude that this device has potential advantages over direct laryngoscopy for difficult intubations.[102]

Rare complications including palatopharyngeal injury have been reported and may be prevented by directly observing tube insertion and advancement, the use of flexible stylets, and avoiding unnecessary force during endotracheal tube insertion.[103, 104] The GlideScope can been used for nasotracheal intubation and, in comparison to direct laryngoscopy, has proven to enable easier and faster intubation, with a better glottic exposure and causing less moderate-to-severe sore throat. The use of Magill forceps were not used, as compared to their high usage (49%) for patients receiving direct laryngoscopy.[105]

Initial experience with the GlideScope in neonates showed some promise for its use, although led to recommendations for modified blades for this small patient size.[106] A subsequent randomized controlled trial comparing the GlideScope to direct laryngoscopy (using a Macintosh blade) in 203 children found that the laryngeal view was improved with the video system, but the time to intubate was longer (36.0 vs. 23.8 s).[107]

Video laryngoscopy would ideally enable the same cervical spine immobility during intubation as a fiberoptic bronchoscope. In this way, it could be of particular use for the trauma patient with potential cervical spine injury, especially as it can be used "easily" in the presence of secretions and blood. Several studies have evaluated cervical spine motion during laryngoscopy and/or intubation with the GlideScope. Turkstra et al.[108] used fluoroscopic video to examine cervical spine motion (occiput-C1 junction, C1-2 junction, C2-5 motion segment, C5-thoracic motion segment) during manual ventilation using bag-mask, laryngoscopy, and intubation with the GlideScope®, a Macintosh 3 blade, and an Intubating Lighted Stylet (Lightwand) in 36 patients with in-line stabilization of the head. The GlideScope® only reduced motion in the C2–5 motion segment (by 50%) compared to direct laryngoscopy, and the time required for laryngoscopy was 62% longer. (The Lightwand produced less movement at all four segments during laryngoscopy). Similarly, although using different motion parameters and cinefluoroscopy, Robitaille et al. found that the GlideScope® produced better glottic visibility but with similar cervical spine motion as that of direct laryngoscopy (Macintosh blade size 3 or 4).[109] Comparing the Lo-Pro GlideScope® to flexible bronchoscopy (video-bronchoscope, Porta-View LF-TP, Olympus Optical Co. Ltd., Japan) during intubation in patients without cervical spine immobilization, Wong et al.[110] found that the GlideScope® produced greater cervical extension throughout the C-spine. In a pathological model consisting of 20 patients with ankylosing spondylitis (12 and 11 of whom were judged as having potentially difficult intubation and laryngoscopy, respectively), the GlideScope® improved laryngeal exposure compared to that provided with a Macintosh size 3 blade and enabled successful nasotracheal intubation in 17/20 patients. [111] These authors conclude that the GlideScope® is a viable option when spontaneous breathing (thus the use of awake FOI) is not possible or desired.

Three studies thus far have compared the use of the GlideScope® to the Macintosh size 3 blade for tracheal intubation by various "inexperienced" personnel in either simulation or clinical settings. Lim et al.[112] found that medical students intubated a human simulator with a difficult (but not standard) airway faster (median 30.5 s vs. 155.5 s) and easier with the GlideScope®. More students (85% vs. 15%) chose it as their intubating device for the difficult airway scenario. Benjamin, Boon, and French[113] evaluated whether the devices enabled 30 anesthesiologists (inexperienced with the GlideScope®) to pass a bougie or stylet through the vocal cords ("intubate") of airway simulators in four scenarios. The GlideScope® only improved the laryngoscopic view of one scenario (pharyngeal obstruction) and failed to improve the ease of intubation in any scenario.

A clinical study of 20 medical personnel inexperienced with intubation found better results for the GlideScope® when intubating 200 healthy elective surgical patients with unanticipated intubation difficulty.[114] Both the success rate (93 vs. 51%) and time for intubation (63 ± 30 vs. 85 ± 35 s) were superior, and these authors concluded that a success rate of more than 90% within 120 s can be achieved by medical personnel even without intubation experience. How do these results compare to evaluation of anesthesiologists' use of these devices? Similar to their study in medical students, as discussed above, Lim et al.[115] also found that the GlideScope® was beneficial during intubation of a difficult airway (requiring less time, with equal or higher success) for experienced anesthesiologists, but of some detriment in the easy airway scenario (requiring more time with similar success and ease).

The design of the GlideScope was intended to enable laryngoscopy and intubation to be performed using less upward force (thus less oropharyngeal stimulation) and neck movement. While some studies have shown that the use of the GlideScope® results in similar cervical spine movement as direct laryngoscopy, there may still be the potential for attenuation of the hemodynamic responses to orotracheal intubation due to less mechanical stimulation.[108,109,116] In a comparison of the hemodynamic responses to orotracheal intubation when using the GlideScope® and both a Macintosh laryngoscope and fiberoptic bronchoscope, Xue and coworkers[116,117] have found similar responses, with no particular benefit from the GlideScope®.

McGrath

The McGrath video laryngoscope (Aircraft Medical, Edinburgh, UK) was the first self-contained (power source, camera, and LCD monitor incorporated) video laryngoscope produced (Fig. 6.26). It contains two light emitting diodes and a small color digital camera at the core of the adjustable-length blade ("camera stick"), and

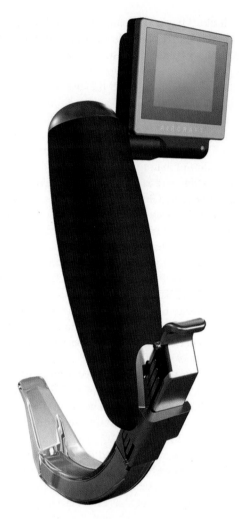

Fig. 6.26 McGrath video-laryngoscope (Copyright 2009 Aircraft Medical Ltd., with permission)

the blade is covered by another acrylic disposable blade. The screen is mounted on the top of the handle and can be tilted and swiveled to allow an optimal view.

In routine intubations of adult airways, Shippey et al.[118] found that the McGrath enabled good Cormack and Lehane grades (grade I 95%; grade II 4%) and high intubation success (98%), both in good insertion times (6.3 s and 24.7 s, respectively). Only minor complications occurred, including reduced oxygen saturation below 92% and small volume blood-stained oropharynx secretions.

This device has shown to be of value in cases of failed laryngoscopy and intubation.[119] Conversely, despite good laryngeal views, the McGrath may not ensure easy intubation, with three of 28 intubations failing in one report.[120] Due to the more anterior view of the larynx provided in general by indirect laryngoscopy, tube passage may be difficult and lead to impingement on the anterior commissure of the glottis.[118, 120] Shippey et al.[118] recommend the use of a thicker more rigid stylet and preshaping of the tracheal tube. If the endotracheal tube cannot be advanced, the stylet can be removed and an Eschmann gum elastic bougie inserted into the tube and advanced into the trachea. The video can then assist railroading of the tube over the bougie.[121]

Airway Scope (AWS-S100)

Koyama and colleagues designed the Airway Scope (AWS, Pentax Corporation, Tokyo, Japan), a rigid video laryngoscope that is portable and incorporates a finely shaped tube-guiding disposable introducer.[122] The charge-coupled device camera and light-emitting diode are attached to the tip of the introducer and the full-color monitor is built into the top of the handgrip (Fig. 6.27). Apart from attaching to the video system, the introducer is composed of two channels for: (1) the passage of the endotracheal tube and (2) suction or application or topical anesthesia.

The device is inserted using a posterior route along the posterior pharyngeal wall, placing the tip posterior to the epiglottis and directly elevating it out of the way. An anterior approach which glides the tip along the tongue may result in endotracheal tube impingement onto the epiglottis.[123] Clinical experience in routine tracheal intubation has shown the AWS to improve the laryngeal view as produced with direct laryngoscopy, while allowing 100% success of intubation quickly (19–42 s) and with ease.[124-126] High success (99.3%) has also been found when evaluating use of the AWS in patients with documented or predicted difficult airways.[127]

Comparing intubation in simulated difficult airway patients (using cervical collars) using either the AWS or the StyletScope (fiberoptic stylet), Komatsu et al.[128] found both to offer high success (AWS 98%; StyletScope 96%), with the AWS faster (19 s vs. 51 s) and causing fewer esophageal intubations. It has offered a full

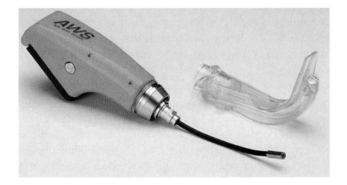

Fig. 6.27 Airway Scope (Copyright 2009 Pentax Canada Inc., with permission)

view of the larynx when viewing, even the epiglottis was limited using a Macintosh laryngoscope in three patients with cervical pathology.[129] Of these three intubations, one was performed with the patient awake. Unique cases where the AWS has been useful include the morbidly obese (the adjustable monitor enabling the semisitting position) and difficult double-lumen tube intubation.[130, 131] While intubation using the AWS has shown to produce similar cardiovascular responses as the Macintosh laryngoscope in patients without intubation difficulty, further study needs to assess whether it may attenuate the stress response in patients with difficult airways.[126]

Maruyama and coworkers[132-134] have performed several investigations to evaluate the amount of cervical spine movement produced during intubation with the AWS. Using radiology to measure angles formed by adjacent vertebrae during intubation, this group found that the AWS resulted in less cumulative upper C-spine movement than the Macintosh laryngoscope in patients with normal (10° less) and immobilized cervical spines (17° less).[132,133] Contrasting results were found for intubation times, with the AWS being slower for the normal spines and of similar speed for the immobilized. In one patient with Halo-Vest Fixation, fluoroscopy confirmed that the AWS allowed intubation while maintaining spine fixation.[134] These results are similar to those found earlier by Hirabayashi's group.[135]

The AWS appears to be successfully used by novice operators and therefore may be beneficial for those who are required to perform tracheal intubation only infrequently in emergency situations outside the operating room. Nonanesthesiology residents have intubated the trachea faster (33 vs. 59 s), with higher first-attempt success, using the AWS than a Macintosh blade.[136,137] The intubation times for novice Advanced Life Support providers are similar to those for experienced personnel (34 vs. 36 s to insert the tube into the trachea).[138] Limited to 30 s, nurses intubated manikins faster (16.7 s vs. 23.2 s) with higher success (91.3% vs. 79.4%) using the AWS over a Macintosh.[139]

Airtraq

The Airtraq (Prodol Medictec, Vizcaya, Spain, or King Systems, Indianapolis, MN) is an optical laryngoscope, somewhat similar to the AWS due to the two side by side channels within the blade, but the optics (contained in one of the channels) consist of a series of lenses, prisms, and mirrors that transfer the image from the tip to a viewfinder (Fig. 6.28). The image can be viewed externally via a clip-on wireless video system.

The procedure uses a similar approach as the Macintosh blade, with the blade tip placed in the vallecula and enabling indirect lifting of the epiglottis when required. Tracheal intubation in patients without risk of difficulty was performed using the Airtraq, with similar success and insertion times to those performed using direct laryngoscopy with a Macintosh blade.[140] In patients with either cervical spine immobilization or high risk for intubation difficulty (three or more risk factors), the Airtraq was superior to the Macintosh for speed of intubation attempts (13.2 s vs.

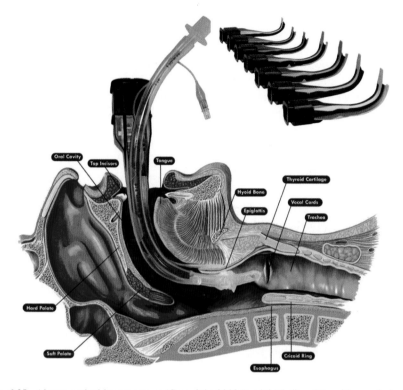

Fig. 6.28 Airtraq optical laryngoscope (Copyright 2009 Prodol Meditec SA, with permission)

20.3 s and 13.4 s vs. 47.7 s, respective to study) and intubation difficulty (0.1 vs. 2.7 and 0.4 vs. 7.7).[141, 142] All of the above studies found the Airtraq to cause less hemodynamic alterations than the Macintosh laryngoscope.

Morbidly obese patients, many of whom may have enlarged tongues, were more quickly intubated (23 s vs. 56 s) using the Airtraq than the Macintosh laryngoscope, and this device prevented similar reductions of arterial oxygen saturation.[143] Moreover, a modified (with a breathing circuit attached and suction catheter inserted through the tracheal tube) Airtraq has been used for awake tracheal intubation of an elderly woman with a history of regurgitation and difficult laryngoscopy.[144] This device may be advantageous over conventional direct laryngoscopy in patients with cervical spine problems, since its use has shown to cause 29% less extension between the occiput and C4, and less anterior vertebral body deviation at most levels.[145] Despite these values, significant movement was still seen during the procedure with the Airtraq. There have been reports of oropharyngeal injuries with the use of the Airtraq, potentially because of poor view of the initial insertion of the blade over the back of the tongue.[146, 147]

Using the Airtraq may improve performance or learning of intubation by novice laryngoscopists or personnel. Medical students with no prior airway management experience more quickly intubated manikins or intubation trainers, using fewer maneuvers and with less teeth clicks, in both easy and difficult airway scenarios when using the Airtraq compared to the Macintosh laryngoscope. In the difficult airway scenario particularly, they had greater success with intubation. Moreover, the students improved their performance with the Airtraq quickly.[148] The Airtraq enabled nonanesthesiology physicians to more quickly secure the airways of patients and with fewer erroneous esophageal intubations than when they were using the Macintosh laryngoscope.[149]

TrachView Intubating Videoscope

The TrachView device (Parker Medical, Highlands Ranch, CO) is a video endoscope, comprised of a detachable, fiberoptic cable and a lightweight, portable case containing a dual light source, camera, LCD screen, and controls (Fig. 6.29).

The scope can be held at a desirable depth within the endotracheal tube by a clip and can be curved sufficiently with a corresponding stylet.[150] After a 10-min demonstration on a manikin, emergency medicine residents obtained a 100% POGO (percent of glottic opening) using the TrachView (vs. 50% using direct laryngoscopy) and medical students obtained 75% POGO (vs. 25%).[151] The majority of the residents (82.1%) and medical students (56.8%) rated the TrachView as improving their intubation attempts.

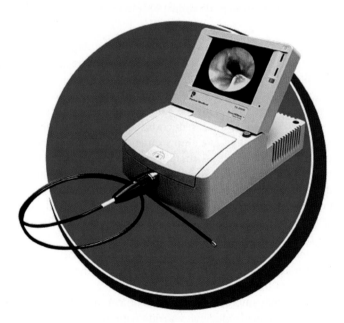

Fig. 6.29 TrachView intubating videoscope (Copyright 2009 Parker Medical, with permission)

Comparisons of Indirect Laryngoscopes

Several investigations have begun to emerge that provide comparative results for many of the indirect laryngoscopy devices manufactured. Compared to the conventional Macintosh laryngoscope, the Glidescope®, Airway Scope, and Truview EVO2 provided better views of the glottis, greater success of tracheal intubation, and ease of device use when used by experienced operators in difficult airway scenarios in manikins. The Airway Scope had the highest success, required less time to perform tracheal intubation, caused less dental trauma, and was easier to use.[152] This device also proved advantageous over the GlideScope® for intubation in easy and difficult situations by medical students, offering faster intubation with greater ease.[153] Similar results were found by experienced anesthesiologists intubating patients with cervical spine immobilization.

While the GlideScope, Truview EVO2, and Airway Scope reduced intubation difficulty, improved glottic views, and reduced the need for optimization maneuvers, the intubation difficulty and the hemodynamic stimulation were the lowest with the Airway Scope. This study showed no difference in intubation success rates with these devices, in comparison to the Macintosh, and found that the indirect laryngoscopes took longer to perform intubation.

The Airtraq has been compared to the Glidescope, McGrath, and Truview. In simulated difficult airway scenarios, anesthesiology providers obtained a better laryngeal exposure with less dental trauma with the use of the indirect laryngoscopes (GlideScope, Airtraq, and McGrath) than the Macintosh. The Airtraq provided the fastest tracheal intubation and the best laryngeal view than the Truview and McGrath laryngoscopes.[154] For intubation of patients undergoing direct microlaryngoscopy, the Airtraq and GlideScope had similar success rates and duration of intubation attempts. Both improved the laryngeal view, although the Airtraq caused more traumatic pharyngeal lesions.[155] The Airtraq performed favorably when compared to the Truview and Macintosh laryngoscopes, in a manikin study of normal and difficult (hard cervical collar) intubations by paramedics. This device required fewer optimization procedures and reduced the potential for dental trauma in both the normal and difficult scenarios. The TruView increased the duration of intubation attempts as compared to the other two devices.[156]

Stylets and Light Wands

Conventional Stylets: Endotracheal Tube Introducers and Exchangers

Gum elastic catheters or bougies (GEB), also known as endotracheal tube introducers, have been used by UK clinicians for years to facilitate difficult intubations, especially when the posterior portion of the larynx is barely visible ("anterior larynx") or the epiglottis cannot be elevated.[157] The use of an introducer is recommended early in cases of unanticipated difficult airways.[158] Many of these catheters are flexible and their distal end may be preformed to allow the tip to be directed beneath the epiglottis and into the airway. A small endotracheal tube is then advanced over the bougie into the glottis, the bougie is then withdrawn and correct placement of the endotracheal tube is confirmed.[159] We recommend using the laryngoscope to elevate the epiglottis as much as possible, lest the tube not pass easily over the bougie (which should be well lubricated before use). There is a characteristic "speed bump" or "click" sensation detected when the bougie is advanced into the trachea as it traverses the tracheal rings. Of course, this sensation will not be detected if the bougie enters the esophagus. For this reason, the bougie may have promise for confirming tube placement.

Bair et al.[160] studied the ability of a GEB for confirmation of endotracheal tube placement in human cadavers undergoing a randomized series of esophageal and tracheal intubations. Ring clicks were 95% specific for tracheal intubation and 95% of esophageal placements were detected. Similar to Kidd et al.'s[161] experience of noting a "holdup" at a certain point as the bougie was advanced into the trachea (usually noted between 24 and 40 cm), presumably due to encroachment on the smaller airways, Bair et al. found that a "hang up" was reported in 100% of tracheal placements.

The Eschmann Healthcare Tracheal Tube Introducer (Sims Portex Ltd., Kent UK, or Keene NH), a reusable GEB, is one of the most popular devices, although Portex has marketed single-use GEBs and other single-use models have been marketed by other manufacturers (e.g., Sun Med, Largo, Fl; Cook Medical, Houston, TX; Proact Medical, and Parker Medical, Englewood, CO) (Fig. 6.30).

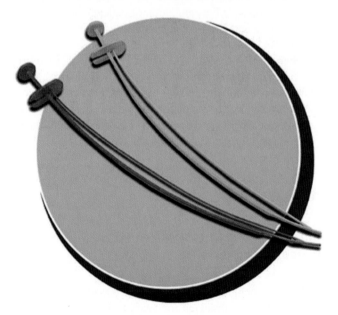

Fig. 6.30 Single-use stylet (Copyright 2009 Parker Medical, with permission)

A recent study, in which emergency medicine physicians and anesthesiologists intubated a simulated difficult airway model with several of the above mentioned currently available GEBs (in the US), found that success was lowest when using the Portex single-use GEB and that there was a preference for the Sun Med model.[162] Anesthesiologists had more success with the GEB than the emergency care physicians. While there have been concerns over the sterility of the reusable Eschmann introducers (particularly since they may be used more than the five times recommended), the single-use introducers produce much more peak force (3–6 times) and may cause more tissue trauma during placement.[163,164]

One study found that the Frova, single-use, introducer (Cook Medical, Houston, TX) afforded greater success than other single-use introducers (Pro-Breathe and Portex) for anesthesiologists intubating a mannequin.[164] Another study found the Frova to be moderately clinically successful (84% first-attempt success rate), but experienced difficulties with this device in hitting the tracheal wall and railroading the tracheal tube.[165] The models by Sun Med and Greenfield provided higher success (both 88%) than the Portex (68%) bougies for intubation of a simulated difficult airway by emergency medicine and anesthesiology residents and physicians, and the Sun Med model was the preferred single-use model.[162] When a difficult airway is encountered, the bougie can be used alone or in conjunction with other devices, such as the LMA.

A bougie can be used to change the endotracheal tube, especially when laryngoscopy is difficult. Otherwise airway exchange catheters (AECs) are useful. The hollow tube exchange catheters may be connected to an oxygen source or to a capnograph and will also facilitate jet ventilation. Bougies or tube changers should be several centimeters longer than the endotracheal tube. They are not foolproof, however, and you may expect occasional failures especially when the airway anatomy is grossly distorted. A number of devices are commercially available. The EndoGuide T (Rusch, Kernen, Germany) is both a tube exchange and intubation stylet (having a stainless steel guidewire in the tube wall). Oxygen insufflation or jet ventilation can be performed through the large lumen of this device. Alternatively, Cook Medical (Bloomington, IN) manufactures a Rapi-Fit adaptor, which can be attached to their intubation catheters (e.g., the Frova Intubating Introducer) to enable jet ventilation during tube exchange. Hagberg[166] lists the following principles when using AECs for jet ventilation:

- Maintain maximal airway patency when jetting through an AEC that is placed inside the trachea rather than inside an endotracheal tube.
- Maintain the AEC above the carina (confirmed by bronchoscopy or limiting the depth to less than 26 cm in the adult) and never advance the AEC through resistance.
- Start with jet ventilation of 25 psi by using an additional in-line regulator, and limit inspiratory time to less than 1 s.
- Use a 1:2 or 1:3 inspiratory:expiratory ratio to allow adequate time for air exit.
- Avoid ventilation during phonation.

Optical Stylets

Fiberoptic optical stylets are generally used as adjuncts to difficult direct laryngoscopy, although they may be used alone in order to perform awake intubation. They typically contain a rigid, semirigid, or malleable shaft containing optical fibers for light and image transmission, a proximal eyepiece and a proximal endotracheal tube connector holder.[167] An endotracheal tube is preloaded onto the stylet, leaving the stylet's distal tip proximal to the end of the tube. The use of these devices avoids the oftentimes difficultly with tube passage experienced with other fiberoptic devices (e.g., GlideScope), although the initial view may be difficult to achieve. These are stiffer than bougies and enable indirect visualization. When used alone, the stylets are generally formed into a J shape, with a distal curvature of 70–90°.

Bonfils Intubation Fibrescope

The Bonfils Intubation Fibrescope (Karl Storz Endoscopy Ltd., Tuttlingen, Germany) is a rigid fiberoptic endoscope that has a long, thin, and straight cylindrical body with a curve of 40° at its distal end (Fig. 6.31). Fiberoptic bundles are contained within the stainless steel body and attached to a moveable eyepiece mounted at the proximal end. Alternatively, a camera can be attached to project the image to a remote monitor or one can purchase a newer version which incorporates a camera (direct coupled interface) that displays the image directly on a video monitor. A battery-powered or standard light source can be attached to the proximal end of the handle. The Bonfils has a locking device to hold the loaded tracheal tube at a point just beyond the scope and (generally outside of the USA) contains

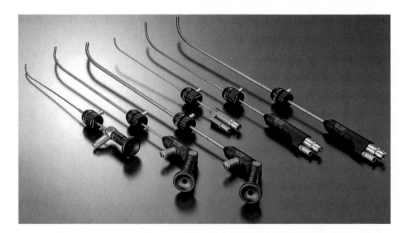

Fig. 6.31 Bonfils intubation endoscope (Copyright 2010 Karl Storz Endoscopy-America, Inc., with permission)

a 1.2-mm working channel (thus is equipped for awake intubation, using a "spray as you go technique").[168] A connector fits to the tracheal tube adapter and also allows for insufflation of oxygen.

Once the laryngeal inlet is located, the operator advances the tracheal tube through the vocal cords under direct vision (rather than the indirect, "offline" vision provided by optical laryngoscopes). After raising the epiglottis and enlarging the retropharyngeal space using a chin lift or chin-and-tongue lift (no direct manipulation of the epiglottis), either a midline or lateral approach can be used for scope advancement; the first aiming the tip of the Bonfils towards the uvula and advancing it towards the epiglottis, and the latter advancing the scope along the pharyngeal wall. A stepwise process can be followed to the extent necessary for placing the tip of the scope under the epiglottis. This process involves a chin lift, chin-and-tongue lift, external jaw thrust with neck extension, and assistance using the Macintosh laryngoscope.[169]

The main difficulties with the use of this device are secretions which may reduce the view (reported as minimal in adults[169] and significant in children[170]) and difficulty getting the scope tip under the epiglottis. In the opinion of Halligan and Charters,[169] the device has a relatively steep learning curve, although clinical experience rather than simulated with manikins is essential for training. The Bonfils is available in adult and pediatric sizes (with an outer diameter as small as 2 mm) and some experience with both has been reported.

The Bonfils has been evaluated in adult patients with normal, anticipated (both clinically predicted and via simulation), and unanticipated difficult airways. Clinical experience with the Bonfils in normal airways by anesthesiologists inexperienced with its use indicates that the device offers high success (98.3% in 60 patients) with efficiency (median time 33 s) and without difficulty.[169] After predicting difficulty in 80 surgical patients, intubation using the Bonfils was compared to that by the intubating LMA (ILMA; see Chap. 5). The Bonfils enabled 97.5% success on first attempt (100% at second; vs. the ILMA 70% and 90% with 5% failure at three attempts) with an intubation time of 40 s (vs. 76 s for the ILMA), without causing clinically significant sore throat or hoarseness (median 0 on a numeric rating scale).[171]

In 75 gynecological patients with simulated airway difficulty via rigid cervical immobilization collars, the Bonfils was compared to the Macintosh laryngoscope for intubation success and insertion times. Higher success within two attempts was obtained for the Bonfils (81.6% vs. 39.5%), although the time to intubate was longer (64 vs. 53 s). In the anticipated difficult airway scenario, these results may not be surprising since awake FOI is recommended over the use of a direct laryngoscopy approach under anesthesia.[168] Moreover, it has been shown in one study that significantly less cervical spine movement was produced with the Bonfils than the Macintosh laryngoscope.[172] The Bonfils has been used successfully for awake intubation by some clinicians and has an advantage over flexible fiberoptic laryngoscop: it enables direct lifting of structures and is more affordable and durable as well as easier to clean.[168, 173]

When difficulty is unanticipated and direct laryngoscopy fails, the Bonfils may be an attractive alternative. In this scenario, Bein et al.[174] found it to offer high success (96% within two attempts) within a reasonable time (median 47.5 s) for 25 patients undergoing coronary artery bypass grafting. This device necessitates adequate mouth opening and, for this reason, it will not compete with flexible fiberoptic devices in these situations.[175]

There have been mixed results regarding the use of the Bonfils in pediatrics. A case report described successful use in a difficult intubation of a newborn who was small for gestational age and presenting with mandibular hypoplasia and a severely enlarged tongue.[176] Conversely, a large case series of 55 children intubated with the Bonfils fiberscope found high first-attempt failure rates in both children receiving ($n=19$, rate 69%) and not receiving ($n=36$, rate 78%) atropine as an antisialagogue. Moreover, the time to intubation in these patients was 60 s and 58 s, respectively. These authors conclude that the use of this device for routine intubation in children may have drawbacks.[170]

Shikani (Seeing) Optical Stylet (SOS)

The SOS (Clarus Medical Inc., Minneapolis MN) is a FOI scope consisting of a malleable stainless steel sheath containing an image fiber bundle, a distal lens, a proximal image fiber connector, several illumination fibers, and a proximal illumination connector (Fig. 6.32). The inner fiberoptic cable can be connected, via the image connector, to a camera and video monitor or to an eyepiece. The stylet fits into endotracheal tubes of size 3.0 mm and up. There is an adjustable tube stop/oxygen port.

Using the stylet as an intubating device, the patient's jaw is lifted to position the mandible anteriorly, the tip of the tongue may be withdrawn by grasping it with the fingers using gauze, and the lubricated stylet (loaded with endotracheal tube) is advanced into the larynx. In cases of difficulty, a laryngoscope blade may be required to retract the base of the tongue. The main advantage of the stylet over a flexible fiberoptic scope is its rigidity, which can better maneuver around the epiglottis. It may be used similar to a light wand, with illumination of the throat after tracheal (but not esophageal) intubation; this will be particularly useful in situations where bloody secretions limit the visibility with fiberoptics. When attached to a video monitor, training will be facilitated.[177] The SOS has been used for anticipated or known difficult airway situations in both adults and children.[178, 179] An awake intubation was possible in an adult patient by an emergency medicine physician.[178] Some investigators report that they use this device for routine intubations at their institutions. After developing their own "left molar approach," they found the SOS to provide favorable hemodynamic responses to the intubation of 80 elective surgery patients compared to direct laryngoscopy.[180]

Levitan FPS (First-Pass Success) Scope

Intended for routine augmentation in emergency laryngoscopy, the Levitan FPS Scope (Clarus Medical, Minneapolis MN) is a streamlined shorter version (30 cm

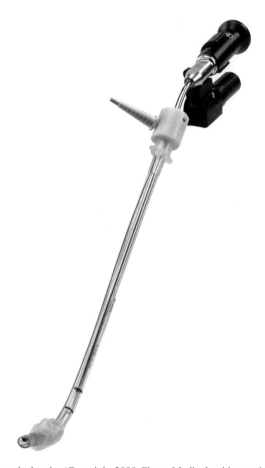

Fig. 6.32 Shikani optical stylet (Copyright 2009 Clarus Medical, with permission)

vs. 38.5 cm) of the Shikani Optical Stylet offering the procedural handling of a standard stylet (Fig. 6.33). Similar to the SOS, it can be either attached to a standard fiberoptic illuminated laryngoscope handle or a dedicated light source. The difference is that this model has a miniature light source which is removable and does not have the moveable tube stop like the SOS. The tracheal tube needs to be larger than 6.0 mm (adult sizes only) and needs to be trimmed to 27.5–28.0 mm to achieve the correct stylet position. A bend of 35° is needed when the device is used as an adjunct to laryngoscopy and gives the tube and stylet better maneuverability within the mouth and hypopharynx.

Under direct vision when the epiglottis can be seen, the tip of the stylet is placed to a point close to, but below and away from, the tip of the epiglottis; the view is then changed to the fiberoptic eyepiece and the stylet is directed under the epiglottis and into the trachea. In comparison to tube introducers, the rigidity of the stylet permits direct lifting of the epiglottis.[181] Two comparisons of the Levitan with single-use bougies have been performed using both manikins and

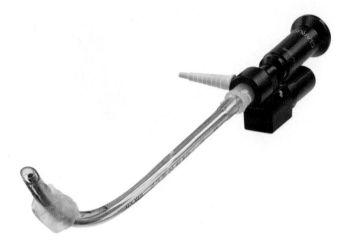

Fig. 6.33 Levitan First-Pass Success scope (Copyright 2009 Clarus Medical, with permission)

patients.[167, 182] In both studies the fiberoptic device offered no additional success in a grade III view, although in manikins it offered greater success in a grade IIIB situation (when the epiglottis was unable to be lifted up and away from the posterior pharyngeal wall). This could be due to the distal bend of the stylet enabling visibility around the relatively acute angle created by a posteriorly displaced epiglottis, as well as its rigidity that enables lifting of the epiglottis.[167] Copious secretions were noted as a major limitation with the use of the Levitan scope.[182]

Airway Pocket Scope

Designed to fit in the lapel pocket for portability, the Airway Pocket Scope (Clarus Medical, Minneapolis, MN) stylet is flexible as it has a nondirectional, atraumatic tip, and is used with an ILMA (Fastrach), a Combitube, or other new supraglottic device to visualize the intubation with as small as a 4.0 ID endotracheal tube (Fig. 6.34). A Clarus light source or any green system laryngoscope handle can be used. This is a newly redesigned version of the Clarus FAST (Flexible Airway Scope Tool) device.

Stylet Scope

Kitamura and colleagues[183] designed this stylet scope (NihonKohden Corp., Tokyo, Japan) in 1999, with an aim to circumvent the problems of predetermined flexion at the distal end of the scope and the need for external light sources and/or time-consuming preparation. The scope uses a plastic fiberoptic system incorporated into the endotracheal tube stylet, with a lens providing a 50° field of view. There is

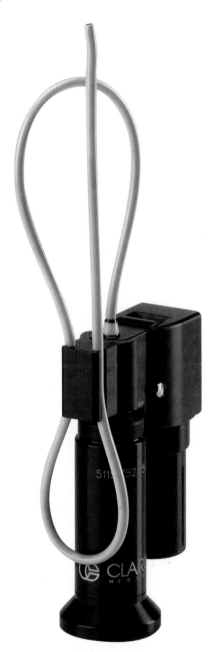

Fig. 6.34 Airway Pocket scope (Copyright 2009 Clarus Medical, with permission)

a lever attached to the handle, which controls the flexion at the distal tip (anterior flexion of 75° is possible to directly view the anterior airway). Similar to other fiberoptic devices, secretions or blood in the airway may limit the use of the StyletScope and the scope cannot be used for nasal intubation.

The intubation procedure when using a laryngoscope can involve lifting the tongue with the laryngoscope and using only the stylet to view the glottic opening and confirm tracheal placement of the tube. This technique (the "insufficient" laryngoscopy technique generating a simulated grade III view) has been shown to be efficient even when used by a resident, thus enabling an intubation success of 100% (94% at first attempt) in 32 general surgery patients within two attempts and within 29 ± 14 s (recorded to when the stylet was removed from the endotracheal tube).[183] The manual adjustment of the tip via the lever has enabled the StyletScope to be used alone during intubation of normal airways and appears to be suitable for use in patients with limited mouth opening. These authors have used techniques with and without an assistant pulling the lower jaw upward.[184]

The StyletScope has been evaluated in patients with simulated difficult airways. Compared to a conventional metal stylet, the StyletScope was more successful (99 vs. 92%) at intubating airways in patients with manual in-line stabilization (producing grades 3–4 in 66% of patients) with significantly fewer attempts.[185] In patients wearing rigid Philadelphia collars, the StyletScope intubated patients with similar success although less quickly (51 s vs. 31 s) to confirmation of intubation by capnography than did the Airway Scope.[128] In these studies, the tube was advanced into the tracheal under direct vision in grades 1 or 2; if the view was grade 3 or 4 (or $\geq 2b$[128]), the tube was advanced to the epiglottis via direct vision or fiberoptically (grade 4) and then further advanced into the trachea after fiberoptic identification of the epiglottis. All of the above studies have reported acceptable hemodynamic changes with the use of the StyletScope. This is similar to what was previously found in two studies comparing hemodynamic changes with use of the StyletScope and direct laryngoscopy.

Kitamura et al.[186] found that the StyletScope, used alone, reduced the increase in heart rate during intubation of normotensive patients. Comparing normo- to hypertensive patients, Kimura and colleagues found that the StyletScope, even with the use of adjuvant direct laryngoscopy, attenuates the hemodynamic changes (SBP, DBP) in comparison with conventional laryngoscopy technique.[187] While these results are encouraging, the small sample size of these studies ($n = 11–15$ per group; no use of sample size calculation) may limit their merit. Kitamura reports that to obtain these results with the StyletScope, one must not use jaw-lifting procedures and should be experienced to perform the intubation quickly.

Illuminating Stylets (Lightwands)

Transillumination of the soft tissues of the neck to blindly intubate the trachea was first suggested by the Japanese, and evaluated clinically and in comparison to direct laryngoscopy in the late 1980s.[188-190] In this "lightwand intubation," a well-circumscribed glow in the anterior neck indicates tracheal location while indiscernible light is produced with esophageal placement. A number of devices have been tested and many improvements made. These devices are now available for both orotracheal and nasotracheal intubation. Early devices were disposable, used poor light sources (thus of limited use in many emergency situations), and often had inadequate lengths which required cutting the endotracheal tube (e.g., with the Tube-Stat [Medtronic ENT, Jacksonville, FL]).

The lighted stylet is a light source on which you can mount an endotracheal tube, and after the stylet's passage beyond the glottis, the endotracheal tube can be railroaded into the trachea.[191] The Trachlight (Laerdal Medical Corp, Long Beach, CA), Lightwand (Vital Signs Inc., Totowa, NJ), and Surch-Lite (Aaron Medical Industries, St. Petersburg, FL) are three of several currently manufactured lighted stylets for use to improve the view during direct laryngoscopy or for transillumination techniques.

Trachlight

The Trachlight is the device for which most literature is available (Fig. 6.35). It is composed of a handle with a locking clamp to accept the endotracheal tube connector, a disposable flexible wand with a bright light bulb distally and proximal connector for adjustable connection to the handle (for accommodating tubes of varying lengths), and a stiff retractable stylet allowing the wand to be shaped into a "hockey-stick" configuration. The wand can become pliable with retraction of the stylet (approximately 10 cm), allowing the tube to be advanced into the trachea with minimal trauma. The device comes with three reusable stylets to accommodate endotracheal tubes 2.5–10 mm. Finally, the light flashes after 30 s to warn of the need to ventilate the patient and to minimize heat production.[191]

The following guidelines are related to transillumination techniques, most specifically when using the Trachlight:

- The shaft of the stylet should be lubricated, as should the wall of the endotracheal tube. The length of the wand should be adjusted to place the light just proximal to the tip of the endotracheal tube. If not manufactured as a preformed stylet, the stylet/tube combination should be preformed into a "hockey stick" configuration.

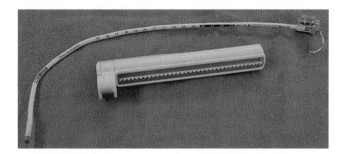

Fig. 6.35 Trachlight

- The patient's head should be placed in the neutral position (or with the neck slightly extended). A jaw-lift maneuver should be used to lift the tongue and epiglottis off the posterior pharyngeal wall.
- The light source is usually bright enough without reducing ambient lighting conditions and may be too bright in thin patients in a dimly lighted room. Dimming the lights should only be used in obese patients, in whom transillumination may not be optimal.
- The lighted stylet may be inserted in the awake or anesthetized patient.
- The Trachlight is inserted in a midline position, a "rocking motion" can be used when resistance is felt (indicating the entrance to the glottic opening), and the tip should be redirected toward the thyroid eminence (indicating positioning at the epiglottic fold) using the glow as a guide. (In a patient with a large chest, the tube should be inserted into the lateral corner of the mouth with repositioning to the midline). Once the circumscribed glow is seen, the stylet is retracted and the wand-endotracheal tube is advanced and the wand is removed from the tube. No force should be used to pass the device against resistance.
- The position of the endotracheal tube should be confirmed with end-tidal CO_2 and auscultation.
- Experience with the light wand should be acquired in patients with a normal airway. The light wand may be a useful approach, especially with the unanticipated difficult intubation in an anesthetized patient.
- The lighted stylet may also be suitable for nasal insertion. Lubricate the nostril as well as the stylet and endotracheal tube. The stylet is removed and the flexible wand is used for guidance. This technique is similar to the oral route, except that flexion of the neck may be used in place of the jaw lift for some patients.

Additionally, a review of lighted stylet tracheal intubation by Davis, Cook-Sather, and Schreiner[192] is a worthwhile read and includes descriptions of basic and advanced ("hybrid") techniques.

Hung et al.[193, 194] have tested the Trachlight in normal and difficult airway situations. Tracheal intubation was successful in 204 of 206 patients (mean time 25.7 ± 20.1 s) who had a history of difficult intubation or were evaluated to have a difficult airway. Moreover, intubation was successful within 19.7 ± 13.5 s in all of the 59 patients with unanticipated difficulty.[193] In 479 patients without known airway difficulty, intubation success was 99%, with 92% after first attempt.[194]

The device may be useful for patients with C-spine instability when use of the flexible fiberoptic bronchoscope is unavailable or technically difficult. After manual in-line stabilization, the Trachlight produced similar maximum segmental motion as the flexible bronchoscope during intubation; both devices produced segmental movements mostly at C0–1 and C1–2 levels and during their introduction.[195] The Trachlight has shown to be effective for reducing the hemodynamic responses during intubation in hypertensive patients, but not healthy or normotensive patients with normal airways.[196, 197] Conversely, in patients undergoing coronary artery bypass grafting, the Trachlight was not associated with significantly different hemodynamics than the use of direct laryngoscopy using a Macintosh blade. While the hemodynamic effects have not been assessed in the anticipated difficult airway patient using the Trachlight, the Surch-Lite has shown to expedite intubation and lower hemodynamic changes as compared to direct laryngoscopy in Mallampati Class III patients.[198]

The Trachlight has also been used in conjunction with alternate techniques besides direct laryngoscopy, including those using the LMA (both classic and intubating [Fastrach, Laryngeal Mask Company North America Inc., CA]) and a retrograde intubation technique.[199] It has proven to help confirm tracheal placement during blind intubation techniques using LMAs, help guide the tube into the trachea with direct laryngoscopy, and help intubate patients for whom retrograde intubation is a likely course (e.g., those with cervical instability). One very recent correspondence piece described its use to facilitate digital intubation of neonates with difficult intubation.

One of the main advantages of lightwand intubation is that insertion of the tracheal tube does not require laryngoscopic instrumentation. Therefore, it is very useful when access to the mouth is limited. It is also useful when there is some risk to dental structures. The main disadvantage is that lightwands are inserted blindly and may damage diseased structures. They may be contraindicated in patients with known abnormal upper airway anatomy or infection of the upper airway.[199,200] If there is accidental partial withdrawal of the Trachlight stylet, there may be difficulties controlling the tip of the device.

Endotracheal Tubes

There is a great variety of endotracheal tubes to choose from. Common types of endotracheal tubes are discussed in Chap. 4 and this chapter will highlight some of those tubes designed for special applications. There are many special types of endotracheal tubes—articulating; armored, or wire-reinforced; double-lumen endobronchial, polar, and uncuffed.

Articulating

The Endotrol (Mallinckrodt, Hazelwood, MO) has the appearance of a regular endotracheal tube, containing a high-volume, low-pressure cuff, but is equipped with a "built-in" stylet. When its "trigger," or ring, is pulled, a thread running through a channel in the tube wall applies traction to the tip of the tube, causing the tube curvature to increase. The currently manufactured tubes (Covidien-Nellcor, Boulder, CO) contain a controllable distal tip.

The Endotrol is used to direct the tip of the endotracheal tube toward the glottis when the glottis is not readily visible or during an attempt at blind nasal intubation.[201] A lightwand (e.g., Trachlight) has been used to assist with blind nasotracheal intubation.[202] It may also be used in a patient with cervical spine injuries. One case report describing tube kinking and occlusion occurring 16 h after its placement suggests that its use for long periods beyond the critical or difficult situation needs to be evaluated.[203] Parker Medical also makes a similar tube called the Easy Curve (Fig. 6.36).

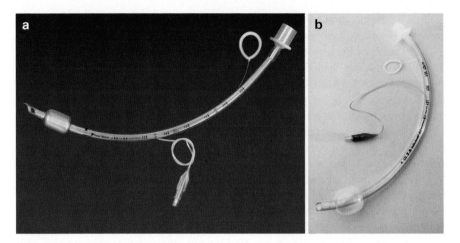

Fig. 6.36 (a) Easy Curve articulating endotracheal tube (Copyright 2009 Parker Medical, with permission) (b) Endotrol tube (copyright 2010 Nellcor Puritan Bennett LLC, Boulder Colorado, part of Covidien, with permission). When the distal ring is pulled, the curvature of the tube increases

Armored or Wire-Reinforced

The wire-reinforced tubes are manufactured with a spiral of metal wire or nylon filament embedded into their wall to prevent kinking or occlusion of the tube when the head or neck is moved (Fig. 6.37). Examples available in the US include the Portex Reinforced Silicone Endotracheal Tube (Smiths Medical International, Watford, UK). As the tube is very flexible in its longitudinal axis, a stylet is needed for intubation. The tube can be used orally, nasally, or through a tracheostomy stoma. The external diameter will be larger than ordinary tube of similar size. Certain manufacturers do not incorporate a bevel or Murphy eye in its tube design. Use of a reinforced tube is indicated when the patient's head is in an extended or flexed position, when the patient will be turned over, or during neurosurgical or head and neck procedures.

Double-Lumen Endobronchial

A double-lumen endobronchial tube is used when differential or selective lung ventilation is desired (Fig. 6.38). Its indications are discussed in Chap. 7. Older designs of this tube include the Gordon-Green, Carlens, White, Bryce-Smith, and Robert-Shaw.[204] Newer, disposable, clear plastic designs are now available (e.g., Broncho-Cath Endobronchial Tube, Covidien-Nellcor, Boulder, CO, the Double-Lumen Endobronchial Tube, Phoenix Medical, Bristol, UK, and Portex Endobronchial Double Lumen, Smiths Medical International, Watford, UK). These are often difficult to insert, however, and can easily occlude the right or left bronchus. An anesthesiologist should always be consulted before they are used.

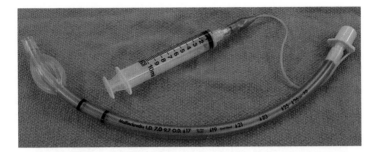

Fig. 6.37 Wire-reinforced endotracheal tube

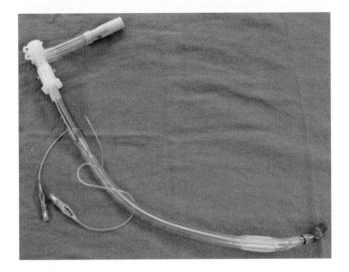

Fig. 6.38 Double-lumen endobronchial tube

Polar RAE (Ring-Adair-Elwyn)

Ring, Adair, and Elwyn developed a polar, preformed, pediatric tracheal tube
(Fig. 6.39), with an acute-angle bend remaining external to the patient, thereby
providing an unobstructed view of the surgical field and preventing injury to the
patient from the pressure of the metal connectors.[205] The tubes can be temporarily
straightened in order to provide suctioning. These tubes (RAE Tubes) are now
available from Mallinkcrodt (Hazelwood, MO) in adult and pediatric sizes for both
oral and nasal intubation. The major drawback for the use of these tubes is the
incidence of accidental bronchial intubation and thus there should be careful assessment of their placement. [206] The use of nasal RAE tubes for orotracheal intubation
has been reported for cases of otolaryngologic procedures requiring a small-sized
(6.0 mm ID) tube.[207]

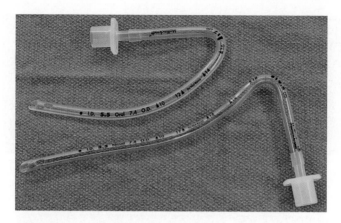

Fig. 6.39   Polar RAE tubes

Uncuffed

Uncuffed tubes are generally inserted in pediatric patients (see Fig. 6.34, Chap. 4). Cuffs are not necessary in most children under 8 years of age because the narrowest portion of a small child's airway is at the cricoid cartilage and an uncuffed tube of appropriate size should afford a reasonable seal at this level. Recent articles document that cuffed endotracheal tubes are safe to use in pediatric patients. The old dogma of using only uncuffed tubes in children is no longer accepted.[208-210]

Parker Flex-Tip

One should consider the orientation and shape of the tip of the endotracheal tube, especially if one has difficulty passing a standard tube through the vocal cords over a fiberoptic scope or a gum bougie. West et al.[211] described an experimental tube that had the bevel reversed and found that it was very easy to pass over a bougie under "simulated" difficult airway conditions. The Parker Flex-Tip (Fig. 6.40) manufactured by Parker Medical (Englewood, CO) comes in a variety of forms including oral and nasal versions in combination with preformed and reinforced walls. This tube has a centered bevel, which points toward the back of the tube. It also has a smooth, "hooded" tip that could facilitate passage of the tube through the glottic opening. The tube is promoted for reducing patient airway trauma, due to less tube tip hang-ups on the airway anatomy. This tracheal tube is useful for use over introducers and for FOIs; the centered, curved tube lies closely against the wall of the fiberscope or introducer.

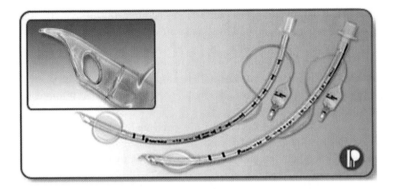

Fig. 6.40 Parker Flex-Tip (Copyright 2009 Parker Medical, with permission)

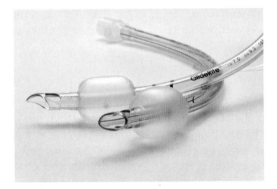

Fig. 6.41 GlideRite endotrachal tube (Copyright 2009 Verathon Inc., with permission)

GlideRite

Designed with the Parker Flex-Tip (Parker Medical, Denver, CO) technology and dual Murphy eyes, the GlideRite tube (Verathon Inc. in partnership with Parker Medical) is promoted for use with the GlideScope Video Larygoscope (Verathon Inc, Bothell, WA) and promises to minimize patient airway trauma and facilitate fast and easy intubation (Fig. 6.41).

Brief Review of Other Tubes

A review article by St. John describes some other interesting equipment for advanced airway management.[212] The Hi-Lo Evac Endotracheal Tube (Mallinckrodt Inc., Hazelwood, MO) incorporates a dedicated suction lumen and channel that can be used to clear secretions below the cords and above the balloon. These secretions may increase the risk of pulmonary infection in long-term intubated patients. St. John also presents a section on endotracheal cuff design and describes an ultrathin-walled tube that has a "no pressure" intraglottic cuff of unique "gill" design. This tube is described by its developers in various articles.[213, 214] Newly designed tubes and cuffs have been introduced that will hopefully make ventilation easier (less airway resistance) and decrease the likelihood of pressure-related trauma and injury to the mouth, larynx, or trachea.

Manufacturers of endotracheal tubes are continually incorporating new materials and design features into their products to make them more useful and safe. An example of one such feature is a cuff impervious to nitrous oxide that could limit pressure buildup in the cuff during an operation. Fujiwara et al.[215] describe the Trachelon (Terumo Co., Ltd., Tokyo, Japan), a gas barrier-type endotracheal tube, with such a cuff design. Comparing this tube with others designed to prevent N_2O diffusion (including the Profile Softseal Cuff (SIMS Portex, Kent, UK)), Karasawa et al.[216] suggest that cuff compliance, rather than N_2O impermeability, may be responsible for lower cuff pressures that develop when N_2O is used.

Cricothyrotomy

Literature supports the standpoint that, because cricothyrotomy is a rarely used technique, familiarity and training with various cricothyrotomy devices is the best predictor of success.[217,218] This section examines both catheter/tube-over-needle and wire-guided techniques and presents potential benefits and drawbacks of devices for each technique. It should also be noted that pediatric versions of several cricothyrotomy devices exist, but there is no evidence base to support their use, particularly in neonates and infants.[219] Detailed information on cricothyrotomy technique can be found in Chap. 12.

Catheter-Over-Needle Technique

Because of their inability to indicate accurate placement in the trachea, catheter or tube-over-needle devices have historically had the disadvantage when compared to wire-guided devices (Seldinger technique). However, a recent study found that, while physicians claimed to prefer wire-guided devices and technique, success rates were similar and insertion times were superior with indicator-guided catheter-over-needle devices.[220] We will examine three such devices and their variances.

PCK Indicator-Guided Device

The PCK indicator-guided instrument kit (Smiths Medical International, Hythe, Kent, UK) was developed for percutaneous emergency cricothyrotomy. The indicator consists of a straight varess needle and a blunt spring-loaded stylet. Guidelines suggest advancing until the red indicator springs back to indicated contact with the posterior wall. At that point, the operator should then redirect and advance the cannula downward. Preliminary in vivo studies are optimistic, provided the operator has received training and practice with the device.[221]

Nu-Trake

The Nu-Trake (Smiths Medical International, Hythe, Kent, UK) system is used for fast emergency airway access. This patented system provides a 4.5, 6.0, and a 7.2-mm I.D. airway within seconds. The integral 15 mm connection allows for immediate ventilation. A suction catheter can be introduced through the Nu-Trake airways. Mattinger et al.[222] suggest that less experienced physicians and residents would benefit from improved time to ventilation with the Nu-Trake kit over the surgical approach (58 ± 18s vs. 106 ± 48 s). However, they, along with Fikkers et al.,[217] also report more complications involving damage to the posterior tracheal wall with this kit.

QuickTrach

The Rusch QuickTrach (Teleflex Medical, Durham, NC) allows quick and safe access for ventilation in the presence of acute respiratory distress with upper airway obstruction. Craven and Vanner[223] point out that unless the occlusion is in the upper airway, the Quicktrach did not perform to satisfaction – a concern that might be alleviated by artificially increasing airway resistance. The kit consists of a preassembled emergency cricothyrotomy unit, with a 10-ml syringe attached to a padded neck strap and a connecting tube (Fig. 6.42). The removable stopper reduces the risk of damage to the posterior wall of the trachea and the conical needle tip guarantees the smallest necessary stoma and reduces bleeding. The syringe allows identification of the trachea by aspirating air.

Wire-Guided Technique

Physicians have stated that they preferred the wire-guided technique to the standard technique and also that it requires a smaller incision than the standard technique.[224] Fikkers et al.[217] warn that less experienced operators should beware of the risk of the guide wire perforating the posterior tracheal wall and the potential difficulty with the extra steps involved in this procedure. Kinking of the guide wire is also a problem reported among less experienced operators.[225] We examine two commonly used wire-guided cricothyrotomy devices.

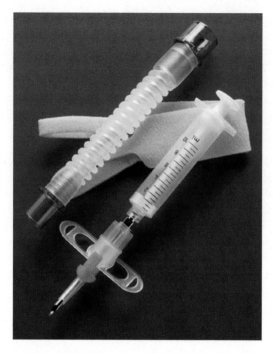

Fig. 6.42 QuickTrach cricothyrotomy set with red removable stopper (copyright © 2009 Teleflex Incorporated, with permission)

Minitrach II

The Seldinger (guidewire) type Minitrach II (Smiths Medical International, Hythe, Kent, UK) allows accurate guidance of the cannula through the cricothyroid membrane. It is reported to be associated with fewer traumas in conscious or partially conscious patients than with the QuickTrach because of the Minitrach's smaller Seldinger needle.[226]

Melker

The new Melker Cricothyrotomy kit (Cook Medical, Bloomington, IN) with cuffed catheter contains equipment necessary for standard wire-guided (Seldinger) technique or surgical technique via the cricothyroid membrane (Fig. 6.43). The Melker is reported to produce fewer and less severe lesions on the posterior wall of the larynx as compared to the PCK kit, likely because no contact between the needle and posterior wall of the larynx is required, as is the case with the PCK. The Melker guidewire allows for confirmation of correct device positioning, which may aid the inexperienced resident in safely performing a cricothyrotomy. Additionally, the curvature of the Melker allows it to be directed caudally, avoiding contact with the

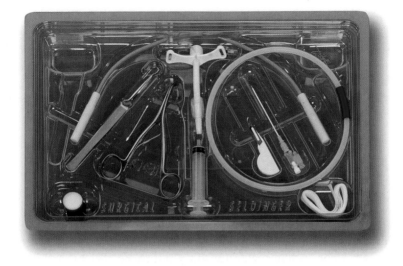

Fig. 6.43 Melker cricothyrotomy kit for wire-guided or surgical technique (Copyright 2009 Cook Medical Incorporated, Bloomington Indiana, with permission)

posterior wall of the trachea, which the more rigid PCK does not.[227, 228] However, the speed with which the Melker was used was questioned in the study of Dimitriadis et al.[229] when they compared the Melker, PCK, QuickTrach, and Minitrach in simulated emergency cricothyrotomy situations. They found the median time to ventilation significantly longer in the Melker as compared to the other three devices. Familiarity with the Seldinger technique has been reported to increase favorable outcomes with the Melker kit.[230]

Ultrasound Imaging of the Airway

Ultrasound technology is becoming more readily available to anesthesiologists due to its success in vascular assessment for regional anesthesia. Ultrasound may serve a supplementary role in clinical examination for assessing the airway both using sublingual or transcutaneous scanning.[231-234] Real-time ultrasound is suitable for evaluating vocal cord mobility in cases of hoarseness and stridor[235-239] and for identifying indirect signs of ventilation.[240] However, its real-time use for facilitating difficult airway management has not been established. This may be because ultrasonographic imaging of airway structures such as the larynx and trachea is limited by the presence of an air–tissue interface which allows little or no transmission of the ultrasound signal. Despite this, the ability of ultrasound to partially visualize the anatomy of the airway may still have a potential role in airway management. The use of this technology is particularly beneficial for pediatric patients due to the lack of radiation exposure or need for sedation, as required during other imaging procedures. In pediatric patients, ultrasound is excellent for identifying airway abnormalities and may aid in determining the presence, nature, and anatomic level of airway compromise.[241]

Portable ultrasound systems make airway imaging more accessible and cost effective. Moreover, they offer similar image resolution as larger systems, even allowing visualization of nerve structures. Following are the highlights of airway ultrasound images that can be obtained with some available systems.

Oral Cavity and Pharynx

Using a sublingual imaging approach, it is possible to obtain a longitudinal view of the oral cavity and pharynx by placing the probe sagittally and longitudinally under the patient's tongue (Fig. 6.44).[233] Excellent probe-tissue contact provides stable images while avoiding contact with the soft palate, thereby circumventing an unpleasant gagging reflex. This technique appears to provide effective imaging for the oral pharynx and bony structures such as the hyoid bone. During swallowing, a dynamic view of the hyoid's movement as it is pulled anteriorly by the geniohyoid muscle is clearly identified due to the bone's distinct hyperechoic (bright) appearance. Sublingual ultrasound images are easily obtained from patients without sedation or topicalization. In a pilot study (unpublished), the absence of the hyoid bone within the ultrasound image (interpreted as indicating a long mandibulohyoid distance which has been associated with difficulties in direct laryngoscopy[242]) was more sensitive and more specific than Mallampatti scoring, thyromental distance, and mouth opening as a predictor of laryngoscopic view.

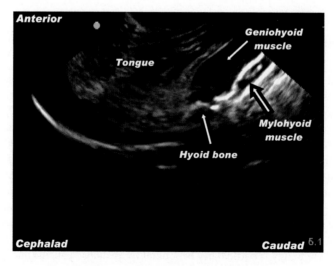

Fig. 6.44 Ultrasound image of the oral cavity and pharynx, with permission[234]

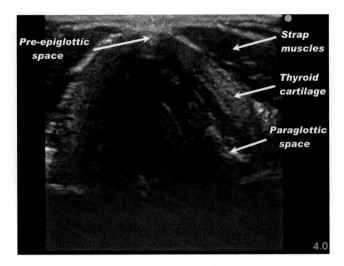

Fig. 6.45 Ultrasound image capturing transverse plane of the larynx

These findings warrant further study to determine whether sublingual ultrasound imaging of the airway can be used in some manner to predict airway difficulties. To achieve sublingual views, a small-footprint, high frequency curved array probe should be used.

Larynx

As shown in the figures, most of the important airway structures of the larynx at the level of vocal cord can be captured using transverse imaging. With the presence of a poor ultrasound medium, such as air, there appears a hyperechoic artifact, which in turn obscures the view of deeper structures (Fig. 6.45). Because a major portion of the epiglottis is suspended in air, and only the caudad portion is in contact with the adipose tissue at the preepiglottic space, intuitively, it should be nearly impossible to obtain a precise ultrasound image of the entire epiglottis (even using an anteroposterior probe orientation) with a transcutaneous approach.

Cervical Trachea

A transverse scan at the lower cervical level reveals the trachea and the location of the esophagus posterior to the trachea. A longitudinal scan at the midline of the anterior neck shows the presence of hypoechoic (dark) tracheal rings along the trachea (Fig. 6.46).

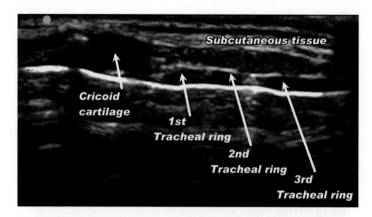

Fig. 6.46 Ultrasound image capturing longitudinal plane of the cervical trachea

Lung

Ultrasound images of the sliding lung sign – sliding of visceral and parietal pleura past each other during intermittent positive pressure ventilation – may be taken on both sides of the chest at the midaxillary line. Studies in a cadaver model[243] and in living subjects[240] show that the identification of a sliding lung sign with ultrasound is an accurate method for confirmation of endotracheal tube placement. Further, the technique may have some utility in differentiating right main stem bronchus from main tracheal intubations. This would allow for diagnosis of correct tube placement at the bedside in emergency situations (respiratory distressed/ventilated patient, cardiac arrest, etc.).[244]

Available Portable Ultrasound Systems

SonoSite (Bothell, WA, USA) makes the M-Turbo for abdominal, vascular, nerve, cardiac, and superficial imaging. It is available with GT and HD technology for enhanced color flow. The newest generation of M-Turbo has greatly improved processing power and is lightweight and portable. The SonoSite Titan is a high-resolution modular system that allows both stationary and mobile use with a Mobile Docking System for operator access to both internal and external information systems. General Electric (Fairfield, CT) combined the technology of their three console systems, the LOGIQ, Vivid, and Voluson, to create a compact, portable version. The LOGIQe is designed specifically for anesthesiologists and would be suitable for obtaining views of the airway. Siemens makes the Acuson line of ultrasound machines (Mountain View, CA) with a variety of models to choose from, including a handheld pocket ultrasound device (Acuson P10) and a device that provides tissue strain analysis, providing a quantitative value measurement of tissue elasticity (Acuson S2000).

Airway Management Training Devices

Airway difficulties are uncommon and the clinician may not receive adequate emergency scenario exposure to confidently handle all stages of the difficult airway algorithm. Alternatives for hands-on training and practice in airway management skills include:[245]

- Task/skills trainers (bench models)
- Simple manikins
- High-fidelity, full-scale simulator manikins and settings
- Animal models
- Cadavers
- Virtual reality simulators

With any of these modalities, annual retraining should be undertaken to maintain knowledge and skills.[246]

Task/Skills Trainers

For specific areas of skill development, instead of entire full-body manikins, anatomy-specific manikins, also called task or skills trainers, are available for use. Studies comparing four of these skills-trainer manikins evaluated ease of insertion of eight types of supraglottic devices,[247] seven types of single-use LMAs,[248] and the teaching methodology of the Difficult Airway Society's (DAS) difficult and advanced airway techniques.[249] The skills-trainer manikins that were studied included Airway Management Trainer (Ambu, UK), Airway Trainer (Laerdal, Norway), Airsim (Trucorp, Northern Ireland), and Bill-1 (VBM, Germany).

When testing ease and accuracy of insertion of the eight supraglottic devices, the Airsim was the overall better performer with all devices, despite acknowledgement that it was the least life-like in appearance. The Airway Trainer also performed significantly better than the other two manikins. Problems with Bill-1 included rigidity of the airway and lack of distinct endpoint, which led to problems with more flexible devices and inserting devices too far. The Airway Management Trainer was noted to have stiff skin and prominent teeth, which made mouth opening difficult.

For the LMA insertion study, researchers found that, while all the manikins studied could be considered adequate for LMA insertion training purposes, the Bill-1 was consistently rated as more life-like in performance and was most often associated with insertion and ventilation success while incorporating measures of clinical and anatomical position (Fig. 6.47).

When comparing the four skills-trainer manikins on their overall performance of DAS-specified airway management techniques, post hoc analysis showed significant differences between manikins, favoring Laerdal's Airway Trainer, followed by

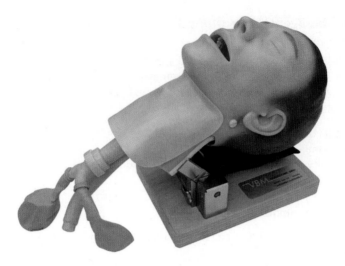

Fig. 6.47 Bill-1 with bayonette connector balloons for practicing endotracheal intubation, bronchoscopy, fiberoptic intubation, cricothyrotomy, transtracheal jet ventilation, mask ventilation, ventilation with laryngeal tube, laryngeal mask, combitube, and Easytube (Copyright 2009 VBM-Medical, with permission)

Trucorp's Airsim. For non-DAS techniques, Laerdal and Trucorp scored at the top with no statistical significance between the two.

In each of these evaluative studies, the authors did note that improvements and modifications to the studied manikin models may have been made since their testing. Also noted was the fact that because only one manikin of each manufacturer was used, unknown variations between individual manikins may exist, and that factors of durability and cost were not assessed, although these would likely affectdecision making on the most appropriate skills-trainer. In their final analysis of all the manikins studied, the authors reported the Laerdal Airway Trainer and the Trucorp Airsim manikins to be suitable for simulating a wide variety of simple and advanced airway management techniques.

Manikins and Simulated Settings

Two full-scale computerized patient simulator manikins are commonly available, one of which is SimMan (Laerdal, Norway), a manikin that provides immediate feedback for interventions. Laerdal also makes SimBaby for airway management, intravenous therapy, defibrillation, and adjustable anatomy to represent conditions such as tongue edema, pharyngeal swelling, laryngospasm, bulging or sunken fontanel, etc. SimNewB features realistic newborn traits and life-like clinical feedback including drug recognition and Advanced Life Support Simulator for training in a wide range of advanced life-saving skills in medical emergencies.

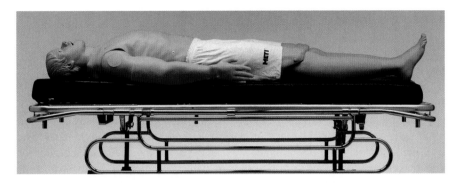

Fig. 6.48 METI human patient simulator (Photo Courtesy of METI© 2009)

SimMan's patented airway system allows simulation of difficult airway management scenarios and realistic practice for chest tube insertion, needle and surgical crico-thyrotomy, and fiberoptic bronchoscopy. The accompanying software with patient monitor allows snapshots of X-rays, ECGs, etc. Instructors can also design and save their own patient cases (Fig. 6.48). John et al.[250] showed that, while all anesthesiologists studied benefitted from practicing cricothyrotomy techniques with SimMan, time to ventilate was increased significantly with the addition of a realistic mock operating theater setting, with standard, noninvasive monitoring and pulse oximeter alarms set at high volume. Psychological stress induced by the realistic situation is likely the cause of increased time to ventilation. Kuduvalli et al.[251] noted that the anatomical characteristics of the SimMan made some of the airway maneuvers more difficult than usual and the degree of obstruction to ventilation may have been unrealistic.

The second full-scale patient simulator is the METI Human Patient Simulator (Medical Education Technologies, Sarasota, FL). METI also makes other models such as the entry-level METI Man, completely wireless iStan, the wired Emergency Care Powerhouse for advanced airway, pulmonary and cardiovascular systems, along with ACLS, and trauma features for emergency training. PediaSIM is calibrated to mirror the parameters and responses of a young patient. BabySIM is a representation of a 3–6-month-old infant for CPR, airway management, drug administration, defibrillation, etc. When one American school of medicine discontinued animal vivisection and switched to using task trainers and the METI ECS full-body patient simulator, students reported increased confidence levels in performing life-saving procedures, including orotracheal intubation and placing a chest tube.[252]

In one recent study,[253] after attending lectures and simulator-based airway management training, the majority of responding attendees reported that the experience gained during simulator-based scenarios in simulated settings helped them to manage difficult airway situations better in their daily clinical practice, more than with lectures and skill stations.

Animal Models

Arguments have been made about the superiority of animal models over manikins. Cho et al.[254] compared a porcine model (made up of larynxes and trachea of freshly slaughtered pigs covered with thinned pigskin, stapled to a wooden board) to the Tracheostomy Trainer and Case manikin (Smith Medical International, Kent, UK). Data on the usefulness of training for the cricothyrotomy technique were compared between the two models. They found that, while there was no difference in degree of difficulty between the two training models, the porcine model scored higher for realistic skin turgor, degree of difficulty with skin penetration, difficulty with landmark recognition, similarity to human anatomy and overall preference. Thus, the porcine model was found to be a more useful training tool than the manikin model for cricothyrotomy with a PCK kit.

Cummings and Getz[255] evaluated a novel animal model for teaching intubation and found that deer heads (over 100,000 of which were harvested in 2004 in the state of Illinois alone) were rated as having more elasticity and realism in tissue and anatomy. Additionally, they were more easily intubated and were preferred as a learning tool by study participants. These findings were compared to Laerdal's Airway Management Trainer, in which participants noted that the esophagus was more easily identified, but that other anatomical structures relevant to the procedure (vallecula, epiglottis, vocal cords, trachea) were more easily identified in the deer model.

Certainly, more realistic tissues, blood, and secretions in animals have advantages over synthetic manikins, but, as with animal studies, it is important to obtain relevant animal ethics approval for training purposes.

Cadaver Models

The most realistic airway management training experience may come from human cadavers, but there is some controversy in this practice, with detractors citing the continual improvement of manikins and other training modalities available.[245] Hatton et al.[256] showed that there was a significant improvement in anesthesiology residents' confidence in performing percutaneous cricothyrotomy and retrograde intubation after training using embalmed cadavers. This does not, however, show that cadaver practice is more effective than other training modalities. Supply issues may also be a problem for ongoing, regular training opportunities.[257]

Virtual Reality Simulators

In patients with anticipated difficult airway, awake FOI offers a higher degree of safety.[258] The value of manikin, task trainer, and simulator-based training in FOI has already been shown[259-261], and virtual reality simulator programs are now showing promise as well.

One such simulator is the AccuTouch Bronchoscopy Simulator (Immersion Medical, Gaithersburg, USA), which comes with its own bench model and accompanying monitor and software. It allows the complex skills associated with FOI to be learned and practiced in virtual reality by presenting realistic bronchoscopy situations. The simulator feels like a realistic bronchoscope and is operated in the same manner. The tension and resistance felt when operating the device in the virtual patient also mimic a realistic scenario (e.g., bleeding if nonanesthetized mucous membranes are hit, causing the "patient" to cough). Goldmann and Steinfeldt[262] showed that viewing a three-dimensional representation of the structures on a two-dimensional monitor allowed residents with no experience to gain the dexterity required to perform a FOI on a cadaver as quickly as an experienced physician, as opposed to residents not exposed to the virtual reality simulator, who required longer to perform a FOI on a cadaver.

Also available is the VFI ("Virtual Fibreoptic Intubation") software (free with a written communication, KarlStorz GMGH). The virtual simulator consists of a single CD-ROM that can be used for self-training on any computer without any additional training or an instructor. This multimedia tool shows reconstructed images of actual patients' computerized tomography and MRI, with disorders ranging from cleft palate to posttracheotomy tracheal stenosis. Patient airway images range from children to adult and unrestricted views are available, allowing the student to navigate the upper airway independently. If students make a mistake, an expert explanation of the correct technique is provided. Boet et al.[263] evaluated this software for its efficacy as an adjunct to instructor-led training by allowing students to acquire airway knowledge through the CD so that they could concentrate on the required psychomotor skills during hands-on practice. They found that, of the students who were given the VFI CD-ROM in addition to didactic teaching on FOI, 81% achieved intubation success in the allotted timeframe, as opposed to the 52% success rate of students who received only the lecture. The VFI group also showed a trend toward higher FOI ability than their non-VFI trained counterparts.

Acknowledgments The author would like to thank Jennifer Pillay, Nikki Stalker, Adam Dryden, and Dr. Pratamaporn Chanthong for their contribution to this chapter.

References

1. Bein B, Scholz J. Supraglottic airway devices. *Best Pract Res Clin Anaesthesiol.* 2005;19:581-593.
2. Miller DM. A proposed classification and scoring system for supraglottic sealing airways: a brief review. *Anesth Analg.* 2004;99:1553–1559.
3. Brain AI. The laryngeal mask–a new concept in airway management. *Br J Anaesth.* 1983;55:801–805.
4. Verghese C. Airway management. *Curr Opin Anaesthesiol.* 1999;12:667–674.
5. Russo SG, Goetze B, Troche S, Barwing J, Quintel M, Timmermann A. LMA-ProSeal for elective postoperative care on the intensive care unit: a prospective, randomized trial. *Anesthesiology.* 2009;111:116–121.
6. Raphael J, Rosenthal-Ganon T, Gozal Y. Emergency airway management with a laryngeal mask airway in a patient placed in the prone position. *J Clin Anesth.* 2004;16:560–561.

7. Bannon L, Brimacombe J, Nixon T, Keller C. Repeat autoclaving does not remove protein deposits from the classic laryngeal mask airway. *Eur J Anaesthesiol.* 2005;22:515–517.

8. Cao MM, Webb T, Bjorksten AR. Comparison of disposable and reusable laryngeal mask airways in spontaneously ventilating adult patients. *Anaesth Intensive Care.* 2004;32:530–534.

9. Brimacombe J, Keller C, Fullekrug B, et al. A multicenter study comparing the ProSeal and Classic laryngeal mask airway in anesthetized, nonparalyzed patients. *Anesthesiology.* 2002;96:289–295.

10. Cook TM, Lee G, Nolan JP. The ProSeal laryngeal mask airway: a review of the literature. *Can J Anesth.* 2005;52:739–760.

11. van Zundert A, Brimacombe J. The LMA Supreme–a pilot study. *Anaesthesia.* 2008;63:209–210.

12. Verghese C, Ramaswamy B. LMA-Supreme–a new single-use LMA with gastric access: a report on its clinical efficacy. *Br J Anaesth.* 2008;101:405–410.

13. Dorges V. Airway management in emergency situations. *Best Pract Res Clin Anaesthesiol.* 2005;19:699–715.

14. Baskett PJ, Parr MJ, Nolan JP. The intubating laryngeal mask. Results of a multicentre trial with experience of 500 cases. *Anaesthesia.* 1998;53:1174–1179.

15. Ferson DZ, Rosenblatt WH, Johansen MJ, Osborn I, Ovassapian A. Use of the intubating LMA-Fastrach in 254 patients with difficult-to-manage airways. *Anesthesiology.* 2001;95:1175–1181.

16. Liu EH, Goy RW, Lim Y, Chen FG. Success of tracheal intubation with intubating laryngeal mask airways: a randomized trial of the LMA Fastrach and LMA CTrach. *Anesthesiology.* 2008;108:621-626.

17. Liu EH, Goy RW, Chen FG. The LMA CTrach, a new laryngeal mask airway for endotracheal intubation under vision: evaluation in 100 patients. *Br J Anaesth.* 2006;96:396–400.

18. Timmermann A, Russo S, Graf BM. Evaluation of the CTrach–an intubating LMA with integrated fibreoptic system. *Br J Anaesth.* 2006;96:516–521.

19. Liu EH, Goy RW, Chen FG. An evaluation of poor LMA CTrach views with a fibreoptic laryngoscope and the effectiveness of corrective measures. *Br J Anaesth.* 2006;97:878–882.

20. Sreevathsa S, Nathan PL, John B, Danha RF, Mendonca C. Comparison of fibreoptic-guided intubation through ILMA versus intubation through LMA-CTrach. *Anaesthesia.* 2008;63:734–737.

21. Mihai R, Blair E, Kay H, Cook TM. A quantitative review and meta-analysis of performance of non-standard laryngoscopes and rigid fibreoptic intubation aids. *Anaesthesia.* 2008;63: 745–760.

22. Dorges V, Ocker H, Wenzel V, Schmucker P. The laryngeal tube: a new simple airway device. *Anesth Analg.* 2000;90:1220–1222.

23. Dorges V, Ocker H, Wenzel V, Steinfath M, Gerlach K. The Laryngeal Tube S: a modified simple airway device. *Anesth Analg.* 2003;96:618–621, table.

24. Cook TM, McKinstry C, Hardy R, Twigg S. Randomized crossover comparison of the ProSeal laryngeal mask airway with the Laryngeal Tube during anaesthesia with controlled ventilation. *Br J Anaesth.* 2003;91:678–683.

25. Cook TM, McCormick B, Asai T. Randomized comparison of laryngeal tube with classic laryngeal mask airway for anaesthesia with controlled ventilation. *Br J Anaesth.* 2003;91:373–378.

26. Asai T, Shingu K. The laryngeal tube. *Br J Anaesth.* 2005;95:729–736.

27. Beylacq L, Bordes M, Semjen F, Cros AM. The I-gel, a single-use supraglottic airway device with a non-inflatable cuff and an esophageal vent: an observational study in children. *Acta Anaesthesiol Scand.* 2009;53:376–379.

28. Levitan RM, Kinkle WC. Initial anatomic investigations of the I-gel airway: a novel supraglottic airway without inflatable cuff. *Anaesthesia.* 2005;60:1022–1026.

29. Bamgbade OA, Macnab WR, Khalaf WM. Evaluation of the i-gel airway in 300 patients. *Eur J Anaesthesiol.* 2008;25:865–866.

30. Wharton NM, Gibbison B, Gabbott DA, Haslam GM, Muchatuta N, Cook TM. I-gel insertion by novices in manikins and patients. *Anaesthesia.* 2008;63:991–995.

31. Hooshangi H, Wong DT. Brief review: the cobra perilaryngeal airway (CobraPLA and the Streamlined liner of pharyngeal airway (SLIPA) supraglottic airways. *Can J Anesth.* 2008;55:177–185.

32. Hein C, Plummer J, Owen H. Evaluation of the SLIPA (streamlined liner of the pharynx airway), a single use supraglottic airway device, in 60 anaesthetized patients undergoing minor surgical procedures. *Anaesth Intensive Care*. 2005;33:756–761.
33. Miller DM, Camporota L. Advantages of ProSeal and SLIPA airways over tracheal tubes for gynecological laparoscopies. *Can J Anesth*. 2006;53:188–193.
34. Miller DM, Light D. Laboratory and clinical comparisons of the Streamlined Liner of the Pharynx Airway (SLIPA) with the laryngeal mask airway. *Anaesthesia*. 2003;58:136–142.
35. Thew M, Paech M. Results of a company designed evaluation of the SLIPA. *Anaesth Intensive Care*. 2008;36:616–617.
36. Brain AI. The development of the Laryngeal Mask–a brief history of the invention, early clinical studies and experimental work from which the Laryngeal Mask evolved. *Eur J Anaesthesiol Suppl*. 1991;4:5–17.
37. Frass M, Frenzer R, Rauscha F, Weber H, Pacher R, Leithner C. Evaluation of esophageal tracheal combitube in cardiopulmonary resuscitation. *Crit Care Med*. 1987;15:609–611.
38. Thierbach AR, Werner C. Infraglottic airway devices and techniques. *Best Pract Res Clin Anaesthesiol*. 2005;19:595–609.
39. Rumball CJ, MacDonald D. The PTL, Combitube, laryngeal mask, and oral airway: a randomized prehospital comparative study of ventilatory device effectiveness and cost-effectiveness in 470 cases of cardiorespiratory arrest. *Prehosp Emerg Care*. 1997;1:1–10.
40. Klein H, Williamson M, Sue-Ling HM, Vucevic M, Quinn AC. Esophageal rupture associated with the use of the Combitube. *Anesth Analg*. 1997;85:937–939.
41. Thierbach AR, Piepho T, Maybauer MO. A new device for emergency airway mangement: the EasyTube. *Resuscitation*. 2004;60:347–348.
42. Thierbach AR, Piepho T, Maybauer M. The EasyTube for airway management in emergencies. *Prehosp Emerg Care*. 2005;9:445–448.
43. Loftus RW, Koff MD, Burchman CC, et al. Transmission of pathogenic bacterial organisms in the anesthesia work area. *Anesthesiology*. 2008;109:399–407.
44. Muscarella LF. Recommendations to resolve inconsistent guidelines for the reprocessing of sheathed and unsheathed rigid laryngoscopes. *Infect Control Hosp Epidemiol*. 2007;28:504–507.
45. Simmons SA. Laryngoscope handles: a potential for infection. *AANA J*. 2000;68:233–236.
46. Skilton RW. Risks of cross infection associated with anaesthesia; cleaning procedures for laryngoscopes–a need for Association guidelines? *Anaesthesia*. 1996;51:512–513.
47. Call TR, Auerbach FJ, Riddell SW, et al. Nosocomial contamination of laryngoscope handles: challenging current guidelines. *Anesth Analg*. 2009;109:479–483.
48. Marks RR, Hancock R, Charters P. An analysis of laryngoscope blade shape and design: new criteria for laryngoscope evaluation. *Can J Anesth*. 1993;40:262–270.
49. McIntyre JW. Tracheal intubation and laryngoscope design. *Can J Anesth*. 1993;40:193–196.
50. Norton ML. Laryngoscope blade shape. *Can J Anesth*. 1994;41:263–265.
51. Relle A. Laryngoscope design. *Can J Anesth*. 1994;41:162–163.
52. Lagade MR, Poppers PJ. Use of the left-entry laryngoscope blade in patients with right-sided oro-facial lesions. *Anesthesiology*. 1983;58:300.
53. McComish PB. Left sided laryngoscopes. *Anaesthesia*. 1965;20:372.
54. Elder J, Waisel DB. Case report of the one-armed anesthesiology resident. *J Clin Anesth*. 2004;16:445–448.
55. Lagade MR, Poppers PJ. Revival of the Polio laryngoscope blade. *Anesthesiology*. 1982;57:545.
56. Bourke DL, Lawrence J. Another way to insert a Macintosh blade. *Anesthesiology*. 1983;59:80.
57. Siker ES. A mirror laryngoscope. *Anesthesiology*. 1956;17:38–42.
58. Bellhouse CP. An angulated laryngoscope for routine and difficult tracheal intubation. *Anesthesiology*. 1988;69:126–129.
59. Mayall RM. The Belscope for management of the difficult airway. *Anesthesiology*. 1992;76:1059–1061.
60. Taguchi N, Watanabe S, Kumagai M, Takeshima R, Asakura N. Radiographic documentation of increased visibility of the larynx with a belscope laryngoscope blade. *Anesthesiology*. 1994;81:773–775.

61. McCoy EP, Mirakhur RK. The levering laryngoscope. *Anaesthesia*. 1993;48:516–519.
62. McCoy EP, Mirakhur RK, McCloskey BV. A comparison of the stress response to laryngoscopy. The Macintosh versus the McCoy blade. *Anaesthesia*. 1995;50:943–946.
63. McCoy EP, Mirakhur RK, Rafferty C, Bunting H, Austin BA. A comparison of the forces exerted during laryngoscopy. The Macintosh versus the McCoy blade. *Anaesthesia*. 1996;51:912–915.
64. Uchida T, Hikawa Y, Saito Y, Yasuda K. The McCoy levering laryngoscope in patients with limited neck extension. *Can J Anesth*. 1997;44:674–676.
65. Chisholm DG, Calder I. Experience with the McCoy laryngoscope in difficult laryngoscopy. *Anaesthesia*. 1997;52:906–908.
66. Gabbott DA. Laryngoscopy using the McCoy laryngoscope after application of a cervical collar. *Anaesthesia*. 1996;51:812–814.
67. Laurent SC, de Melo AE. exander–Williams JM. The use of the McCoy laryngoscope in patients with simulated cervical spine injuries. *Anaesthesia*. 1996;51:74–75.
68. Sugiyama K, Yokoyama K. Head extension angle required for direct laryngoscopy with the McCoy laryngoscope blade. *Anesthesiology*. 2001;94:939.
69. Tewari P, Gupta D, Kumar A, Singh U. Opioid sparing during endotracheal intubation using McCoy laryngoscope in neurosurgical patients: the comparison of haemodynamic changes with Macintosh blade in a randomized trial. *J Postgrad Med*. 2005;51:260–264.
70. Aoyama K, Nagaoka E, Takenaka I, Kadoya T. The McCoy laryngoscope expands the laryngeal aperture in patients with difficult intubation. *Anesthesiology*. 2000;92:1855–1856.
71. Asai T, Matsumoto S, Shingu K. Use of the McCoy laryngoscope or fingers to facilitate fibrescope-aided tracheal intubation. *Anaesthesia*. 1998;53:903–905.
72. Randell T, Maattanen M, Kytta J. The best view at laryngoscopy using the McCoy laryngoscope with and without cricoid pressure. *Anaesthesia*. 1998;53:536–539.
73. Ochroch EA, Levitan RM. A videographic analysis of laryngeal exposure comparing the articulating laryngoscope and external laryngeal manipulation. *Anesth Analg*. 2001;92:267–270.
74. Usui T, Saito S, Goto F. Arytenoid dislocation while using a McCoy laryngoscope. *Anesth Analg*. 2001;92:1347–1348.
75. Benham SW, Gale L. A new hinged tip laryngoscope. *Anaesthesia*. 1997;52:869–871.
76. Iohom G, Franklin R, Casey W, Lyons B. The McCoy straight blade does not improve laryngoscopy and intubation in normal infants. *Can J Anesth*. 2004;51:155–159.
77. Gerlach K, Wenzel V, von Knobelsdorff G, Steinfath M, Dorges V. A new universal laryngoscope blade: a preliminary comparison with Macintosh laryngoscope blades. *Resuscitation*. 2003;57:63–67.
78. Sethuraman D, Darshane S, Guha A, Charters P. A randomised, crossover study of the Dorges, McCoy and Macintosh laryngoscope blades in a simulated difficult intubation scenario. *Anaesthesia*. 2006;61:482–487.
79. Leung YY, Hung CT, Tan ST. Evaluation of the new Viewmax laryngoscope in a simulated difficult airway. *Acta Anaesthesiol Scand*. 2006;50:562–567.
80. Barak M, Philipchuck P, Abecassis P, Katz Y. A comparison of the Truview blade with the Macintosh blade in adult patients. *Anaesthesia*. 2007;62:827–831.
81. Miceli L, Cecconi M, Tripi G, Zauli M, Della RG. Evaluation of new laryngoscope blade for tracheal intubation, Truview EVO2: a manikin study. *Eur J Anaesthesiol*. 2008;25:446–449.
82. Singh R, Singh P, Vajifdar H. A comparison of Truview infant EVO2 laryngoscope with the Miller blade in neonates and infants. *Pediatr Anesth*. 2009;19:338–342.
83. Bjoraker DG. The Bullard intubating laryngoscopes. *Anesthesiol Rev*. 1990;17:64–70.
84. Borland LM, Casselbrant M. The Bullard laryngoscope. A new indirect oral laryngoscope (pediatric version). *Anesth Analg*. 1990;70:105–108.
85. Dyson A, Harris J, Bhatia K. Rapidity and accuracy of tracheal intubation in a mannequin: comparison of the fibreoptic with the Bullard laryngoscope. *Br J Anaesth*. 1990;65:268–270.
86. Mendel P, Bristow A. Anaesthesia for procedures on the larynx and pharynx. The use of the Bullard laryngoscope in conjunction with high frequency jet ventilation. *Anaesthesia*. 1993;48:263–265.

87. Wu TL, Chou HC. A new laryngoscope: the combination intubating device. *Anesthesiology*. 1994;81:1085–1087.
88. O'Neill D, Capan LM, Sheth R. Flexiguide intubation guide to facilitate airway management with WuScope system. *Anesthesiology*. 1998;89:545.
89. Sprung J, Weingarten T, Dilger J. The use of WuScope fiberoptic laryngoscopy for tracheal intubation in complex clinical situations. *Anesthesiology*. 2003;98:263–265.
90. Wu TL, Chou HC. WuScope versus conventional laryngoscope in cervical spine immobilization. *Anesthesiology*. 2000;93:588–589.
91. Bucx MJ, Veldman DJ, Beenhakker MM, Koster R. The effect of steam sterilisation at 134 degrees C on light intensity provided by fibrelight Macintosh laryngoscopes. *Anaesthesia*. 1999;54:875–878.
92. Tousignant G, Tessler MJ. Light intensity and area of illumination provided by various laryngoscope blades. *Can J Anesth*. 1994;41:865–869.
93. Fletcher J. Laryngoscope light intensity. *Can J Anesth*. 1995;42:259–260.
94. Kaplan MB, Ward DS, Berci G. A new video laryngoscope-an aid to intubation and teaching. *J Clin Anesth*. 2002;14:620–626.
95. Kaplan MB, Hagberg CA, Ward DS, et al. Comparison of direct and video-assisted views of the larynx during routine intubation. *J Clin Anesth*. 2006;18:357–362.
96. Jungbauer A, Schumann M, Brunkhorst V, Borgers A, Groeben H. Expected difficult tracheal intubation: a prospective comparison of direct laryngoscopy and video laryngoscopy in 200 patients. *Br J Anaesth*. 2009;102:546–550.
97. Wald SH, Keyes M, Brown A. Pediatric video laryngoscope rescue for a difficult neonatal intubation. *Pediatr Anesth*. 2008;18:790–792.
98. Fiadjoe JE, Stricker PA, Hackell RS, et al. The efficacy of the Storz Miller 1 video laryngoscope in a simulated infant difficult intubation. *Anesth Analg*. 2009;108:1783–1786.
99. Cooper RM, Pacey JA, Bishop MJ, McCluskey SA. Early clinical experience with a new videolaryngoscope (GlideScope) in 728 patients. *Can J Anesth*. 2005;52:191–198.
100. Neustein SM. The GlideScope-specific rigid stylet to facilitate tracheal intubation with the Glidescope. *Can J Anesth*. 2008;55:196–197.
101. Rai MR, Dering A, Verghese C. The Glidescope system: a clinical assessment of performance. *Anaesthesia*. 2005;60:60–64.
102. Sun DA, Warriner CB, Parsons DG, Klein R, Umedaly HS, Moult M. The GlideScope video laryngoscope: randomized clinical trial in 200 patients. *Br J Anaesth*. 2005;94:381–384.
103. Cooper RM. Complications associated with the use of the GlideScope videolaryngoscope. *Can J Anesth*. 2007;54:54–57.
104. Leong WL, Lim Y, Sia AT. Palatopharyngeal wall perforation during Glidescope intubation. *Anaesth Intensive Care*. 2008;36:870–874.
105. Jones PM, Armstrong KP, Armstrong PM, et al. A comparison of glidescope videolaryngoscopy to direct laryngoscopy for nasotracheal intubation. *Anesth Analg*. 2008;107:144–148.
106. Trevisanuto D, Fornaro E, Verghese C. The GlideScope video laryngoscope: initial experience in five neonates. *Can J Anesth*. 2006;53:423–424.
107. Kim JT, Na HS, Bae JY, et al. GlideScope video laryngoscope: a randomized clinical trial in 203 paediatric patients. *Br J Anaesth*. 2008;101:531–534.
108. Turkstra TP, Craen RA, Pelz DM, Gelb AW. Cervical spine motion: a fluoroscopic comparison during intubation with lighted stylet, GlideScope, and Macintosh laryngoscope. *Anesth Analg*. 2005;101:910–915, table.
109. Robitaille A, Williams SR, Tremblay MH, Guilbert F, Theriault M, Drolet P. Cervical spine motion during tracheal intubation with manual in-line stabilization: direct laryngoscopy versus GlideScope videolaryngoscopy. *Anesth Analg*. 2008;106:935–941, table.
110. Wong DM, Prabhu A, Chakraborty S, Tan G, Massicotte EM, Cooper R. Cervical spine motion during flexible bronchoscopy compared with the Lo-Pro GlideScope. *Br J Anaesth*. 2009;102:424–430.
111. Lai HY, Chen IH, Chen A, Hwang FY, Lee Y. The use of the GlideScope for tracheal intubation in patients with ankylosing spondylitis. *Br J Anaesth*. 2006;97:419–422.

112. Lim Y, Lim TJ, Liu EH. Ease of intubation with the GlideScope or Macintosh laryngoscope by inexperienced operators in simulated difficult airways. *Can J Anaesth.* 2004;51:641–642.
113. Benjamin FJ, Boon D, French RA. An evaluation of the GlideScope, a new video laryngoscope for difficult airways: a manikin study. *Eur J Anaesthesiol.* 2006;23:517–521.
114. Nouruzi-Sedeh P, Schumann M, Groeben H. Laryngoscopy via Macintosh blade versus GlideScope: success rate and time for endotracheal intubation in untrained medical personnel. *Anesthesiology.* 2009;110:32–37.
115. Lim TJ, Lim Y, Liu EH. Evaluation of ease of intubation with the GlideScope or Macintosh laryngoscope by anaesthetists in simulated easy and difficult laryngoscopy. *Anaesthesia.* 2005;60:180–183.
116. Xue FS, Zhang GH, Li XY, et al. Comparison of hemodynamic responses to orotracheal intubation with the GlideScope videolaryngoscope and the Macintosh direct laryngoscope. *J Clin Anesth.* 2007;19:245–250.
117. Xue FS, Zhang GH, Li XY, et al. Comparison of haemodynamic responses to orotracheal intubation with GlideScope videolaryngoscope and fibreoptic bronchoscope. *Eur J Anaesthesiol.* 2006;23:522–526.
118. Shippey B, Ray D, McKeown D. Case series: the McGrath videolaryngoscope–an initial clinical evaluation. *Can J Anesth.* 2007;54:307–313.
119. Shippey B, Ray D, McKeown D. Use of the McGrath videolaryngoscope in the management of difficult and failed tracheal intubation. *Br J Anaesth.* 2008;100:116–119.
120. O'Leary AM, Sandison MR, Myneni N, Cirilla DJ, Roberts KW, Deane GD. Preliminary evaluation of a novel videolaryngoscope, the McGrath series 5, in the management of difficult and challenging endotracheal intubation. *J Clin Anesth.* 2008;20:320–321.
121. Budde AO, Pott LM. Endotracheal tube as a guide for an Eschmann gum elastic bougie to aid tracheal intubation using the McGrath or GlideScope videolaryngoscopes. *J Clin Anesth.* 2008;20:560.
122. Koyama J, Aoyama T, Kusano Y, et al. Description and first clinical application of AirWay Scope for tracheal intubation. *J Neurosurg Anesthesiol.* 2006;18:247–250.
123. Suzuki A, Abe N, Sasakawa T, Kunisawa T, Takahata O, Iwasaki H. Pentax-AWS (Airway Scope) and Airtraq: big difference between two similar devices. *J Anesth.* 2008;22:191–192.
124. Hirabayashi Y, Seo N. Airway Scope: early clinical experience in 405 patients. *J Anesth.* 2008;22:81–85.
125. Suzuki A, Toyama Y, Katsumi N, et al. The Pentax-AWS((R)) rigid indirect video laryngoscope: clinical assessment of performance in 320 cases. *Anaesthesia.* 2008;63:641–647.
126. Suzuki A, Toyama Y, Katsumi N, Kunisawa T, Henderson JJ, Iwasaki H. Cardiovascular responses to tracheal intubation with the Airway Scope (Pentax-AWS). *J Anesth.* 2008;22:100–101.
127. Asai T, Liu EH, Matsumoto S, et al. Use of the Pentax-AWS in 293 patients with difficult airways. *Anesthesiology.* 2009;110:898–904.
128. Komatsu R, Kamata K, Hamada K, Sessler DI, Ozaki M. Airway scope and StyletScope for tracheal intubation in a simulated difficult airway. *Anesth Analg.* 2009;108:273–279.
129. Liu EH, Poon KH, Ng BS, Goh EY, Goy RW. The Airway Scope, a new video laryngoscope: its use in three patients with cervical spine problems. *Br J Anaesth.* 2008;100:142–143.
130. Suzuki A, Terao M, Aizawa K, Sasakawa T, Henderson JJ, Iwasaki H. Pentax-AWS airway Scope as an alternative for awake flexible fiberoptic intubation of a morbidly obese patient in the semi-sitting position. *J Anesth.* 2009;23:162–163.
131. Poon KH, Liu EH. The Airway Scope for difficult double-lumen tube intubation. *J Clin Anesth.* 2008;20:319.
132. Maruyama K, Yamada T, Kawakami R, Hara K. Randomized cross–over comparison of cervical-spine motion with the AirWay Scope or Macintosh laryngoscope with in-line stabilization: a video-fluoroscopic study. *Br J Anaesth.* 2008;101:563–567.
133. Maruyama K, Yamada T, Kawakami R, Kamata T, Yokochi M, Hara K. Upper cervical spine movement during intubation: fluoroscopic comparison of the AirWay Scope, McCoy laryngoscope, and Macintosh laryngoscope. *Br J Anaesth.* 2008;100:120–124.

134. Maruyama K, Yamada T, Hara K, Nakagawa H, Kitamura A. Tracheal intubation using an AirWay Scope in a patient with Halo-Vest Fixation for upper cervical spine injury. *Br J Anaesth*. 2009;102:565–566.
135. Hirabayashi Y, Fujita A, Seo N, Sugimoto H. Cervical spine movement during laryngoscopy using the Airway Scope compared with the Macintosh laryngoscope. *Anaesthesia*. 2007;62:1050–1055.
136. Hirabayashi Y, Seo N. Tracheal intubation by non-anaesthetist physicians using the Airway Scope. *Emerg Med J*. 2007;24:572–573.
137. Hirabayashi Y. Airway Scope: initial clinical experience with novice personnel. *Can J Anesth*. 2007;54:160–161.
138. Sadamori T, Kusunoki S, Otani T, et al. Airway Scope for emergency intubations: usefulness of a new video-laryngoscope. *Hiroshima J Med Sci*. 2008;57:99–104.
139. Miki T, Inagawa G, Kikuchi T, Koyama Y, Goto T. Evaluation of the Airway Scope, a new video laryngoscope, in tracheal intubation by naive operators: a manikin study. *Acta Anaesthesiol Scand*. 2007;51:1378–1381.
140. Maharaj CH, O'Croinin D, Curley G, Harte BH, Laffey JG. A comparison of tracheal intubation using the Airtraq or the Macintosh laryngoscope in routine airway management: a randomised, controlled clinical trial. *Anaesthesia*. 2006;61:1093–1099.
141. Maharaj CH, Buckley E, Harte BH, Laffey JG. Endotracheal intubation in patients with cervical spine immobilization: a comparison of macintosh and airtraq laryngoscopes. *Anesthesiology*. 2007;107:53–59.
142. Maharaj CH, Costello JF, Harte BH, Laffey JG. Evaluation of the Airtraq and Macintosh laryngoscopes in patients at increased risk for difficult tracheal intubation. *Anaesthesia*. 2008;63:182–188.
143. Ndoko SK, Amathieu R, Tual L, et al. Tracheal intubation of morbidly obese patients: a randomized trial comparing performance of Macintosh and Airtraq laryngoscopes. *Br J Anaesth*. 2008;100:263–268.
144. Suzuki A, Toyama Y, Iwasaki H, Henderson J. Airtraq for awake tracheal intubation. *Anaesthesia*. 2007;62:746–747.
145. Hirabayashi Y, Fujita A, Seo N, Sugimoto H. A comparison of cervical spine movement during laryngoscopy using the Airtraq or Macintosh laryngoscopes. *Anaesthesia*. 2008;63:635–640.
146. Dhonneur G, Ndoko SK, Amathieu R, et al. A comparison of two techniques for inserting the Airtraq laryngoscope in morbidly obese patients. *Anaesthesia*. 2007;62:774–777.
147. Holst B, Hodzovic I, Francis V. Airway trauma caused by the Airtraq laryngoscope. *Anaesthesia*. 2008;63:889–890.
148. Maharaj CH, Costello JF, Higgins BD, Harte BH, Laffey JG. Learning and performance of tracheal intubation by novice personnel: a comparison of the Airtraq and Macintosh laryngoscope. *Anaesthesia*. 2006;61:671–677.
149. Hirabayashi Y, Seo N. Airtraq optical laryngoscope: tracheal intubation by novice laryngoscopists. *Emerg Med J*. 2009;26:112–113.
150. Parker Medical. Parker TrachView: Product User Guide. [Internet]. Highlands Ranch (CO): Parker Medical Inc.; [Updated 2010, cited 2009 Dec 15]. Available from www.parkermedical.com/pdf/Parker_TrachView.pdf.
151. Roppolo L, Hatten B, Brockman C, et al. A prospective study comparing standard laryngoscopy to the TrachView videoscope system for orotracheal intubation by emergency medical residents and medical students. *Ann Emerg Med*. 2004;44(4):S117.
152. Malik MA, O'Donoghue C, Carney J, Maharaj CH, Harte BH, Laffey JG. Comparison of the Glidescope, the Pentax AWS, and the Truview EVO2 with the Macintosh laryngoscope in experienced anaesthetists: a manikin study. *Br J Anaesth*. 2009;102:128–134.
153. Tan BH, Liu EH, Lim RT, Liow LM, Goy RW. Ease of intubation with the GlideScope or Airway Scope by novice operators in simulated easy and difficult airways–a manikin study. *Anaesthesia*. 2009;64:187-190.

154. Savoldelli GL, Schiffer E, Abegg C, Baeriswyl V, Clergue F, Waeber JL. Comparison of the Glidescope, the McGrath, the Airtraq and the Macintosh laryngoscopes in simulated difficult airways. *Anaesthesia*. 2008;63:1358–1364.

155. Lange M, Frommer M, Redel A, et al. Comparison of the Glidescope and Airtraq optical laryngoscopes in patients undergoing direct microlaryngoscopy. *Anaesthesia*. 2009;64: 323–328.

156. Nasim S, Maharaj CH, Butt I, et al. Comparison of the Airtraq and Truview laryngoscopes to the Macintosh laryngoscope for use by Advanced Paramedics in easy and simulated difficult intubation in manikins. *BMC Emerg Med*. 2009;9:2.

157. MacIntosh RR. An aid to oral intubation. *BMJ*. 1949;1:28.

158. American Society of Anesthesiologists Task Force on Management of the Difficult Airway. Practice guidelines for management of the difficult airway: an updated report. *Anesthesiology*. 2003;98:1269–1277.

159. Nolan JP, Wilson ME. An evaluation of the gum elastic bougie. Intubation times and incidence of sore throat. *Anaesthesia*. 1992;47:878–881.

160. Bair AE, Laurin EG, Schmitt BJ. An assessment of a tracheal tube introducer as an endotracheal tube placement confirmation device. *Am J Emerg Med*. 2005;23:754–758.

161. Kidd JF, Dyson A, Latto IP. Successful difficult intubation. Use of the gum elastic bougie. *Anaesthesia*. 1988;43:437–438.

162. Braude D, Ronan D, Weiss S, Boivin M, Gerstein N. Comparison of available gum-elastic bougies. *Am J Emerg Med*. 2009;27:266–270.

163. Hodzovic I, Latto IP, Wilkes AR, Hall JE, Mapleson WW. Evaluation of Frova, single-use intubation introducer, in a manikin. Comparison with Eschmann multiple-use introducer and Portex single-use introducer. *Anaesthesia*. 2004;59:811–816.

164. Janakiraman C, Hodzovic I, Reddy S, Desai N, Wilkes AR, Latto IP. Evaluation of tracheal tube introducers in simulated difficult intubation. *Anaesthesia*. 2009;64:309–314.

165. Hodzovic I, Wilkes AR, Stacey M, Latto IP. Evaluation of clinical effectiveness of the Frova single-use tracheal tube introducer. *Anaesthesia*. 2008;63:189–194.

166. Hagberg CA. Special devices and techniques. *Anesthesiol Clin North America*. 2002;20: 907–932.

167. Kovacs G, Law JA, McCrossin C, Vu M, Leblanc D, Gao J. A comparison of a fiberoptic stylet and a bougie as adjuncts to direct laryngoscopy in a manikin-simulated difficult airway. *Ann Emerg Med*. 2007;50:676–685.

168. Liao X, Xue FS, Zhang YM. Tracheal intubation using the Bonfils intubation fibrescope in patients with a difficult airway. *Can J Anesth*. 2008;55:655–656.

169. Halligan M, Charters P. A clinical evaluation of the bonfils intubation fibrescope. *Anaesthesia*. 2003;58:1087–1091.

170. Bein B, Wortmann F, Meybohm P, Steinfath M, Scholz J, Dorges V. Evaluation of the pediatric Bonfils fiberscope for elective endotracheal intubation. *Paediatr Anaesth*. 2008;18:1040–1044.

171. Bein B, Worthmann F, Scholz J, et al. A comparison of the intubating laryngeal mask airway and the Bonfils intubation fibrescope in patients with predicted difficult airways. *Anaesthesia*. 2004;59:668–674.

172. Rudolph C, Schneider JP, Wallenborn J, Schaffranietz L. Movement of the upper cervical spine during laryngoscopy: a comparison of the Bonfils intubation fibrescope and the Macintosh laryngoscope. *Anaesthesia*. 2005;60:668–672.

173. Abramson SI, Holmes AA, Hagberg CA. Awake insertion of the Bonfils Retromolar Intubation Fiberscope in five patients with anticipated difficult airways. *Anesth Analg*. 2008;106:1215–1217, table.

174. Bein B, Yan M, Tonner PH, Scholz J, Steinfath M, Dorges V. Tracheal intubation using the Bonfils intubation fibrescope after failed direct laryngoscopy. *Anaesthesia*. 2004;59:1207–1209.

175. Rudolph C, Schlender M. Clinical experiences with fiber optic intubation with the Bonfils intubation fiberscope. *Anaesthesiol Reanim*. 1996;21:127–130.

176. Caruselli M, Zannini R, Giretti R, et al. Difficult intubation in a small for gestational age newborn by bonfils fiberscope. *Paediatr Anaesth*. 2008;18:990–991.

177. Shikani AH. New "seeing" stylet–scope and method for the management of the difficult airway. *Otolaryngol Head Neck Surg*. 1999;120:113–116.
178. Kovacs G, Law AJ, Petrie D. Awake fiberoptic intubation using an optical stylet in an anticipated difficult airway. *Ann Emerg Med*. 2007;49:81–83.
179. Shukry M, Hanson RD, Koveleskie JR, Ramadhyani U. Management of the difficult pediatric airway with Shikani Optical Stylet. *Paediatr Anaesth*. 2005;15:342–345.
180. Yao YT, Jia NG, Li CH, Zhang YJ, Yin YQ. Comparison of endotracheal intubation with the Shikani Optical Stylet using the left molar approach and direct laryngoscopy. *Chin Med J (Engl)*. 2008;121:1324–1327.
181. Levitan RM. Design rationale and intended use of a short optical stylet for routine fiberoptic augmentation of emergency laryngoscopy. *Am J Emerg Med*. 2006;24:490–495.
182. Greenland KB, Liu G, Tan H, Edwards M, Irwin MG. Comparison of the Levitan FPS Scope and the single-use bougie for simulated difficult intubation in anaesthetised patients. *Anaesthesia*. 2007;62:509–515.
183. Kitamura T, Yamada Y, Du HL, Hanaoka K. Efficiency of a new fiberoptic stylet scope in tracheal intubation. *Anesthesiology*. 1999;91:1628–1632.
184. Kitamura T, Yamada Y, Du HL, Hanaoka K. An efficient technique for tracheal intubation using the StyletScope alone. *Anesthesiology*. 2000;92:1210–1211.
185. Kihara S, Yaguchi Y, Taguchi N, Brimacombe JR, Watanabe S. The StyletScope is a better intubation tool than a conventional stylet during simulated cervical spine immobilization. *Can J Anesth*. 2005;52:105–110.
186. Kitamura T, Yamada Y, Chinzei M, Du HL, Hanaoka K. Attenuation of haemodynamic responses to tracheal intubation by the styletscope. *Br J Anaesth*. 2001;86:275–277.
187. Kimura A, Yamakage M, Chen X, Kamada Y, Namiki A. Use of the fibreoptic stylet scope (Styletscope) reduces the hemodynamic response to intubation in normotensive and hypertensive patients. *Can J Anesth*. 2001;48:919–923.
188. Yamamura H, Yamamoto T, Kamiyama M. Device for blind nasal intubation. *Anesthesiology*. 1959;20:221.
189. Ellis DG, Jakymec A, Kaplan RM, et al. Guided orotracheal intubation in the operating room using a lighted stylet: a comparison with direct laryngoscopic technique. *Anesthesiology*. 1986;64:823–826.
190. Mehta S. Transtracheal illumination for optimal tracheal tube placement. A clinical study. *Anaesthesia*. 1989;44:970–972.
191. Hung OR, Stewart RD. Lightwand intubation: I–a new lightwand device. *Can J Anesth*. 1995;42:820–825.
192. Davis L, Cook-Sather SD, Schreiner MS. Lighted stylet tracheal intubation: a review. *Anesth Analg*. 2000;90:745–756.
193. Hung OR, Pytka S, Morris I, Murphy M, Stewart RD. Lightwand intubation: II–Clinical trial of a new lightwand for tracheal intubation in patients with difficult airways. *Can J Anesth*. 1995;42:826–830.
194. Hung OR, Pytka S, Morris I, et al. Clinical trial of a new lightwand device (Trachlight) to intubate the trachea. *Anesthesiology*. 1995;83:509–514.
195. Houde BJ, Williams SR, Cadrin-Chenevert A, Guilbert F, Drolet P. A comparison of cervical spine motion during orotracheal intubation with the trachlight(r) or the flexible fiberoptic bronchoscope. *Anesth Analg*. 2009;108:1638–1643.
196. Kihara S, Brimacombe J, Yaguchi Y, Watanabe S, Taguchi N, Komatsuzaki T. Hemodynamic responses among three tracheal intubation devices in normotensive and hypertensive patients. *Anesth Analg*. 2003;96:890–895, table.
197. Takahashi S, Mizutani T, Miyabe M, Toyooka H. Hemodynamic responses to tracheal intubation with laryngoscope versus lightwand intubating device (Trachlight) in adults with normal airway. *Anesth Analg*. 2002;95:480–484, table.
198. Rhee KY, Lee JR, Kim J, Park S, Kwon WK, Han S. A comparison of lighted stylet (Surch-Lite) and direct laryngoscopic intubation in patients with high Mallampati scores. *Anesth Analg*. 2009;108:1215–1219.

199. Agro F, Hung OR, Cataldo R, Carassiti M, Gherardi S. Lightwand intubation using the Trachlight: a brief review of current knowledge. *Can J Anesth*. 2001;48:592–599.
200. Lavery GG, McCloskey BV. The difficult airway in adult critical care. *Crit Care Med*. 2008;36:2163–2173.
201. Asai T. Endotrol tube for blind nasotracheal intubation. *Anaesthesia*. 1996;51:507.
202. Asai T, Shingu K. Blind intubation using the endotrol tube and a light wand. *Can J Anesth*. 2000;47:478–479.
203. Spiller JD, Noblett KE. Endotracheal tube occlusion following blind oral intubation with the Endotrol (trigger) endotracheal tube: a case report. *Am J Emerg Med*. 1998;16:276–278.
204. Miller RD. *Anesthesia*. New York: Churchill Livingstone; 1981.
205. Ring WH, Adair JC, Elwyn RA. A new pediatric endotracheal tube. *Anesth Analg*. 1975;54:273–274.
206. Black AE, Mackersie AM. Accidental bronchial intubation with RAE tubes. *Anaesthesia*. 1991;46:42–43.
207. Chee WK. Orotracheal intubation with a nasal Ring-Adair-Elwyn tube provides an unobstructed view in otolaryngologic procedures. *Anesthesiology*. 1995;83:1369.
208. Brambrink AM, Braun U. Airway management in infants and children. *Best Pract Res Clin Anaesthesiol*. 2005;19:675–697.
209. Deakers TW, Reynolds G, Stretton M, Newth CJ. Cuffed endotracheal tubes in pediatric intensive care. *J Pediatr*. 1994;125:57–62.
210. Khine HH, Corddry DH, Kettrick RG, et al. Comparison of cuffed and uncuffed endotracheal tubes in young children during general anesthesia. *Anesthesiology*. 1997;86:627–631.
211. West MR, Jonas MM, Adams AP, Carli F. A new tracheal tube for difficult intubation. *Br J Anaesth*. 1996;76:673–679.
212. St John RE. Advances in artificial airway management. *Crit Care Nurs Clin North Am*. 1999;11:7–17.
213. Kolobow T, Tsuno K, Rossi N, Aprigliano M. Design and development of ultrathin-walled, nonkinking endotracheal tubes of a new "no-pressure" laryngeal seal design. A preliminary report. *Anesthesiology*. 1994;81:1061–1067.
214. Reali-Forster C, Kolobow T, Giacomini M, Hayashi T, Horiba K, Ferrans VJ. New ultrathin-walled endotracheal tube with a novel laryngeal seal design. Long-term evaluation in sheep. *Anesthesiology*. 1996;84:162–172.
215. Fujiwara M, Mizoguchi H, Kawamura J, et al. A new endotracheal tube with a cuff impervious to nitrous oxide: constancy of cuff pressure and volume. *Anesth Analg*. 1995;81:1084–1086.
216. Karasawa F, Mori T, Okuda T, Satoh T. Profile soft-seal cuff, a new endotracheal tube, effectively inhibits an increase in the cuff pressure through high compliance rather than low diffusion of nitrous oxide. *Anesth Analg*. 2001;92:140–144.
217. Fikkers BG. van VS, van der Hoeven JG, van den Hoogen FJ, Marres HA. Emergency cricothyrotomy: a randomised crossover trial comparing the wire-guided and catheter-over-needle techniques. *Anaesthesia*. 2004;59:1008–1011.
218. Stringer KR, Bajenov S, Yentis SM. Training in airway management. *Anaesthesia*. 2002;57:967–983.
219. Cote CJ, Hartnick CJ. Pediatric transtracheal and cricothyrotomy airway devices for emergency use: which are appropriate for infants and children? *Pediatr Anesth*. 2009;19(suppl 1):66–76.
220. Assmann NM, Wong DT, Morales E. A comparison of a new indicator-guided with a conventional wire-guided percutaneous cricothyroidotomy device in mannequins. *Anesth Analg*. 2007;105:148–154.
221. Aneeshkumar MK, Jones TM, Birchall MA. A new indicator-guided percutaneous emergency cricothyrotomy device: in vivo study in man. *Eur Arch Otorhinolaryngol*. 2009;266:105–109.
222. Mattinger C, Petroianu G, Maleck W, Bergler W, Hormann K. [Emergency tracheotomy in Gottingen minipigs. Comparison: standard technique versus Nu-Trake cricothyrotomy set]. *Laryngorhinootologie*. 2000;79:595–598.
223. Craven RM, Vanner RG. Ventilation of a model lung using various cricothyrotomy devices. *Anaesthesia*. 2004;59:595–599.

224. Chan TC, Vilke GM, Bramwell KJ, Davis DP, Hamilton RS, Rosen P. Comparison of wire-guided cricothyrotomy versus standard surgical cricothyrotomy technique. *J Emerg Med.* 1999;17:957–962.

225. Eisenburger P, Laczika K, List M, et al. Comparison of conventional surgical versus Seldinger technique emergency cricothyrotomy performed by inexperienced clinicians. *Anesthesiology.* 2000;92:687–690.

226. Fikkers BG, van Vugt S, van der Hoeven JG, van den Hoogen FJA, Marres HAM. A response to 'Emergency cricothyrotomy: a randomised crossover trial comparing the wire-guided and catheter-over-needle techniques.' *Anaesthesia.* 2004;59:1008-1011; *Anaesthesia.* 2005;60:105.

227. Benkhadra M, Lenfant F, Nemetz W, Anderhuber F, Feigl G, Fasel J. A comparison of two emergency cricothyroidotomy kits in human cadavers. *Anesth Analg.* 2008;106:182–185, table.

228. Melker JS, Gabrielli A. Melker cricothyrotomy kit: an alternative to the surgical technique. *Ann Otol Rhinol Laryngol.* 2005;114:525–528.

229. Dimitriadis JC, Paoloni R. Emergency cricothyroidotomy: a randomised crossover study of four methods. *Anaesthesia.* 2008;63:1204–1208.

230. Vadodaria BS, Gandhi SD, McIndoe AK. Comparison of four different emergency airway access equipment sets on a human patient simulator. *Anaesthesia.* 2004;59:73–79.

231. Lakhal K, Delplace X, Cottier JP, et al. The feasibility of ultrasound to assess subglottic diameter. *Anesth Analg.* 2007;104:611–614.

232. Prasad A, Singh M, Chan VW. Ultrasound imaging of the airway. *Can J Anesth.* 2009;56: 868–869.

233. Tsui BC, Hui CM. Sublingual airway ultrasound imaging. *Can J Anesth.* 2008;55:790–791.

234. Tsui BC, Hui CM. Challenges in sublingual airway ultrasound interpretation. *Can J Anesth.* 2009;56:393-394.

235. Friedman EM. Role of ultrasound in the assessment of vocal cord function in infants and children. *Ann Otol Rhinol Laryngol.* 1997;106:199–209.

236. Ma G, Davis DP, Schmitt J, Vilke GM, Chan TC, Hayden SR. The sensitivity and specificity of transcricothyroid ultrasonography to confirm endotracheal tube placement in a cadaver model. *J Emerg Med.* 2007;32:405–407.

237. Park SC, Ryu JH, Yeom SR, Jeong JW, Cho SJ. Confirmation of endotracheal intubation by combined ultrasonographic methods in the Emergency Department. *Emerg Med Australas.* 2009;21:293–297.

238. Sustic A. Role of ultrasound in the airway management of critically ill patients. *Crit Care Med.* 2007;35:S173–S177.

239. Werner SL, Smith CE, Goldstein JR, Jones RA, Cydulka RK. Pilot study to evaluate the accuracy of ultrasonography in confirming endotracheal tube placement. *Ann Emerg Med.* 2007;49:75–80.

240. Marciniak B, Fayoux P, Hebrard A, Krivosic-Horber R, Engelhardt T, Bissonnette B. Airway management in children: ultrasonography assessment of tracheal intubation in real time? *Anesth Analg.* 2009;108:461–465.

241. Eslamy HK, Newman B. Imaging of the pediatric airway. *Pediatr Anesth.* 2009;19(suppl 1): 9–23.

242. Chou HC, Wu TL. Mandibulohyoid distance in difficult laryngoscopy. *Br J Anaesth.* 1993;71:335–339.

243. Weaver B, Lyon M, Blaivas M. Confirmation of endotracheal tube placement after intubation using the ultrasound sliding lung sign. *Acad Emerg Med.* 2006;13:239–244.

244. Razzaq QM. Use of the 'sliding lung sign' in emergency bedside ultrasound. *Eur J Emerg Med.* 2008;15:238–241.

245. Goldmann K, Ferson DZ. Education and training in airway management. *Best Pract Res Clin Anaesthesiol.* 2005;19:717–732.

246. Nargozian C. Teaching consultants airway management skills. *Paediatr Anaesth.* 2004;14:24–27.

247. Jackson KM, Cook TM. Evaluation of four airway training manikins as patient simulators for the insertion of eight types of supraglottic airway devices. *Anaesthesia*. 2007;62:388–393.
248. Cook TM, Green C, McGrath J, Srivastava R. Evaluation of four airway training manikins as patient simulators for the insertion of single use laryngeal mask airways. *Anaesthesia*. 2007;62:713–718.
249. Jordan GM, Silsby J, Bayley G, Cook TM. Difficult Airway Society. Evaluation of four manikins as simulators for teaching airway management procedures specified in the Difficult Airway Society guidelines, and other advanced airway skills. *Anaesthesia*. 2007;62: 708–712.
250. John B, Suri I, Hillermann C, Mendonca C. Comparison of cricothyroidotomy on manikin vs. simulator: a randomised cross-over study. *Anaesthesia*. 2007;62:1029–1032.
251. Kuduvalli PM, Jervis A, Tighe SQ, Robin NM. Unanticipated difficult airway management in anaesthetised patients: a prospective study of the effect of mannequin training on management strategies and skill retention. *Anaesthesia*. 2008;63:364–369.
252. Shukla A, Kline D, Cherian A, et al. A simulation course on lifesaving techniques for third-year medical students. *Simul Healthc*. 2007;2:11–15.
253. Russo SG, Eich C, Barwing J, et al. Self-reported changes in attitude and behavior after attending a simulation-aided airway management course. *J Clin Anesth*. 2007;19:517-522.
254. Cho J, Kang GH, Kim EC, et al. Comparison of manikin versus porcine models in cricothyrotomy procedure training. *Emerg Med J*. 2008;25:732–734.
255. Cummings AJ, Getz MA. Evaluation of a novel animal model for teaching intubation. *Teach Learn Med*. 2006;18:316–319.
256. Hatton KW, Price S, Craig L, Grider JS. Educating anesthesiology residents to perform percutaneous cricothyrotomy, retrograde intubation, and fiberoptic bronchoscopy using preserved cadavers. *Anesth Analg*. 2006;103:1205–1208.
257. Friedman Z, You-Ten KE, Bould MD, Naik V. Teaching lifesaving procedures: the impact of model fidelity on acquisition and transfer of cricothyrotomy skills to performance on cadavers. *Anesth Analg*. 2008;107:1663–1669.
258. American Society of Anesthesiologists. Practice Guidelines for Management of the Difficult Airway: an updated report by the American society of anesthesiologists task force on management of the difficult airway. *Anesthesiology*. 2003;98:1269–1277.
259. Naik VN, Matsumoto ED, Houston PL, et al. Fiberoptic orotracheal intubation on anesthetized patients: do manipulation skills learned on a simple model transfer into the operating room? *Anesthesiology*. 2001;95:343–348.
260. Ovassapian A, Dykes MH, Golmon ME. A training programme for fibreoptic nasotracheal intubation. Use of model and live patients. *Anaesthesia*. 1983;38:795–798.
261. Ovassapian A, Yelich SJ, Dykes MH, Golman ME. Learning fibreoptic intubation: use of simulators v. traditional teaching. *Br J Anaesth*. 1988;61:217-220.
262. Goldmann K, Steinfeldt T. Acquisition of basic fiberoptic intubation skills with a virtual reality airway simulator. *J Clin Anesth*. 2006;18:173–178.
263. Boet S, Bould MD, Schaeffer R, et al. Learning fiberoptic intubation with a virtual computer program transfers to 'hands on' improvement. *Eur J Anaesthesiol*. 2010;27:31–35.

Chapter 7
Indications and Preparation of the Patient for Intubation

Contents

B.T. Finucane et al., *Principles of Airway Management*,
DOI 10.1007/978-0-387-09558-5_7, © Springer Science+Business Media, LLC 2011

Introduction

Endotracheal intubation has been a recognized technique in anesthesia for more than 100 years. It was first performed clinically in 1880 by MacEwan[1] in Glasgow, who blindly introduced a metal tube into the trachea of a patient using the oral route. Sixty years or so ago, as techniques and equipment became more refined, endotracheal intubation evolved into a routine procedure for adults and children undergoing general anesthesia, resuscitation, and respiratory care. Nevertheless, the decision to intubate the trachea should not be made lightly. You must always weigh the risks of the procedure against those of nonintervention. If intubation is necessary, select the most appropriate route as well as the type of sedation or anesthesia required.

The indications for tracheal intubation in anesthesia have changed considerably since the introduction of supraglottic devices in the 1980s. Prior to that time, we tracheally intubated patients more frequently because the task of mask anesthesia was far more cumbersome, and limited our ability to do anything else but maintain the airway and anesthesia. With the introduction of the laryngeal mask airway (LMA), the need for tracheal intubation is greatly reduced. We can also speculate that because of this innovation we see fewer difficult airways. These devices can also be used when we encounter difficult airways. We have now reached the point in the development of supraglottic devices that in the very near future tracheal intubation will be obsolete in most cases. However, we have not quite reached that point yet (refer to Chap. 5 for in depth discussion on this topic).

General Indications for Intubation

As a technique, endotracheal intubation is one of the most common lifesaving procedures performed today. However, the decision whether to intubate or not is not always clear-cut and ethical issues surrounding the initiation of advanced life support in some cases, are being raised more frequently. The indications for intubation are outlined in Box 7.1 and will be discussed in detail in this chapter.

Ventilatory Support

Respiratory failure requiring mechanical ventilation and/or oxygen therapy is a common indication for endotracheal intubation. The tube provides a conduit through

Box 7.1 Indications for Intubation

Ventilatory support (assisted or mechanical)
Protection of the airway
Ensuring airway patency
Anesthesia and surgery
Suctioning

which you can apply various modalities of ventilatory support – intermittent mandatory ventilation (IMV), control mode ventilation (CMV), and in certain cases, high frequency ventilation (HFV). Furthermore, you can institute various end-expiratory maneuvers (e.g., positive end-expiratory pressure [PEEP] or continuous positive airway pressure [CPAP]) to enhance oxygenation, increase the functional residual capacity (FRC), improve lung compliance, and decrease the work of breathing in selected patients (see Chap. 13 for more complete details on ventilatory support.)

Once you have determined the etiology of the pulmonary pathology, you can determine whether ventilatory support should be directed toward primarily treating an oxygenation problem, a ventilation problem, or both (as commonly occurs). When treating ventilated patients, it helps to direct your efforts toward specific goals (Box 7.2). The remainder of this section discusses the various conditions that necessitate ventilatory support, most of which fall under the heading hypoxia.

Box 7.2 Objectives in Ventilatory Support

1. Make the correct etiological diagnosis
2. Institute therapy to treat pathology

   (a) Pneumonia: antibiotics
   (b) Cardiogenic pulmonary edema: cardiac support and diuretics
   (c) Status asthmaticus: bronchodilators

3. Oxygenation goals

   (a) Wean $FiO_2 \leq 50\%$
   (b) Oxyhemoglobin saturation $\geq 90\%$
   (c) $PaO_2 \geq 60$ mmHg
   (d) Pulmonary shunt fraction $\leq 18\%$

4. Ventilation goals

   (a) Adjust the minute ventilation to achieve pH homeostasis (provided there is no profound metabolic acidosis) $7.35 \leq pH \leq 7.45$

5. Be prepared to react to complications and problems

Hypoxia

Hypoxia, as an inadequate supply of oxygen to meet physiologic demands of the tissues,[2] can be arbitrarily subdivided into six categories (Box 7.3). The most common cause, requiring ventilatory support or oxygen supplementation, is *hypoxic hypoxia*; thus, in this chapter, considerable emphasis will be placed on this category. The term *hypoxic hypoxia* is synonymous with *hypoxemia*.

Box 7.3 Classification of Hypoxia

1. Hypoxic
   $\downarrow$ PaO_2, hypoxemia
2. Anemic
   $\downarrow$ O_2 carrying capacity, anemia
3. Histotoxic
   Impaired O_2 utilization (e.g., cyanide poisoning)
4. Stagnant
   Inadequate tissue perfusion (e.g., shock, cardiac failure, pulmonary embolus)
5. Hypermetabolic
   $\uparrow$ O_2 demand (e.g., septicemia, hyperthyroidism, MH)
6. Interference with O_2 transport mechanisms (e.g., carbon monoxide poisoning, methemoglobin, hemoglobinopathies)

Hypoxemia

Hypoxemia is defined as a reduced partial pressure of oxygen in arterial blood (P_aO_2). The normal P_aO_2 varies with age and can be estimated using the following formula:

$$P_aO_2 (mmHg) = 102 - 0.33 \text{ Age (in years)}.$$

Hypoxemia *per se* is not an indication for intubation and ventilation. Supplemental oxygen can be administered to patients via a face mask or nasal prongs. However, intubation should be considered if:

1. The patient cannot maintain an oxyhemoglobin saturation of at least 90% or a P_aO_2 of at least 60 mmHg on a concentration of inspired oxygen less than 50%.
2. The disease causing the hypoxemia is expected to persist and signs of exhaustion are observed.

During this observation period you need to assess the patient carefully for signs of further deterioration and be ready to intubate immediately if necessary.

Box 7.4 Common Causes of Hypoxemia

1. Decreased inspired oxygen concentration
2. Hypoventilation
3. Decreased diffusion capacity
4. Ventilation/perfusion inequality
5. True or anatomical shunt

The ensuing discussion covers the five general causes of hypoxemia (Box 7.4): decreased inspired oxygen concentration, hypoventilation, ventilation/perfusion inequality, decreased diffusion capacity, and anatomical shunt.

Decreased Oxygen Content of Inspired Air

Atmospheric pressure at sea level is about 760 mmHg. Thus, the partial pressure of inspired oxygen at sea level is about 150 mmHg:

$$P_IO_2 = (P_b - P_{H_2O}) \times F_IO_2$$
$$= (760 - 47) \times 0.21$$
$$= 149.72 \text{ mmHg}$$

where P_IO_2 is the partial pressure of inspired oxygen, P_b the barometric pressure (760 mmHg at sea level), P_{H_2O} the water vapor pressure (47 mmHg at 37°C), and F_IO_2 the concentration of inspired oxygen in room air (0.21).

On ascending to high altitudes, the partial pressure of oxygen in inspired air decreases; at 30,000 ft., for example, it is only about 40 mmHg. Low oxygen content may occur during the administration of anesthesia (e.g., selection of hypoxic gas mixtures, plumbing accidents involving oxygen delivery systems, or faulty equipment). Oxygen analyzers are a valuable means of detecting the delivery of hypoxic gas mixtures to patients.

Hypoventilation

Respiration is rigorously regulated by a complex feedback system in the CNS. The rhythmic movements of the diaphragm and other respiratory muscles are controlled by impulses originating in the brain stem that reach the motor units peripherally through the phrenic, vagus, and intercostal nerves. Central chemoreceptors in the medulla are exquisitely sensitive to even small changes in carbon dioxide tension in the arterial blood. Likewise, peripheral chemoreceptors (in the carotid and aortic bodies) are very sensitive to falling oxygen tensions, especially when the P_aO_2 falls below 60 mmHg.

Numerous disease processes and medications may interfere with normal respiratory function, leading to respiratory pump failure or hypoventilation.

Hypoventilation occurs when the movement of air in and out of the lungs in a given period is insufficient to meet the oxygen demands and carbon dioxide excretory requirements of the organism. Its causes are legion, but they may be broadly divided into two main categories: central and peripheral.

The hallmark of hypoventilation is an elevation in the alveolar carbon dioxide tension ($P_A CO_2$). The relationship between $P_A CO_2$ and alveolar ventilation is best expressed by the Alveolar Air equation[3]:

$$\dot{V}_A = \dot{V}_{CO_2} / P_A CO_2 \times K.$$

Therefore:

$$P_A CO_2 = \dot{V}_{CO_2} / \dot{V}_A \times K.$$

When $\dot{V}_A$ is alveolar ventilation (L/min), $\dot{V}_{CO_2}$ is CO_2 production (L/min), $P_A CO_2$ is alveolar CO_2 tension (mmHg) (note that this is nearly identical to the arterial CO_2 tension [$P_a CO_2$] in normal subjects), and K is 0.863 (conversion factor relating $\dot{V}_A$ at BTPS and $\dot{V}_{CO_2}$ STPD and correcting for alveolar P_{H_2O}). $\dot{V}_A$ and $\dot{V}_{CO_2}$ are the only determinants of $P_A CO_2$, and ultimately of $P_a CO_2$.

If an individual hypoventilates while breathing room air, the space occupied by carbon dioxide in the alveoli expands, to the detriment of the space available for the other respiratory gases (including oxygen). This is a simple way of explaining why hypoxemia occurs when patients hypoventilate. This phenomenon may be clarified by studying the clinically useful alveolar air equation:

$$P_A O_2 = F_I O_2 (P_B - P_{H_2O}) - P_A CO_2 / R.$$

When $P_A O_2$ is the alveolar oxygen tension (mm Hg), $F_I O_2$ the concentration of inspired oxygen, $P_A CO_2$ the alveolar carbon dioxide tension (mm Hg), and R the respiration quotient (usually assumed to be 0.8). For example, if $F_I O_2$ is 0.2, P_b 760 mmHg, P_{H_2O} 47 mmHg, $P_A CO_2$ 40, and R 0.8, then the $P_A O_2 = 100$.

Hypoventilation is a common cause of hypoxemia usually seen in patients with chronic obstructive lung disease and in individuals who have received excessive doses of opioids and other respiratory-depressant drugs. In addition to causing hypoxemia, it can seriously interfere with acid/base balance. Hypoventilation caused by respiratory depressant drugs may require only supplemental oxygen therapy. However, hypoventilation caused by respiratory pump failure (e.g., Guillain–Barre syndrome) may require urgent and prolonged mechanical ventilatory support.

Decreased Diffusion Capacity

There are two major causes of decreased diffusion capacity: *loss of lung tissue* following surgery or disease that decreases the surface area available for gas exchange, and *failure of equilibrium* between the alveolar oxygen tension ($P_A O_2$)

and the alveolar carbon dioxide tension (P_ACO_2). Diffusion impairment also occurs if equilibrium is not reached between the alveolar oxygen tension (P_AO_2) and the arterial oxygen tension (P_aO_2). Diseases that cause a change in the thickness of the respiratory membrane fall into this category. Hypoxemia may not manifest itself unless the patient is exercised. Hypoxemia caused by diffusion impairment may be corrected by administering a high F_IO_2 to the patient.

Ventilation/Perfusion Inequality

Ventilation/perfusion inequality occurs when the normal relationships of ventilation and perfusion in the lung are mismatched as a result of various disease processes. A simple description of ventilation/perfusion ratios in Riley's in a three-compartment model of the lung consists of three zones:

1. Ventilated but unperfused alveoli (dead space)
2. Perfused but unventilated alveoli (shunt or venous admixture)
3. Ideally ventilated and perfused alveoli

The institution of an end-expiratory maneuver (e.g., PEEP or CPAP) may improve oxygenation in patients with diseases that cause venous admixture: atelectasis, acute respiratory distress syndrome (ARDS), and pneumonia.

True or Anatomic Shunt

A shunt is produced when blood passes through an unventilated portion of the lung or bypasses the lung altogether. A physiologic shunt may be the result of any disease that causes a venous admixture. However, there are other causes. In patients with congenital heart disease, blood may bypass the lungs through an atrial or ventricular defect or a patent ductus arteriosus. One form of intrapulmonary shunt may result from an arteriovenous fistula in a tumor. In contrast to the other causes of hypoxemia, increasing the F_IO_2 in these patients will not increase the P_aO_2 to levels seen in normal subjects. Once the etiology of the hypoxemic condition is determined, the underlying defect must be corrected as soon as possible. The moment hypoxemia is detected, patients must receive immediate supplemental oxygen, preferably 100% until the exact quantification of the hypoxemia has been established.

Protection of the Airway in a Patient with Impaired Laryngeal Reflexes

One of the most important indications for intubation is protection of the airway in patients who have depressed laryngeal reflexes. These reflexes may be impaired because of stupor and coma (e.g., anesthesia, encephalopathy, cerebrovascular accident (CVA), drug overdose, ethanol intoxication, cardiac arrest, seizures, postictal state, airway burns, tracheoesophageal fistula, and partial paralysis of the laryngeal musculature). These patients are at great risk for aspiration of gastric contents, which can result in aspiration pneumonitis. In most instances, endotracheal intubation with a cuffed endotracheal tube prevents regurgitated material from entering the trachea.

Ensuring Airway Patency in a Patient with Abnormal Pathology or Depressed Level of Consciousness

Comatose patients may not be able to breathe adequately because of airway obstruction by the tongue or by any encroachment on the airway. Tumors of the larynx are among the most common cause, but other diseases and conditions can also interfere – acute epiglottitis, croup, airway burns, foreign-body aspiration, vascular trauma to the neck, anaphylaxis. The passage of an endotracheal tube in these persons may be lifesaving.

Anesthesia and Surgery

Endotracheal intubation is required during surgery whenever the site of the operation will interfere with the ability to safely administer an anesthetic. Most operations on the head, neck, and face fall into this category, for without an endotracheal tube the surgeon simply does not have sufficient access to the operative site. In addition, there is a risk of aspiration of blood or other materials during surgery. Furthermore, contamination of the surgical field may occur because of proximity of the anesthesiologist and equipment to the surgical site. If a patient is at risk from aspiration of gastric contents, a cuffed endotracheal tube should be inserted during general anesthesia (e.g., emergency surgery).

Endotracheal intubation should be performed whenever neuromuscular blocking drugs are used (with some rare exceptions e.g., ECT therapy), because the protective reflexes are significantly impaired during paralysis. It is called for also when elective surgical procedures are likely to last more than 2 h, to facilitate the delivery of oxygen and anesthetic gases and reduce the risk of aspiration. Intubation is also indicated when the patient is in an operative position that will interfere with ventilation (e.g., prone, sitting, lateral, head down, or extreme lithotomy). The above statements may be considered by some to be overly conservative, particularly in view of the experience anesthesiologists have gained with the LMA. (For a more complete discussion on this topic please refer to Chapter 5).

Positive-pressure ventilation is usually required during thoracic and upper abdominal surgical procedures and it is best achieved with an endotracheal tube in place. Occasionally mask anesthesia can fail because of the inability to maintain an adequate mask seal, especially if the patient is edentulous, obese, large, or bearded.

Specific Indications

The following specific circumstances call for endotracheal intubation during the administration of anesthesia:

Surgery on the head, face, neck, shoulder, or thorax
In patients at increased risk of regurgitation/aspiration

Muscle paralysis
Lengthy surgery
Upper abdominal or any major abdominal surgery
Failure of mask anesthesia
Abnormal positions
Limited access to the airway
Morbid obesity

Suctioning

An endotracheal tube allows access to the tracheobronchial tree to suction secretions. Occasionally a patient will produce large quantities of secretions during surgery, especially surgery in the vicinity of the airway. This can be prevented by the administration of anticholinergic drugs preoperatively, such as atropine, scopolamine, or glycopyrrolate. The administration of succinylcholine, however, is often associated with excessive secretions, especially if anticholinergic drugs are not used. Any surgical patient who has recently had a cold will produce an excessive quantity of secretions, which may necessitate intubation. If secretions cannot be readily handled through an endotracheal tube, the patient undergoing prolonged ventilation may require a tracheostomy.

Selecting the Route of Intubation

Once the decision has been made to intubate a patient, you need to select the appropriate route – orotracheal, nasotracheal, or transtracheal. Although orotracheal is by far the most common, the other routes are preferable in selected circumstances.

Orotracheal Intubation

Except in the specific clinical situations, the oral route is routinely selected for intubation. General indications are listed in Box 7.1. Orotracheal intubation is used in most surgical patients undergoing general anesthesia. It is especially necessary for avoiding contamination of the surgical field. This latter issue is important from a historical perspective. Formerly, surgeons were limited in their ability to operate on lesions in the mouth or in the vicinity of the airway while the patient was receiving anesthesia by mask. It was this particular problem that motivated MacEwan in 1880 to introduce the technique of endotracheal intubation, and today surgical field avoidance remains one of the most common indications for oral intubation.

Contraindications

There are very few absolute contraindications to oral intubation. And, quite simply, these are the usual indications for nasotracheal intubation:
Surgical field avoidance

Poor oral access
Prolonged ventilation

Nasotracheal Intubation

In selected circumstances, the nasotracheal route is preferred to orotracheal. Its indications include surgical field avoidance, poor oral access, and prolonged ventilation.

Surgical Field Avoidance

Otolaryngologists, plastic surgeons, neurosurgeons, head and neck surgeons, dentists, and oral surgeons often require access to the mouth and plastic and oral surgeons occasionally wire the maxilla and mandible together. Although an oral endotracheal tube may suffice in most situations, occasionally it will obscure the operative site. Accordingly, nasotracheal intubation is selected. When dealing with specialists in this area, it is best to discuss their preferences before proceeding.

Poor Oral Access

Gaining access to the mouth may be difficult in patients with trismus, tetanus, status epilepticus, fractured mandible, or arthritis of the TMJ or cervical spine. In these situations, nasotracheal intubation is the method of choice. Also, if you are unable to elevate the epiglottis when attempting oral intubation, the nasal route is often successful because the tube, upon emerging from the nasopharynx, tends to point beneath the epiglottis toward the vocal cords.

Prolonged Ventilation

Specialists generally agree that the nasal route is more comfortable than the oral route for patients requiring prolonged intubation. Nasal tubes are also easier to stabilize. In addition, patients tend to salivate less, and there is no danger of damage to the tube from dental occlusion.

Contraindications

Nasotracheal intubation is contraindicated in the following circumstances:

Bleeding disturbances
Nasal pathology (epistaxis, polyps, septal deviation, infections)
Basal skull fracture

CSF leakage
Chronic sinusitis
Nasal stenosis

Transtracheal Intubation

An endotracheal tube can be readily inserted into the trachea via an existing tracheostomy stoma.

Endobronchial Intubation

Endobronchial intubation is employed when ventilation of only one lung is desired. The indications are listed in Box 7.5.

Box 7.5 Indications for Endobronchial Intubation

Absolute

1. Isolation of one lung

   (a) Unilateral infection
   (b) Massive hemorrhage

2. Control of the distribution of ventilation

   (a) Bronchopleural fistula
   (b) Bronchopleural cutaneous fistula
   (c) Giant unilateral lung cyst

3. Unilateral bronchopulmonary lavage

Relative

1. Surgical exposure
2. Upper lobectomy
3. Aortic aneurysm resection

Preparation of the Patient for Intubation Outside the Operating Room[4]

Anesthesiologists are occasionally called upon to assist in airway problems that occur outside the operating room. General anesthesia is not usually required in these situations because the patient is already obtunded or even comatose. Many patients, however, are far from comatose and require airway intervention because of respiratory failure. The following preparatory measures are recommended in these cases:

Patient interview
Sedation
Topical anesthesia
Nerve block
General anesthesia

Patient Interview

When possible, it is strongly recommended that a few moments be spent with the patient before "awake" intubation to explain the reasons for the intervention and what to expect *vis-à-vis* pain and discomfort. All too often clinicians, eager to solve a life-threatening problem, forge ahead with intubation and fail to pay attention to these all-important and humane aspects of medical care.

Sedation

When It Is Needed

Most conscious patients presenting for intubation benefit from sedation; they are anxious about the procedure, and the application of topical anesthesia and nerve blocks can cause discomfort. In an emergency there may not be time, but in elective situations you should take the time to provide adequate sedation. Effective sedation requires patience and a good knowledge of the pharmacology of sedative and hypnotic drugs.[4] Sedation is associated with impaired reflex activity, and therefore patients who have recently eaten are at increased risk from aspiration. Adults presenting for elective surgery should refrain from food for 6 h and clear liquids for at least 3 h before the operation. Regurgitation and pulmonary aspiration is a real risk during attempts at intubation in sedated patients because they are supine, somewhat restrained, and partially obtunded.

How It Is Done

The best way to sedate a patient is first to obtain reliable venous access, and to select an appropriate combination of agents (a benzodiazepine and an opioid are optimal). Of the benzodiazepines, one of the most effective is midazolam.[5] This water-soluble compound appears to have all the benefits of diazepam without

Table 7.1 Recommended doses of sedative/analgesic/topical anesthetic/vasoconstrictor/reversal agents

Indication	Medication	Dosage increments[a]
Opioid	Fentanyl	50–100 μg
	Alfentanil	500–1,000 μg
	Remifentanil	100–200 μg
	Morphine	3–5 mg
	Meperidine	25–50 mg
Sedative/hypnotic	Midazolam	0.5–3 mg
	Propofol	20–30 mg
Topical anesthesia	Lidocaine 2%	7 mg/kg
Spray/nebulizer	Cocaine 4%	2 mg/kg
Topical/vasoconstrictors	Phenylephrine (0.5%)	Up to 3 sprays/nostril
	Oxymetazoline (0.05%)	Up to 3 sprays/nostril
Opioid reversal	Naloxone	0.1–0.4 mg
Benzodiazepine Reversal	Flumazenil	0.5–1.0 mg

Doses should be titrated carefully to effect. Doses should be reduced when used in combination with other centrally acting medications. These doses are recommended for adults only
[a] Suggested doses when these medications are used alone. These doses may be modified at the discretion of the physician prescribing them

the problems (Table 7.1). It also has a much shorter half-life (2–4 h) than other benzodiazepines, and the incidence of venous thrombosis appears to be insignificant. It is 2–4 times more potent than diazepam on a milligram-per-milligram basis, and thus no more than 1.0 mg increments should be used at a time and even less than 1.0 mg is recommended in the elderly and infirm.

In preparing a patient for intubation, opiates such as fentanyl and morphine or meperidine are often injected with a benzodiazepine. They not only provide analgesia but also suppress the cough reflex, enabling the patient to better tolerate the intubation procedure. Morphine is usually administered in 3 mg increments intravenously, and its effects may persist for 1–2 h. In contrast, fentanyl, which is administered in a dose of 25–50 μg intravenously, has a much shorter duration of action, 30–60 min and remifentanil even shorter again (1–5 min). The most serious side effect of opioids is respiratory depression. Additional side effects include hypotension, bradycardia, nausea, vomiting, pruritus, and sleep disturbances. The effects of opioid overdose can be reversed by the opiate antagonist naloxone, 0.1–0.4 mg intravenously. Since naloxone has a short duration of action (30–60 min) repeat doses may be necessary. Propofol is a very effective sedative/hypnotic when given in small increments (10–20 mg); however, it is associated with pain on injection. This pain can be alleviated by adding a small dose of lidocaine (up to 40 mg) to the solution.

The combination of benzodiazepine and opioid is synergistic and has powerful depressant effects on the respiratory center; therefore, caution must be used at all times when using this combination. This combination also shifts the CO_2 response curve to the right and alters the slope of the curve in an adverse (downward) direction. Benzodiazepine/morphine and benzodiazepine/fentanyl are combinations commonly used. Recommended increments are as follows: midazolam, 0.5 mg; morphine, 3 mg; fentanyl, 25 μg and remifentanil 50 μg. These drugs should only be used if the person administering them is fully familiar with their properties, side effects, and dosage.

How the Patient Should Be Monitored

Vital signs (blood pressure, pulse, respirations) should be monitored at regular intervals (at least every 5 min) while you are sedating a patient. Electrocardiogram monitoring, pulse oximetry, and arterial blood gases, if available, provide the clinician with additional information that may help assess the effects of sedation.

When It Is Adequate

Small increments of sedative drugs are injected, and sufficient time is allowed to assess their effects. Some patients require large quantities; others very little. Sedation is adequate when the patient appears to be sleeping quietly yet is responsive to oral commands. Other indicators include slurred speech, decreased respiratory rate (<12 breaths per minute), and a lowered blood pressure. Snoring, retractions, and unresponsiveness are signs of oversedation and airway obstruction.

Local Anesthetic Techniques

If, when using these end points, you feel that the patient is adequately sedated, a topical anesthetic should be applied to the nose or oropharynx, depending upon the route of intubation. If the patient appears disturbed by this intervention, more sedation may be necessary. It must be clearly understood, however, that sedation of patients for intubation can result in significant cardiovascular and respiratory depression, and therefore, life-sustaining equipment must always be immediately available. Local anesthetic techniques have been described in detail in Chap. 11.

General Anesthesia

Few patients require general anesthesia for intubation outside the operating room. If a patient must be restrained to the degree that a general anesthetic is required for intubation, you should seriously question the indication for intubation. However, situations do exist in which general anesthesia is necessary – for example, in patients with cerebral injury and when the patient is totally uncooperative.

Cerebral Injury

Occasionally a patient who is quite responsive will present in the emergency room with serious cerebral damage requiring hyperventilation to reduce intracranial pressure. In this situation, a poorly performed awake intubation can aggravate the intracranial injury. However, general anesthesia administered by a competent anesthesiologist allows the intubation to be performed with skill and alacrity. Furthermore, the intravenous medication used during induction of anesthesia helps reduce intracranial pressure and cerebral oxygen consumption.

Acute Epiglottitis

When a child presents with acute epiglottitis, no attempt should be made to confirm the diagnosis by examining the airway. Instrumentation of these children in the conscious state is strictly contraindicated. Ideally, they should be brought to the operating room, where general anesthesia can be induced. Premature intubation of a child in the awake or semianesthetized state may lead to laryngospasm and complete airway obstruction. Occasionally, however, time does not permit the benefit of general anesthesia. If bag/valve/mask ventilation fails under these circumstances, "awake" intubation or a tracheostomy may be the only option.

Uncooperative Patient

On occasion, patients present in the emergency room with life-threatening airway compromise that requires urgent intervention but are uncooperative. Rarely, general anesthesia may be the only option for safe intubation. Hypoxia, alcohol ingestion, and the use of mind-altering substances all cause a person to behave abnormally or erratically, forcing you to employ a general anesthetic. The new inhalation anesthetic Sevoflurane can be used to suppress an otherwise agitated patient and may be an alternative to intravenous anesthesia in a patient with an abnormal airway or when you are having problems obtaining venous access.

However, once this course of action is decided upon, remember: you are responsible for sustaining the patient's life; if difficulty is anticipated in securing the airway, it may be preferable to restrain the patient physically and attempt an awake intubation.

Neuromuscular Blocking Drugs

Neuromuscular blocking drugs, introduced into anesthesia practice by Griffith and Johnson[6] in 1941, have revolutionized the practice of anesthesia and surgery. Up to that time, muscle relaxation was achieved by deepening the level of inhalation anesthesia, with the consequent prolongation of recovery. Following the introduction of neuromuscular blocking drugs, the concept of balanced anesthesia – consisting of hypnosis, analgesia, and muscle relaxation – was developed and it was no longer necessary to expose patients to deep levels of inhalation agents for long periods in order to achieve adequate muscle relaxation. Furthermore, the technique of endotracheal intubation was greatly facilitated by the muscle relaxants.

These drugs may be divided into two classes depending upon their mechanism of action. *Depolarizing* agents (mainly succinylcholine) act as acetylcholine receptor agonists and depolarize the motor end plate; since they are not hydrolyzed by acetylcholinesterase, they remain at the neuromuscular junction, preventing repolarization (and mimicking the effects of excessive acetylcholine). The *nondepolarizing, competitive* agents (e.g., pancuronium, atracurium, vecuronium) act as antagonists and compete with acetylcholine for receptor sites on the motor end plate. All striated muscle groups, including respiratory muscles, are affected; smooth muscle is not. When using any neuromuscular blocking agent, therefore, it is advisable to monitor the degree of muscle paralysis with a nerve stimulator.[7]

Since these drugs cause respiratory paralysis, the implications of their use are enormous. They should never be prescribed for patients outside the operating room without consulting an anesthesiologist or another physician who is fully familiar with their pharmacology. Also, they are rarely administered unless intubation and mechanical ventilation are anticipated. (*Note:* Use of the term *muscle relaxant* can be deceptive. Physicians not fully familiar with these drugs might construe *relaxant* to mean a relaxer or sedative so we must be very clear in our terminology when using these medications.)

It should be clearly understood that neuromuscular blocking drugs have no inherent sedative effects. Although the lack of movement gives the impression that a patient is resting quietly, he or she may actually be quite anxious. It is inhumane to paralyze and mechanically ventilate an alert patient without providing an adequate level of sedation.

Depolarizing Drug: Succinylcholine

Unless there are contraindications to its use, succinylcholine is the drug of choice when rapid intubation is required. Its neuromuscular blocking effects (first described by Bovet et al.[8]) are widely utilized, and the compound has been the "gold standard" since Foldes et al.[9] reported using it in 1952 for muscular relaxation in patients undergoing surgery.

The drug has a rapid onset of action (about 30 s) and a relatively short duration. In the average adult a 1 mg/kg dose lasts 5–20 min. Within about 30 s of injection, there is a marked muscle fasciculation of varying intensity followed by a profound flaccid paralysis lasting 5–20 min, depending upon the dose and the patient. Succinylcholine is rapidly hydrolyzed by plasma pseudocholinesterase.

One serious side effect (Box 7.6), however, is life-threatening hyperkalemia – which can occur following an injection in patients with burns, muscle injury, upper or

Box 7.6 Disadvantages of Succinylcholine (Classified by Mechanism of Action)

Depolarization (end plate and muscle)
  Fasciculation and increased abdominal pressure
  Contracture
    Denervated, extraocular, and jaw muscles
  Potassium efflux and cardiac consequences
  Muscle pain
  Changing nature of block
    Tachyphylaxis and slow recovery
Other agonist actions
  Tachycardia and hypertension, other dysrhythmias
  Sinus bradycardia and arrest
Idiosyncratic responses
  Failure to metabolize succinylcholine
    Atypical plasma cholinesterase
  Exaggerated multisystem reactions
  Malignant hyperthermia
  Muscular dystrophies
Active metabolites
Drug interactions and complicating medical conditions
  Cardiac dysrhythmias
    Hyperkalemia in burns, renal failure, etc.
    Other electrolyte imbalances
    Cardiac glycosides
  Contractures and cardiac dysrhythmias
    Major neurological lesions
    Muscular dystrophies
  Reduced metabolism of succinylcholine
    Physiological (e.g., pregnancy, obesity, age extremes)
    Cholinesterase inhibition
  Increased metabolism of succinylcholine
  Increased neuromuscular sensitivity (e.g., magnesium, myasthenia gravis [nondepolarizing agents])
  Reduced neuromuscular sensitivity (e.g., myasthenia gravis [depolarizing agent])

lower motor neuron disease, or a number of other conditions – owing to the massive potassium efflux during prolonged muscle depolarization.[10] In a few susceptible individuals, succinylcholine can trigger malignant hyperthermia. Bradycardia often follows a repeat dose, especially in children, and can be prevented by administering atropine.

The duration of action of succinylcholine is determined by the degree of pseudo-cholinesterase activity in the plasma, which may be influenced by hereditary factors, disease states, pregnancy, or concurrently used medications. Hereditary factors are most often responsible for delayed recovery.[11] In these cases, the deficiency is due not so much to the quantity of the enzyme present but as to the atypical nature of the enzyme. Patients with this hereditary defect may remain apneic and paralyzed for up to 8 h. A typical homozygous pseudocholinesterase deficiency occurs in approximately 1 out of every 2,500 patients. Deficient quantities of the enzyme are most commonly found in patients receiving echothiophate eyedrops and cyclophosphamide (Cytoxan) therapy, but there may also be deficiencies in patients who are suffering from severe liver disease or have recently undergone plasmapheresis and in women who are pregnant. One of the major advantages of succinylcholine is its rapid onset and short duration of action. It is ideal when profound relaxation is required for a short time, as for intubation. The usual intravenous dose in adults is 1.5 mg/kg, and in children, 2 mg/kg. In children, it should be preceded by atropine or another suitable anticholinergic drug that blocks the undesirable muscarinic effects of acetylcholine (e.g., salivation, bronchial secretions, and bradycardia). (*Note:* Anticholinesterase agents do not reverse, but rather *potentiate*, the effects of succinylcholine.) The use of succinylcholine has been restricted in children to emergency use only because of potential risks associated with its use.

Nondepolarizing Drugs

In contrast to depolarizing neuromuscular drugs, which are few (and, practically speaking, there is just one), there are several nondepolarizing drugs to choose from.[12-14] A number of new neuromuscular blocking drugs has been introduced in the past 15 years, but it is not necessary for you to be familiar with all of them. Nondepolarizing drugs are most frequently used in anesthesia to provide muscle relaxation during surgery. They are also used to facilitate mechanical ventilation in some cases. Table 7.2 shows a classification of nondepolarizing drugs.

Nondepolarizing neuromuscular blocking drugs are predominantly used by anesthesiologists and critical care specialists in patients who require neuromuscular blockade during surgery or to facilitate mechanical ventilation in critical care units. Curare is now considered obsolete and the only long-acting agent in frequent use is pancuronium. Side effects of pancuronium include tachycardia and hypertension, which are dose-dependent and may be undesirable in patients with limited cardiac reserve. Neuromuscular blocking effects of pancuronium tend to persist long after reversal.

Table 7.2 Classification of nondepolarizing NMBs

Long-acting	Intermediate	Short-acting
Pancuronium	Atracurium	Rocuronium
Vecuronium	*Cis*-atracurium	Mivacurium

Chapter 8
Techniques of Intubation

Contents

B.T. Finucane et al., *Principles of Airway Management*,
DOI 10.1007/978-0-387-09558-5_8, © Springer Science+Business Media, LLC 2011

Introduction

This chapter provides the necessary information to successfully perform tracheal intubation. Individuals who are proficient at intubation can usually complete the procedure in less than 30 s.

In learning intubation, some hands-on experience is vital. Patients scheduled for elective surgery under general anesthesia and requiring intubation are ideal for teaching clinicians the technique. Allowing the clinician to get his or her feet wet can be stressful for everyone involved. The teacher must allow for the novice's lack of expertise and speed and must, simultaneously, protect the patient from trauma and hypoxia. Also, there is a (small) risk of aspiration of gastric contents. Patients should be preoxygenated before intubation. The traditional method of preoxygenation is 3 min of tidal volume breathing at 5 L/min using 100% oxygen.[1] Alternatively, Baraka et al.[2] have shown equally good results when breathing 8 deep breaths within 60 s at 10 L/min. Nimmagadda et al.[3] concurred with Baraka's approach and suggested that maximal preoxygenation was achieved when deep breathing at high flows (10 L/min) was extended for 1.5–2 min.

Current technology allows the continuous monitoring of a patient's oxygenation during intubation by use of a pulse oximeter. This noninvasive monitoring device – attached to a digit, an earlobe, or the nasal septum – relays information about the patient's oxygen saturation and pulse rate to a receiver that electronically displays this information on a screen. Falling oxygen saturations are signaled by a warning sound. Pulse oximetry has revolutionized the teaching of intubation because it provides an excellent intervention end point. Previously, clinical methods or simply timed intervention was used, but neither was entirely satisfactory. It is important to remember that there is a time lag before the monitor actually detects a falling oxygen saturation, therefore it is important to observe the patient for evidence of cyanosis at all times.

When teaching medical and other students airway skills, it is more important to teach them how to competently perform bag/valve/mask ventilation as opposed to intubation. However, bag/valve/mask ventilation is more difficult to learn. How quickly do students learn to perform these tasks? There is some information on medical students learning endotracheal intubation. Following didactic lectures and practice on a mannequin, 30 medical students performed intubation on 90 patients. One third of the students correctly intubated patients on their first attempt. However, 47% of these students incorrectly identified the position of the endotracheal tube. Ninety-three percent of the students correctly intubated patients after the third attempt, but of these, 20% failed to recognize incorrect tube placement. It seems unlikely that students obtain sufficient training in airway management in a 1- to 2-week rotation in anesthesia.[4]

Although there are no good yardsticks for determining when a clinician is competent to perform intubation, in simplest terms, an individual is probably competent if he or she can place a tube within the trachea in 30 s or less and complete all the preliminary and follow-up steps required within 1 min. Konrad et al.[5] completed a study on 11 first year anesthesia trainees who had little, if any, exposure to common

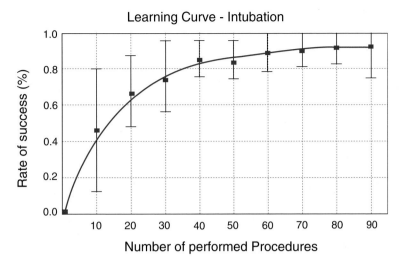

Fig. 8.1 Intubation learning curve

technical anesthesia tasks such as the performance of spinal, epidural, and brachial plexus anesthesia, the insertion of an arterial line, and the performance of tracheal intubation. They generated learning curves for these various procedures and noted that epidural anesthesia was the most difficult task to learn and tracheal intubation was the easiest. Residents achieved a 90% success rate after 57 orotracheal intubations using a Macintosh blade (Fig. 8.1). However, improvement was readily seen even after 10 intubations. Nasal intubation was not included in this study. One can estimate therefore that perhaps 100 intubations including both oral and nasal tubes would be required to have an acceptable success rate (100%) with tracheal intubation. The consequences of failure of tracheal intubation are far more serious than failure of epidural or spinal anesthesia. Safar[6] suggests using a checklist to measure competence in learners (Fig. 8.2).

Intubation Methods

The vast majority of intubations are performed using direct vision; however, there are also indirect or blind methods, which may be used in specific situations.

Orotracheal Intubation by Direct Vision in an Adult (Macintosh Blade)

Direct vision is the most common method employed in the performance of oral endotracheal intubation in adult patients.

Student's name	Date	Evaluator's name

☐ Passed
☐ Failed

Measures	Technique	Time
	☑ Check if correct performance	☑ Check if within correct time lapse

Measures	Technique	Time
Tracheal intubation of *adult* manikin	☐ Checked laryngoscope light before use	sec.
	☐ Checked tube patency before use	
	☐ Held laryngoscope correctly	
	☐ Used no grossly traumatic manoeuvre during intubation attempt	
	☐ Inserted tube into trachea rapidly . . . . . . ☐ < 30	
	☐ Gave first lung inflation rapidly via tube by bag-valve or mouth . . . . ☐ < 60	
	☐ Inflated cuff of tube correctly (with helper)	
	☐ Used bite-block, secured tube and connected ventilation device correctly	
	☐ Checked to rule out bronchial intubation	
Tracheal intubation of *infant* manikin	☐ Checked laryngoscope light before use	
	☐ Checked tube patency before use	
	☐ Held laryngoscope correctly	
	☐ Used no grossly traumatic manoeuvre during intubation attempt	
	☐ Inserted tube into trachea rapidly . . . . . . ☐ < 30	
	☐ Gave first lung inflation rapidly via tube (by mouth) . . . . ☐ < 60	
	☐ Used bite-block, secured tube and connected ventilation device correctly	
	☐ Checked to rule out bronchial intubation	
Tracheal suctioning (curved-tipped catheter)	☐ Used correct technique to suction each lung separately . . . . ☐ < 60	

Fig. 8.2 Checklist for testing intubation competence (from Safar,[6] with permission)

Preparation

The first task is to perform an equipment check. It is essential that one be able to deliver 100% oxygen at high flows (up to 10 L/min) using a bag and mask. Other mandatory equipment includes: (1) a suction apparatus connected via clear, plastic tubing to a rigid tonsil sucker capable of drawing a negative pressure of 25 cm H_2O, and (2) an intubation tray containing the following items (Fig. 8.3):

Two laryngoscope handles and a MAC 3 and 4 blade
Oral airways
Variety of endotracheal tubes
Stylet
K-Y Jelly or other suitable lubricant

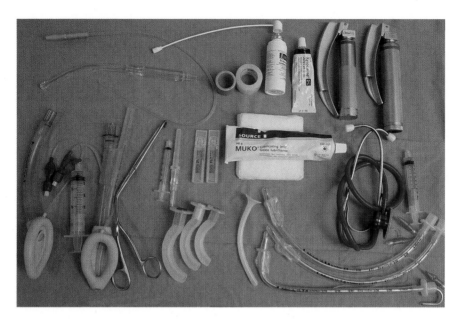

Fig. 8.3 An intubation tray

Tonsil sucker (Yankauer) and flexible suction catheter
Magill forceps
Tape
Towels
Local anesthetic spray
Laryngeal mask airways
Syringes (20 and 10 mL)
Stethoscope

Both laryngoscopes should be functioning, and the endotracheal tube cuff should be checked for leaks. The tube should be well lubricated and some specialists also recommend lubricating the blade up to the bulb with lubricant.

Positioning

An otolaryngologist name Kirstein[7] was among the first to suggest that neck flexion and extension of the atlantooccipital joint improved the view of the larynx when performing direct laryngoscopy. This observation was further supported by Chevalier Jackson,[8] who performed some clinical studies on this matter. Sir Ivan Magill[9] was given credit for coining the phrase *sniffing position* in relation to optimal head and neck position for direct laryngoscopy as it resembles the posture of the head and neck when sniffing the morning air. In 1944, Bannister and MacBeth et al.[10] published a paper in the *Lancet* in which they proposed the three axis theory for optimal positioning of the head and neck when performing laryngoscopy.

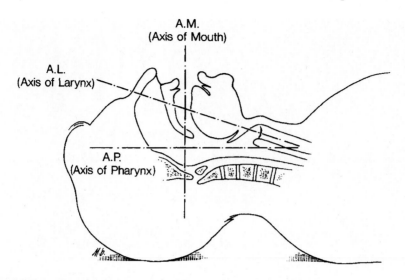

Fig. 8.4 Poor alignment of the axes of the larynx, pharynx, and mouth

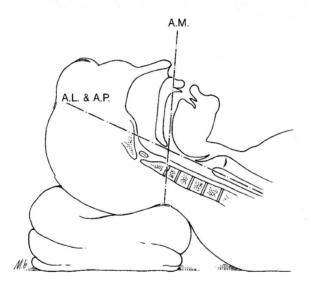

Fig. 8.5 Cervical flexion

They suggested that the axes of the mouth, the larynx, and pharynx must be in alignment in order to improve the view of the larynx during laryngoscopy.

In Fig. 8.4, the head is in the neutral position and the axes of the larynx (AL), pharynx (AP), and mouth (AM) are poorly aligned. By flexion of the cervical spine, the axes of the larynx and pharynx are brought into unison (Fig. 8.5). By extension of the atlantooccipital joint, the axis of the mouth is aligned close to the axes of the larynx and pharynx (Fig. 8.6). With proper positioning, all three axes are close to unison with laryngoscopy (Fig. 8.7).

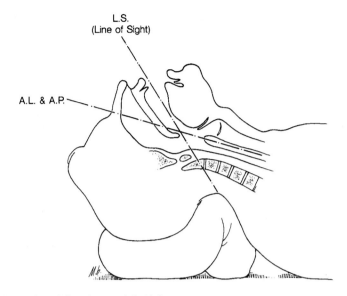

Fig. 8.6 Extension of the atlantooccipital joint

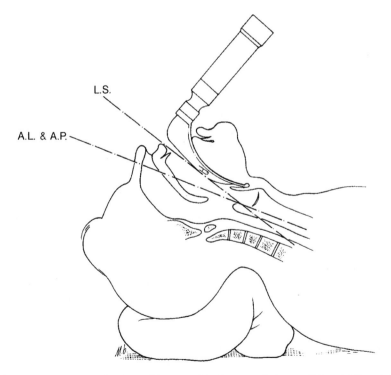

Fig. 8.7 Final exposure. Alignment of the axes of the larynx and pharynx (AL and AP) and showing the line of sight (LS)

The three axes alignment theory went unchallenged for close to 60 years. Using MRI, Adnet et al.[11] recently demonstrated that it was not possible to align the three axes into one by adopting the sniffing position. However, they did demonstrate that the *sniffing position* significantly improved the angle associated with the best laryngoscopic view. They also showed an improved laryngoscopic view by just extending the atlantooccipital joint, and there was no significant difference in the angles observed when these two maneuvers were compared.

Chou[12] recently contributed to the discussion by suggesting that Bannister and MacBeth failed to indicate start and finish points for the three axes theory and only mentioned the direction of the axes. Chou proposed a modified theory. He suggested that direct laryngoscopy involved two axes, the pharynx, and the mouth and tongue. Before the laryngoscope is introduced, the angle between the incisors and the pharynx and glottis is approximately 90°. Head extension converts this angle to approximately 125° and then the advancement of the tongue with the laryngoscope makes this angle approach 180°. However, there are other elements that do not always make it possible to achieve 180° line of sight. These elements are the mobility and size of the soft tissues and bony structures and the size of the oropharyngeal space in relation to the tongue and other soft tissues. The cervical spine cannot be readily extended in arthritic conditions, thereby limiting one's ability to open the 90° angle between the mouth and glottis. Temporomandibular joint disease limits one's ability to move the tongue forward, and those with a hypoplastic mandible or large tongue have a reduced oropharyngeal space. It is with some reluctance that we debunk the theories of old masters, but it is difficult to refute what Adnet et al. and Chou and others have observed. However, although the three axis theory has been challenged, there is still general agreement that the *sniffing position* facilitates exposure of the glottis during direct laryngoscopy

There is one other point worth discussing about positioning. In recent years, we have seen an epidemic of obesity in the developed world, which is related to the rapid expansion of the fast food industry and the excessive consumption of soft drinks. Obesity per se is not an automatic indicator of difficult intubation or mask ventilation. However, statistics do indicate that overweight patients make up a large percentage of those with problem airways and, because of their size, pulmonary reserves are reduced and we do not have as much time as usual to deal with issues like hypoxemia or hypercarbia. There have been a number of studies recently dedicated to optimizing head and chest position of obese patients prior to intubation. In addition to the usual recommendations about aligning the axes of the larynx and pharynx in preparation for intubation, we also read that a 25° elevation of the upper torso and shoulders, such that the external auditory meatus and the sternal notch are in the same horizontal plane, facilitates tracheal intubation in obese patients.[13] This makes complete sense. This position facilitates not only tracheal intubation, but also mask ventilation. Functional residual capacity (FRC) must increase on the basis of gravity and the risk of passive gastric regurgitation is reduced. Perhaps all patients undergoing anesthesia should be induced in this position. There are two ways of achieving this position: one is by placing blankets or other padding behind the patient's back and shoulders and the other far more practical method is by adjusting the operating table at the thigh-trunk hinge.

Exposure

The final exposure is achieved by opening the mouth and anteriorly displacing the mandible and soft tissues of the oral cavity and neck with the laryngoscope blade (Fig. 8.7).

To perform the final exposure, stand directly behind the patient's head and take the laryngoscope handle in the left hand (right-handed laryngoscopes are available for left-handed people) as you would a paddle. With the right hand, open the mouth using the *scissors maneuver* (Fig. 8.8a), depressing the lower teeth with the thumb and elevating the upper teeth with the index or middle finger or both. Pressing upon the upper teeth will automatically extend the atlantooccipital joint. Alternatively, you may introduce the laryngoscope using the *no-touch technique* (Fig. 8.8b). In paralyzed patients, the mandible usually descends, allowing room for insertion of the laryngoscope blade without inserting a finger into the mouth. These maneuvers should allow good exposure of the airway. (Gloves are strongly recommended when performing any airway maneuver)

Visualization

At this stage, the laryngoscope blade is introduced into the mouth with the concave portion arching over the tongue in the midline (Fig. 8.9). If the blade is introduced at the side, it is more likely to tear the mucous membrane near the tonsillar folds on the right. It is always a good idea to make sure that the upper lip is not trapped between the laryngoscope blade and the teeth before advancing the laryngoscope. Failure to do so can cause unsightly bruising of the upper lip and can be the source of discomfort and annoyance to patients afterwards.

Advance the blade over the tongue until the uvula and the tonsillar folds are seen. Then move it to the right side of the mouth so it lies between the aryepiglottic folds and the tongue. This maneuver displaces the tongue to the left (Fig. 8.10). Advance the blade further until its tip lies in the vallecula (Fig. 8.11) and then pull it forward and upward using firm but steady pressure without rotating the wrist (Fig. 8.12). If possible, avoid leaning on the upper teeth with the blade, since damage to the teeth may occur. In most situations, the vocal cords should become visible at this stage (Fig. 8.13). If not, exert gentle pressure over the cricoid area to help bring them into view.

Insertion

The endotracheal tube is usually inserted at the right corner of the mouth, below, and to the right of the laryngoscope blade, with its concave portion facing toward the ceiling. Occasionally, it is necessary to rotate the tube 90° to the right or left before insertion.

Once the cuff has passed beyond the vocal cords, advance the tube another 3 cm. However, remember that there is a tendency to advance the tube further than necessary

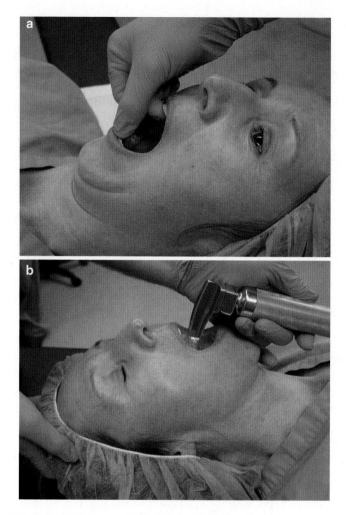

Fig. 8.8 (**a**) The scissors maneuver. (**b**) The no-touch technique

when learning this technique. To facilitate placement, have the assistant retract the right corner of the mouth. Occasionally, teeth may damage the cuff of the tube *en route* to the trachea.

Cuff Inflation

When reasonably satisfied that the endotracheal tube is correctly placed, inflate the cuff with the required amount of air. This is best determined by connecting the tube to the oxygen source and manually applying pressure to the reservoir bag until 20 cm H_2O registers on the airway pressure monitor. Then listen for a leak at the

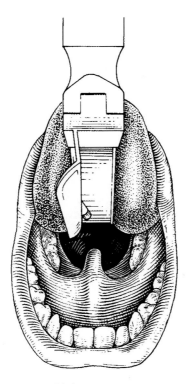

Fig. 8.9 Introducing the laryngoscope blade

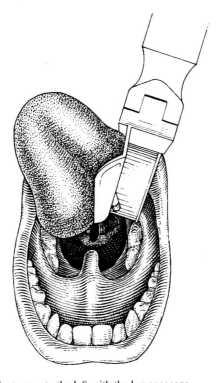

Fig. 8.10 Displacing the tongue to the left with the laryngoscope

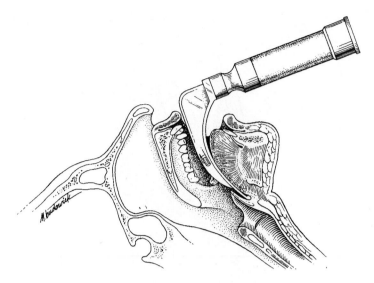

Fig. 8.11 Direct laryngoscopy with the blade in the vallecula

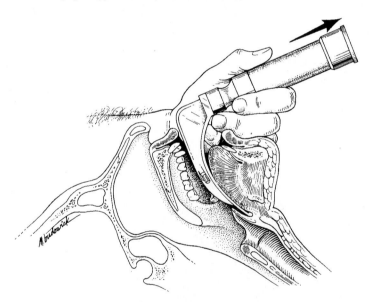

Fig. 8.12 Forward-upward lift. The wrist should be straight

patient's mouth and inflate the cuff until there is no longer an audible leak at 20 cm H_2O pressure. Remember: overinflation of the cuff can lead to ischemia of the tracheal mucosa surrounding to the cuff.

If the cuff continues to leak despite large quantities of injected air, two possibilities exist: (1) the cuff may have been damaged during intubation, or (2) the tube may not be down far enough (i.e., the tip of the tube may be below the level of the vocal cords, but a portion of the cuff may be lying above it). This problem can be

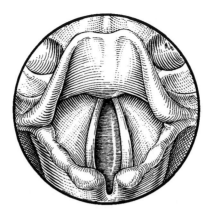

Fig. 8.13 Direct exposure of the larynx

verified by looking into the patient's mouth with a laryngoscope and identifying the inflated cuff.

Confirmation

Endotracheal intubation is a technique readily learned by physicians and other health care personnel. Laryngoscopy and insertion of the tube are usually considered to be the most interesting part of the task, but confirmation of correct tube placement, though perhaps less interesting, is even more important and can never be taken for granted. Auscultatory methods alone can no longer be relied upon to confirm placement of the tube in the trachea. The anesthesia literature is replete with reports of deaths and serious injuries resulting from undetected esophageal intubation. It is even more sobering to note that "even a conscientious, careful anesthesiologist may be unable to differentiate between tracheal and esophageal intubation by the commonly employed methods."[14] In a review of 29 cases of esophageal intubation by the ASA[1] confirmation of correct endotracheal tube placement was entered in the anesthesia record in only 18 of the cases.

Twenty-five years or so ago, continuous carbon dioxide monitoring of exhaled gases or capnometry became a standard of care in operating rooms in most developed countries in the world, and it is now considered the most reliable method of detecting extratracheal tube placement. Capnometry (the measurement of CO_2 concentrations during a respiratory cycle) is different from capnography (the display of wave forms on a screen or a printout) (Fig. 8.14).

It is important to recognize that CO_2 may be detected in the esophagus when exhaled gases enter the esophagus during mask ventilation.[15] Furthermore, CO_2 can be released from the stomach, in varying quantities, from carbonated beverages and antacids.[16] However, the wave forms do not follow the usual patterns. It is also important to point out that capnometry/capnography is not foolproof. There have

---

[1] ASA Committee on Professional Liability in relation to esophageal intubation.

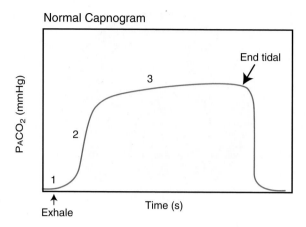

Fig. 8.14 The normal capnogram. *1* Anatomic deadspace. *2* Anatomic+alveolar spaces. *3* Alveolar plateau

been a few isolated cases of failure, although most clinicians[17] agree that this technology is still the most reliable method of detecting unrecognized esophageal intubation in elective situations. Capnography alone is not totally reliable in emergency medical situations. A recent meta-analysis of over 2,000 emergency room intubations showed an aggregate sensitivity of 93% and specificity of 97% of capnography. These data indicate a 10% inaccuracy rate in emergency medical situations, which is unacceptable.[18] Therefore, one should not totally rely on capnography in emergency medical situations. We should also extend that philosophy to elective situations. Why is capnography so unreliable in emergency medicine? Capnography depends on the presence of carbon dioxide. If pulmonary blood flow is impaired, carbon dioxide will not be readily detected. The following box provides a list of false-negative and false-positive results leading to capnography misinterpretation (Boxes 8.1 and 8.2).

Not only must you confirm that the endotracheal tube is in the trachea, but also ascertain that it is correctly placed within the trachea and not in a mainstem bronchus. Furthermore, there is no guarantee that once the tube is correctly placed within the trachea, it will remain there.

In addition to using capnometry and other methods of continuously monitoring exhaled CO_2, you must confirm that the endotracheal tube is correctly positioned in the trachea. This is best achieved by auscultatory methods in an operating room setting and radiologically in an intensive care unit (ICU) setting. Immediately following intubation, the tracheal placement of the tube is confirmed by capnometry and then the centimeter marking on the tube is noted at the level of the teeth. The distance from the teeth to midtrachea in the average adult is about 22 cm with the head in neutral position. If the centimeter marking is greater than 22 or less than 20, the tube should be adjusted before auscultation.

Auscultation is best performed by listening in the axillae while simultaneously ventilating the patient manually. In addition, you should observe chest wall

> **Box 8.1** False/Negative Results (Tube in Trachea, Capnogram Suggests
> That Tube Is in Esophagus)
>
> 1. Concurrent PEEP with ETT cuff leak
> 2. Severe airway obstruction
> 3. Low cardiac output
> 4. Severe hypotension
> 5. Pulmonary embolus
> 6. Advanced pulmonary disease

> **Box 8.2** False-Positive Results (Tube Not in Trachea, Capnogram Suggests
> Tube Is in Trachea)
>
> 1. Bag/valve/mask ventilation prior to intubation
> 2. Antacids in stomach
> 3. Recent ingestion of carbonated beverages
> 4. Tube in pharynx

movements (which are symmetrical when both lungs are being ventilated). Pulmonary compliance may appear diminished if the tube enters a mainstem bronchus, and peak inspiratory pressures will usually be well above the normal range of 15–25 cm because the complete tidal volume (normally shared by both lungs) is being forced into one lung (Fig. 8.15). These signs are not totally reliable, however, because they can also be observed in the presence of bronchospasm or pneumothorax. Nevertheless, auscultation remains the most practical method of confirming correct positioning of an endotracheal tube. Of course, fiberoptic bronchoscopy is a reliable method for confirming correct positioning of an endotracheal tube, especially when difficulties arise, and should be available in every operating suite.

Pulse oximetry has become another indispensable monitoring device during airway intervention. Although it does not confirm correct or incorrect tube placement, it does act as a warning device and is particularly useful when teaching students airway management techniques. If during the course of endotracheal intubation the patient becomes hypoxic, you must strongly suspect incorrect tube placement or malfunction of a correctly placed tube; if there is any doubt about tube placement, remove the tube and ventilate by mask using 100% oxygen. Modern technology makes some of these decisions more difficult because the data obtained from capnography are very reliable. However, when faced with a crisis, you must revert to basic principles; and always remember the old adage "If in doubt, take it out." The longer you delay this process, the less time you will have to correct a problem; thus, be decisive and intervene early.

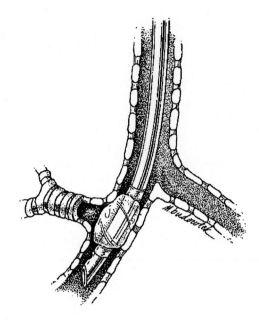

Fig. 8.15 Right mainstem intubation

In most circumstances involving airway management, there should be little hesitation about extubating a patient with suspected esophageal intubation. However,
when an intubation has been especially difficult or the patient is extremely obese,
there may be more reluctance than usual to extubate.

An alternative is to pass a tube changer or bougie, then extubate, and then perform mask ventilation with the tube changer or bougie in place. If the patient's
condition improves with mask ventilation, you will have time to perform direct
laryngoscopy again. The tube changer itself may be used to confirm whether the
tube has been correctly placed. When a tube changer is advanced into the trachea,
resistance is usually felt as its tip encounters the carina or mainstem bronchus,
which in adults is usually at about 30 cm.[19] No such resistance is encountered at
30 cm when the changer is advanced into the esophagus. If, indeed, it was in the
trachea initially, you may "railroad" another tube over it. Alternatively, you can
apply mask ventilation with a "cutoff" tube in place.[20] If the patient's condition
improves after mask ventilation over an endotracheal tube, esophageal intubation is
to be suspected. A number of other strategies may be used under these circumstances[21] (Boxes 8.3 and 8.4).

Although the technique of endotracheal intubation becomes quite routine with
practice, you should never undertake it lightly. The consequences of incorrect
placement are devastating. The patient's cerebral function may be impaired for life,
or life ended altogether. It would appear that the practice of auscultation of the chest
following intubation is diminishing at least in the operating room setting. This is
regrettable because there is no other reliable, practical way to detect endobronchial

Box 8.3 Suspicion of Esophageal Intubation: Indications for Extubation

1. Decreasing oxygen saturation
2. Minimal or absent chest movement
3. CO_2 not detected by capnograph
4. Cyanosis
5. Increasing abdominal distension
6. Absence of condensation in the expired gas
7. Gurgling sound from ETT

Source: Data from Clyburn and Rosen[21]

Box 8.4 Actions for Suspected Esophageal Intubation

1. When in doubt remove the tube
2. Bag/mask ventilation
3. Reevaluate the head and neck position
4. Select a smaller tube
5. Implement difficult airway algorithm

Source: Data from Clyburn and Rosen[21]

intubation. The most reliable method of confirming endotracheal tube placement in the trachea is to continuously monitor the concentration of CO_2 in exhaled gases. All other methods are either unreliable or impractical.

Following is a list of the various methods used to verify tube placement in the trachea:

End-tidal CO_2 monitoring
Auscultation
Movement of the chest and epigastrium
Direct vision
Vital signs
Condensation in the tube
Videostethoscope
Negative pressure tests
Tube markings
Movement of the reservoir bag
Vocal silence ("awake" intubation)
Pulse oximetry

Fiberoptic bronchoscopy
Chest X ray
Tube changer
Cuff palpation
Transtracheal illumination
Sternal compression
Acoustic reflectometry

There are a number of other devices available to detect esophageal intubation, but they are not used by anesthesiologists and these include The SCOTI device (sonomatic confirmation of tracheal intubation), acoustic reflectometry, esophageal detector bulb, electronic esophageal detectors, and colorimetric detection of end-tidal carbon dioxide. These devices are mostly used in Emergency Departments and prehospital settings and are not discussed in this text as we have little experience with them.

Stabilization

Some novices are so overjoyed at successfully intubating a patient that they fail to secure the tube properly. Securing tubes may sound easier than it is. In an anesthetized patient it is easy, but on the ward it can be quite difficult. Often, when reoxygenated, a once comatose patient becomes revitalized and is distraught at finding a large plastic tube in his larynx. Patients have been known to bite the tube in half or to occlude it completely, preventing air from entering or leaving. Be prepared for this possibility. A combination of morphine and midazolam is usually quite effective in sedating such patients. If you are not planning to ventilate the patient, the dose of these drugs must be chosen very carefully. As a guide, morphine should be given in 2.5-mg increments and midazolam in 1-mg increments. As much as 15 mg of morphine and 10 mg of midazolam intravenously may be required for initial sedation in the average adult, but there is considerable variation. In securing the endotracheal tube, always use highly adhesive tape. The mandible is quite mobile; therefore, it is preferable to stabilize the tube to the maxilla. If the tube is to be left in for some time, apply benzoin to the upper lip and recheck tube position after it has been stabilized.

Tape may not be adequate to secure the endotracheal tube under certain circumstances (e.g., oral, dental, or plastic surgery or burn debridements in the perioral region). There are a number of ways to secure it in these circumstances. You may wire it to a stable lower tooth or suture it to the tongue. If it is sutured, however, be sure to use strong suture material and to introduce it horizontally through the median raphe of the tongue which is made up of sturdy fibrous tissue.

Movement of the head and neck may alter the position of endotracheal tubes in both adults and children. Flexing the head results in movement of the tip of the endotracheal tube toward the larynx and extension of the head does the opposite. Rotation of the head to the right results in withdrawal of the tube in most cases in adults. Head rotation to the left leads to unpredictable results. Head rotation to the right and left in children results in withdrawal in all cases.[22]

Orotracheal Intubation by Direct Vision in an Adult (Miller Blade)

The Macintosh laryngoscope blade is widely used all over the world. The straight blade, better known as the Miller blade, is quite popular in the United States. There is general agreement that the novice finds the Macintosh blade easier to use, which may explain its popularity. However, we are unable to see the larynx in up to 8% of cases when we use the Macintosh blade.[23] The curvature of the Macintosh blade impairs your vision when laryngoscopy is difficult. This deficiency led to the modification described in (Fig. 8.16) (improved-vision Macintosh blade). The Macintosh laryngoscope blade tends to compress the tongue distally, causing posterior displacement of the epiglottis, thereby creating a soft tissue obstruction of the larynx.[24] There is a shallower learning curve with the Miller laryngoscope, but when you become familiar with its use, the ability to see the larynx improves. Your view is not obstructed by the curvature of the blade and, because the tip of the blade is placed beneath the epiglottis, one usually has a better view of the larynx (Fig. 8.17). In a recent study comparing views obtained with the Macintosh and Miller blades, laryngoscopy using the Miller blade allowed 100% of the vocal cords to be visualized in 78% of cases, whereas this was achieved in only 53% of cases with the Macintosh blade ($p=0.0014$).[25] The straight blade is very useful in cases of micrognathia and when the epiglottis is elongated and floppy. However, there are some limitations to the Miller blade. It is rather narrow and, if used incorrectly, the tongue tends to overlap it. It is also sometimes difficult to pass the endotracheal tube when it is used. Henderson[26] has addressed some of these problems with a newly designed laryngoscope. The key to successful use of the straight laryngoscope blade is to introduce the blade at the right side of the mouth and keep it lateral to the tongue at all times (paraglossal approach).[27] Traditional teaching of laryngoscopy with the straight blade recommended introducing the blade in the midline, which invariably resulted in a difficult exposure because the tongue had a tendency to overlap the blade. New trainees should learn to perform laryngoscopy using both blades, bearing in mind that it is more difficult to master the straight blade.

Nasotracheal Intubation by Direct Vision in an Adult (Macintosh Blade)

Endotracheal tubes can also be introduced under direct vision through either nostril. This is slightly more difficult, however, and usually takes longer than orotracheal intubation. It is also more traumatic, and bleeding is quite common.

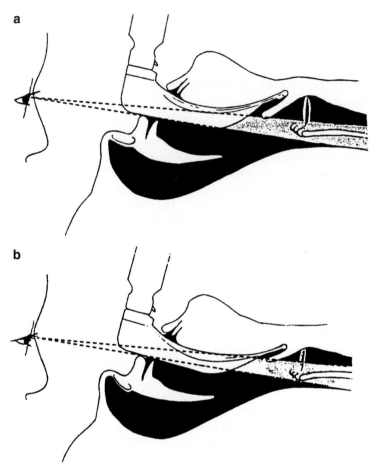

Fig. 8.16 (**a**) Regular Macintosh. (**b**) Improved-vision Macintosh blade (from Racz,[42] with permission from Wiley)

Preparation

In terms of equipment, the preparation for nasal intubation is basically the same as for orotracheal intubation. For emphasis, it should be restated that you should not perform nasotracheal intubation unless oxygen and suction are immediately available. Intubation trays should contain the same items. In addition, a Magill forcep is absolutely necessary for guiding the tube toward the glottis. Also, 0.25% phenylephrine, lidocaine, and a nebulizer should be available.

Before beginning nasal intubation, perform a cursory airway examination, paying specific attention to the nostrils. If the patient is conscious, check the patency of the nostrils and question him about any clotting abnormality. In some cases, the septum may be deviated or nasal polyps may be a problem. These factors will influence your choice. Spray both nostrils with a combination of 2% lidocaine and

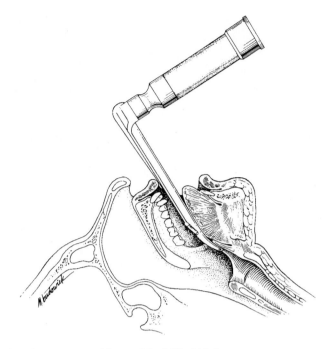

Fig. 8.17   Direct laryngoscopy with a straight (Miller) blade

0.25% phenylephrine or 4% cocaine. Sedation may or may not be required, depending upon the situation. Select an endotracheal tube with an internal diameter that is one-half size less than would normally be used for an oral intubation. Lubricate the tube and selected nostril with a suitable lubricant.

Positioning

Position the head and neck as for orotracheal intubation, standing immediately behind the supine patient and extending his neck with your left hand.

Tube Insertion

Insert the tube, which should be connected to an oxygen source, into the nostril with the bevel pointing toward the septum (Fig. 8.18). Direct it vertically downward, at a right angle to the horizontal, until it reaches the oropharynx (Fig. 8.19). Inexperienced practitioners sometimes direct the tube toward the cribriform plate and, in at least one case, this faulty direction led to the introduction of a nasogastric tube into the cranial cavity in a traumatized patient.[28]

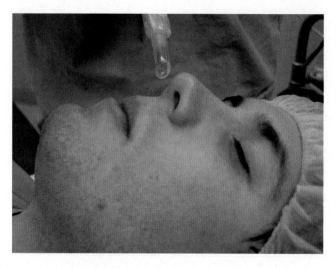

Fig. 8.18 Nasotracheal intubation. Note that the bevel is pointing toward the septum

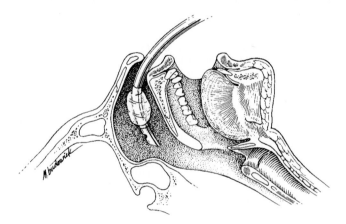

Fig. 8.19 Introduction of the nasal endotracheal tube

Exposure

Open the mouth widely using the methods already described for orotracheal intubation.

Visualization

You can readily see the vocal cords in an average-sized patient using a Macintosh 3 laryngoscope blade.

Tube Placement

It is possible, in many instances, to direct the endotracheal tube toward and past the vocal cords manually by manipulating the tube from the top. More often than not, however, Magill forceps will be required to direct it toward the glottis.

Hold the forceps in your right hand and position, as shown in Fig. 8.20. Grip the tube toward its tip, above the point of attachment of the cuff (if possible), to avoid damaging the cuff. It can then be advanced by the assistant while you point it in the direction of the rima glottidis.

The tube should enter the trachea without difficulty. Occasionally, however, it will reach the vocal cords and not advance any further. In this situation, its distal end is probably impinging upon the anterior commissure, which lies nearly perpendicular to the axis of the trachea. The problem can be remedied by acutely flexing the cervical spine (Fig. 8.21). Another approach is to gently rotate the tube so that its concavity points toward the posterior trachea wall. If earlier attempts at nasotracheal intubation have been unsuccessful, do not withdraw the tube altogether, but merely extract it far enough into the oropharynx to connect it to an oxygen source. This will allow adequate oxygenation without undue trauma to the nasal mucosa. (In fact, the oxygen should be hooked up at all times during any intubation attempt.) The average distance from the nose to midtrachea is 25 cm in an individual with normal proportions weighing about 70 kg (154 lb) (Fig. 8.22).

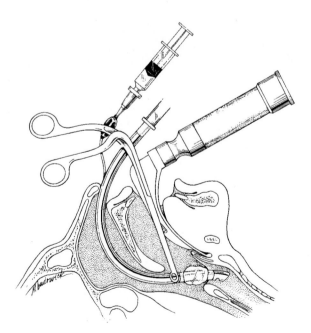

Fig. 8.20 Nasotracheal intubation with Magill (straight) forceps

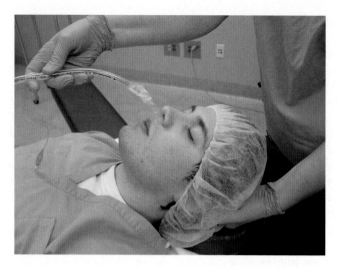

Fig. 8.21 Flexion of the cervical spine facilitates nasotracheal intubation

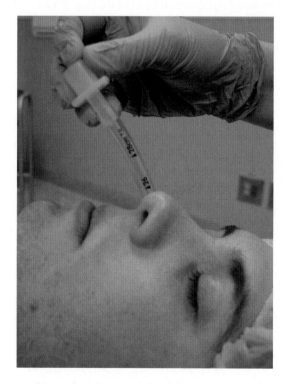

Fig. 8.22 The average distance from the nose to the midtracheal region in an adult is about 25 cm

Confirmation

The same rules apply for nasotracheal as for orotracheal intubation.

Stabilization

In addition to following previous advice about securing the tube, be particularly careful about securing one in an unconscious patient. The cartilaginous tip of the nose, because of its meager blood supply, is particularly vulnerable to pressure necrosis from an endotracheal tube. This problem can be allayed to some degree by using specifically designed tubes (nasal ring adhere Elwin [RAE]) and connectors that do not lean on the nasal rim during surgery.

Blind Nasotracheal Intubation

The technique of blind nasotracheal intubation, pioneered by Magill and Rowbotham[27, 29] during World War I, has been replaced by improved direct and indirect methods, but in certain situations it remains invaluable. It is indicated when direct visualization of the airway is difficult or impossible because the mouth cannot be opened, or the instrumentation might damage teeth or other structures in the oropharynx. The preparation and equipment are identical to those used for the direct visualization approach.

Technique

The technique can be performed on an awake, sedated, or anesthetized patient. The only strict requirement is that the patient be capable of breathing spontaneously – although the use of succinylcholine has also been described.[30]

When performing the technique on an awake, sedated patient, spend a few moments explaining the procedure. It is usually performed with the patient supine, but when serious airway obstruction is present, it may be performed in the sitting position.

Spray both nostrils with 4% cocaine or a mixture of lidocaine and phenylephrine. The chosen nostril should be well lubricated. Place the tube, connected to an oxygen source, in the nostril and advance it into the oropharynx. More local anesthetic solution may be sprayed down the tube, whose tip should be pointing toward the glottis. Flex the cervical spine by placing a folded towel beneath the patient's head. Then extend the head and pull the mandible upward with your left hand. Occlude the mouth and free nostril at this time.

Next, to make the breath sounds more audible, disconnect the oxygen tubing. By lowering your left ear over the endotracheal tube, you will be able to hear and feel the breath sounds and can use them as an indicator of how close the tube tip is to the airway. Slowly advance the tube with the right hand. When it enters the airway, the patient usually coughs and a definite tubular sound replaces the harsher breath sound previously heard. A number of reports[31,32] refer to the use of a simple whistle, which can be attached to the tube connector during intubation attempts.

Blind nasal intubation is not always achieved on the first attempt and, in some cases, may require several attempts. If the tube does not enter the larynx, *the tube* is *either* above the glottic opening, below it in the esophagus, or on either side of it in the piriform sinus. When the tube is excessively curved or when the patient's cervical spine is overextended, the tip of the tube tends to abut the anterior commissure. This can be remedied by withdrawing it slightly, flexing the neck, and advancing the tube slowly into the airway. The tube can also enter the esophagus if the patient's head is excessively flexed or the tube is too straight.

Occasionally, the tube will fail to go beneath the epiglottis and instead enter the vallecula. This problem can be remedied by withdrawing it slightly, pulling the mandible forward, and rotating the tube through 90°. An attempt should then be made to advance the tube into the glottis. One report[33] describes extrusion of the tongue as an aid to blind nasal intubation.

Finally, the tube may be deflected laterally toward either piriform sinus. Palpation of the neck will usually reveal to which side it is pointing. The tube should then be withdrawn slightly and rotated medially, its point directed toward the glottis.

Successful blind nasal intubation is usually heralded by a harsh "bovine" cough followed by vocal silence. However, other evidence of correct placement is also sought as described for orotracheal intubation.

In modern times the art of blind nasotracheal intubation is being rapidly replaced by fiberoptic laryngoscopy and bronchoscopy. Despite this new trend, however, physicians involved in airway management should be encouraged to learn the blind technique.

Summary

Nasotracheal intubation is usually more difficult to perform, more traumatic, and more time-consuming than orotracheal intubation. However, it has one important advantage – the presence of the tube in the nasopharynx provides a conduit through which oxygenation and sometimes ventilation can occur during laryngoscopy while attempting intubation. (Complications of nasotracheal intubation are discussed in Chap. 15.)

Airway Maneuvers

Anesthesiologists and other experts in airway management employ various maneuvers to facilitate intubation or to protect patients against aspiration. Some of these maneuvers will now be described.

BURP

The BURP maneuver was first described by Knill[34] and is now a well-recognized aid to improve visualization of the airway during routine and difficult intubation. The maneuver has three distinct components:

1. Posterior pressure on the larynx against the cervical vertebrae (Backward)
2. Superior pressure on the larynx as far as possible (Upward)
3. Lateral pressure on the larynx to the right (Right)

By adding (Pressure) to the preceding terms, Knill came up with a memorable acronym, BURP.

The efficacy of this maneuver has been tested in 630 patients by Takahata et al. and they concluded that it was a worthwhile maneuver and should be used routinely during attempts at laryngoscopy.[35] However, the BURP maneuver does not always work and, in some cases, impedes an optimal view of the larynx.[36]

OELM

Benumof et al.[37] described a variation of the BURP maneuver referred to as Optimal External Laryngeal Manipulation, and it implies that one should experiment to find the optimal maneuver on the larynx to improve visualization.

Sellick's Maneuver (Cricoid Pressure)

Sellick's maneuver[38] is the name assigned to cricoid pressure applied during rapid sequence induction (RSI) of anesthesia to prevent passive regurgitation of gastric contents and aspiration. This maneuver has now become a standard of care in anesthesia in any situation in which patients are considered at risk for aspiration. It is not a universally accepted maneuver and its use has never been validated. The original experimental work was carried out on cadavers. There are many concerns about cricoid pressure. First of all, it is frequently applied incorrectly. It may distort one's view of the airway. It may damage the airway. It may increase the risk of regurgitation, and there are other issues as well. In a recent study conducted in healthy volunteers, investigators showed that the esophagus was displaced laterally in 52% of healthy volunteers when using MRI and in greater than 90% of cases when cricoid pressure was applied.[39] Brimacombe et al.[40] recently published an extensive review of this topic.

Cricoid pressure is usually applied by an informed assistant during RSI of anesthesia. The single-handed method involves placing the thumb and middle finger on either side of the cricoid cartilage and the index finger above to prevent movement of the cricoid. A pressure of 20 N should be applied until loss of consciousness, at which time it is increased to 30 N.[41] The assistant is instructed to maintain pressure on the cricoid until instructed to release. Clearly, the operator must be assured that the endotracheal tube is in the trachea and is able to manually ventilate the patient, and that there is no leak.

Failed Intubation (Normal Anatomy)

Failed intubation in a patient with normal anatomy is most often caused by poor positioning of the head. Novices seem to have difficulty opening the mouth wide enough, and considerable time is lost trying to place the laryngoscope in the mouth. When they do succeed, they allow the tongue to overlap the laryngoscope blade, and this blocks their vision. Practitioners learning the technique often flex the wrist of their left hand in a pivoting motion, exerting excessive pressure on the patient's upper teeth. This does not help visualize the airway and it may damage the upper teeth. Instead, a firm but steady upward and forward motion should be used without flexing the wrist. Beginners are generally aware of the relative urgency of the situation and therefore rush. In contrast, some individuals are too timid in their approach and do not apply enough force.

The common causes of failed intubation in a patient with normal anatomy are as follows:

Incorrect positioning of the patient's head
Poor oral access
Tongue overlapping the laryngoscope blade
Pivoting laryngoscope against the upper teeth
Rushing
Being overly cautious
Inappropriate equipment

Summary

As with most endeavors, it becomes easier to manage orotracheal intubation when the technique is broken down into its component steps. To intubate a patient, flex the cervical spine, extend the atlantooccipital joint, open the mouth, insert a laryngoscope blade, displace the tongue, elevate the epiglottis, expose the vocal cords (preferably without chipping the patient's upper teeth), and guide the endotracheal tube through the rima glottidis – all within 30 s. Once the tube is inserted, confirm that it is in the proper place; ideally the tip should lie at the midtracheal level. Gurgling sounds in the epigastrium or asymmetry of breath sounds and chest wall excursion are poor prognostic signs that necessitate repositioning of the tube. If there are any doubts about tube placement, they must be dealt with immediately. First, observe the end-tidal CO_2 monitor, then listen for breath sounds over the chest and epigastrium. If you are still not satisfied, immediately perform direct laryngoscopy. If doubt still remains, remove the tube and ventilate the patient by mask, using 100% oxygen. When the tube is placed properly, inflate the cuff with sufficient pressure to seal off the trachea, but not so much that you damage the cuff or cause tracheal ischemia. (The pressure exerted by the cuff on the tracheal mucosa should not exceed capillary pressure and devices are available for measuring that pressure). In addition, you must secure the endotracheal tube with adhesive tape, since tubes and patients have a natural tendency to become separated from each other.

The procedure for nasotracheal intubation via direct visualization is similar, except that you insert the tube into the nostril and then perform laryngoscopy to direct it through the rima glottidis. In blind nasotracheal intubation, which is used in patients who cannot undergo direct laryngoscopy, you must rely on the loudness of the breath sounds to guide the tube into the trachea.

There are numerous pitfalls in learning how to intubate, and most novices stumble into a few of them. It is of little consolation for the beginner to know that failure to intubate is usually the result of faulty technique rather than a faulty patient. (Nevertheless, as discussed in Chap. 9, intubating patients with structural anomalies or certain diseases may prove difficult even for experienced anesthesiologists.)

References

1. Berthoud M, Read DH, Norman J. Preoxygenation: how long? *Anaesthesia.* 1983;38:96–102.
2. Baraka AS, Taha SK, Aouad MT, El-Khatib MF, Kawkabani NI. Preoxygenation: comparison of maximal breathing and tidal volume breathing techniques. *Anesthesiology.* 1999;91:612–616.
3. Nimmagadda U, Chiravuri SD, Salem MR, et al. Preoxygenation with tidal volume and deep breathing techniques: the impact of duration of breathing and fresh gas flow. *Anesth Analg.* 2001;92:1337–1341.
4. Flaherty DO, Adams AP. Endotracheal intubation skills of medical students. *J R Soc Med.* 1992;85:603–604.
5. Konrad C, Schüpfer G, Wietlisbach M, Gerber H. Learning manual skills in anesthesiology: is there a recommended number of cases for anesthetic procedures? *Anesth Analg.* 1998;86:635–639.
6. Safar P. *Cardiopulmonary Cerebral Resuscitation.* 1st ed. Philadelphia: WB Saunders; 1981.
7. Kirstein A. Autoskopie des larynx und der trachea. *Arch Laryngol Rhinol.* 1895;3:156–164.
8. Jackson C. The technique of insertion of intratracheal insufflation tubes. *Surg Gynecol Obstet.* 1913;17:507–509.
9. Magill IW. Endotracheal anesthesia. *Am J Surg.* 1936;34:450–455.
10. Bannister PB, MacBeth RG. Direct laryngoscopy and tracheal intubation. *Lancet.* 1944;1:651–654.
11. Adnet F, Borron SW, Dumas JL, Lapostolle F, Cupa M, Lapandry C. Study of the "sniffing position" by MRI. *Anesthesiology.* 2001;94:83–86.
12. Chou HC. Rethinking the three axis alignment theory for direct laryngoscopy. *Acta Anaesthesiol Scand.* 2001;45:261–264.
13. Rao SL, Kunselman AR, Schuler SG, Des Harnais S. Laryngoscopy and tracheal intubation in the head-elevated position in obese patients: a randomized, controlled equivalence trial. *Anesth Analg.* 2008;107:1912–1917.
14. Solazzi RW, Ward RJ. The spectrum of medical liability cases. *Int Anesth Clin.* 1984;22:43–59.
15. Linko K, Paloheimo M, Tammsto T. Capnography for detection of accidental esophageal intubation. *Acta Anaesthiol Scand.* 1983;27:199–202.
16. Sum Ping ST, Mehta MP, Symreng T. Reliability of capnography in identifying esophageal intubation with carbonated beverage or antacid in the stomach. *Anesth Analg.* 1991;73:333–337.

17. Deluty S, Turndorf H. The failure of capnography to properly assess endotracheal tube location. *Anesthesiology*. 1993;78:783–784.
18. Li J. Capnography alone is imperfect for endotracheal tube placement confirmation. *J Emerg Med*. 2001;20:223–229.
19. Kidd JF, Dyson A, Latto IP. Successful difficult intubation: use of gum elastic bougie. *Anaesthesia*. 1988;43:437–438.
20. Howells TH, Riethmuller RJ. Signs of endotracheal intubation. *Anaesthesia*. 1980;35:984–986.
21. Clyburn P, Rosen M. Accidental oesophageal intubation. *Br J Anaesth*. 1994;73:55–63.
22. Kim J-T, Kim H-J, Ahn W, et al. Head rotation, flexion and extension alter endotracheal tube position in adults and children. *Can J Anesth*. 2009;56:751–756.
23. Crosby ET, Cooper RM, Douglas MJ, et al. The unanticipated difficult airway with recommendations for management. *Can J Anaesth*. 1998;45:757–776.
24. Horton WA, Fahy L, Charters P. Factor analysis in difficult tracheal intubation: laryngoscopy-induced airway obstruction. *Br J Anaesth*. 1990;65:801–805.
25. Achen B, Terblanche OC, Finucane BT. View of the larynx obtained using the Miller blade and paraglossal approach, compared to that with the Macintosh blade. *Anaesth Intensive Care*. 2008;36:1–5.
26. Henderson JJ. Solutions to the problem of difficult tracheal tube passage associated with the paraglossal straight laryngoscopy technique. *Anaesthesia*. 1999;54:601–602.
27. Magill IW. Technique in endotracheal anaesthesia. *Ann Surg*. 1910;52:23–29.
28. Temple AP, Katz J. Management of acute head injury. *AORNJ*. 1987;46:1068.
29. Rowbotham ES, Magill IW. Anesthetics in the plastic surgery of the face and jaws. *Proc R Soc Med*. 1921;14:17.
30. Collins PD, Godkin RA. Awake blind nasal intubation: a dying art. *Anaes Int Care*. 1992;20:225–227.
31. Jantzen JP. Tracheal intubation – blind but not mute. *Anesth Analg*. 1985;64:646–653.
32. Dyson A, Saunders PR, Giesecke AH. Awake blind nasal intubation: use of a simple whistle. *Anaesthesia*. 1990;45:71.
33. Adams AL, Cane RD, Shapiro BA. Tongue extrusion as an aid to blind nasal intubation. *Crit Care Med*. 1982;5:335–336.
34. Knill RL. Difficult laryngoscopy made easy with a BURP. *Can J Anaesth*. 1993;40:279–282.
35. Takahata O, Kubota M, Mamiya K, et al. The efficacy of the "BURP" maneuver during a difficult laryngoscopy. *Anesth Analg*. 1997;84:419–421.
36. Snider DD, Clarke D, Finucane BT. The "BURP" maneuver worsens the glottis view when applied in combination with cricoids pressure. *Can J Anesth*. 2005;52(1):100–104.
37. Benumof JL, Cooper SD. Quantitative improvement in laryngoscopic view by optimal external laryngeal manipulation. *J Clin Anesth*. 1996;8:136–140.
38. Sellick BA. Cricoid pressure to control regurgitation of stomach contents during induction of anesthesia. *Lancet*. 1961;2:404.
39. Smith K, Dobranowski J, Yip G, Dauphin A, Choi P. Cricoid pressure displaces the esophagus: an observational study using MRI. *Anesthesiology*. 2003;99:60–64.
40. Brimacombe JR, Berry A. Cricoid pressure. *Can J Anaesth*. 1997;44:414–425.
41. Vanner RG. Mechanisms of regurgitation and its prevention with cricoid pressure. *Int J Obst Anes*. 1993;2:207–215.
42. Racz GB. Improved vision modification of the Macintosh laryngoscope. *Anaesthesia*. 1984;39:1249–1250.

Suggested Reading

Hagberg CA. *Benumof's Airway Management*. Philadelphia: Mosby/Elsevier; 2007.

Chapter 9
The Difficult Airway

Contents

Introduction

The key tenet in the practice of medicine is that physicians must not perform procedures on patients unless they are capable of dealing with the complications. Every clinician must be prepared to establish a surgical airway if conventional means fail. When airway problems occur and the oxygen supply is removed, every second counts. There is only a limited amount of time before substantial injury occurs while waiting for the arrival of a surgeon to perform a tracheostomy. Clinicians must be prepared to deal with this problem themselves. Residents in training should, therefore, be exposed to the necessary equipment and should practice the techniques needed to establish a surgical airway. Ideally, they should be allowed to perform these procedures on animals during their training. A difficult intubation needs to be managed in an organized fashion as it is a true medical emergency. Most clinicians respond robotically to a cardiac arrest and quickly move through the ABCs of resuscitation without even thinking – a similar attitude must be adopted when dealing with difficult intubations.

In any busy operating room (OR) with patients undergoing routine elective surgery, there are usually one or two difficult intubations each week. However, over a 1-year period, even anesthesiologists who deal with airway management daily will be exposed to this emergency only a few times and a resident in training may encounter it even less frequently. Duncan et al.[1] have estimated that a resident in training needs to be exposed to this emergency about 29 times before competency can be achieved. Few residency training programs are capable of providing this kind of experience. The problem is even greater in obstetrics, in which the need for general anesthesia has decreased dramatically during the past 25 years because the pattern of practice has changed predominantly to regional anesthesia (which is considered safer). Therefore, groups who work solely in obstetric anesthesia get very little exposure to difficult intubations and may not perform well when confronted with one. For this reason, it is crucial that difficult airway drills be incorporated into routine practice guidelines and into residency training curricula.

This chapter provides basic information about the difficult airway. There is a comprehensive look at the American Society of Anesthesiologists' (ASA) practice guidelines, including the Difficult Airway Algorithm. The importance of mask ventilation is emphasized, with guidelines for effective use and predicting difficulties. A structured approach to the difficult airway following different scenarios is outlined and there is some information related to special circumstances that may arise in which there will likely be a higher prevalence of difficulty.

Definitions

When discussing incidences, clinical strategies, and outcomes with respect to airway difficulties, it is important to have consensus on the applicable terminology. What does the *difficult airway* mean? To some, it means spending 10 or 15 min trying to intubate the trachea; to others it means difficult mask ventilation (DMV) or failure to intubate. The American Society of Anesthesiologists (ASA) Task Force on Management of the Difficult Airway[2] defines the difficult airway as "the clinical situation in which a conventionally trained anesthesiologist experiences difficulty with face mask ventilation of the upper airway, difficulty with tracheal intubation, or both." They describe difficult face mask ventilation as the following:

"It is not possible for the anesthesiologist to provide adequate face mask ventilation due to one or more of the following problems: inadequate mask seal, excessive gas leak, or excessive resistance to the ingress or egress of gas. b) Signs of inadequate face mask ventilation include (but are not limited to) absent or inadequate chest movement, absent or inadequate breath sounds, auscultatory signs of severe obstruction, cyanosis, gastric air entry or dilatation, decreasing or inadequate oxygen saturation (SpO_2), absent or inadequate exhaled carbon dioxide, absent or inadequate spirometric measures of exhaled gas flow, and hemodynamic changes associated with hypoxemia or hypercarbia."

According to the previous report by this task force,[3] oxygen saturation should remain above 90% using 100% oxygen and positive pressure mask ventilation in a patient whose saturation was greater than 90% before the anesthetic intervention. Difficult laryngoscopy is currently described by the task force as follows: "It is not possible to visualize any portion of the vocal cords after multiple attempts with conventional laryngoscopy."[2] The description of difficult tracheal intubation is, "...tracheal intubation requires multiple attempts, in the presence or absence of tracheal pathology," and the description of failed intubation is "... placement of the endotracheal tube fails after multiple intubation attempts."[2] What is meant by *conventional laryngoscopy*? Clearly, conventional laryngoscopy could apply to those who predominantly use a Macintosh or a Miller blade. There is some suggestion that the incidence of difficult laryngoscopy is less with the Miller blade.

The task force's original definition of *difficult intubation,* stipulating that the intubation should be complete within three attempts and 10 min,[3] was challenged by at least one group on the basis that it should not be *time* nor *attempt* based because successful intubation can be achieved in less than 10 min or in less than three attempts in some cases, even when presented with a grade 4 laryngoscopic view.[4] Furthermore, the laryngoscopist, when presented with a grade 4 view, may immediately use an airway adjunct and successfully intubate the patient on the first attempt. They offered an alternative definition for difficult tracheal intubation as follows: "...when an experienced laryngoscopist, using direct laryngoscopy, requires (1) more than one attempt with the same blade; (2) a change in blade or an adjunct to a direct laryngoscope (i.e., bougie); or (3) use of an alternative device or technique following failed intubation with direct laryngoscopy." Many studies define difficult intubation as it relates to difficult laryngoscopy (grade III or IV Cormack and Lehane grade[5]), alone[6] or in combination with a multiple attempt criterion.[7] Unfortunately, we will not obtain accurate data on this topic until we all agree on a universal definition.

Mask Ventilation

The importance of mask ventilation has been overshadowed over the years by the inherently more attractive technique of intubation. The average anesthesiologist in full-time clinical practice may intubate as many as 500 patients per year. Mask ventilation is a component of the intubation process and is frequently used before intubation. It is also, in fact, one of the first contingencies called upon when difficulties arise. Thus, your ability to perform mask ventilation must be assessed before attempting endotracheal intubation. This may in fact help predict that difficulties in intubation may ensue, since many of the same predisposing factors apply to both. One study has found a discerning result that 25% of those patients for whom mask ventilation was impossible also had difficult intubations; fortunately the large majority were managed without a surgical airway.[7] Alternatively, intubation has been successful in many patients in whom mask ventilation was difficult or impossible, and has even been recommended as a prudent option in cases of impossible mask ventilation. Noteworthy, the ASA difficult airway algorithm does not include how to manage a patient who is difficult or impossible to mask ventilate before tracheal intubation attempts. Different underlying mechanisms may account for difficulty with mask ventilation, including: errors in technique, equipment malfunction, suboptimal head position, side effects of certain drugs, and pathological partial or complete airway obstruction. A recent review can be referred to for a more comprehensive explanation.[8] Some guidelines for the use of mask ventilation are:

- A high-flow oxygen source (approximately 10 L/min) allows compensation for facemask leaks and the generation of sufficient positive pressure to overcome resistance to gas flow.
- A patent airway will be best attained by way of a jaw thrust and neck extension.
- The size of the mask should be chosen to fit over the nose at the level of the nose bridge and the mouth just above the chin.
- Difficulty with obtaining a seal (e.g., in the obese patient) may be circumvented by lifting the chin pad while applying the jaw thrust.
- Effective techniques to position the tongue (especially if large) in a way to improve ventilation include early insertion of a plastic oral airway and lateral tilt of the head while ventilating.
- In cases of difficulty, either a 2-person technique or a one-person 2-handed technique can be used. In the latter, the provider can use both hands to obtain a seal and use the ventilator to apply the appropriate tidal volume. The operator can use their hands to advance the mandible while using the head straps to improve the mask seal. Additionally, the reservoir can even be compressed between the knees, under the axilla or even under the foot.[9] The use of either the binasopharyngeal airway system[10] or an intraoral device (to advance the mandible)[11] may improve mask ventilation.[12]
- Alternatively, alternative devices such as the laryngeal mask airway (LMA) may be used as a substitute airway, or intubation (using direct or indirect laryngoscopy) may be attempted.

Training and experience are critical to enable provision of sufficient and safe mask ventilation. An increased risk of gastric inflation with regurgitation and pulmonary aspiration may occur with poor performance.[13] Other complications which may ensue include: injury to the eyes, trauma or necrosis to the nose and chin, nasal bleeding (if using nasopharyngeal airway), and airway obstruction or trauma to the oropharyngeal airway (if using oropharyngeal airways).[8] Chapter 4 includes step-by-step instructions in the use of a bag/valve/mask. Effective mask ventilation in many cases requires much more practice than intubation and a number of factors can interfere with your ability to do it efficiently (Table 9.1[14-16]).

The ability to predict difficult or impossible mask ventilation is significant in that it will allow the clinician to prepare for potential complications by securing the presence of a second anesthesia provider or preparing for the provision of an alternative method of ventilation. One group has developed a four-point grading scale that defines factors that will assist in predicting mask ventilation success or difficulty, with grade 3 (inadequate, unstable or requiring two providers) defining difficulty and grade 4 (impossible to ventilate with or without muscle relaxant) defining failure.[17] Independent predictors of DMV (grade 3 MV) from a prospective study of 22,660 attempts at mask ventilation by this group included a body mass index (BMI) $\geq$30 kg/m^2, a beard, age $\geq$57 years, severely limited jaw protrusion and snoring.[14] The only immediately modifiable factor of these is presence of a beard, suggesting that patients – especially those in whom other risk factors exist – should be made aware of this risk factor and should consider shaving before surgery. Predictions for impossible mask ventilation (although without statistical power) were history of snoring and thyromental distance of less than 6 cm, and predictors of grade 3 or 4 DMV together with difficult intubation were severely limited mandibular protrusion, thick/obese neck anatomy, sleep apnea, snoring, and BMI $\geq$30 kg/m^2.[2-14] If a patient has two or more risk factors, there may be a heightened risk of difficulty.[4] More recent work by this group's review of 53,041 attempts at mask ventilation has defined independent predictors of impossible mask ventilation (incidence in this study of 0.15%) to be: neck radiation changes, male sex, sleep apnea, Mallampati III or IV (as modified by Samsoon and Young[18]), and presence of beard.[7] Table 9.2[14, 15, 19-26] includes a mnemonic to aid in the recall of the factors that will help in predicting DMV and other airway management difficulties. The importance of mask ventilation cannot be overemphasized. In fact, it is the determining factor between difficult intubation being an urgent matter and a life or death medical emergency.

Incidence of the Difficult Airway

There have been several reports of the incidences of difficult or failed mask ventilation, difficult laryngoscopy, and difficult intubation. The data from several reports of difficulties in general surgical patients is included in Table 9.3.[7, 14-16, 27-36]

Considering all general anesthesia patients, the incidences of difficult laryngoscopy and intubation are similar, at approximately 1.5–8.5%[4,6], especially

Table 9.1 Difficult mask ventilation (DMV)

Study characteristics	Incidence of DMV	Potential predictive risk factors for DMV from univariate analysis	Independent risk factors for DMV from multivariate analysis (odds ratios)
Langeron et al.[15] 1,502 Patients undergoing surgery with GA	(5%) DMV 1 Case IMV 30% of DMV patients had DI	Body mass index (BMI) Age Macroglossia Beard Lack of teeth History of snoring Increased Mallampati grade Lower thyromental distance	Presence of beard (3.18) BMI $\geq$26 kg/m^2 (2.75) Lack of teeth (2.28) Age $\geq$55 years (2.26) History of snoring (1.84)
Yildiz et al.[16] 576 Patients undergoing elective surgery under GA	75.5% Easy MV 16.7% Awkward MV 7.8% Difficult MV 15.5% of DI patients had DMV Awkward is not considered difficult by other definitions and includes use of oral airway, 1-operator maneuvers, or 1–2 uses of oxygen flush valve	Height Weight Age Male gender Increased Mallampati grade History of snoring Lack of teeth Beard	Mallampati grade 4 (9.69) Male gender (3.54) History of snoring (2.18) Age (1.03) Weight (kg) (1.02)
Kheterpal et al.[14] 22,660 Adult patients undergoing GA Used 4-point scale for ease or difficulty with MV	1.4% Grade 3 MV (inadequate to maintain oxygenation, unstable MV, or MV requiring 2 providers) 0.16% Grade 4 MV (impossible MV noted by absence of carbon dioxide measurement and lack of chest wall movement during PPV attempts) 0.37% Grade 3 or 4 and DI	Mallampati grade 3 or 4 Abnormal cervical spine Thick/obese neck Abnormal neck anatomy Edentulous dentition Thyromental distance <6 cm Mouth opening <3 cm Limited mandibular protrusion test Beard Cough COPD Asthma Snoring Sleep apnea BMI $\geq$25 kg/m^2 Age $\geq$55 years Emergent operation Resident anesthetist	*For grade 3 MV* BMI $\geq$30 Beard Mallampati 3 or 4 Age $\geq$57 year Jaw protrusion – severely limited Snoring *Grade 3 or 4 MV & DI*: Jaw protrusion – limited or severely limited Thick/obese neck anatomy Sleep apnea Snoring BMI $\geq$30 kg/m^2

DMV difficult mask ventilation; *IMV* impossible mask ventilation; *DI* difficult intubation; *GA* general anesthesia

Table 9.2 Mnemonics for predicting difficulties in airway management

MOANS difficult mask ventilation (DMV)

M   Mask seal: Adequate mask seal can be difficult to achieve with the presence of abundant
     facial hair, encrusted blood, or lower facial abnormalities

O   Obesity: This includes obese patients (BMI >26–30 kg/m^2 was the threshold range that
     maximized sensitivity and specificity between Langeron et al.[15] and Kheterpal et al.[14]),
     as well as near-term parturients and patients with upper airway obstruction or abscesses,
     angioedema, or epiglottitis. The difficulty may arise from reduced chest compliance and
     increased intraabdominal pressure, with resistance to diaphragmatic excursion by the
     abdominal contents. There also may be resistance to airflow in the supraglottic airway.
     Obese individuals and parturients also have the tendency to desaturate more quickly,
     which may also cause DMV

A   Age: Patients over 57 years of age[14] are associated with DMV. This may be partly due to loss
     of muscle and tissue tone in the upper airway

N   No teeth: Obtaining a good seal may be difficult in edentulous patients. Dentures may be left
     in during bag mask ventilation, as long they are removed for intubation

S   Snores or stiff: Sleep apnea and history of snoring is an important consideration.
     Significantly increased airway resistance or decreased pulmonary compliance can
     hinder the ability to bag mask ventilate

LEMON difficult laryngoscopy and intubation

L   Look externally: Many of the physical features which have been associated with a difficult
     laryngoscopy and intubation include small or large mandible, short neck, bull neck,
     lower facial disruption, and large breasts are some indications of possible difficulty

E   Evaluate 3-3-2: This rule ensures adequate assessment of the upper airway geometry
     3 – Can patient place three fingers breadths into their mouth (adequacy of oral access)?
     3 – Can patient accommodate three fingers breadths between the tip of the mentum and the
     mandible-neck junction (capacity to accommodate the tongue on laryngoscopy)
     2 – Can patient fit three fingers breadths between the mandible-neck junction and the thyroid
     notch (optimal distance of the larynx to the base of tongue)

M   Mallampati class: Classification of visibility of the posterior oropharyngeal structures.
     Classes III and IV are associated with more failures than Classes I and II; failure rates
     with Class IV may exceed 10%. Best used for information about the access to the oral
     cavity and potential of difficult glottic visualization

O   Obstruction: Look for three cardinal signs: muffled voice, difficulty swallowing secretions,
     and stridor

N   Neck mobility: Cervical flexion and head extension are staring points for obtaining the
     best possible view of the larynx on oral laryngoscopy. Bannister et al. added that the
     ears should be anterior to (or at least level with) the sternum.[20] The main analogy which
     has been used is "sniffing the morning air," although some feel that this analogy is not
     ideal[19,21,23]

RODS difficulty with extraglottic devices (EGD)

R   Restricted mouth opening: This will depend upon the particulars of each EGD

O   Obstruction: The EGD will not bypass an upper airway obstruction at the level of the larynx
     or below

D   Disrupted or distorted airway: To the extent that the "seat and seal" of the EGD be
     compromised[22]

S   Stiff lungs or cervical spine: Large increases in airway resistance or decreases in pulmonary
     compliance may make ventilation with an EGD difficult or impossible. A fixed flexion
     deformity of the neck may limit the seal. LMA insertion may be difficult in patients with
     limited neck movement[24]

(continued)

Table 9.2 (continued)

SHORT difficult cricothyrotomy

S   Surgery/disrupted airway: Previous surgery may have left the neck distorted

H   Hematoma or infection: These should not be considered contraindications to a life-
        threatening situation, but may make the cricothyrotomy incision technically
        difficult

O   Obese/access problem: Obesity may make percutaneous access to the neck difficult.
        Fixed flexion deformities or halo traction may also limit the access to the anterior
        neck

R   Radiation: There may be tissue distortion from the tissue changes caused by past
        radiation

T   Tumor: There may either be access problems or bleeding complications

This table was adapted from Murphy and Walls[25] and Murphy and Doyle[26], with data added from
references.[14, 15, 19–24] Prediction of impossible mask ventilation has shown to be different, with
independent risk factors being: neck radiation changes, male sex, sleep apnea, Mallampati III or
IV, and presence of a beard[7]

Table 9.3 Incidence of difficult airway in the general surgical population

Study (population)	Difficult/failed mask ventilation	Difficult laryngoscopy[a]	Difficult intubation[a]	Failed intubation
Kheterpal et al.[7] (53,041)	2.2% Difficult 0.15% Failed	10.4% of failed mask ventilations	25% of failed mask ventilations	
Kheterpal et al.[14] (22,660)	1.4% Difficult 0.16% Failed			
Yildiz et al.[16] (576)	7.8% Difficult			
Koh et al.[29] (605)		5.1%	6.9%	
Langeron et al.[15] (1,502)	5% Difficult 0.07% Failed		30% of difficult mask ventilations	
Suyama et al.[33] (476)			5.5%	
Arne et al.[27] (1,200)		9.0%	4.2%	0%
Ulrich et al.[35] (1,993)		4.7%		0%
Yamamoto et al.[36] (6,184)		1.3%		
el-Ganzouri et al.[28] (10,057)	0.08% Difficult	6.1		
Rose and Cohen[32] (3,325)		10.1%	1.9%	
Rose and Cohen[30] (6,477)		1.5%	1.7%	0.3%
Tse et al.[34] (471)		13%		0%
Rose and Cohen[31] (18,558)	0.9% Failed		1.8%	0.3%

[a] If the results indicated the incidence of Cormack and Lehane Grades 3 and 4, this was recorded
here as difficult laryngoscopy irrespective of whether the individual study defined this as difficult
laryngoscopy or intubation. If additional or alternative criteria were used for difficult intubation,
an additional incidence was recorded in this column

considering that many studies use a Cormack and Lehane grade of 3^5 as a primary criterion for defining difficult intubation. One metaanalysis reported 6–27% difficult laryngoscopy and 6–13% difficult intubation, although the authors note a high prevalence in those studies which included patients with airway pathologies and diabetes.[37] Failed intubation occurs in approximately 0.13–0.3% of attempts. An accepted incidence of DMV is 1.4%.[8,14] As well, impossible mask ventilation (incidence 0.15%) is associated with difficult intubation.[7] Some studies have isolated those cases where there was difficulty in intubation from direct laryngoscopy as compared to those cases where alternate (e.g., indirect) intubation approaches have been undertaken from the outset.[31] Similar to difficult or failed mask ventilation, there have been evaluations of the predisposing and predictive factors associated with intubation difficulties; one such example is that of Rose and Cohen from their review of 18,558 intubations (Table 9.4).[31]

Table 9.4 Significant differences[a] between rates of easy and difficult intubation in terms of demographics/patient factors and results from preoperative airway examination

	Easy intubation $n = 17,129$	Difficult intubation (>2 laryngoscopies) $n = 326$
Demographic/patient factors (%)		
Male sex	41.6	56.4
Age 40–59 year	30.2	44.5
Age <40 year	41.8	23.6
ASA 3/4	22.8	31.1
Overweight (female >120 kg, male >120 kg)	2.4	5.5
Preoperative airway exam results (total number[b], number/rate of easy and difficult)		
Normal (8,953)	8,523/95.2	113/1.3
Incomplete data (3,153)	2,967/94.1	53/1.7
Missing data (4,596)	4,326/94.1	48/1.0
Limited mouth opening only (93)	58/62.4	9/9.7
Restricted neck movement only (556)	418/75.1	18/3.2
Thyromental distance <3 fingers only (265)	194/73.2	28/10.6
Decreased visibility of hypopharynx (406)	332/81.8	21/5.2
2 Abnormalities (409)	254/62.1	28/6.8
≥3 Abnormalities (127)	57/44.9[c]	8/6.3

Table compiled from data in Rose and Cohen[31]

[a] Results are significantly different to <0.01 in all cases between easy and difficult cases

[b] Total number includes those cases where intubation with direct laryngoscopy was graded as "awkward" or where intubation was performed with an alternative means (i.e., not considered easy or difficult intubation). In total, there were 18,558 patients, with 448 having awkward intubation and 353 having an alternative intubation approach

[c] An alternative means of intubation was performed in many (37%) patients in whom there were three or more abnormalities

Reports of difficult laryngoscopy and difficult intubation may vary depending upon the population studied. Difficult laryngoscopy has been shown to occur more frequently in patients with cervical disease.[38] There is conflicting data with respect to whether the incidence is higher for obstetrics (see the related section of this chapter) or for the pediatric patient. A study of pediatric ENT surgical patients reported a higher incidence of difficult intubation (26%) than with other populations studied, but the small sample size (100 patients) should be taken into account.[39] Despite this, it is generally thought the incidence of difficult intubation is less in children than in adults.[40] Rose and Cohen[31] have also shown that the incidence of difficult intubation is greater in males than females and in the 40–59 age group.

Etiology of Difficult Intubation

The causes of difficult intubation are discussed in some detail in Chap. 7. Instead of presenting a long list of diseases and syndromes that may cause problems, the difficult intubation is divided arbitrarily here into three broad categories: limited access to the oropharynx or nasopharynx; poor visualization of the larynx; and diminished cross-sectional area of the larynx or trachea.

Limited Access to the Oropharynx or Nasopharynx

Conventional methods of endotracheal intubation require the insertion of a laryngoscope blade into the oropharynx as a primary step. Any disease or condition that limits access to the oropharynx or nasopharynx may impair your ability to perform endotracheal intubation.

Inability to See the Larynx

Having gained access to the oropharynx, you must next move the soft tissues forward to allow the laryngeal opening to come into view. Failure to do so will make intubation difficult.

Diminished Cross-Sectional Area of the Larynx or Trachea

Finally, in some cases, although there may be no problems opening the mouth or seeing the larynx, for some reason you are unable to advance the endotracheal tube far enough into the trachea. Narrowing of the larynx and trachea may necessitate the insertion of a much smaller tube.

Practice Guidelines and the ASA Difficult Airway Algorithm

Routine endotracheal intubation for anesthesia has been in vogue for close to 50 years and the need for practice guidelines has been raised numerous times. Tunstall et al.[41] were among the first to suggest an algorithm for the difficult airway in obstetric anesthesia. Benumof[42] advanced this issue further in 1991 and this, together with a report of the high number of perioperative respiratory adverse events during airway management,[43] created so much interest in the topic that the ASA commissioned a task force in 1992 to establish practice guidelines for managing the difficult airway.

Their guidelines, including an algorithm, were published in 1993,[3] modified further in 1996[44], and the ASA published an updated report with changes to the algorithm in 2003.[2] These guidelines are required reading by any serious student of airway problems, and although they do not give comprehensive details about each possible airway problem, they are extremely useful.

The updated ASA guidelines stress on continual application of oxygen during management, an early attempt at insertion of the LMA if face mask ventilation is not adequate, and an early "call for help" (Fig. 9.1).

Guidelines for management of the difficult airway have been published by other national societies, including those from Canada (Canadian Airway Focus Group),[4] the United Kingdom (Difficult Airway Society [DAS]),[45] France,[46] Italy[47], and Germany[48] (Table 9.5). The guidelines from the DAS are concerned with the unanticipated difficult airway only and include a series of flow-charts rather than one comprehensive algorithm like that of the ASA. The society emphasizes that their series of simple and definitive charts narrow the choices offered at each stage, thus perhaps making the charts more useful for airway emergencies. Their simplicity may also make the flow-charts more suitable for training and practice.[49]

The Canadian guidelines on the difficult airway do not differ remarkably from those published by the ASA, although they focus on the unanticipated difficult airway and include considerations on the obstetric and pediatric airway. Although there are numerous practice guidelines which can be practiced, the guidelines for anticipated difficult airways usually focus on awake techniques (e.g., flexible fiberoptic intubation), while those for the unanticipated difficult intubation recommend various attempts, often using different blades, and alternative supraglottic techniques.

The most critical elements of all the guidelines should be adhered to, including an early call for help and maintenance of oxygenation throughout the entire procedure. Regardless of choice of algorithm in practice, having immediate availability of the equipment (see the following section on the "Difficult Airway Kit") is of utmost importance. Attempts to awaken the patient at various steps should always be considered and, of course, an individualized approach will be important.[49]

Most guidelines (including those from the ASA and Canadian Airway Focus Group) place an emphasis on the importance of careful preoperative evaluation of the airway in order to reduce the number of unanticipated difficult intubations. Unfortunately, compliance among anesthesiologists is poor despite these warnings. Rose and Cohen[31]

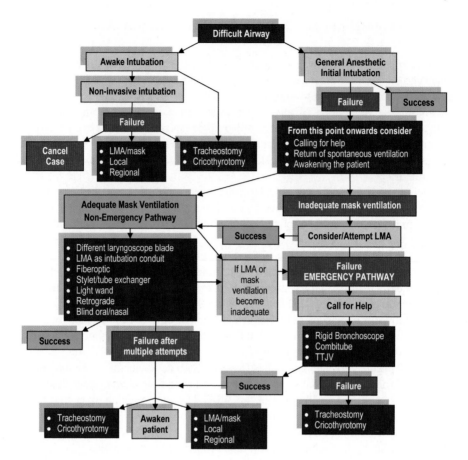

Fig. 9.1 Algorithm for the difficult airway

noted inadequate preoperative evaluation of the airway in 50% of cases in their large series of 18,500 cases. Furthermore, even when difficult airways are identified, there seems to be a great reluctance to perform awake intubations.

Duncan et al.[1] have estimated that residents in training need to be exposed to 29 separate difficult airway scenarios in order to become proficient. Few training programs can offer that kind of experience to trainees on a random basis and reducing the amount of time residents spend in the OR, limits the chances of exposure to challenging airway cases.[50] Koppel et al.[51] noted that only 27% of 143 programs in the United States offered formal training in the difficult airway and, when training was offered, it mostly consisted of didactic lectures.

A survey by Hagberg et al.[52] noted 19% of responding American anesthesiology residency training programs (79 out of 132 surveyed) had a case number requirement regarding the use of airway devices. It seems ironic that we have neglected to tackle this problem more vigorously in view of the number of airway-related anesthetic deaths that have occurred. While current data is limited, a 1986–2000 closed claim analysis of the ASA reported 503 respiratory-related damaging

Table 9.5 Comparison of recommendations for difficult airway management from various National Societies

National Society algorithm

Clinical Scenario	USA[2] (ASA)	Canada[4] (CAFG)	UK[45] (DAS)	Italy[47] (SIAARTI)	France[46]	Germany[48] (DGAI)
Anticipated difficult airway	Awake intubation Decision between noninvasive & invasive airway access	No recommendations	No recommendation	Awake intubation in severe cases Use fiberoptic or retrograde intubation	Awake technique	Maintain spontaneous breathing, awake technique (e.g., fiberoptic intubation, LMA)
Unanticipated difficult tracheal intubation	Consider calling for help, returning to spontaneous ventilation, and awakening patient. Ventilate using face mask; if not possible use LMA, fiberoptic intubation, stylet etc	Awaken patient or consider adjuncts to laryngoscopy or alternatives to laryngoscopy (light stylet, scope)	Make no more than four attempts then consider LMA or ILMA, reverting to face mask or awaken patient	After two attempts, optimize laryngoscopy, use two more attempts, then LMA or Combitube, or awaken patient	Use no more than two attempts, then use LMA, fiberoptic scope or different blades for up to two more attempts, awaken patient	Choose: alternative intubation techniques (e.g., ILMA, fiberoptic intubation), use LMA, return to spontaneous ventilation, awaken patient
Difficult mask ventilation	Consider/attempt LMA	Use laryngoscopy & intubation, LMA or Combitube, or awaken patient	Maintain oxygenation with face mask then use LMA	Maintain oxygenation with face mask then use LMA or Combitube	Use LMA	Maintain oxygenation using a face mask
Cannot intubate, cannot ventilate	Call for helpTry noninvasive airway ventilation (rigid bronchoscope, Combitube, transtracheal jet ventilation). If not successful, use invasive airway access (tracheostomy or cricothyroidotomy)	Transtracheal airway	Transtracheal catheter or surgical cricothyroidotomy	Tracheal puncture or surgical cricothyroidotomy	Cricothyroidotomy or tracheostomy	Try LMA or Combitube, then transtracheal jet ventilation, then surgical cricothyroidotomy, then tracheostomy

events associated with death and permanent brain damage.[53] Of these claims, 64% were attributed to "less-than-appropriate anesthesia care," with difficult intubation, inadequate ventilation/oxygenation, esophageal intubation, and premature extubation making up the majority.

These results are likely equally poor if not worse in other countries. Therefore, there must be a continual campaign within each institution to avoid taking unnecessary chances when dealing with the airway, and promotion of formal airway training programs is paramount.[43] A structured approach for training in airway management is favorable and the ability to follow and use a difficult airway algorithm (i.e., develop good decision-making skills) should be started from the onset.[50]

Difficult Airway Kit

Each operating or emergency suite should have a dedicated difficult airway kit. Operating and emergency suites all over the world have their own airway management culture and traditions; therefore, it would be impossible to come up with a generic kit that satisfies all groups. Ideally, the kit should include specific tools with which the clinician is familiar and experienced, rather than contain merely an abundance of tools.[4] The following items are considered essential and then individual preferences can be added (additional information regarding airway equipments is discussed in Chaps. 4 and 11):

Basic Essentials of an Airway Kit

- A variety of straight and curved laryngoscope blades
- A gum elastic catheter or bougie and an airway exchange catheter
- A fiberoptic bronchoscope
- An illuminating stylet or Bullard laryngoscope
- An LMA or Combitube
- A transtracheal airway kit

A jet ventilation apparatus and cricothyrotomy Seldinger kit would be prudent additions.

Structured Approach to the Difficult Airway in the Operative Room

The importance of preoperative evaluation in detecting the difficult airway has already been discussed. Even though there is no absolutely reliable way to detect all difficult airway cases, the vast majority can be detected by making a few simple observations. It is then possible to safely secure the airway in most of these cases by performing awake or asleep intubation under controlled circumstances.

Failed Awake Intubation for Elective Surgery

Occasionally, it is impossible to perform awake intubation due to a lack of preparation, an uncooperative patient, equipment failure, or anatomic limitations. In elective situations the options are postponement and further evaluation. It is very important to place a time limit on efforts to secure the airway in all circumstances, not just for humane reasons but also for safety reasons. As a general rule, efforts should be abandoned after a maximum of 30 min or at any time that adequate oxygenation or ventilation of the patient is unachievable. Efforts to secure the airway should also be aborted if the patient is endangered in any way from the intervention.

Inducing general anesthesia should be considered if patient cooperation is an issue. Before doing so, however, it is necessary to attain reasonable assurance that mask ventilation will be easy. Difficult airways are invariably managed under general anesthesia in children. The LMA is a useful crutch in some situations, leaving the clinician's hands free to solve the problem while allowing the patient to breathe an inhalation agent spontaneously. There are several options open at this time, and individuals usually select the airway adjunct that they are most familiar with. Following are some of these options:

- Direct laryngoscopy using a straight or curved blade
- Bougie with direct laryngoscopy
- The Bullard laryngoscope
- Illuminating stylets
- Fiberoptic-assisted intubation
- Intubating laryngeal mask
- Retrograde catheter techniques

Regional anesthesia may also be an option in the event of failed awake intubation; however, these techniques should never be used to sidestep a difficult airway. If there is even a remote possibility that airway intervention may be required, the airway should be secured first. It would be unwise to embark on major abdominal, thoracic, or vascular surgery under regional anesthesia if there was a problem with the airway. Regional anesthesia can be safely performed in patients with difficult airways as long as the procedure can be easily terminated or completed with local anesthesia supplementation in the event of intraoperative failure of regional anesthesia. There will always be the need for a preformulated strategy for intubation of the difficult airway. A surgical airway may be the first option in some cases with anticipated difficult intubation. An example of this would be a patient presenting with a laryngeal tumor scheduled for a radical neck dissection.

Unanticipated Difficult Airway in Elective Surgery

This is one of the most common airway emergencies encountered in the OR (Fig. 9.2).

The usual scenario is as follows: On induction of general anesthesia and the administration of a muscle relaxant, the vocal apparatus is not visible. The priority at this point is maintenance of adequate oxygenation. Assuming that ventilation and oxygenation are possible, the next priority is to maintain anesthesia and relaxation. At this point the difficult airway cart should be requested, as well as an assistant if one is not already present. The clinician should try to figure out why the vocal apparatus is not visible. Is the appropriate size and type of laryngoscope blade being used? As the clinician tries to determine what the problem is, it is important

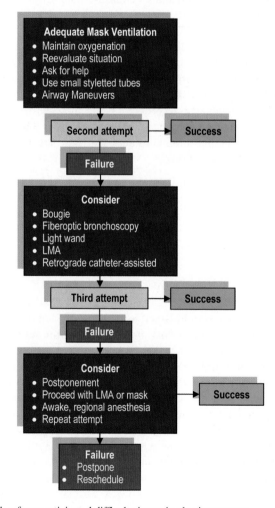

Fig. 9.2 Algorithm for unanticipated difficult airway in elective surgery

to do something different with every new attempt. There is a tendency to keep doing the same thing over and over. Before making a second attempt, the clinician should do the following:

1. Check suction
2. Try a smaller styletted tube
3. Check the head position
4. Ask the assistant to be ready to apply pressure on the larynx
5. Repeat laryngoscopy
6. Attempt to place a bougie or ventilating stylet

With each failed attempt, the risk of trauma increases and the presence of blood in the mouth interferes with the recognition of structures. Furthermore, laryngeal edema with repeated attempts can lead to DMV. Most difficult intubations are successful on the second attempt because initial failures are often due to inadequate preparation or head position.

Some airway experts suggest the use of airway adjuncts after the first failure. It is difficult to argue against that approach, but from a practical point of view, it usually takes some time before the difficult airway cart becomes available and by then most impatient clinicians would have made a second attempt. It would be reasonable to attempt to pass a bougie at this stage. Should failure occur on the second attempt, help should be sought. Once again, it is important to go back to the basics ensuring that oxygenation and ventilation of the patient are still possible, and to prepare to proceed with the next step. At this stage, abandonment of conventional laryngoscopy should be considered in favor of one of the following devices:

- Illuminating stylet
- Bullard laryngoscope
- Intubating laryngeal mask
- Fiberoptic-assisted intubation
- Retrograde catheter device

Most of these techniques have all been discussed in other chapters. The majority of anesthesia departments will stock some if not all of the equipment needed. Each department tends to have its own culture, and there are also international differences. Bougie techniques, for example, are traditionally more popular in the UK as a first-line approach. Fiberoptic techniques are more popular in North America. Consideration should be given to using some of these techniques as a *first-line* of approach when confronted with a difficult airway.

If the airway cannot be secured after three or four good attempts by an experienced person in a purely elective situation, it is advisable to postpone the case. Few would argue with this philosophy. The longer the clinician persists, the greater the likelihood of morbidity. Spontaneous ventilation and consciousness should be allowed to return, and the patient should be informed of the circumstances. Some clinicians will have difficulty accepting failure, but the ego should never be allowed to stand in the way of good medical practice. What is best for the patient should always be the foremost consideration.

Unanticipated Difficult Intubation in Emergency Surgery

An unanticipated difficult intubation will occasionally be encountered in a patient scheduled for emergency surgery. The same rules apply (Fig. 9.3). But, in addition, this patient presents the risk of aspiration of gastric contents. The option to postpone no longer exists.

A more aggressive approach must be taken from the outset. Regurgitation must be prevented while the patient is unconscious by applying continuous cricoid pressure. An awake fiberoptically-assisted intubation must be considered. Either flexible or rigid intubation fiberscopes can be used, although the rigid fiberscope may require less expertise. The rigid Bonfils intubation fiberscope in conjunction with indirect laryngoscopy may be very useful in these cases. If the option for regional anesthesia exists, it should be given every consideration. In life-threatening emergencies (e.g., difficult intubation in the face of massive hemorrhage), a surgical approach may be required from the outset.

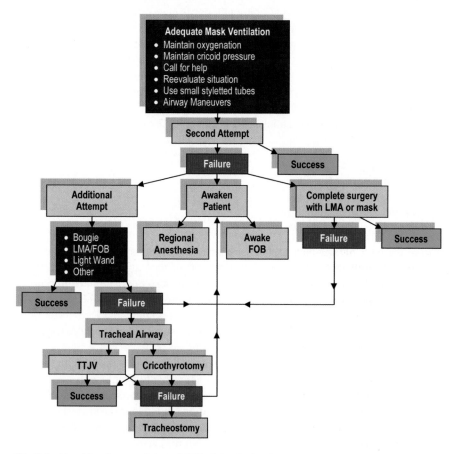

Fig. 9.3 Algorithm for unanticipated difficult intubation in emergency surgery

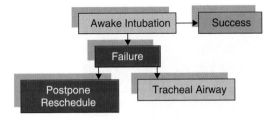

Fig. 9.4 Algorithm for anticipated difficult airway in elective or emergency surgery

Anticipated Difficulty in Elective or Emergency Surgery

Awake techniques are usually recommended if difficult intubation is anticipated in an elective or emergency situation, the exception being in pediatric practice where general anesthesia is often induced while the ability to breathe spontaneously is not interfered with (Fig. 9.4). If the clinician is in doubt as to their ability to intubate a patient, neuromuscular blocking drugs should be avoided. However, if for some reason they must be used, only short-acting agents (10–20 mg succinylcholine IV/70 kg) should be selected and the dose should be kept small so that adequate ventilation can recur within a minute.

Loss of the Airway: "Cannot Intubate, Cannot Ventilate"

Fortunately, "cannot intubate, cannot ventilate" (CICV) situations are rare. A survey of 971 Canadian anesthesiologists showed that only 57% had personally experienced the CICV scenario.[54] Ironically, this places anesthesiologists at a bit of a disadvantage in that few have had much experience treating this serious problem. Clinicians must be prepared to aggressively manage CICV. This means sufficient training using manikins, airway simulators, and animal models is paramount. Familiarity with the patient's history and the equipment, techniques, and drugs administered prior to the CICV scenario may help to diagnose the problem and formulate a course of action.

If two-handed mask ventilation fails, four-handed ventilation should be attempted (two hands holding the mask, two compressing the bag). The difficult airway kit should be immediately available. Insertion of an LMA, Combitube or another extraglottic device should be considered. In emergency situations, clinicians are frequently guilty of continuing to retry the same nonsurgical attempts at tracheal intubation. If these methods fail, cannula or scalpel cricothyrotomy, followed by transtracheal jet ventilation (TTJV) or low pressure ventilation (respectively) must be performed immediately (Fig. 9.5) (these techniques are described in detail in Chap. 12). However, there is little data on the safety and efficacy of these techniques in emergency airway management. Complications rates have been reported at approximately 40% when performed under emergency conditions.[55] Besides

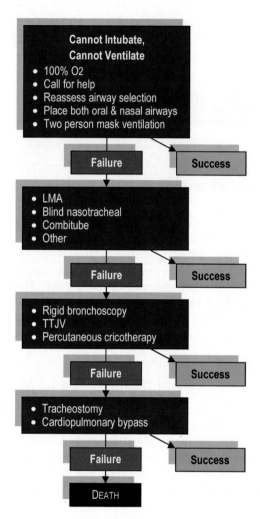

Fig. 9.5 Cannot intubate, cannot ventilate algorithm

acute complications including failure, long-term complications include subglottic stenosis, infections, and dysphonia.[56] In the past, the authors conducted a survey on the use of TTJV in emergency situations within their institution. Receiving data on 16 patients, the success rate was 25%, with 75% failure and a death rate of 25% (unpublished data). Subcutaneous air was a serious and frequent complication.

Although many clinicians have relied heavily on their surgical colleagues to establish a surgical airway in the past, most practitioners are now of the opinion that time does not permit this luxury. Heard et al.[57] suggest that the anesthesiologist's familiarity with using a cannula at the end of a syringe – as opposed to the surgeon's skill with a scalpel blade – may help direct the choice of device and technique applied in a CICV situation (i.e., cannula cricothyrotomy vs. scalpel cricothyrotomy).

Difficult Airway in Special Circumstances

Emergency Room

The same basic rules apply to managing difficult airways regardless of geography. Emergency room (ER) intubations are usually more challenging because invariably there is a greater sense of urgency. ER physicians occasionally require assistance from other airway experts, such as anesthesiologists, to deal with challenging airway problems. However, it is important to point out that the anesthesiologist is usually not familiar with the personnel, equipment, or surroundings outside the OR. Patients usually have injuries that need urgent attention and may be uncooperative because of hypoxemia, mind-altering substances, or head injuries. There is rarely sufficient time to do a thorough evaluation of the airway, and quite often uncertainty exists about treatment because of a lack of information.

An algorithm for emergency airway management should be followed.[58] Oxygenation is of critical importance and any intubation attempts should be halted after 40 s to ventilate the patient. There are no contraindications for tracheal intubation in an emergency. An awake intubation should be chosen for patients with an anticipated difficult airway provided the patient is cooperative, stable and spontaneously breathing. General anesthesia may be considered if the patient is uncooperative/combative, although spontaneous ventilation should be maintained if possible.[59]

Surgical airway control may be in the best interest of the trauma patient in certain situations, due to their risk of hemorrhagic shock, aspiration, and head trauma.[60] The situation is often dynamic and can change within minutes. In the next few pages, examples of challenging airway problems in the ER will be discussed. In addition to the airway management requirements of the emergent scenarios described here, complicating factors such as obesity, pregnancy, or obstructive sleep apnea (OSA) may need to be considered. See the following section on "Operating Room" for more on these situations.

Difficult Airway Prediction: Mnemonics to Use in Emergency Situations

In addition to the ASA definitions of difficult airway situations, a more comprehensive view of the difficult airway includes consideration of five dimensions:[25,26]

1. Difficult bag mask ventilation
2. Difficult laryngoscopy
3. Difficult intubation
4. Difficult placement of an extraglottic device
5. Difficult cricothyrotomy

In an emergency situation, expeditious evaluation of these dimensions can be supported by use of mnemonics which have been developed for predicting the difficulty with the associated technical operations.[25] Table 9.2 summarizes the mnemonics available for prediction of: difficult bag-mask ventilation (BMV; MOANS), difficult laryngoscopy and intubation (LEMON), difficult placement of an extraglottic device (EGD; RODS), and difficult cricothyrotomy (SHORT).

The results from Kheterpal et al.[14] should also be kept in mind for anticipation of difficulty with both ventilation and intubation; the independent risk factors for difficulty/failure with ventilation (grade 3 or 4 as per their grading scale) and intubation were limited mandibular protrusion, thick/obese neck anatomy, sleep apnea, snoring, and a BMI ≥ 30 kg/m^2. Conversely, when this same group evaluated patient characteristics associated with impossible mask ventilation, the independent predictors were neck radiation changes, male sex, sleep apnea, Mallampati III or IV, and presence of a beard.[7]

Head and Neck Injury

Incidence and Etiology

Cervical spine injuries occur in 1.5–3% of all major trauma victims and in up to 3% of all head injuries in adults.[61-65] Therefore, this matter should be considered when general anesthesia is being administered to these patients. A patient presenting with head and neck injuries may require the expertise of the anesthesiologist. The second most common cause of death associated with head and neck trauma is obstructive airway injury.[60] Although aerodigestive tract injury (including the larynx and trachea) only occurs after approximately 5% of blunt and penetrating neck injuries,[66] many of these patients will require airway management. Injuries in the neck after trauma include: disruption of tracheal continuity, obstruction of the airway from larynx/cricoid fractures, compression or obstruction of the airway from hematoma formation caused by major arterial or venous bleeding, and cervical spine injury (CSI) causing perforation of the esophagus or apnea or neurogenic shock.[60]

Management

Securing the airway is the highest priority for patients who have sustained penetrating and blunt neck trauma. The more commonly seen injuries, including stab wounds and low-velocity gun shots, do not usually require prehospital or ER intubation.[60] In a life-threatening situation, emergency intubation is usually required because of inadequate oxygenation/ventilation. A surgical airway may need to be performed in cases where the oxygen saturation is poor or airway obstruction is imminent. More frequently, however, intubation is required to reduce the risk of aspiration of gastric contents in a patient who is semicomatose. Early or even prophylactic tracheal intubation may be performed if the patient is to be transferred to less safe environments, such as that for diagnostic imaging, partly because signs of airway compromise may be nonexistent or subtle right up to the point of total obstruction.[67]

Occasionally, hyperventilation will be required to reduce intracranial pressure. Sometimes, general anesthesia is necessary because the patient is so uncooperative that appropriate diagnostic work cannot be performed. General anesthesia is preferable in a patient with serious head injury (unless difficult intubation is anticipated) because the intracranial pressure increases dramatically during attempts at awake intubation. Thiopental and lidocaine are frequently used as induction drugs, and both decrease intracranial pressure.

Time-permitting and with stable hemodynamics, evaluating the airway visually using a flexible naso or oropharyngoscope, will determine if the airway is aligned and will help decide if a rapid-sequence technique is suitable for intubation. This route is contraindicated in patients suspected to have laryngotracheal discontinuity. If attempted, there should be: (1) fiberoptic confirmation of the proper tube position, and (2) thorough planning for alternative techniques, for example intubation using a rigid fiberoptic laryngoscope or videolaryngoscope, or performing a surgical airway. Blind intubation attempts may be performed but are generally ill advised.[68] In addition, extraglottic devices may not be dependable in cases where the obstructing lesion cannot be circumvented.

Cervical Spine Injury

Incidence and Etiology

Approximately, 6,000 people die from CSI and 5,000 new quadriplegics are reported in the United States each year.[69] Most victims are males ranging in age from 15 to 35 years. CSI is most frequently associated with accidents involving motor vehicles, diving, contact sports, riding horses, falls, and blunt head and neck trauma.The incidence of CSI due to blunt head trauma is 1.8%,[70] and the incidence of CSI is higher among those with low Glasgow Coma Scores (e.g., initial scores below 8).[71] Most patients with CSI have stable injuries.[72] Injuries occur primarily at one of three levels of the cervical spine: C2, C6, or C7.[73] If you encounter an accident anywhere, how do you decide who needs cervical spine precautions? Alert victims, devoid of neck pain and tenderness, numbness, or weakness in the arms or legs, should not require cervical spine evaluation or special precautions. Any victim who reports even the slightest symptom of neck discomfort or anyone who is not fully alert should have cervical spine precautions. Motor vehicle accidents with speeds in excess of 35 mph and accidents with a headfirst fall are considered higher risk than injuries from contact sports or nonheadfirst falls.[74]

Management

The trauma victim's neck should be immobilized as soon as possible after injury and remain so until neck injury has been excluded or definitive management for CSI has been initiated.[75] Despite this, prolonged immobilization especially in patients of low risk for CSI, is costly and may itself pose a risk to the patient.[76] The most reliable method of immobilizing the neck is to secure the victim on a hard board. If possible, a rigid collar is placed around the neck with sandbags at each side. These measures will reduce movement significantly, though not completely. All airway maneuvers, including cricoid pressure, widen the disc space to some degree. When performing intubation using direct laryngoscopy, the view obtained may be improved when using manual in-line immobilization rather than collars because of improved mouth opening.[77]

If there is a need for rapid airway establishment and oxygenation in the CSI patient, the Combitube may be very useful. Flexion of the neck is not required, so that this device can be safely inserted in these patients. Patients with unstable C_1C_2 fractures seem most vulnerable to neurological damage from intubation. Despite the potential for serious neurological deficit during airway manipulation, the actual incidence is extremely rare. Few reports have appeared dealing with serious injury after intubation and they are rarely published.[78]

The patient is at greatest risk of neurological injury when CSI is not recognized. Reid et al.[79] found that new neurological deficits were 7.5 times more common if an injury went unrecognized. It is important to remember that up to 8% of C-spine fractures are not recognized radiologically, even when three views are taken. Radiological clearance may give a false sense of security. In one study involving 128 patients with suspected CSI, both the senior radiologist and emergency medicine physician missed the diagnosis of CSI in 25% of cases.[80] It has been suggested that the anesthesiologist should be able to read the ABCs of cervical spine films as well. This interpretation requires knowledge of the alignment of the vertebrae (Fig. 9.6), the condition of the bones and cartilage, and the width of the soft tissue and intervertebral spaces. Therefore, when obtaining a history, even if there is only the remotest hint of neck injury, handle the patient with extreme care if airway manipulation is required. In managing CSI patients, clinicians must carefully address both cervical spine clearance and airway management techniques.

Cervical Spine Clearance

While radiological study is often performed for trauma patients suspected of having CSI, the use of radiological assessment in asymptomatic patients (approximately one-third of trauma patients) has been raised. According to the National Emergency X-Radiography Utilization Study (NEXUS) low risk criteria, patients who are asymptomatic include those who meet all of the following: are neurologically normal, not intoxicated, do not have neck pain or midline tenderness, and do not have an associated injury that is distracting to the patient.[81, 82]

While these criteria are adopted in recent neurosurgical guidelines,[81] a more sensitive and specific assessment protocol is the C-Spine Rule developed and studied by the Canadian CT Head and Cervical Spine Study Group, which incorporates 20 standardized clinical findings.[83, 84] In those patients who are symptomatic, radiological clearance should be obtained before allowing airway manipulation to take place. Each center should ideally have their own protocol for deciding which patients require radiological clearance for clearing of the cervical spine (thus

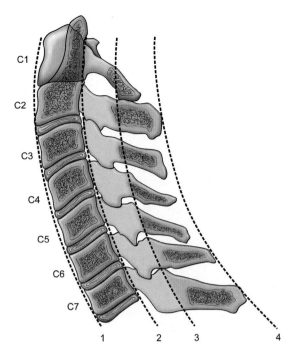

Fig. 9.6 Diagram of the lateral view of the cervical spine demonstrating normal alignment. Lines drawn through the anterior (*1*) and posterior (*2*) margins of the vertebral border, the junction between the lamina and spinous processes (*3*), and the tips of the spinous processes (*4*) should be smooth curves. Lines (*2*) and (*3*) are the approximate boundaries of the spinal canal

removing the necessity of spine immobilization). Patients who present with significant facial trauma, brain injury and/or with multiple injuries will be hard to clear through clinical findings. A three-view clinical series (anteroposterior, lateral, and open-mouth odontoid peg) of which all seven vertebrae are visible (Fig. 9.7) is usually recommended[81] for patients who are symptomatic after traumatic injury, although these views may only identify about 90% of cervical spine injuries.[84]

It is moderately prevalent for centers to use a five-view series in response to specific scenarios.[85] The "swimmer's view" (axillary view) may be necessary to view the cervicothoracic junction. The craniocervical junction will be better visualized by high-resolution computed tomography (CT) than radiography. It is also recommended that areas that are suspicious, or not well-visualized, should be supplemented with a CT scan.[86] In addition, helical CT of the entire cervical spine will be sensitive and specific enough to allow clearance of the cervical spine in patients who are unresponsive.[87]

Widening of the cervical soft tissue space may be the only evidence of an injury at C_1C_2 and should alert the anesthesiologist to the possibility of difficult intubation caused by airway encroachment (Fig. 9.8).[88, 89] Full clearance of the cervical spine should ideally include exclusion of isolated ligamentous injury, which may not be diagnosed with plain films or CT scan. Several imaging techniques

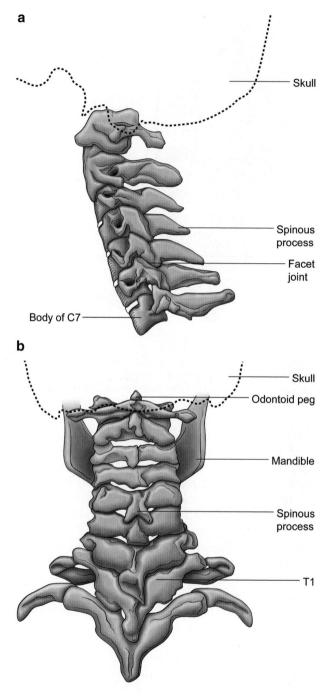

Fig. 9.7 Cervical spine line drawings. (**a**) Lateral, (**b**) anterior–posterior, (**c**) through-the-mouth Showing C1, C2

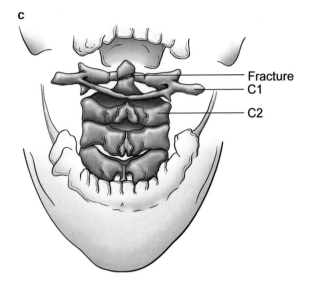

Fig. 9.7 Continued

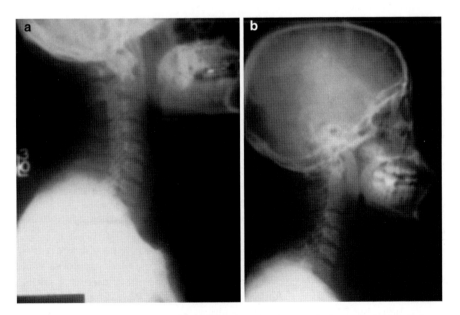

Fig. 9.8 Cervical spine soft tissue films. (**a**) Normal with cervical prevertebral soft tissue. (**b**) Abnormal swelling of cervical prevertebral soft tissue

(i.e., MRI and dynamic fluoroscopy) have been used for diagnosing ligamentous injury, although these are not routinely performed. In each patient, clearance will depend on a risk–benefit decision, considering the likelihood of spinal injury and the morbidity and mortality associated with prolonged immobility.

Airway Management

Airway management in the presence of CSI is often a challenging prospect. In emergency situations, the clinician may be forced to intervene without information about the cervical spine. It has been demonstrated over and over again that intubation even in the presence of CSI is safe – provided proper precautions are taken, which include in-line stabilization (without traction forces)[76] and appropriate caution during laryngoscopy.

The debates continue about the optimal way to handle a patient with CSI (e.g., awake vs. general anesthesia, nasotracheal vs. orotracheal intubation). There is no published evidence regarding the superiority of any one intubation option, yet there are recommendations and standards of care that are followed to a large extent.[76] Intuitively, it would appear that awake fiberoptically assisted oral or nasal intubation is the ideal method because head or neck movement is limited. Furthermore, in patients who are not overly sedated, neurological assessment can be performed after intubation using awake techniques.[90]

In emergency situations, direct laryngoscopy may be heavily relied upon. There may be less cervical manipulation with the use of the McCoy laryngoscope blade and bougie.[91] The use of standard or intubating LMAs may produce posterior displacement of the upper cervical spine, although the clinical relevance of this has not been determined.[92,93]

Surgical cricothyrotomy is an option if nasal or oral routes cannot be used or are unsuccessful.[76] The relative safety of various airway intervention techniques cannot be studied easily. Since the incidence of neurologic deterioration after any intervention is so rare, an overwhelming number of subjects would need to be studied.[76]

The most important consideration is that the anesthesiologist secures the airway using the most familiar techniques. Having limited skills with the bronchoscope will preclude safe and successful awake fiberoptic intubation regardless of prevailing opinions of its merit. There is no room for dogma in dealing with these cases. Direct laryngoscopy is perfectly safe provided reasonable precautions are taken, including appropriate spine immobilization. Awake intubation may be dangerous in an uncooperative patient or one who is semicomatose. There is a suggestion that neck muscles act as a splint in the awake state and this is lost when general anesthesia is used with muscle relaxants.

A difficult intubation in the presence of CSI is probably the ultimate airway challenge faced by anesthesiologists. Cricothyrotomy is an obvious option, while tracheostomy generally is considered inappropriate in the emergency setting. Retrograde catheter-assisted techniques may also help. TTJV is valuable in desperate situations, but it does not protect the airway against aspiration. The laryngeal mask may also be a useful temporizing measure in some cases. Training with the insertion of the LMA will be essential to avoid cervical movement.

In summary, CSIs present some unique challenges. No one technique of airway management appears to be any better than another. In view of the multiple disciplines involved, it would make sense to establish clinical guidelines for optimal management of these cases.

Airway Burns

Incidence and Etiology

The 2009 Annual Report from the American National Burn Repository stated that the presence of inhalation injury, among other predictive factors, increased the chance of death from thermal burn by 15 times. Furthermore, pneumonia and respiratory failure resulting from airway burns were more frequent in patients who had undergone mechanical ventilation for more than 4 days.[94]

One study reported physical examination findings in patients with inhalation injury and found that 65% had burns to the face, 48% had carbonaceous sputum, 44% had soot in the mouth and nose, and 31% wheezed; but fewer coughed (9%), or evinced stridor (5%) or dyspnea (3%).[95] Thus, the clinician cannot depend on the classic signs of airway obstruction (stridor, voice change, dyspnea) to indicate airway injury. Patients presenting with airway burns may have carbon monoxide poisoning, which can be difficult to diagnose clinically because the usual clinical signs (pallor, clamminess) are masked by carbonaceous material staining the skin. Carboxyhemoglobin (CO) levels should be determined and treatment is required if quantities around 15% are detected. Levels near 50% are usually fatal. Oxygen therapy (100%) via an endotracheal tube or nonrebreathing bag rapidly reduces the half-life of CO from about 4 h in room air to 40 min.

A patient with burns around the head and neck is at risk of developing upper airway obstruction. Thermal injury causes obstruction by way of progressive swelling and may also be complicated by skin sloughing. Coughing episodes and hoarseness in the presence of singed facial and nasal hair are often symptomatic of airway burns, but these are not the only signs to look for, as previously noted. Even if there are no external signs, one should be suspicious of airway swelling and inhalation injury. Early airway intervention is fundamental. Bag mask ventilation (BMV) with positive pressure manual ventilation may be able to overcome the upper airway obstruction if started early. An airway that appears normal on first evaluation may well progress to become obstructed by edema via increased microvascular permeability of the tissues and the fluid requirements of burn patients.[96]

Management

The most reliable way to assess the airway is to perform fiberoptic bronchoscopy following topical anesthesia and sedation. Alternatively, an evaluation of the likelihood of vocal cord visibility may be undertaken in the awake patient using a laryngoscope. In either method of assessment, the level of sedation provided will need to be high, since cooperation may be minimal in the patient with excruciating pain and respiratory distress. Ketamine may be ideal, with its analgesic properties. Likely there may be anatomical changes (e.g., from edema) affecting airway patency, resistance and compliance, as well as bronchospasm – both complicating the ability to deliver effective BMV or use of an extraglottic device. Intubation is likely to proceed and anticipation of difficulty will be evident. The anatomy of the airway becomes grossly distorted following fluid resuscitation, making intubation extremely difficult at times. Facial burns, particularly if there are scars from chronic burns, may limit skin elasticity and therefore restrict mouth opening, jaw movement, and access to the nasal passages, as well as limit flexion and extension of the neck. These consequences may make endotracheal intubation very difficult. Eschar formation may limit chest expansion and compromise ventilation.

The route of intubation will partly depend on whether there is the ability to have the patient remain awake.

- If flexible fiberoptic bronchoscopy was undertaken for airway evaluation, one may consider passing the endotracheal tube over the scope.
- Rapid sequence induction may be undertaken if difficulty is not anticipated during laryngoscopy and intubation, if an awake technique was not achieved, or if it is warranted by the urgency of the situation.

It is imperative to have rescue devices (e.g., Trachlight, Combitube, rigid fiberoptic or Bullard laryngoscope) and a surgical airway kit immediately available. With the imminent progression of airway obstruction and in the face failed intubation and ventilation, one may need to perform cricothyrotomy or tracheostomy. Open cricothyrotomy will be preferable to a percutaneous technique if there are significant burns on the anterior neck.

Ventilation Considerations in the Patient with Airway Burns

Failure with ventilation in the burn patient may be related to various factors: heat-induced upper airway obstruction, inhalation injury, and the restrictive defects associated with chest eschars. Inhalation injury leads to various effects as mentioned above (e.g., edema, capillary leak, bronchospasm, small airway occlusion due to mucosal debris and impaired ciliary clearance). Any of these outcomes can cause air trapping, decreased lung and chest wall compliance, and intrapulmonary shunting. Considerations for ventilating airway burn patients are listed below:

- Adequate expiratory times should be permitted due to air trapping
- Inhaled β_2-agonists may help alleviate bronchospasm
- Endobronchial debris, alveolar fluid, and infection will necessitate aggressive pulmonary toilet
- Alveolar collapse may be overcome (thus improving gas exchange) with positive end-expiratory pressure (PEEP) – patients with acute lung injury will require a PEEP of at least 15 cm H_2O[97]
- Excessive inflation pressures should be avoided so as not to exacerbate lung injury
- Permissive hypercapnia (ventilation using low inspiratory volume and pressure [e.g., initial tidal volume of 6 mL/kg and a plateau pressure of 30 cm H_2O or less]) may improve outcomes by attenuating mechanical stress and its associated inflammatory effects.[98] Hypercapnia may worsen intracranial pressure, therefore should be avoided in trauma patients when brain injury is suspected or confirmed

- Constricting eschars leading to fixed flexion in the anterior neck may require release through vertical incision

Airway burns are among the most challenging airway problems in medicine. If there is no trauma requiring immediate attention, the priorities with these patients are early airway control, fluid resuscitation, and pain control. Attention to underlying medical conditions will need to be considered at all times.

Facial Trauma

Incidence and Etiology

In a facial trauma victim, the airway reflexes may be impaired by associated head injuries or inebriation, and aspiration of vomitus, blood, teeth, or bony fragments is a real possibility. Although significant injury to the upper airway is uncommon (0.3–2.8%), edema and swelling in the vicinity of the airway may lead to airway obstruction even in the presence of intact airway reflexes.[60] Close and repeated evaluation for airway-threatening swelling should be performed since significant swelling can occur despite an absence of fractures, and swelling can take several hours to develop.[87] After craniofacial trauma, injuries to the spine, particularly cervical spine, should be assumed until excluded. The need and urgency for securing the airway with anesthesia and intubation should be decided upon quickly. An anesthesiologist or other clinician trained in advanced emergency airway management should make these decisions on a case-by-case basis, keeping in mind that, on one hand, clinical assessment for other injuries or systems effects (e.g., neurological deterioration) will be hindered by anesthesia and/or intubation; while, on the other hand, delaying securement of the airway may delay life-saving intervention or may complicate the intubation itself.

Management

High-flow oxygen and pulse oximetry monitoring should be performed in all trauma patients.[87] If the patient is immobilized in the supine position, the mouth, nose, and pharynx should be cleared through high-volume suctioning and care should be taken not to induce vomiting. With suspected CSI, excessive manipulation of the spine (e.g., atlanto-axial extension and cervical flexion) should be avoided; a jaw thrust and chin lift may be performed with counter support of the head. Blood loss may be reduced by certain maneuvers, such as reduction of displaced fractures. Consider an oropharyngeal (not nasopharyngeal) airway if the patient is deeply unconscious and obstructing. "Clearing" of the spine should be undertaken as soon as possible, either through radiological or clinical evaluation (depending on symptoms). The reader is referred to the section on "Cervical Spine Injury" for a discussion on cervical spine clearing.

Securing and Maintaining the Airway

A patent airway without ventilation may be managed through two-person manual ventilation with a mask, or placement of a supraglottic airway device. In order to maintain a secure airway, though, a definitive airway will need to be placed. Intubation and ventilation are recommended in the following circumstances[87,99]:

- Bilateral mandibular fractures – this recommendation may result in unnecessary anesthetics[87]
- Copious bleeding into the mouth
- Loss of protective laryngeal reflexes
- A GCS 8 or less
- Seizures
- Deteriorating blood gases
- If gross swelling is anticipated
- In "significant" facial injuries where a long interhospital transfer is required

The preferred method for tracheal intubation in a trauma patient is usually rapid sequence intubation with cervical in-line immobilization.[60] Blind nasotracheal and fiberoptically-assisted oro-or nasotracheal intubation are controversial, but not contraindicated in the presence of severe maxillofacial or skull injuries, provided proper technique is used.[100] Nasotracheal intubation may be difficult in a patient with Lefort II or III fractures of the maxilla because bony fragments may encroach on the nasal airway. Tears in the dura mater along with leakage of cerebrospinal fluid occur in 25% of all Le Fort II and III fractures as well as basilar skull fractures.[101] Leakage of cerebrospinal fluid is a contraindication to nasotracheal intubation because of the risk of meningitis. Awake fiberoptic intubation may be helpful in the spine injured patient, but is burdened by poor visualization in the presence of bleeding and edema. Trauma to the mandible, especially in the region of the condyle, limits a person's ability to open the mouth because of disruption of temporomandibular joint function. Mouth opening may also be limited by trismus associated with mandibular fractures. Access to the oropharynx may be impeded by a knife impaled in the vicinity of the airway. Endotracheal intubation may also be difficult in these cases because the anatomy is distorted or concealed by blood and secretions.

It is advisable to discuss the preferred route of intubation, if and when it is required, with the surgeon. In maxillary and mandibular fractures, the surgeon frequently wires the mandible and maxillae together; thus oral intubation would be contraindicated. When intubation or ventilation is not possible, the LMA may be a very useful adjunct. Cricothyrotomy is associated with a 90% success rate and its early performance may improve outcomes as compared to repeated intubation attempts.[56] Surgical cricothyrotomy is recommended over needle cricothyrotomy because a larger airway can be introduced thus allowing positive pressure ventilation and reliable expiration.[87] Although tracheostomy is generally considered inappropriate in the emergency setting, occasionally the degree of destruction and swelling is so great that the surgeon will elect to perform a tracheostomy.

Cardiac Arrest

Cardiac arrest is the most common indication for emergency intubation outside the OR.[58] Oxygenation and ventilation are priorities and are achieved best by endotracheal intubation. Bag mask ventilation cannot be reliably carried out during chest compressions (synchronization with the ventilation is required) and regurgitation of gastric contents is very common during cardiac arrest. The decreased pulmonary compliance and lower esophageal sphincter pressure during cardiac arrest can lead to larger volumes of air being directed towards the stomach rather than lungs during CPR.

Intensive Care Unit (ICU)

Incidence and Etiology

All invasive airway maneuvers can be considered difficult in the ICU.[102] In contrast to the OR setting, there is a challenge to secure a safe airway as well as secure and manage the airway over a prolonged period. There are numerous factors which contribute to difficulty of ventilation or intubation in this setting.[103,104]

- Patients in the ICU often have limited physiologic reserve and usually require respiratory and/or hemodynamic support.
- The physician's expertise in airway management in the ICU may be variable; outcomes improve as the skill set of the operator increase.[105]
- Cardiac arrest is more common (2%) in the ICU than in the OR (0.068%).[106]
- Positioning can be difficult on an ICU bed; furthermore, the environment is often overcrowded with equipment and specialized apparatus such that additional room is limited for airway management equipment.
- Previous airway instrumentation or the presence of an endotracheal tube can lead to an edematous airway.
- Immobilization or the need for avoiding neck mobility in the potentially unstable cervical spine is paramount.
- The effectiveness of preoxygenation may be reduced in ICU patients with poor gas exchange. Furthermore, the critically ill adult can experience pronounced oxygen desaturation due to intolerance to a brief interruption in oxygen delivery.[107]
- Patients with cardiovascular instability may have hypotension, hypoperfusion, and erroneous oximetry readings.
- Induction doses which are recommended for the ambulatory population are excessive and dangerous in most ICU patients.
- There is a rate (4–12%)[108] of reintubation in the ICU setting and previous difficulty may make these attempts more difficult.
- Only a portion of ICUs maintain difficult airway kits or routinely use devices to confirm tracheal intubation and detect esophageal intubation.[103]

In addition to these considerations, obesity and OSA may further exacerbate the difficult airway scenario. These situations are addressed in the "Operating Room" section.

Management

There is a need to select appropriate drugs and dosages, particularly when there is coexistent hepatic or renal dysfunction. The practitioner should use the lowest amount of drug possible while allowing intubation in a comfortable patient. Suitable choices for induction may be ketamine and etomidate, which have more favorable cardiovascular profiles for patients as compared to propofol, which causes significant hypotension.[109] It should be noted that during awake airway examination, ketamine may precipitate laryngospasm. If an opioid is used for intubation, to attenuate the hemodynamic responses to laryngoscopy, fentanyl and sufentanil are choices which may be used even in the presence of liver disease. Pharmacologic adjuncts, including sedative hypnotics and muscle relaxants, may compromise the ability to oxygenate and ventilate these patients and therefore should only be used by those skilled with a variety of rescue airway techniques.

Methods to preoxygenate patients in order to build their oxygen reserve and tolerance to apnea have been investigated, although effective techniques have yet to be elucidated. Extending the oxygenation period from 4 to 8 min failed to improve arterial oxygen levels in a clinically significant manner.[110] Other methods, including adding PEEP, may also be helpful but need to be studied.[111] When planning for airway management in the critically ill patient, it is incumbent on the practitioner to carefully consider five separate issues, and incorporate their evaluation into a plan which follows the ASA difficult airway algorithm (the algorithm alone will be of limited use in the ICU setting). The issues include:

- Is airway management necessary?
- Will direct laryngoscopy and tracheal intubation be straightforward?
- Can supralaryngeal ventilation be used?
- Is there an aspiration risk?
- In the event of airway failure, will the patient tolerate an apneic period?

Rosenblatt[107] argues that the difficult airway algorithm can be used for any patient undergoing general anesthesia with tracheal intubation. Ideally, there will be recognition of difficulty before it occurs so that the difficult airway algorithm can be entered at the stage of anticipated difficult airway.

Without anticipated or encountered difficulty, rapid sequence intubation will be the safest and most successful technique. Dosing of drugs and the patient's functional residual capacity need to be considered in addition to the fact that alternative rescue techniques may also be difficult in certain patients. Extraglottic devices (e.g., LMA, Combitube) may be lifesaving so long as they are available and familiar to the practitioner. Topical anesthesia, anxiolysis, and sedation (the latter from judicious use of benzodiazepines and opioids) can facilitate awake intubation if difficulty with laryngoscopy and/or intubation is anticipated.

Difficult airway management may also be considered when planning extubation, since reintubation may also be difficult. An endotracheal tube exchange catheter may be particularly helpful for these patients. A trial of extubation over the tube exchanger is incorporated as a core aspect of one extubation algorithm.[112]

Operating Room

Obesity

Incidence and Etiology

The high prevalence of obesity (BMI >30 kg/m^2) today in many countries (36–41% in the US and 23% in Canada according to the World Health Organization[113]) will lead to management changes in many areas of anesthesia, including airway management and pharmacokinetics considerations. While some investigations report that BMI alone may not account for or predict a difficult airway,[114,115] others have found a BMI of $\geq$30 kg/m^2 (as well as a thick/obese neck) to be an independent predictor of DMV or difficulty with ventilation and intubation.[14] In addition, there are commonly associated factors beyond body mass in these individuals which may lead to difficulty.

Obese patients, particularly the morbidly obese (BMI >35 kg/m^2), have several anatomic and physiologic factors which may predispose the difficult management of their airways, including difficulty with BMV,[15] laryngoscopy and intubation, use of extraglottic devices, and cricothyrotomy (see Table 9.2 – mnemonics).

Anatomical Factors

- Large breasts
- Short neck
- Large tongue
- Redundant pharyngeal tissue with smaller pharyngeal area
- Superior and anterior larynx
- Limited mouth opening and cervical spine mobility

Physiological Factors

- Increased intraabdominal and intrathoracic pressures
- Reduced tolerance to apnea (via reduced respiratory reserve and increased metabolic demand) which correlates to the degree of obesity. There is a 50% reduction in observed functional residual capacity in the obese anesthetized patient, as compared to a 20% reduction in the nonobese patient[116]
- Restrictive lung defect with decreased lung compliance (associated with an increased pulmonary blood volume), total respiratory compliance, vital capacity, functional residual capacity, expiratory reserve volume, and inspiratory capacity[117]

- Higher work of breathing due to increase in chest wall resistance, increased airway resistance, and higher minute ventilation from increased metabolic demands

Management

Preparation, Medicating, and Securing the Airway

Morbidly obese patients should receive prophylaxis against aspiration, usually in the form of an H_2 blocker and a prokinetic.[118] Access to the mouth and performance of direct laryngoscopy will be difficult in these patients when they lie supine with their head resting on a regular pillow.[119] Furthermore, the patient's already reduced functional residual capacity falls further in the supine position. Prior to induction of anesthesia, positioning the patient in a "ramped" position (with sheets or towels placed under the shoulders, head and neck) to obtain an adequate "sniffing position" may improve the laryngoscopic view,[120] reduce the apnea time required for intubation and increase the oxygen reserve.[119]

Physiologic changes brought on by obesity can affect the distribution, binding, and elimination of anesthetic drugs.[118] The percentage increase of fat tissue surpasses that of lean tissue (20–40% of the excess weight is lean) in obesity, mainly affecting the apparent volume of distribution and tissue diffusion of anesthetic drugs according to their lipid solubility. The pharmacokinetic profile of anesthetic drugs can also be affected by other obesity-related changes, such as the absolute increase in total blood volume and cardiac output and the alterations in plasma protein binding.[121] Changes in drug elimination may occur in the obese patient. Hepatic clearance is usually normal, whereas renal clearance (and creatinine clearance) increases as long as there is no chronic renal disease.

Although there are no documented/regulated recommendations for scaling drug dosing to weight, there has been some research supporting scaling to either ideal/lean or not scaling (using total body weight) depending upon the drugs pharmacokinetics in the obese vs. nonobese patient. Calculations may be made based on total body weight, ideal body weight (IBW) or adjusted/lean body weight (ABW). An ABW calculation accounts for the additional lean body mass in the obese and will be more appropriate than IBW at times:

$$IBW = 50kg + 2.3kg \ (\# \, inches \, over \, 60) \ (Men)$$
$$= 45.5kg + 2.3kg \ (\# \, inches \, over \, 60) \ (Women).$$

An estimation of IBW is: IBW = height (cm) − x (x is 100 in males and 105 in females)[118]

$$ABW = IBW + 0.25 \ (TBW − IBW).$$

Below are some specific considerations according to particular drugs:

- For *thiopental*, the volume of distribution is larger, clearance similar and elimination half-life longer in obesity vs. normal weight patients[122] – a dose proportional to lean body mass has been suggested.[123]

- For *propofol*, both the volume of distribution and clearance are correlated to total body weight, thus the elimination half-life is similar to patients of normal weight[124] – an induction or maintenance dose using total/actual body weight is appropriate but there might be a need for consideration of the cardiovascular effect of very large doses.[117]

- Highly lipophilic *benzodiazepines* have an increased volume of distribution and elimination half-life, with a similar total clearance in obesity – a single dose of any benzodiazepine should be increased in proportion to the total body weight, while a continuous infusion dose should reflect the ideal or lean weight.

- *Desflurane* and *sevoflurane* have much less lipid solubility than older inhalation anesthetics, and they are beneficial for this population due to their more rapid and consistent recovery profile.

- *Atracurium, vecuronium,* and *rocuronium* pharmacokinetics are similar in the obese and nonobese patient. Duration of action may be longer if the dosing is made based on total body weight, thus calculations should be made based on IBW.

- *Succinylcholine*, often used for muscle relaxation in obese patients, should be used based on total body weight since the level of pseudocholinesterase activity (determining the duration of action of succinylcholine) increases in relation to body weight.

- Synthetic opioids (e.g., *sufentanil, fentanyl, remifentanil*) are highly lipophilic drugs. In obese patients, sufentanil has an increased volume of distribution and elimination half-life, with a similar plasma clearance when used in nonobese patients. Loading doses of sufentanil and fentanyl should account for total body weight, whereas infusion/maintenance doses should be reduced to account for the slower elimination in the face of increased risk of postoperative hypoxemia.

- Doses of renally excreted drugs must be adjusted according to the measured creatinine clearance if there is renal dysfunction.

Generally, doses for bolus drug regimes will depend largely on the volume of distribution of the drug (larger volume requires larger dose), while doses for continuous infusions will depend more on the clearance of the drug (larger clearance allows larger dose). Furthermore, hyposensitivity or hypersensitivity to the anesthetic effect may require further changes to the drug dosing regime. Further study is warranted for defining clear recommendations on when drug scaling is required and whether the scaling should be based on ideal or adjusted weight.

Predicting difficult intubation in obese patients may be challenging, since some standard clinical tests for predicting difficulty (e.g., Mallampati scoring) have not proven useful among obese patients.[115,125] A greater difficulty with intubation may largely result from the predisposition to desaturation (largely due to reduced functional residual capacity) and anatomical alterations within the upper airway, rather than bony anatomical factors. One group has developed a standardized test which may be more clinically relevant for determining intubation difficulty, yet the standardized methods to predict difficulty have not been developed.[126] Despite some increase in intubation difficulty, some report 100% success with tracheal intubation by direct laryngoscopy.[115] One issue which may be a factor is the large variation in anatomical and physiological changes between obese and morbidly obese individuals.

Bag mask ventilation will be difficult in morbidly obese patients, usually requiring a 2-person technique with both oral and nasopharyngeal airways in place.[127] Ventilation prior to induction and intubation may be augmented by applying continuous positive airway pressure (CPAP; 5–15 cm H_2O pressure) or PEEP. Intubation will be complicated by a reduction in the pharyngeal area. One should consider using awake laryngoscopy or a fiberoptic approach with topical anesthesia and systemic sedation. Alternatively, rapid sequence induction using succinylcholine after preoxygenation should be attempted. During rapid sequence induction, the reduced pharyngeal area may lead to the need for oral and nasal airways to overcome the collapse of the soft-walled pharynx upon relaxation of the upper airway muscles. A short-handled laryngoscope may be helpful if there is excessive chest tissue. If only the epiglottis is visualized during direct laryngoscopy, a gum elastic bougie may help enable the tracheal intubation. The LMA can be an effective rescue device in obese patients and may be used successfully as a conduit for flexible fiberoptic bronchoscopy. An intubating LMA and lighted stylet may both be useful. Cricothyrotomy will be very challenging due to anatomic changes brought on by increased adipose tissue, and will often require assistance to identify landmarks and deeper and longer incisions.[127] During postintubation ventilation, the initial tidal volume should be calculated according to the patient's IBW, to avoid excessive airway pressures. Using PEEP may help prevent end-expiratory airway closure, but at the expense of cardiac output and oxygen delivery.[128]

Where possible, clinicians should employ regional anesthesia techniques in place of general anesthesia for the morbidly obese in order to reduce the risks from difficult intubation and to provide safe and effective postoperative analgesia. Alternatively, regional techniques can be used in combination with general anesthesia, for example during thoracotomy, to improve outcomes related to intra and postoperative opioid administration, timing of extubation, and postoperative analgesia. Neuraxial techniques may be challenging to perform due to difficulty in identifying bony landmarks. Another consideration during neuraxial technique is the potential for a reduced epidural space in obesity. This is due to fatty infiltration and increased blood volume, which may reduce the predictability of the local anesthetic spread and block height. Ultrasound imaging may be beneficial for determining a successful puncture location during these blocks in order to visualize and mark the midline and appropriate intervertebral space prior to performing the block in a blind manner. Performing a thorough evaluation of the block prior to surgery will be paramount.

Obstructive Sleep Apnea

Incidence and Etiology

Patients with OSA have soft, pliable, and narrow pharyngeal airways with a predisposition to collapse (via relaxation of the pharyngeal dilator muscles) during sleep; this is characterized by turbulent airflow and snoring.[129] The apnea continues until the sleep is disrupted, via increased inspiratory effort in response to hypoxia and hypercapnia, and the individual regains pharyngeal muscle tone.[130] Airway patency may be very difficult to maintain during sleep in patients who have received sedatives or who have enlarged pharyngeal soft tissue. Those who suffer OSA may also have hypertension, polycythemia, hypoxemia/hypercapnia, and right ventricular hypertrophy. Diagnosis requires polysomnography in a sleep laboratory. The mechanism of obstruction may be different in obese vs. nonobese individuals; pharyngeal airway tissue enlargement is relatively specific to the obese population, whereas bony abnormalities are a large part of the etiology in those of normal weight.

The prevalence of moderately severe OSA in the general population is 11.4% in men and 4.7% in women, although higher prevalence has been seen in the surgical population.[131] Main predisposing factors include: male gender, middle age, and obesity (e.g., 42–55% of men with a BMI >40 kg/m^2 had moderately severe OSA, being >15 episodes of apnea or hypopnea per hour of sleep), although the majority of patients with OSA may not be obese.[132] Most (80–90%) patients with OSA in North America have not been clinically diagnosed,[133] making preoperative screening for OSA critical. It is clear that not only obese patients should be questioned about OSA. Patients at a greater risk for OSA are those: who smoke, who have diabetes, older women with congestive heart failure, who are in the acute phase of their first-ever stroke, with hypothyroidism or alcoholism, and those with head and neck cancer.[131] A patient who has had corrective airway surgery should be assumed to be at risk for OSA complications.[134]

Signs

OSA is characterized largely by:

- Frequent episodes of apnea or hypopnea (lasting more than 10 s) during sleep
- Snoring
- Daytime hypersomnolence, impaired concentration, memory problems, and potentially morning headaches
- Physiologic changes including episodic hypoxemia and hypercapnia, and pulmonary and systemic vasoconstriction

Management

The ASA has published practice guidelines regarding perioperative management of patients with OSA,[134] but due to the limited strength of evidence most of the recommendations came from consultants' opinions. There is a lack of strong evidence-based perioperative management strategies for patients with OSA. A recent systemic review was performed, partly to determine the anesthetic implications for surgical patients with OSA.[131] The following discussion is therefore largely open to revision based on future research.

Preoperative Evaluation

- Preprocedure identification of a patients' OSA status (including presumptive diagnosis) improves perioperative outcomes.
- Evaluation should ideally be performed long enough prior to surgery to enable decisions related to whether preoperative management or sleep studies are necessary to further evaluate the patient.
- Considerations should be made for the severity of the OSA, the invasiveness of the procedure, and the requirement for postoperative analgesics.

Preoperative Management

- While various preoperative strategies may be undertaken to help improve outcomes, there is little support for their impact.
- The efficacy of perioperative CPAP use has not been established; nevertheless, the ASA guidelines suggest that preoperative initiation of CPAP should be considered, especially for patients with severe OSA.

Intraoperative Management

- There is little evidence-based support for basing decisions regarding intraoperative anesthetic technique, airway management, and patient monitoring.
- Regional anesthesia techniques should be considered for surgical anesthesia, especially for peripheral surgical approaches. Perioperative placement of peripheral or neuraxial nerve blocks, in order to provide postoperative analgesia, will help reduce risks of respiratory compromise from administration of opioids and other drugs with central respiratory effects.
- General anesthesia with a secured airway may be preferable to moderate or deep sedation during superficial procedures as well as those involving the upper airway.
- Intra and postoperative respiratory compromise should be considered when choosing sedatives, opioids, and inhaled anesthetics. There are no evidence-based strategies that can minimize the impact of the anesthesia or sedation on OSA. Dexamedetomidine's lack of respiratory depression and ability to spare opioid use may make this drug useful for sedation and anesthesia in OSA patients. Propofol anesthesia has been shown to be better than isoflurane for postoperative oxygen saturation and recovery time of spontaneous breathing in sleep apnea patients undergoing uvulopalatopharyngoplasty.[135]

- Patients may have upper airway obstruction, thus continuously monitoring ventilation during moderate sedation is recommended.

Postoperative Management

- Extubation should be performed using a semiupright position, only when the patient is fully awake, without neuromuscular blockade. An oro- or nasopharyngeal airway should be in situ if possible and personnel should be ready to perform two-person mask ventilation.[136] The tracheal tube should be removed over an airway exchange catheter or fiberscope if there is doubt about the ability of the patient to breathe adequately or of the practitioner to reintubate.[137]
- The supine position is generally avoided during recovery, although not all patients show positional dependence. A recent study by Saigusa et al.[138] showed that patients with positional OSA have wider airways in the lateral parts, lower facial height, and a more backward position of the lower jaw.
- Oxygen saturation should be monitored continuously in the ICU or step down unit.
- Opioid sparing, or avoidance, should be considered for postoperative analgesia, either through regional anesthesia using local anesthetics, through administration of nonsteroidal antiinflammatory agents, or avoiding background infusions of opioids during patient-controlled systemic opioid use. Multimodal approaches seem most appropriate, using various analgesics from different classes and different sites of administration.[131,139]
- There are reports of the need for rescue airway management in the postoperative period. Both drug-induced and deep-sleep induced life-threatening apnea can occur in the first week after surgery, due to, initially, the need for large analgesic doses and, later, the return of deep REM sleep.[136]

Specifics of Tracheal Intubation

Many airway management strategies used for OSA patients will be similar to those for obese patients, particularly since many OSA patients will also be obese and present with pharyngeal airway tissue enlargement. Snoring and obesity are both risk factors for DMV (Table 9.1). OSA is a risk factor for difficult intubation,[131] although the method often used to determine difficulty with intubation (e.g., Cormack and Lehane classification) may be more reflective of difficult laryngoscopy.[140] The excess pharyngeal tissue which is typically present in obese OSA patients may not be evident on routine examination. The expectation of DMV and intubation warrants an awake approach to intubation.

Prior to performing an awake technique, nerve block anesthesia of the upper airway may be useful in addition to topical anesthesia. A technique that permits visualization of the structures in an atraumatic manner is one which places a flexible fiberscope through a rigid oropharyngeal conduit. If general anesthesia is used, preoxygenation is important in the obese OSA patient to help reduce the risk of desaturation. Laryngoscopy should be performed with the patient in the optimal position and while applying external laryngeal manipulation if the view of the larynx is poor.[141] Options must be immediately available for the case of "cannot ventilate, cannot intubate."

Obstetrical Airway

Incidence and Etiology

Anesthesia in the past has been a major primary or associated factor in maternal death, and thus is the premise for the Reports of the Confidential Enquiries into Maternal Deaths in England and Wales which have found airway emergencies a common feature.[142] On one occasion anesthetic deaths were ranked as the third most frequent cause of mortality. It has been estimated that 10–13 obstetrical deaths occurred annually in the UK up until 1981 as a result of complications of anesthesia, and airway problems feature prominently in most of these disasters. Fortunately, the incidence of maternal death related to anesthesia has declined significantly, with only 1–2 deaths per annum between 1985 and 1996 and 6 deaths in total between 2000 and 2002. However, the majority are still airway related. Hawkins and colleagues[143] compiled the US experience of anesthesia-related maternal mortality from 1979 to 1990. The results were somewhat similar to those in the UK. Anesthesia complications were the sixth most common cause of maternal death in the United States. Most of the deaths were linked with cesarean section (82%). From 1979 to 1981 there were 4.3 anesthesia-related maternal deaths per million live births, and from 1988 to 1990 there were 1.7 anesthesia-related maternal deaths per million live births. The decline in maternal mortality rates in the US was credited to the increased use of regional anesthesia (with its reduced risk of mortality) for operative obstetrics. Unfortunately, the number of deaths related to general anesthesia remained the same. A report covering the years 1991–1996 found a further reduction of the relative risk for mortality with general as compared to regional anesthesia, partly attributed to the use of pulse oximetry and capnometry and to more structured guidelines.[144] Several authors have reported maternal mortality data from localized regions within the US; these have generally found similar results; although anesthetic-related deaths are rare, airway problems account for a large proportion of the etiology.

Whether the incidence of failed intubation is higher in obstetrics than in the general surgical population is controversial and accurate information is unknown due to lack of prospective comparative studies. Some literature suggests that the incidence of failed obstetrical intubation may be approximately ten times that in surgical patients.[18,145] Reviewing the obstetric airway literature and comparing the results to those reported by the Canadian Airway Focus Group,[4] Goldszmidt[146] summarizes that the incidence of difficult intubation ranges from approximately 1–6% in obstetrical patients and 1.5–8.5% in the general population, and failed intubation occurs in 0.1–0.6% of obstetrical patients compared to 0.13–0.3% in the general population. Nevertheless, most clinicians agree that difficult intubation in an obstetrical patient carries with it far greater risk of morbidity and mortality in both mother and fetus because of their diminished oxygen reserves (leading to early desaturation) and the other physiological changes associated with pregnancy.

Besides the usual anatomical airway abnormalities which may be seen in non-pregnant women, obstetrical patients have some added risk factors. Elevated estrogen levels stimulate the development of mucosal edema and hypervascularity in the upper airways. Nasal breathing may become difficult due to capillary engorgement causing nasal congestion, and the efficacy of mask ventilation may be hindered.[147] The caliber of the airway may be smaller and anatomical structures may be difficult to identify because of edema, especially if the woman is preeclamptic.[148] Pilkington et al.[149] reported an increased Mallampati classification with advancing pregnancy, probably related to fluid retention. The Mallampati classification may also advance further during bearing down, due to progression of the edema of the lower pharynx.[150] The metabolic demands of the growing fetus, uterus, and placenta lead to a 30–60% increase in oxygen consumption in the parturient. Anatomical changes, including a displaced diaphragm secondary to the enlarged gravid uterus, lead to a 20% decrease in functional residual capacity. These two main respiratory changes may accelerate the onset of desaturation during hypoventilation and apnea.[151] Furthermore, weight gain is a common feature of late pregnancy, adding further to diminished respiratory reserves and poor visualization of the airway (there is a much greater chance that the oropharyngeal structures will be obliterated in the obese parturient).[152]

Management

Advances in regional anesthesia within the past 20 years have been such that general anesthesia is infrequently used for operative obstetrics in the developed world. Consequently, individuals who subspecialize in obstetrical anesthesia are exposed to difficult airways even less frequently than most anesthesiologists.[153] This clearly has training implications for both residents and staff, who must find other ways to maintain their skills.

The ASA and other groups have published guidelines for the management of difficult airways, but these are quite generic and do not address specific problems. Tunstall and Sheikh[41] have suggested guidelines in obstetrics that are well worth reading. However, a number of important advances have taken place since and are worthy of discussion.

The obstetric care team should "be alert" for the general anesthesia risk factors when admitting patients to the labor floor and consult a specialist in certain cases in order to evaluate the airway or place a "prophylactic" epidural in early labor. Anticipated difficulties in airway management should be addressed to the patient early in labor. All patients presenting for operative obstetrics should be carefully evaluated by an anesthesiologist and undergo thorough scrutiny of the airway. Whenever possible, regional anesthesia should be selected. The main reasons for general anesthesia are: patient preference, sepsis, coagulopathy, fetal distress, fixed cardiac output states, and maternal hemorrhage. The only absolute contraindications to regional anesthesia are patient refusal and coagulopathy.[151] Patients who demand general anesthesia should clearly understand the implications. Fetal distress per se is *not* necessarily an indication for general anesthesia. In fact, an anesthesiologist skilled in modern regional anesthesia techniques can administer a spinal anesthetic as quickly as a general. The risks of hemorrhage and fixed cardiac output states are also *not* necessarily considered absolute contraindications to regional anesthesia, especially in patients with a known difficult airway. In elective situations with a known difficult airway, some clinicians feel more comfortable securing the airway first, whereas others will elect to use regional anesthesia. The technique that the clinician is most comfortable with should be selected.

If general anesthesia is planned or required, responsibility for the administration of general anesthesia should be delegated to an individual with specialty qualifications in anesthesia. Although a resident may actually administer the anesthetic, an attending anesthesiologist should be present. A difficult airway kit must be immediately available and should be checked daily. The LMA should be part of the kit and may be used as a rescue maneuver. Careful planning regarding the method of ventilation and oxygenation will include whether a difficult airway is anticipated. Rapid sequence induction will normally be used in obstetrics when there is no anticipation of difficulty, in order to minimize the risk of aspiration. Awake intubation using flexible fiberoptic bronchoscopy is commonly used if there is anticipation of difficulty. Care must be taken with topicalization of the edematous airway. A drying agent will be necessary.

Prophylaxis against aspiration, a potential consequence of difficult intubation, should be administered. Numerous strategies can be considered, including nonparticulate antacids, H_2 receptor antagonists, or proton-pump inhibitors and prokinetics.[154,155] Application of cricoid pressure should be used during rapid sequence induction. Intake of solids is usually restricted. The first attempt at intubation is always the best chance, so it should not be squandered by lack of preparation. Each time intubation is attempted following a previously failed attempt, the patient is exposed to increased risk. During laryngoscopic intubation, the patient needs to be properly positioned. The neck needs to be flexed at the cervico-thoracic junction and extended at the antlanto-occipital joint and pillows should be used to exaggerate the position.[151] Ramping (raising the thorax, shoulders, neck and head) may be required in obese parturients, in order to properly align their airway axes.[156]

How does the clinician proceed if, while administering a general anesthetic to an obstetrical patient, intubation is unsuccessful (Fig. 9.9)? Obstetrical patients desaturate rapidly. Oxygenation is the top priority, and positive pressure ventilation while maintaining cricoid pressure should be administered without hesitation. Remember: inappropriately applied cricoid pressure may interfere with visibility of the larynx, and thus temporary cricoid pressure release may be of benefit. It is also possible to apply cricoid pressure and backward/upward right pressure (BURP) simultaneously. Edema of the airway is quite common in late pregnancy, so a *small* endotracheal tube for the first attempt (7.0 mm ID) should always be selected.

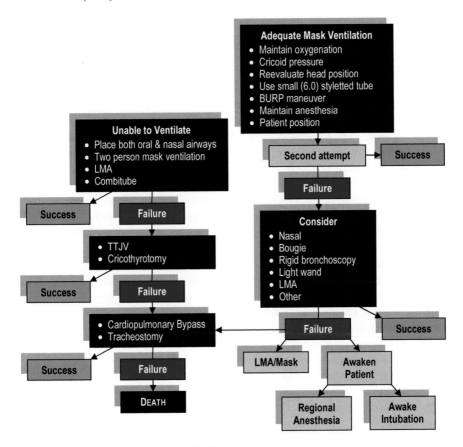

Fig. 9.9 Failed obstetrical intubation algorithm

A styletted 6.0-mm ID cuffed tube also should be used following a failed first attempt. If after two attempts at intubation (including use of alternative positions and blades and the use of a bougie) there is failure, further steps will depend on the ability to ventilate with 100% oxygen and whether there is fetal distress.

With successful ventilation, an alternative anesthetic technique (awake intubation or regional anesthesia) may be considered if there is no fetal distress. With ventilation and fetal distress, an attempt to continue the case may be taken using BMV or an external glottic device (LMA or Combitube). Regurgitation and aspiration should be prevented as much as possible when using an LMA as the airway.[157] The LMA should be inserted without hesitation, following a failed second attempt at intubation. The ProSeal LMA offers some additional advantages over the LMA Classic; however, its value compared to LMA Classic on maternal morbidity remains unknown.[158] An alternative to the LMA which may be beneficial in obstetrics includes the GlideScope videolaryngoscope, which may improve the glottic view.[146,159] The LMA functions optimally when patients are adequately anesthetized.

An intubating LMA can serve as a conduit through which blind (tube size 6.0 mm ID) or fiberoptically-assisted intubation is performed. Alternatively, a bougie may be passed through the LMA into the airway and an endotracheal tube may be advanced over that.

If there is a problem at any time with ventilation, oral and nasal airways should be inserted and two-handed mask ventilation attempted with the aid of an assistant. Without ventilation, the patient is allowed to wake up. If necessary, rescue techniques, including the placement of a LMA or Combitube, or a surgical airway should be performed. Intubation may be attempted through an intubating LMA (e.g., LMA Fastrach).[147]

A failed airway will necessitate a surgical airway. While an option, TTJV is difficult to perform in obstetrical patients and catastrophes have been reported to occur during emergency situations.[147] Open or percutaneous cricothyrotomy can usually be performed successfully in the obstetrical patient. A cuffed tracheal device is mandatory in the kit located in the labor and delivery suite.[156] The anesthesiologist must be prepared to perform these procedures and not rely on surgical colleagues who might not be familiar with either the circumstances or the equipment. With TTJV, high airway pressure may be necessary to overcome the pregnancy-related decrease in lung compliance.[151] If TTJV or needle cricothyrotomy is successful, tracheostomy will be required to protect the airway from aspiration. If TTJV or cricothyrotomy is not successful, cardiopulmonary bypass may be necessary and must be considered if and when facilities are available.

In summary, airway problems in the parturient are among the most challenging. When problems ensue, there is even less time than usual to act, and the lives of both mother and her infant are at stake. The consequences of failure to secure the airway may be loss of life, and in some, permanent brain damage in mother and child.

Summary

There are no clear-cut guidelines that can be applied to all difficult intubations. Each case is different. Obviously, a failed intubation in a patient with rapidly progressive airway obstruction is a much more urgent problem than a failed attempt in elective surgery. The only requirement common to all cases is that oxygenation must be maintained at all times. The experience of the individual dealing with the problem is also important. Experienced practitioners tend to be more aggressive from the outset. Do not underestimate the value of vigorous manipulation of the airway by an experienced colleague. We have not emphasized this aspect sufficiently in algorithms. Unfortunately, we frequently do not have good assistance when we encounter difficult airways.

In recent years, bougies have become much more popular and are often used as a first-line of defense when difficulties arise. We endorse this approach, especially since one of the drawbacks of fiberoptic techniques is the fact that preparation time is invariably needed.

Also remember the old adage, "a difficult oral is often an easy nasal intubation." However, if you do attempt nasal intubation during a failed oral intubation, you must take appropriate precautions to prevent nasal bleeding. Most anesthesiologists are reluctant to follow this course because of the risk of hemorrhage. A brisk nasal hemorrhage not only makes it impossible to see the airway but may also precipitate a "CICV" scenario.

The most important advance in airway management in recent years is the introduction of the LMA and its many modifications. The LMA has a particular value in the difficult airway situation for a number of reasons. In some cases, the problem may be solved by placing an LMA. One can only speculate on the number of difficult intubations that have been preemptively avoided as a result of the introduction of the LMA. The LMA is a noninvasive approach to the difficult airway and allows time to regroup and reevaluate a difficult situation. The LMA may also act as a conduit for subsequent endotracheal intubation. The ProSeal variation of the LMA comes close to a replacement for endotracheal intubation.

Your must always be prepared to deal with *complete airway obstruction*. Many centers have special "difficult intubation" trays complete with all the necessary equipment. Certainly do not attempt intubation unless the ability to deliver oxygen and apply suction is immediately at hand.

We have seen a tremendous increase in the number of technical devices that have become available to facilitate difficult intubation and mask ventilation in the past two decades. Each department of anesthesia across the globe seems to develop its own culture when it comes to using these devices. It would be difficult to attain competence in the use of all of these devices; however, one should strive to master at least two or three of them.

Ultimately, knowledge and competence in handling difficult intubations will be acquired only by managing patients. As an astute observer once said, "Good judgment comes from experience, and experience comes from bad judgment."

Acknowledgements The author would like to thank Jennifer Pillay, Nikki Stalker, and Adam Dryden for their contribution to this chapter.

References

1. Duncan PG, Cohen MM, Yip R. Clinical experiences associated with anaesthesia training. *Ann R Coll Physicians Surg Can.* 1993;26:363–367.
2. American Society of Anesthesiologists Task Force on Management of the Difficult Airway. Practice guidelines for management of the difficult airway: an updated report. *Anesthesiology.* 2003;98:1269–1277.
3. American Society of Anesthesiologists Task Force on Management of the Difficult Airway. Practice guidelines for management of the difficult airway. *Anesthesiology.* 1993;78:597–602.
4. Crosby ET, Cooper RM, Douglas MJ, et al. The unanticipated difficult airway with recommendations for management. *Can J Anesth.* 1998;45:757–776.

5. Cormack RS, Lehane J. Difficult tracheal intubation in obstetrics. *Anaesthesia.* 1984;39:1105–1111.
6. Shiga T, Wajima Z, Inoue T, Sakamoto A. Predicting difficult intubation in apparently normal patients: a meta-analysis of bedside screening test performance. *Anesthesiology.* 2005;103:429–437.
7. Kheterpal S, Martin L, Shanks AM, Tremper KK. Prediction and outcomes of impossible mask ventilation: a review of 50,000 anesthetics. *Anesthesiology.* 2009;110:891–897.
8. El-Orbany M, Woehlck HJ. Difficult mask ventilation. *Anesth Analg.* 2009;109:1870–1880.
9. Benyamin RM, Wafai Y, Salem MR, Joseph NJ. Two-handed mask ventilation of the difficult airway by a single individual. *Anesthesiology.* 1998;88:1134.
10. Elam JO, Titel JH, Feingold F, Weisman H, Bauer RO. Simplified airway management during anesthesia or resuscitation. A binasal pharyngeal system. *Anesth Analg.* 1969;48:307–316.
11. Kuna ST, Woodson LC, Solanki DR, Esch O, Frantz DE, Mathru M. Effect of progressive mandibular advancement on pharyngeal airway size in anesthetized adults. *Anesthesiology.* 2008;109:605–612.
12. Salem MR, Ovassapian A. Difficult mask ventilation: what needs improvement? *Anesth Analg.* 2009;109:1720–1722.
13. Stone BJ, Chantler PJ, Baskett PJ. The incidence of regurgitation during cardiopulmonary resuscitation: a comparison between the bag valve mask and laryngeal mask airway. *Resuscitation.* 1998;38:3–6.
14. Kheterpal S, Han R, Tremper KK, et al. Incidence and predictors of difficult and impossible mask ventilation. *Anesthesiology.* 2006;105:885–891.
15. Langeron O, Masso E, Huraux C, et al. Prediction of difficult mask ventilation. *Anesthesiology.* 2000;92:1229–1236.
16. Yildiz TS, Solak M, Toker K. The incidence and risk factors of difficult mask ventilation. *J Anesth.* 2005;19:7–11.
17. Han R, Tremper KK, Kheterpal S, O'Reilly M. Grading scale for mask ventilation. *Anesthesiology.* 2004;101:267.
18. Samsoon GL, Young JR. Difficult tracheal intubation: a retrospective study. *Anaesthesia.* 1987;42:487–490.
19. Adnet F, Baillard C, Borron SW, et al. Randomized study comparing the "sniffing position" with simple head extension for laryngoscopic view in elective surgery patients. *Anesthesiology.* 2001;95:836–841.
20. Bannister PB, MacBeth RG. Direct laryngoscopy and tracheal intubation. *Lancet.* 1944;1:651–654.
21. Brindley PG. "Win with your chin": an alternative to the "sniffing position" analogy for teaching optimal head-positioning with intubation (letter to the editor). *Resuscitation.* 2008;78:242.
22. Buckham M, Brooker M, Brimacombe J, Keller C. A comparison of the reinforced and standard laryngeal mask airway: ease of insertion and the influence of head and neck position on oropharyngeal leak pressure and intracuff pressure. *Anaesth Intensive Care.* 1999;27:628–631.
23. Cattermole GN. Sniff the morning air or drink a pint of beer? *Anaesthesia.* 2002;57:411.
24. Ishimura H, Minami K, Sata T, Shigematsu A, Kadoya T. Impossible insertion of the laryngeal mask airway and oropharyngeal axes. *Anesthesiology.* 1995;83:867–869.
25. Murphy M, Walls RM. Identification of the difficult and failed airway. In: Walls RM, Murphy MF, Luten R, eds. *Manual of Emergency Airway Management.* Philadelphia: Lippincott Williams & Wilkins; 2004:70–81.
26. Murphy MF, Doyle DJ. Airway evaluation. In: Hung O, Murphy MF, eds. *Management of the Difficult and Failed Airway.* New York: McGraw Hill; 2008:3–14.
27. Arne J, Descoins P, Fusciardi J, et al. Preoperative assessment for difficult intubation in general and ENT surgery: predictive value of a clinical multivariate risk index. *Br J Anaesth.* 1998;80:140–146.
28. el-Ganzouri AR, McCarthy RJ, Tuman KJ, Tanck EN, Ivankovich AD. Preoperative airway assessment: predictive value of a multivariate risk index. *Anesth Analg.* 1996;82:1197–1204.

29. Koh LK, Kong CE, Ip-Yam PC. The modified Cormack-Lehane score for the grading of direct laryngoscopy: evaluation in the Asian population. *Anesth Intensive Care*. 2002;30:48–51.
30. Rose DK, Cohen MM. Predicting difficult laryngoscopy (reply). *Can J Anesth*. 1996;43:1082.
31. Rose DK, Cohen MM. The airway: problems and predictions in 18,500 patients. *Can J Anesth*. 1994;41:372–383.
32. Rose DK, Cohen MM. The incidence of airway problems depends on the definition used. *Can J Anesth*. 1996;43:30–34.
33. Suyama H, Tsuno S, Takeyoshi S. The clinical usefulness of predicting difficult endotracheal intubation. *Masui*. 1999;48:37–41. Abstract in English.
34. Tse JC, Rimm EB, Hussain A. Predicting difficult endotracheal intubation in surgical patients scheduled for general anesthesia: a prospective blind study. *Anesth Analg*. 1995;81:254–258.
35. Ulrich B, Listyo R, Gerig HJ, Gabi K, Kreienbuhl G. [The difficult intubation. The value of BURP and 3 predictive tests of difficult intubation]. *Anaesthesist*. 1998;47:45–50. Abstract in English.
36. Yamamoto K, Tsubokawa T, Shibata K, Ohmura S, Nitta S, Kobayashi T. Predicting difficult intubation with indirect laryngoscopy. *Anesthesiology*. 1997;86:316–321.
37. Lee A, Fan LT, Gin T, Karmakar MK, Ngan Kee WD. A systematic review (meta-analysis) of the accuracy of the Mallampati tests to predict the difficult airway. *Anesth Analg*. 2006;102:1867–1878.
38. Calder I, Calder J, Crockard HA. Difficult direct laryngoscopy in patients with cervical spine disease. *Anaesthesia*. 1995;50:756–763.
39. Wrightson F, Soma M, Smith JH. Anesthetic experience of 100 pediatric tracheostomies. *Pediatr Anesth*. 2009;19:659–666.
40. Valois T. The pediatric difficult airway. In: Astuto M, ed. *Basics: Anesthesia, Intensive Care and Pain in Neonates and Children*. Italy: Springer; 2009:31–48.
41. Tunstall ME, Sheikh A. Failed intubation protocol: oxygenation without aspiration. *Clin Anaesthesiol*. 1986;4:171–187.
42. Benumof JL. Management of the difficult adult airway. With special emphasis on awake tracheal intubation. *Anesthesiology*. 1991;75:1087–1110.
43. Caplan RA, Posner KL, Ward RJ, Cheney FW. Adverse respiratory events in anesthesia: a closed claims analysis. *Anesthesiology*. 1990;72:828–833.
44. Benumof JL. Laryngeal mask airway and the ASA difficult airway algorithm. *Anesthesiology*. 1996;84:686–699.
45. Henderson JJ, Popat MT, Latto IP, Pearce AC. Difficult Airway Society guidelines for management of the unanticipated difficult intubation. *Anaesthesia*. 2004;59:675–694.
46. Boisson-Bertrand D, Bourgain JL, Camboulives J, et al. [Difficult intubation. French Society of Anesthesia and Intensive Care. A collective expertise]. *Ann Fr Anesth Reanim*. 1996;15:207–214.
47. SIAARTI Task Force on Difficult Airway Management. L'intubazione difficile e la difficolta di controllo delle vie aeree nell'adulto. *Minerva Anestesiol*. 1998;64:361–371.
48. Braun U, Goldmann K, Hempel V, Krier C. Airway management. Leitlinie der deutschen gesellschaft fur anasthesiologie und intensivmedizin. *Anaesthesiol Intensivmed*. 2004;45:302–306.
49. Heidegger T, Gerig HJ, Henderson JJ. Strategies and algorithms for management of the difficult airway. *Best Pract Res Clin Anaesthesiol*. 2005;19:661–674.
50. Goldmann K, Ferson DZ. Education and training in airway management. *Best Pract Res Clin Anaesthesiol*. 2005;19:717–732.
51. Koppel JN, Reed AP. Formal instruction in difficult airway management. A survey of anesthesiology residency programs. *Anesthesiology*. 1995;83:1343–1346.
52. Hagberg CA, Greger J, Chelly JE, Saad-Eddin HE. Instruction of airway management skills during anesthesiology residency training. *J Clin Anesth*. 2003;15:149–153.
53. Cheney FW, Posner KL, Lee LA, Caplan RA, Domino KB. Trends in anesthesia-related death and brain damage: a closed claims analysis. *Anesthesiology*. 2006;105:1081–1086.
54. Wong DT, Lai K, Chung FF, Ho RY. Cannot intubate-cannot ventilate and difficult intubation strategies: results of a Canadian national survey. *Anesth Analg*. 2005;100:1439–1446. table.

55. Helm M, Gries A, Mutzbauer T. Surgical approach in difficult airway management. *Best Pract Res Clin Anaesthesiol*. 2005;19:623–640.
56. Leibovici D, Fredman B, Gofrit ON, Shemer J, Blumenfeld A, Shapira SC. Prehospital cricothyroidotomy by physicians. *Am J Emerg Med*. 1997;15:91–93.
57. Heard AM, Green RJ, Eakins P. The formulation and introduction of a 'can't intubate, can't ventilate' algorithm into clinical practice. *Anaesthesia*. 2009;64:601–608.
58. Dorges V. Airway management in emergency situations. *Best Pract Res Clin Anaesthesiol*. 2005;19:699–715.
59. Wilson WC. Trauma airway management. ASA difficult airway algorithm modified for trauma -and five common trauma intubation scenarios. *ASA Newsl*. 2005;69:9–16.
60. Pierre EJ, McNeer RR, Shamir MY. Early management of the traumatized airway. *Anesthesiol Clin*. 2007;25:1–11. vii.
61. Bachulis BL, Long WB, Hynes GD, Johnson MC. Clinical indications for cervical spine radiographs in the traumatized patient. *Am J Surg*. 1987;153:473–478.
62. Bayless P, Ray VG. Incidence of cervical spine injuries in association with blunt head trauma. *Am J Emerg Med*. 1989;7:139–142.
63. Bryson B, Mulkey M, Mumford B, Schwedhelm M, Warren K. Cervical spine injury, incidence and diagnosis. *J Trauma*. 1986;26:669.
64. Cadoux CG, White JD, Hedberg MC. High-yield roentgenographic criteria for cervical spine injuries. *Ann Emerg Med*. 1987;16:738–742.
65. Kreipke DL, Gillespie KR, McCarthy MC, Mail JT, Lappas JC, Broadie TA. Reliability of indications for cervical spine films in trauma patients. *J Trauma*. 1989;29:1438–1439.
66. Vassiliu P, Baker J, Henderson S, Alo K, Velmahos G, Demetriades D. Aerodigestive injuries of the neck. *Am Surg*. 2001;67:75–79.
67. Murphy MF. Airway management of a patient with a stab wound to the neck. In: Hung O, Murphy MF, eds. *Management of the Difficult and Failed Airway*. New York: McGraw Hill; 2008:265–268.
68. Weitzel N, Kendall J, Pons P. Blind nasotracheal intubation for patients with penetrating neck trauma. *J Trauma*. 2004;56:1097–1101.
69. Ivy ME, Cohn SM. Addressing the myths of cervical spine injury management. *Am J Emerg Med*. 1997;15:591–595.
70. Crosby ET, Lui A. The adult cervical spine: implications for airway management. *Can J Anesth*. 1990;37:77–93.
71. Holly LT, Kelly DF, Counelis GJ, Blinman T, McArthur DL, Cryer HG. Cervical spine trauma associated with moderate and severe head injury: incidence, risk factors, and injury characteristics. *J Neurosurg*. 2002;96:285–291.
72. Crosby ET. Considerations for airway management for cervical spine surgery in adults. *Anesthesiol Clin*. 2007;25:511–533. ix.
73. Goldberg W, Mueller C, Panacek E, Tigges S, Hoffman JR, Mower WR. Distribution and patterns of blunt traumatic cervical spine injury. *Ann Emerg Med*. 2001;38:17–21.
74. Hastings RH, Marks JD. Airway management for trauma patients with potential cervical spine injuries. *Anesth Analg*. 1991;73:471–482.
75. Hadley MN. Guidelines for the management of acute cervical spine and spinal cord injuries. Cervical spine immobilization before admission to hospital. *Neurosurgery*. 2002;50:S7–S17.
76. Crosby ET. Airway management in adults after cervical spine trauma. *Anesthesiology*. 2006;104:1293–1318.
77. Heath KJ. The effect of laryngoscopy of different cervical spine immobilisation techniques. *Anaesthesia*. 1994;49:843–845.
78. Hastings RH, Kelley SD. Neurologic deterioration associated with airway management in a cervical spine-injured patient. *Anesthesiology*. 1993;78:580–583.
79. Reid DC, Henderson R, Saboe L, Miller JD. Etiology and clinical course of missed spine fractures. *J Trauma*. 1987;27:980–986.
80. Blahd WH Jr, Iserson KV, Bjelland JC. Efficacy of the posttraumatic cross table lateral view of the cervical spine. *J Emerg Med*. 1985;2:243–249.

81. Hadley MN. Guidelines for the management of acute cervical spine and spinal cord injuries. Radiographic assessment of the cervical spine in asymptomatic trauma patients. *Neurosurgery*. 2002;50:S30–S35.
82. Hoffman JR, Mower WR, Wolfson AB, Todd KH, Zucker MI. Validity of a set of clinical criteria to rule out injury to the cervical spine in patients with blunt trauma. National Emergency X-Radiography Utilization Study Group. *N Engl J Med*. 2000;343:94–99.
83. Stiell IG, Wells GA, Vandemheen KL, et al. The Canadian C-spine rule for radiography in alert and stable trauma patients. *JAMA*. 2001;286:1841–1848.
84. Stiell IG, Clement CM, McKnight RD, et al. The Canadian C-spine rule versus the NEXUS low-risk criteria in patients with trauma. *N Engl J Med*. 2003;349:2510–2518.
85. Grossman MD, Reilly PM, Gillett T, Gillett D. National survey of the incidence of cervical spine injury and approach to cervical spine clearance in U.S. trauma centers. *J Trauma*. 1999;47:684–690.
86. Hadley MN. Guidelines for the management of acute cervical spine and spinal cord injuries. Radiographic assessment of the cervical spine in symptomatic trauma patients. *Neurosurgery*. 2002;50:S36–S43.
87. Perry M, Morris C. Advanced trauma life support (ATLS) and facial trauma: can one size fit all? Part 2: ATLS, maxillofacial injuries and airway management dilemmas. *Int J Oral Maxillofac Surg*. 2008;37:309–320.
88. Biby L, Santora AH. Prevertebral hematoma secondary to whiplash injury necessitating emergency intubation. *Anesth Analg*. 1990;70:112–114.
89. Gopalakrishnan KC, el Masri W. Prevertebral soft tissue shadow widening–an important sign of cervical spinal injury. *Injury*. 1986;17:125–128.
90. Chesnut RM. Management of brain and spine injuries. *Crit Care Clin*. 2004;20:25–55.
91. Gabbott DA. Laryngoscopy using the McCoy laryngoscope after application of a cervical collar. *Anaesthesia*. 1996;51:812–814.
92. Keller C, Brimacombe J, Keller K. Pressures exerted against the cervical vertebrae by the standard and intubating laryngeal mask airways: a randomized, controlled, cross-over study in fresh cadavers. *Anesth Analg*. 1999;89:1296–1300.
93. Kihara S, Watanabe S, Brimacombe J, Taguchi N, Yaguchi Y, Yamasaki Y. Segmental cervical spine movement with the intubating laryngeal mask during manual in-line stabilization in patients with cervical pathology undergoing cervical spine surgery. *Anesth Analg*. 2000;91:195–200.
94. American Burn Association. Chicago: National Burn Repository Report of data From 1999–2008. National Burn Repository 2009 Version 5.0, 12. http://www.ameriburn.org/. [Updated 2009; cited 12 Nov 2009].
95. Cancio LC. Airway management and smoke inhalation injury in the burn patient. *Clin Plast Surg*. 2009;36:555–567.
96. Vissers RJ. Airway management in the patient with burns to the head, neck, upper torso, and the airway. In: Hung O, Murphy MF, eds. *Management of the Difficult and Failed Airway*. New York: McGraw Hill; 2008:269–273.
97. Cereda M, Foti G, Musch G, Sparacino ME, Pesenti A. Positive end-expiratory pressure prevents the loss of respiratory compliance during low tidal volume ventilation in acute lung injury patients. *Chest*. 1996;109:480–485.
98. Rogovik A, Goldman R. Permissive hypercapnia. *Emerg Med Clin North Am*. 2008;26:941–949.
99. The Association of Anaesthetists of Great Britain and Ireland. London: Recommendations for the Safe Transfer of Patients with Brain Injury. http://www.aagbi.org/publications/guidelines/docs/braininjury.pdf#search="braininjury". [Updated May 2006, cited 12 Nov 2009].
100. Walls MW. Blind nasotracheal intubation in the presence of facial trauma – is it safe? *J Emerg Med*. 1997;15:243–244.
101. Dutton RP, McCunn M. Anesthesia for trauma. In: Miller RD, ed. *Miller's Anesthesia*. Philadelphia: Churchill Livingstone; 2005:2451–2459.

102. Schwartz DE, Matthay MA, Cohen NH. Death and other complications of emergency airway management in critically ill adults. A prospective investigation of 297 tracheal intubations. *Anesthesiology*. 1995;82:367–376.

103. Beed S. Airway Management in the Intensive Care Unit. In: Hung O, Murphy MF, eds. *Management of the Diffiuclt and Failed Airway*. New York: McGraw Hill; 2008:289–296.

104. Lavery GG, McCloskey BV. The difficult airway in adult critical care. *Crit Care Med*. 2008;36:2163–2173.

105. Dorman T, Angood PB, Angus DC, et al. Guidelines for critical care medicine training and continuing edical education. *Crit Care Med*. 2004;32:263–272.

106. Olsson GL, Hallen B. Cardiac arrest during anaesthesia. A computer-aided study in 250,543 anaesthetics. *Acta Anaesthesiol Scand*. 1988;32:653–664.

107. Rosenblatt WH. Preoperative planning of airway management in critical care patients. *Crit Care Med*. 2004;32:S186–S192.

108. Demling RH, Read T, Lind LJ, Flanagan HL. Incidence and morbidity of extubation failure in surgical intensive care patients. *Crit Care Med*. 1988;16:573–577.

109. Reves J, Glass P, Lubarsky DA, McEvoy MD. Intravenous non-opioid anesthetics. In: Miller RD, ed. *Miller's Anesthesia*. New York: Elsevier; 2005:323.

110. Mort TC, Waberski BH, Clive J. Extending the preoxygenation period from 4 to 8 mins in critically ill patients undergoing emergency intubation. *Crit Care Med*. 2009;37:68–71.

111. Mort TC. Preoxygenation in critically ill patients requiring emergency tracheal intubation. *Crit Care Med*. 2005;33:2672–2675.

112. Miller KA, Harkin CP, Bailey PL. Postoperative tracheal extubation. *Anesth Analg*. 1995;80:149–172.

113. World Health Organization. WHO Global Infobase [Internet]. WHO Global Infobase. https://apps.who.int/infobase/report.aspx?rid=114&iso=USA&ind=BMI. [Updated 2008, cited 12 Nov 2009].

114. Brodsky JB, Lemmens HJ, Brock-Utne JG, Vierra M, Saidman LJ. Morbid obesity and tracheal intubation. *Anesth Analg*. 2002;94:732–736.

115. Juvin P, Lavaut E, Dupont H, et al. Difficult tracheal intubation is more common in obese than in lean patients. *Anesth Analg*. 2003;97:595–600. table.

116. Damia G, Mascheroni D, Croci M, Tarenzi L. Perioperative changes in functional residual capacity in morbidly obese patients. *Br J Anaesth*. 1988;60:574–578.

117. Casati A, Putzu M. Anesthesia in the obese patient: pharmacokinetic considerations. *J Clin Anesth*. 2005;17:134–145.

118. Adams JP, Murphy PG. Obesity in anaesthesia and intensive care. *Br J Anaesth*. 2000;85:91–108.

119. Pytka S, Carroll I. Airway management of a morbidly obese patient suffering from a cardiac arrest. In: Hung O, Murphy MF, eds. *Management of the Difficult and Failed Airway*. New York: McGraw Hill; 2008:233–238.

120. Collins JS, Lemmens HJ, Brodsky JB, Brock-Utne JG, Levitan RM. Laryngoscopy and morbid obesity: a comparison of the "sniff" and "ramped" positions. *Obes Surg*. 2004;14:1171–1175.

121. Cheymol G. Effects of obesity on pharmacokinetics implications for drug therapy. *Clin Pharmacokinet*. 2000;39:215–231.

122. Jung D, Mayersohn M, Perrier D, Calkins J, Saunders R. Thiopental disposition in lean and obese patients undergoing surgery. *Anesthesiology*. 1982;56:269–274.

123. Wada DR, Bjorkman S, Ebling WF, Harashima H, Harapat SR, Stanski DR. Computer simulation of the effects of alterations in blood flows and body composition on thiopental pharmacokinetics in humans. *Anesthesiology*. 1997;87:884–899.

124. Servin F, Farinotti R, Haberer JP, Desmonts JM. Propofol infusion for maintenance of anesthesia in morbidly obese patients receiving nitrous oxide. A clinical and pharmacokinetic study. *Anesthesiology*. 1993;78:657–665.

125. Gaszynski T. Standard clinical tests for predicting difficult intubation are not useful among morbidly obese patients. *Anesth Analg*. 2004;99:956.

126. Adnet F, Borron SW, Racine SX, et al. The intubation difficulty scale (IDS): proposal and evaluation of a new score characterizing the complexity of endotracheal intubation. *Anesthesiology.* 1997;87:1290–1297.

127. Zane RD. The morbidly obese patient. In: Walls RM, Murphy MF, eds. *Manual of Emergency Airway Management.* 2nd ed. Philadelphia, PA: Lippincott Williams & Wilkins; 2004:302–306.

128. Pelosi P, Ravagnan I, Giurati G, et al. Positive end-expiratory pressure improves respiratory function in obese but not in normal subjects during anesthesia and paralysis. *Anesthesiology.* 1999;91:1221–1231.

129. Douglas NJ, Polo O. Pathogenesis of obstructive sleep apnoea/hypopnoea syndrome. *Lancet.* 1994;344:653–655.

130. Kessler R, Chaouat A, Weitzenblum E, et al. Pulmonary hypertension in the obstructive sleep apnoea syndrome: prevalence, causes and therapeutic consequences. *Eur Respir J.* 1996;9:787–794.

131. Chung SA, Yuan H, Chung F. A systemic review of obstructive sleep apnea and its implications for anesthesiologists. *Anesth Analg.* 2008;107:1543–1563.

132. Nieto FJ, Young TB, Lind BK, et al. Association of sleep-disordered breathing, sleep apnea, and hypertension in a large community-based study. Sleep Heart Health Study. *JAMA.* 2000;283:1829–1836.

133. Young T, Evans L, Finn L, Palta M. Estimation of the clinically diagnosed proportion of sleep apnea syndrome in middle-aged men and women. *Sleep.* 1997;20:705–706.

134. American Society of Anesthesiologists Task Force on Perioperative Management of Patients with Obstructive Sleep Apnea. Practice guidelines for the perioperative management of patients with obstructive sleep apnea. *Anesthesiology.* 2006;104:1081–1093.

135. Hendolin H, Kansanen M, Koski E, Nuutinen J. Propofol-nitrous oxide versus thiopentone-isoflurane-nitrous oxide anaesthesia for uvulopalatopharyngoplasty in patients with sleep apnea. *Acta Anaesthesiol Scand.* 1994;38:694–698.

136. Benumof JL. Obstructive sleep apnea in the adult obese patient: implications for airway management. *Anesthesiol Clin North Am.* 2002;20:789–811.

137. Benumof JL. Airway exchange catheters: simple concept, potentially great danger. *Anesthesiology.* 1999;91:342–344.

138. Saigusa H, Suzuki M, Higurashi N, Kodera K. Three-dimensional morphological analyses of positional dependence in patients with obstructive sleep apnea syndrome. *Anesthesiology.* 2009;110:885–890.

139. Joshi GP. Multimodal analgesia techniques for ambulatory surgery. *Int Anesthesiol Clin.* 2005;43:197–204.

140. Siyam MA, Benhamou D. Difficult endotracheal intubation in patients with sleep apnea syndrome. *Anesth Analg.* 2002;95:1098–1102. table.

141. Benumof JL, Cooper SD. Quantitative improvement in laryngoscopic view by optimal external laryngeal manipulation. *J Clin Anesth.* 1996;8:136–140.

142. Cooper GM, McClure JH. Maternal deaths from anaesthesia. An extract from Why Mothers Die 2000–2002, the Confidential Enquiries into Maternal Deaths in the United Kingdom: Chapter 9: Anaesthesia. *Br J Anaesth.* 2005;94:417–423.

143. Hawkins JL, Koonin LM, Palmer SK, Gibbs CP. Anesthesia-related deaths during obstetric delivery in the United States, 1979–1990. *Anesthesiology.* 1997;86:277–284.

144. Hawkins JL, Chang J, Callaghan W. Anesthesia-related maternal mortality in the United States, 1991–1996. An Update. *Anesthesiology.* 2002;96:A1046.

145. Hawthorne L, Wilson R, Lyons G, Dresner M. Failed intubation revisited: 17-yr experience in a teaching maternity unit. *Br J Anaesth.* 1996;76:680–684.

146. Goldszmidt E. Principles and practices of obstetric airway management. *Anesthesiol Clin.* 2008;26:109–125. vii.

147. Ross BK. What is unique about the obstetrical airway? In: Hung O, Murphy MF, eds. *Management of the Difficult and Failed Airway.* New York: McGraw Hill; 2008:423–431.

148. Izci B, Riha RL, Martin SE, et al. The upper airway in pregnancy and pre-eclampsia. *Am J Respir Crit Care Med.* 2003;167:137–140.
149. Pilkington S, Carli F, Dakin MJ, et al. Increase in Mallampati score during pregnancy. *Br J Anaesth.* 1995;74:638–642.
150. Farcon EL, Kim MH, Marx GF. Changing Mallampati score during labour. *Can J Anesth.* 1994;41:50–51.
151. Vasdev GM, Harrison BA, Keegan MT, Burkle CM. Management of the difficult and failed airway in obstetric anesthesia. *J Anesth.* 2008;22:38–48.
152. Rocke DA, Murray WB, Rout CC, Gouws E. Relative risk analysis of factors associated with difficult intubation in obstetric anesthesia. *Anesthesiology.* 1992;77:67–73.
153. Bucklin BA, Hawkins JL, Anderson JR, Ullrich FA. Obstetric anesthesia workforce survey: twenty-year update. *Anesthesiology.* 2005;103:645–653.
154. American Society of Anesthesiologists' Task Force on Obstetrical Anesthesia. Practice guidelines for obstetrical anesthesia: a report. *Anesthesiology.* 1999;90:600–611.
155. O'Sullivan GM, Guyton TS. Aspirartion: risk, prophylaxis and treatment. In: Chestnut DH, ed. *Obstetric Anesthesia Principles and Practice.* Philadelphia: Elsevier Mosby; 2004:523–534.
156. Olufolabi AJ, Muir HA. Unanticipated difficult airway in an obstetrical patient requiring an emergency cesarean section. In: Hung O, Murphy MF, eds. *Management of the Difficult and Failed Airway.* New York: McGraw Hill; 2008:437–441.
157. McClune S, Regan M, Moore J. Laryngeal mask airway for caesarean section. *Anaesthesia.* 1990;45:227–228.
158. Brain AI, Verghese C, Strube PJ. The LMA 'ProSeal'–a laryngeal mask with an oesophageal vent. *Br J Anaesth.* 2000;84:650–654.
159. Cooper RM, Pacey JA, Bishop MJ, McCluskey SA. Early clinical experience with a new videolaryngoscope (GlideScope) in 728 patients. *Can J Anesth.* 2005;52:191–198.

Chapter 10
Pediatric Airway Management

Contents

B.T. Finucane et al., *Principles of Airway Management*,
DOI 10.1007/978-0-387-09558-5_10, © Springer Science+Business Media, LLC 2011

Section A: Basic and Difficult Airway Management

Introduction

Pediatric airway problems are among the most difficult challenges clinicians may face in their medical careers. Those unaccustomed to dealing with children tend to approach pediatric airway problems with a disproportionate amount of fear – which, often engendered by inexperience, can interfere with performance. This chapter provides the knowledge necessary to deal with common airway problems occurring in children, as well as some advanced devices and their applications.

The Pediatric Airway: Anatomy and Function

The anatomical differences between the infant, child, and adult airways have been described in Chap. 1 (see Figs. 1.24–1.26 in Chap. 1). Generally, by the age of 8 years, the airways of children and adults are very similar.[1] Differences in the pediatric airway can lead to airway obstruction, susceptibility to respiratory failure (including rapid desaturation), and to difficulty during endotracheal intubation.

Susceptibility to Obstruction

Susceptibility to airway obstruction in children arises mainly due to:

- The predominance of nasal breathing to the age of 12–18 months, due to the larynx locking into the pharynx during quiet respiration (see below), leading to nasal obstruction or congestion.
- A smaller larynx (the larynx of the neonate is approximately one-third of the size of those in adults) with an average anteroposterior subglottic diameter of 6 mm, which approaches the critical diameter of 4 mm for subglottic stenosis.[2]

- The relatively larger occiput which results in neck flexion (a pillow should be placed under a neonate or premature child's shoulders during resuscitation).
- Flexible trachea leading to pressure on the tracheal rings (the trachea's ability to resist external compression is weak).
- The proportionally larger and caudally situated (close to laryngeal inlet) tongue. Anterior pressure on the angle of the mandible to shift the tongue anteriorly often helps during induction or mergence of anesthesia.[3]
- The larger and broader epiglottis can readily cause airway obstruction when it becomes swollen.

A face mask must be carefully positioned onto an infant's face, covering the nose and mouth without impeding the nostril. Placing the fingers on the base of the tongue during face mask use can force the tongue against the palate and cause obstruction, especially due to the edentulous nature of an infant.[4] An additional consideration is that infants have highly viscous mucus which can rapidly obstruct the endotracheal tube (ETT).

Distinct Relationship Between the Tongue, Pharynx, and Larynx in the Infant

In infancy and early childhood, the key developmental feature related to the anatomical airway is the positional change of the larynx as it descends into the neck and thus places the opening of the larynx into the inferior aspect of the pharynx. This and other changes are essential to a variety of important functions including breathing, swallowing, and vocalization.[5, 6]

The tongue of the newborn is short and broad (4.0 cm long, 2.5 cm wide and 1.0 cm thick with the mouth closed), is larger in proportion to the rest of the oral cavity, and its base sits entirely within the oral cavity. When the newborn's mouth is closed, the tongue comes into contact with the gums laterally and the roof the mouth above. The pharynx (4 cm) is about twice as long as the larynx (2 cm), with the latter being widest at its upper margin. Humans are the only air-breathing vertebrates in which the posterior portion (1/3) of the tongue descends into the neck after birth to become a part of the anterior wall of the oropharynx. Together with the tongue, the larynx (also positioned high in the newborn) begins its descent during the first year after birth and completes this course during the 4th–5th year of life.[5]

The developmental and functional anatomy of the newborn larynx is similar to that of other mammals, above the egg-laying species.[7, 8] While the tongue is positioned cephalad, it is attached to the epiglottis of the larynx, thus placing the opening of the larynx directly below the oral cavity. The elongated epiglottis passes up behind and contacts the soft palate to guide a locking of the larynx directly into the nasopharynx, thus providing for a direct air channel while maintaining a separate path for food (Fig. 10.1). The soft palate becomes a flap, or velum, of striated muscle, which can either close off the nasopharynx (completely separating the nasal cavity from the oral cavity and larynx) or fit tightly against the front and sides

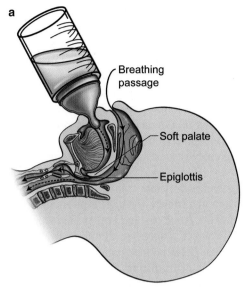

Swallowing milk simultaneously through faucium channels formed laterally by interlocking of soft palate and epiglottis

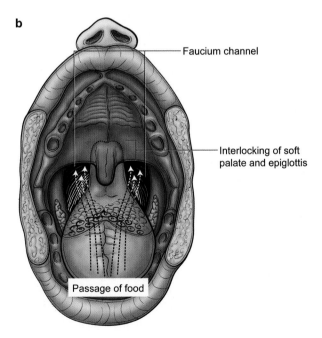

Fig. 10.1 Elevation of the larynx in the infant and young child enables simultaneous breathing and swallowing. (**a**) The epiglottis and soft palate are functionally interlocked and (**b**) lateral faucium channels are formed to allow for the passage of milk

of the larynx when it is inserted into the nasopharynx.[9] When the larynx is locked up within the nasopharynx (snuggly encircled by the pharyngeal wall posteriorly and the soft palate anteriorly and laterally), the wide continuation of the oral cavity is divided with the oropharynx, the isthmus faucium, into two channels or clefts (faucium channels), one on each side of the larynx (Fig 10.1b). The milk flows within these clefts, passes through the pharynx and enters the esophagus, without interfering with the passage of air into the larynx and trachea.

This function of the epiglottis in mammals has been considered as subserving the sense of smell, signaling an approaching enemy during eating. In humans, this "obligatory" nasal breathing enables suckling while breathing (Fig. 10.1). In addition, since the airway resistance contributed by the nasal passages of human newborn infants is slightly less than half of that contributed by adult human passages, obligate nasal breathing is a more efficient form of respiration.[10]

While frequent contact of the epiglottis and soft palate occurs throughout the first 6 months of life, palatal contact is only typical during swallowing for up to 18 months and no contact can made between the epiglottis and soft palate in cadavers of children beyond 4 years of age.[7] This distinct feature may also provide an explanation for why the epiglottis is elongated, wider, and omega-shaped. More recently, observations of infant breathing patterns demonstrated that even infants can switch from nasal to oral breathing, via elevation of the soft palate, in response to nasal occlusion. This finding has modified the term from "obligatory" to "preferential," or "predominant breathing." Beyond youth, the function of the epiglottis for protection of the larynx is not obligatory, and even trauma or destruction leads to no untoward effects in adults.[11]

A disadvantage of the infant's highly-located larynx is that their phonetic repertoire is greatly limited.[5] Thus, the newborn could not produce complex articulated sound even if they had the necessary maturity in their central nervous systems. It is necessary for the larynx to descend in such a manner to locate the laryngeal opening lower into the pharynx, thus enabling the pharyngeal and tongue muscles to produce the rapid alterations in pharyngeal size and shape necessary for the production of complex speech sounds.

Susceptibility to Respiratory Failure

The susceptibility to respiratory failure stems from:

- A different composition of muscle fibers with a predisposition to early fatigue (fewer type I [slow twitch, high oxidative] skeletal muscle fibers and less storage of glycogen and fat in their respiratory muscles).
- A flatter diaphragm, more horizontal ribs, and a higher respiratory rate, all leading to less reserve.
- A functional residual capacity when awake that is 40% of an adults[12] and when in deep sleep is even less, leading to reduced oxygen reserve to meet their high metabolic rates (which are two times that of an adult).

- Increased airway resistance due to their relatively small airway. During periods of apnea, infants desaturate much more rapidly than adults due to their higher metabolic rate.[1]

The pulmonary functional differences between adults and children are the greatest for neonates.[13]

Difficulty During Tracheal Intubation

There are many contributors to difficulty in airway visualization and ETT manipulation during endotracheal intubation. Some examples are the relatively large pediatric tongue, the high and anterior airway (epiglottis lies at C1 and the larynx lies at C3-C4 at birth [C4-5 and C7 by 6 and 13 years of age, respectively[14]]), and the more acute angle between the epiglottis and the tracheal opening (due to the attachment of the hyoid bone to the thyroid in the infant). The tongue may be difficult to move out of the visual field due to the relatively superior larynx. Enlarged tonsils may obscure the laryngeal view or may interfere with BMV.[15]

The trachea in infants is short and narrow and angled posteriorly, which may result in accidental endobronchial intubation with changes in head position. Difficulty passing the ETT during routine or fiberoptic intubation may result from the anterior slant of the vocal cords.[16] Finally, the shallow vallecula epiglottis may lead to difficulty in lifting the epiglottis during laryngoscopy. These factors are all attributed to infants with normal airways, and clearly more considerations will ensue if there are malformations or other factors involved. The sections on the Difficult Pediatric Airways and Upper Airway Obstruction in the Child will discuss several of these issues.

Basic Airway Management and CPR in Infants and Children

The principles of airway management in infants and children are similar to those in adults, with some exceptions. Airway obstruction can be avoided by careful positioning of the head of the child and keeping the child's nostrils unobstructed, with or without mouth opening during mask ventilation. Extension of the infant cervical spine during the head-tilt maneuver tends to flatten the airway, causing some degree of obstruction, thus should always be done gently, especially in children with Downs or Hurler syndrome (in which significant instability of the atlantoaxial joint has been reported).[17]

Inflation pressures required to ventilate an infant or child satisfactorily are much less than those required in an adult. Thus, much smaller breaths should be used during mouth-to-mouth respiration or positive-pressure ventilation (PPV) of any type, lest pulmonary barotrauma might occur. Cardiac arrest in an infant or child is usually secondary to respiratory insufficiency causing hypoxia or asphyxia.

Following are the most common causes of respiratory insufficiency in otherwise healthy children:

- Trauma
- Accidental poisoning
- Foreign-body aspiration
- Drowning
- Airway infections
- Unexplained (e.g., sudden infant death syndrome)
- Burns

Opening the Airway

Despite the pediatric patient's preference for nasal breathing, it is possible to maintain a patent oral airway.[18, 19] Several simple techniques should not be overlooked in favor of more invasive procedures. For example, in spontaneously breathing, unconscious patients, simple lateral positioning may help maintain the airway.[20] Applying chin lift and jaw-thrust maneuvers with the patient in the lateral position also improves outcomes.[21] There is some debate in the literature as to whether the open-mouthed chin lift or the jaw thrust is the more effective maneuver, but because both techniques push the hyoid bone anteriorly, they displace the epiglottis and open the pharynx.[22] Both maneuvers should be performed with the minimum necessary head tilt when cervical spine trauma is a concern.

In addition to widening the airway through the jaw-thrust/chin-lift techniques, continuous positive air pressure (CPAP) can improve air flow below the glottis through pneumatic stiffening of the pharynx during inspiration.[23] The less experienced practitioner should use the self-inflating bags over the flow-inflating type bags to apply CPAP. A two-person BMV technique may be more effective in generating sufficient tidal volumes in apneic pediatric patients.[24] One operator applies the jaw thrust and creates a tight seal between mask and face, while the other operator compresses the bag and applies cricoid pressure where necessary.[25] More strategies to overcome difficult mask ventilation (DMV) are a focus of this section's discussion on Difficult Pediatric Airways.

Use of Airway Adjuncts

In addition to these simple and sometimes overlooked methods of opening and maintaining the airway, both the nasopharyngeal and oropharyngeal airways provide efficient airway adjuncts. In the conscious child, the nasopharyngeal airway is better tolerated, particularly when the tube is warmed in water, sufficiently lubricated, and directed posteriorly.[18, 19] The flange shape of the nasopharyngeal airway prevents loss of the tube in the nostril and a variety of sizes are available to precisely fit the patient. See the discussion on Airway Equipment in this section for more details on oral and nasal airways.

Basic Life Support

Effective CPR saves lives. The recent evidence points towards variable quality of both basic and advanced life support (ALS), and the quality of CPR could be improved with effective education. Applying educational concepts to resuscitation training, Hunt et al.[26] provided the following principles which must be followed to improve training:

- Encourage instructors to adapt mock scenarios to learners' practice settings to make the learning relevant to them.
- Align the context of learning to the context in which those skills will be applied.
- Provide learners with an opportunity to accurately assess their competency level and help them achieve a conscious level of competence through targeted feedback and deliberate practice in resuscitation.
- Enhance levels of self-efficacy congruent with actual competency by way of mastery experiences in mock resuscitations.
- Actively engage all learners in deliberate practice until they achieve a predetermined mastery level of performance assessed through rigorous outcomes measures.

Compliance to guidelines set through evidence-based resuscitation evaluation should be strengthened. In accordance with this, the following discussion focuses on the recent guidelines set forth by the American Heart Association (AHA).

Based on the 2005 International Consensus Conference on Cardiopulmonary Resuscitation and Emergency Cardiovascular Care Science With Treatment Recommendations (developed by the International Liaison Committee on Resuscitation [ILCOR]),[27] the AHA has revised their guidelines, including those for pediatric basic and ALS and neonatal resuscitation.[28] The guidelines from 2000 have changed, with explicit attention to improving the quality of CPR as well as modifications related to several areas of controversy. The new mantra for basic pediatric CPR is, "push hard, push fast, minimize interruptions; allow full chest recoil and don't hyperventilate." The major changes of 2010 AHA guidelines will also be included in the following discussion.

The chain of survival in pediatrics includes:

- Prevention of cardiopulmonary arrest
- Basic CPR
- Prompt access to emergency medical services (EMS) system
- Prompt pediatric ALS
- Effective pediatric postresuscitation and rehabilitative care

"Phone fast" for infants and children under 8 years of age, and "phone first" for children over 8 years old, and adults was retained as a guideline, although the etiology of cardiac arrest may be considered rather than age in some cases. Sudden collapse may be attributed to ventricular fibrillation in some infants and children (7–15%, which is higher than previously thought) and calling for help first, before providing some CPR immediately may improve outcomes.

The definitions of infant and children have been changed and vary depending on whether the resuscitator is a lay person or health care (HC) provider; much of the basis for this is retention of knowledge in the lay person in order to increase the performance of bystander CPR in out-of-hospital settings. An "infant" is less than 1 year of age, except for newborns which is specific to the infant's initial hospitalization. For lay rescuers, the child basic life support guidelines should be used for a child between approximately 1 and 8 years of age; for HC providers, the pediatric ("child") guidelines should apply from 1 year of age to the start of puberty (presence of secondary sexual characteristics).

Recommended Sequence for Basic Life Support

The 2005 recommended CPR sequence (ABC) for use in an infant or child is included below, with an algorithm for HC provide found in Fig. 10.2. It is important to note that the 2010 guidelines rearranged the order of CPR steps to from ABC to CAB.

1. Ensure safety of rescuer and victim.
2. Check for response.
3. Activate the EMS and get the automated external defibrillator (AED) if the child is 1 year of age or older. The AHA recommends five cycles of CPR (2 min) on an unresponsive child before calling EMS if a single rescuer is present. If the arrest was witnessed and sudden, the EMS should be activated immediately.
4. Position the patient supine on a hard flat surface.
5. Open the airway and check breathing. Use the head tilt-chin lift procedure if there is no evidence of head or neck trauma. Use the jaw trust without head tilt if there is a suspected cervical spine injury. Take no more than 10 s to see whether the victim is breathing – *look, listen, and feel*.
6. Give rescue breaths. Give two breaths (each over 1 s) and ensure that the chest rises. In an infant use mouth-to-mouth-and-nose technique (Fig. 10.3); in children use mouth-to-mouth technique. If not successful, reposition the victim's head and attempt to ventilate. (Improper head position is the most common cause of inability to ventilate.) If out-of-hospital, BMV should be used instead of endotracheal intubation if the transport time is short. Use a self-inflating bag of at least 450–500 mL and attach an oxygen reservoir of 10–15 L/min. Avoid delivering excessive ventilation.
7. Assess the circulation. Lay rescuers should look, listen, and feel for breathing or coughing and look for movement. If none of these signs are present, compressions should be started. HC workers should assess the circulation by looking for a pulse (brachial in infants and carotid or femoral in children aged 1–8 years). HC workers should spend no more than 10 s looking for a pulse. If there is a pulse, but no breathing, 12–20 breaths per minute should be provided and the pulse rechecked every 2 min. If no pulse is detected, or if the pulse rate is less than 60 beats per minute (bpm) and perfusion seems inadequate, compressions should be started.

The compression-ventilation ratio for lay rescuers (for infants, children and adults) and lone HC providers has changed to 30:2. HC providers performing 2-person CPR

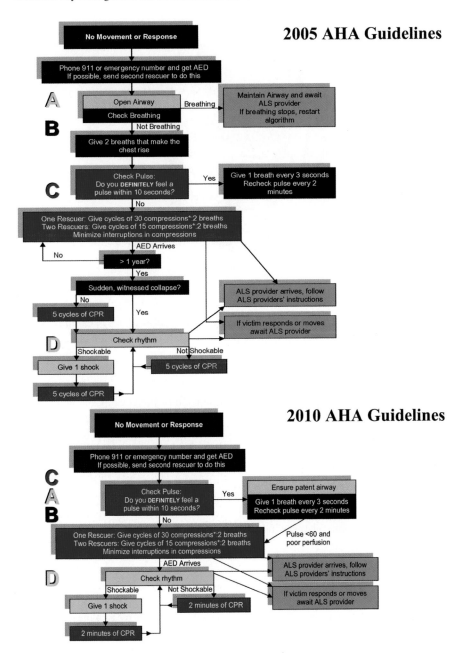

Fig. 10.2 Basic life support of the child by the health care provider. Flow chart based on (*Top*) 2005 and (*Bottom*) 2010 AHA guidelines[28a, b]

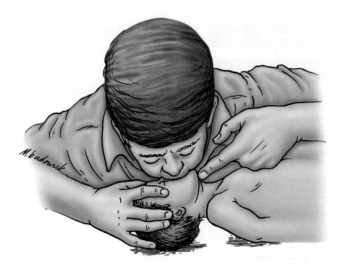

Fig. 10.3 Mouth-to-mouth/nose ventilation

in children beyond the newborn period should use a ratio of 15:2. Compressions should be performed quickly (100 times per minute). If there is an advanced airway placed, compressions should not be interrupted for ventilations, and ventilations should be provided 8–10 times per minute. Compression should be provided over the lower half of the sternum, enough to compress the chest approximately one-third to one half of the anterior–posterior dimension of the chest. Complete recoil should be allowed with minimal interruptions. In an infant, lay rescuers should use two-fingers below the intermammary line (see the following section on Resuscitation of the Neonate for more details on performing compressions on infants). When 2 HC rescuers are present, the thumb-encircling hand technique is recommended since it produces higher coronary artery perfusion pressure. In a child, the heel of one or two hands should be used to compress the lower half of the sternum. Table 10.1 presents an overview of the rates of compressions, ventilations, and depth of compressions. (also see Table 3.1)

Resuscitation of the Neonate

Neonatal resuscitation is one of the most important tasks in a medical practitioner's career. About 10% of newborns require some help to begin breathing at birth, and 1% require extensive resuscitation efforts.[27] The consequences of inadequately performed resuscitation not only are devastating to the newborn and family, they place a huge financial burden on the health system. Thus, the task should be delegated only to highly responsible and well-trained individuals. The Apgar scoring system was devised to assess the immediate outcome of neonatal resuscitation.[29] (Table 10.2)

Table 10.1 CPR in infants and children[a]

	Compression rate (per minute)	Ventilation rate (breaths per min) in victim with pulse	Compression-to-ventilation ratio	Depth of compressions	Hand/finger position
Infant	At least 100	20	30:2	1/3–1/2 anteroposterior diameter of chest	Use 2 fingers just below the intermammary line
Child	At least 100	20	30:2	1/3–1/2 anteroposterior diameter of chest	Place 1 or 2 hands 2 fingers-breadths above xiphoid
Adult (for comparison)	At least 100	10–12	30:2	At least 2 in.	Place 2 hands 2 finger-breadths above xiphoid

[a] This resuscitation sequence is to be used *outside* the hospital by lay rescuers and lone HC providers, where there is little if any equipment.
Source: Data from the American Heart Association Guidelines for Cardiopulmonary Resuscitation (CPR) and Emergency Cardiovascular Care (ECC)[28]

Table 10.2 Apgar scoring system

Parameter	0	1	2
Heart rate	Absent	<100	>100
Respiration	Absent	Slow	Crying
Muscle tone	Limp	Some tension	Active
Reflex activity	Absent	Grimace	Cough
Color	Blue or gray	Mostly pink	All pink

Asphyxiation of the neonate has been carefully studied in animal models and is characterized by a brief period of vigorous respiratory effort during which the heart rate and blood pressure rise and the PaO_2 falls. Then a primary apnea with reduced heart rate and blood pressure occurs that lasts for 1–5 min. If active resuscitation is not performed during this phase, the infant enters a gasping phase that eventually results in secondary apnea characterized by profound asphyxiation (PaO_2 <50 and $PaCO_2$ ~ 100 mmHg, pH <7.0) and quickly leads to the death of the infant unless there is some intervention. Apnea at birth should be treated as secondary apnea of unknown duration, thus assuming it began in utero, and resuscitation should begin immediately. Features of primary and secondary apnea are listed below:[30]

- Primary apnea – blue color, heart rate 40–100 bpm, and muscle tone may be present, simple resuscitation sufficient, and will respond with gasps before turning pink.
- Secondary apnea – pale or gray color, heart rate <40 bpm, muscle tone is absent, vigorous resuscitation required, and victim will turn pink before gasping.

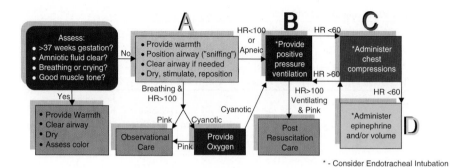

Fig. 10.4 Resuscitation of the Neonate (data from ref.[31])

2005 and 2010 American Heart Association Neonatal Resuscitation Guidelines[28, 31]

Careful assessment of all newborns must be performed in addition to dry and keep warm prior to place on their mother's chest. The assessments should consider their gestation age (born at term or not), amniotic fluid appearance (free of meconium and infection evidence), physical states (breathing or crying) and strength (good muscle tone). If the preceding categories are not all present, the infant should receive one or more of the following, in sequence:

(a) Initial steps in stabilization (clearing the airway, positioning, stimulating)
(b) Ventilation
(c) Chest compressions
(d) Medications or volume expansion

Figure 10.4 contains the 2005 neonatal flow algorithm. This algorithm remains unchanged for 2010 AHA guidelines. Progression from one step to another should be based on assessment of vital signs: respiration, heart rate, and color. A summary of important recommendations related to each step is included below.

Initial Steps in Stabilization

Temperature control

- Very low birth weight infants should be provided with additional warming using plastic wrapping or radiant heat. Careful monitoring should be performed to prevent hyperthermia.

Clearing the airway of meconium

- It is no longer advised to perform routine intrapartum suctioning of the airway (suctioning after delivery of the head but before delivery of the shoulders). While it was once routine to perform ETT intubation in infants with meconium staining of the amniotic fluid, and to provide suctioning from the ETT during tube withdrawal, this practice was shown to be of no significant benefit in otherwise vigorous infants (i.e., strong respiratory efforts, good muscle tone and a heart rate > 100 bpm).[32,33] ETT suctioning should be performed immediately after birth if signs of vigor do not accompany meconium staining.

Supplementary oxygen

- Supplementary oxygen is recommended whenever positive-pressure ventilation is indicated for resuscitation, while free-flow oxygen should be administered to infants who are breathing but have central cyanosis.
- There is not enough evidence to specify the concentration of oxygen to be used at initiation of resuscitation. If room air is administered, supplementary oxygen should be available to use if there is no appreciable improvement within 90 s after birth. The ability to achieve normoxia may be expedited by providing a variable concentration of oxygen while monitoring with pulse oximetry.

Ventilation

PPV should be administered if:

- The infant remains apneic or gasping.
- The heart rate remains <100 bpm 30 s after the initial steps, or
- The infant continues to have persistent central cyanosis despite receiving supplementary oxygen.

Initial breaths

- Assisted ventilation should be delivered at a rate of 40–60 breaths per minute to promptly achieve or maintain a heart rate >100 bpm. Prompt improvement in heart rate is the primary measure of adequate initial ventilation. If monitored, initial peak inflation pressure should be individualized; 20 cm H_2O may be effective in most infants but 30–40 cm H_2O may be required for some without spontaneous ventilation.

Ventilation devices

- A self-inflating, a flow-inflating bag, or a T-piece can be used to ventilate a newborn.
- Laryngeal mask airways (LMA) that fit over the laryngeal inlet have shown to be effective for ventilating newly born near-term and full-term infants. There is not enough evidence to support the routine use of LMAs as a primary airway device during resuscitation in cases where there is meconium-stained amniotic fluid, when chest compressions are required, in very low birth weight infants, or for delivery of emergency intratracheal medications.

Assisted ventilation of preterm infants

- Large-volume lung inflations should be avoided; these may be indicated through excessive chest wall movement and may be avoided with monitoring of pressure.

- If PPV is required, most preterm infants can be ventilated with an initial inflation pressure of 20–25 cm H_2O; higher pressures may be needed if there is no
  prompt improvement in heart rate or chest movements.
- BMV requires considerable practice before competency is achieved. Neonatal
  resuscitation is frequently done by individuals who are not exposed to BMV
  often enough to maintain their skills. In these cases, using the LMA may be a
  suitable alternative method of providing PPV.

ETT placement

Endotracheal intubation may be indicated:

- When tracheal suctioning for meconium is required.
- If BMV is ineffective or prolonged.
- When chest compressions are performed.
- When endotracheal administration of medications is desired.
- For special circumstances such as extremely low birth weight (<1,000 g) or
  congenital diaphragmatic hernia.

ETT placement must be assessed visually during intubation and by confirmatory
methods after intubation (e.g., exhaled CO_2 detection) if the heart rate remains low
or is not rising.

Chest Compressions

If the heart rate remains <60 bpm after adequate ventilation with supplementary
oxygen for 30 s, chest compressions are indicated. Optimal assisted ventilation
should be delivered prior to starting chest compressions.

- The compressions should be delivered on the lower third of the sternum to a
  depth of approximately one-third to one half the anterior–posterior diameter of
  the chest. The 2 thumb-encircling hands technique (Box 10.1 and Fig. 10.5) (the
  fingers encircling the chest and supporting the back) is recommended because it
  may generate higher peak systolic and coronary perfusion pressure.
- A 3:1 ratio of compressions to ventilations (120 events per minute) is recommended; there should not be simultaneous delivery and the chest should fully
  reexpand without removing the thumbs from the chest.

Medications or Volume Expansion

Administration of epinephrine or volume expansion may be indicated if the heart
rate remains <60 bpm despite adequate ventilation with 100% oxygen and chest
compressions.

- The IV route of epinephrine (1:10,000 [0.1 mg/ml]) should be used as soon as
  venous access is established; the recommended IV dose is 0.01–0.03 mg/kg per

Box 10.1

Thumb Method
The chest is encircled by both hands and the thumbs are applied side by side on the sternum on an imaginary line between the nipples. The fingers of both hands support the back. Only the *tips* of the thumbs should be used for compression lest rib fractures occur. In premature babies the thumbs may be superimposed upon one another.

Two-Finger Method
This may be used if the resuscitator's hands are too small or if access to the umbilicus is required. The tips of the index and middle fingers are applied to the sternum on an imaginary line between the nipples. The other hand supports the back (see Fig. 10.5).

Source: Data from American Heart Association[29]

dose. While access is being obtained, administration through an ETT (dose up to 0.1 mg/kg) may be considered.

- When blood loss is suspected or the infant appears to be in shock (while not responding to other resuscitative measures), volume expansion should be considered. An isotonic crystalloid (10 mg/kg) is preferred to albumin;[34, 35] its administration may need to be repeated and caution should be taken with respect to rate of expansion in premature infants (giving them too fast can lead to intraventricular hemorrhage).

These are the main recommendations outlined in the latest AHA guidelines. The guidelines should be read carefully with respect to the scientific background and details of the above recommendations and the additional guidelines with respect to postresuscitative care (including glucose monitoring and induced hypothermia) and withholding and discontinuing resuscitation.

The Neonatal Resuscitation Program

The neonatal resuscitation program (NRP) is a structured learning package and workshop supported by the American Heart Association and American Academy of Pediatrics (in Canada by the AHA and Heart and Stroke Foundation) to provide delivery-room care-providers a set of neonatal resuscitation guidelines. The NRP program workshops offer experience through simulations of the resuscitation steps, including endotracheal intubation. The modules are geared towards the entire HC team, although certain steps (i.e., administration of medications) will

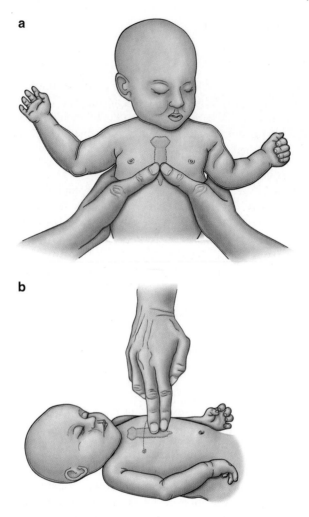

Fig. 10.5 Chest compression technique

only be performed by physicians. The syllabus is divided into six educational modules, each emphasizing a particular skill necessary for resuscitation success:

1. Preparation for delivery
2. Initial stabilization
3. Ventilation (BVM)
4. Chest compressions
5. Tracheal intubation
6. Medications

Airway Equipment

Most of the airway equipment used in adults is also available in pediatrics. The routine equipment is very similar to that used in adults except it is proportionally smaller. A comprehensive discussion of airway management equipment, including ultrasound imaging, can be found in Chap. 6. Following, is a brief explanation for pediatric versions of several airway devices.

The LMA is used routinely in pediatric practice now and is being incorporated into pediatric difficult airway algorithms. The cuffed oropharyngeal airway (COPA) is also available in pediatric sizes and adds a new dimension to the oropharyngeal airway (uncuffed and cuffed ETT are acceptable in infants and children). Fiberoptic-assisted intubation is being used more frequently in pediatric practice now that smaller-gauge fiberscopes (2.1 mm) have become available. Lighted stylets are now being used in difficult airway cases in pediatrics. A Bullard laryngoscope, adapted for pediatric use, is now available for challenging airways. The equipment discussed below will be used for resuscitation, as well as, routine and difficult endotracheal intubation during anesthesia.

Face Masks

Self-inflating bags of suitably reduced size are used in infants and children, although bags with at least 450–500 ml capacity are required for CPR to deliver an effective tidal volume and longer inspiratory times required by full-term neonates or infants. Using the right size mask is imperative and should be individualized to the patient. The mask must fit the patient's nasal bridge, include the mouth, and not obstruct the eyes of the patient. It should also provide a tight seal. Masks such as the Rendell-Baker, which was designed to fit the facial contours of children, will eliminate the mechanical dead space and thus optimize oxygenation.[36] Masks of several sizes should be available for all anesthetic procedures. Specially designed clear plastic face masks are recommended for fiberoptic intubation.[37]

Airways

Airways are used to displace the tongue in order to achieve ventilation without causing trauma to the oral cavity. Having access to an oropharyngeal airway (Guedel airways) of an appropriate size is important. An airway cart should contain two of each size of airway. Generally, the correct size of oral airway can be estimated as the distance from the angle of the mandible to the corner of their mouth. If too small, the airway may worsen obstruction by pushing the base of tongue against the posterior pharyngeal wall. Conversely, obstruction can result and ventilation can worsen if the airway is too big that it pushes the tip of the epiglottis;

laryngospasm may even result. While nasopharyngeal airways are generally tolerated in conscious children, oral airways will mostly require adequate anesthetic
depth prior to their insertion. In children under 8 years of age, the oropharyngeal
airway should be inserted from either corner of the mouth and rotated 90° as it is
inserted or by using a tongue depressor to hold the tongue while the airway is
inserted anatomically with the curvature of the patient's airway.

Nasopharyngeal airways of sizes 12–32 French should be available for use in
emergency life support as well as during anesthetic procedures (i.e., contained in
the difficult airway cart) in those cases of difficult access to the mouth. The length
of the device can be estimated by the distance between the angle of the mandible
and the nostrils. The tip of the tube is placed at the posterior pharynx, at least 1 cm
from the epiglottis; if placed lower, coughing and vomiting will be stimulated and
gases may be passed into the esophagus.

Laryngeal Mask Airway (LMA) and Other Supraglottic Devices

There are numerous devices for use as an option to the tracheal tube and the face
mask. Of these the LMA is the most commonly used, partly due to the availability
of evidence supporting its efficacy and safety. Additionally, this device allows for
hands-free technique as compared to using the face mask. While a significant benefit
for ventilation as compared to face masks has not been shown, their decreased invasiveness compared to the tracheal tube may be beneficial in certain situations (e.g.,
respiratory tract infection).[38] The supraglottic devices may not only be used during
routine anesthesia, but also for airway rescue after failed intubation, as a conduit for
tracheal intubation, and as an emergency airway device used by primary rescuers.

Use of the Classic LMA in children has demonstrated high first-time (90%) and
overall (99–100%) insertion rates and a fairly low rate (<11%) of serious complications.[38] The Classic, Proseal, and Flexible LMAs will be most suitable for use in
children and are available in sizes, i.e., sizes 1–3, for use in infants and children.
The Proseal contains an esophageal drainage tube for enabling protection from
aspiration, and the Flexible version (both reusable and single-use) is wire-reinforced
to enable head and neck surgery without losing a tight seal. The Proseal LMA has
been noted for facilitating good fiberoptic views of the larynx and has higher
oropharyngeal leak pressures compared to the Classic LMA. Its overall reception
in clinical use has been very promising.[39,40]

After preoxygenation and induction to a deep state (propofol is suitable in doses
of at least 4 mg/kg and analgesic coinduction is preferable), the LMA is inserted.
The original Brain Technique can be used for the Classic LMA insertion; guidance
of the Proseal LMA includes mounting it onto a gastric tube, introducing the gastric
tube with a laryngoscope and then letting the LMA slip in place via the gastric
tube.[41] Gum elastic bougie or suction catheter guided techniques may also be used.
Bite blocks are recommended to use with an LMA which does not integrate them
into their construction (except the Proseal LMA). The LMA can be used for resuscitation as well as in the normal and difficult airway populations for anesthesia.

Their use for anesthesia in neonates and infants may be associated with more complications, such as gastric insufflation (due to gas leakage) and laryngospasm, than in older children.[42,43] While outcomes appear positive with pediatric LMA use, there is some evidence of complications when using the smaller sizes, including postinsertion impingement of the epiglottis on the LMA bars.[44] Other complications associated with LMA use are easy displacement, partial or complete airway obstruction, laryngospasm (if insufficient anesthesia), and uvular, pharyngeal, and laryngeal trauma. It will be difficult to use in patients who have malformations of the oral cavity, copious secretions, or hypertrophied tonsils.

In patients for whom intubation is difficult due to facial malformations, the use of an LMA may be very useful for the blind passage of the ETT or during fiberoptic intubation. The intubating LMA (Fastrach LMA) allows blind insertion of a tracheal tube in children over 25 kg (available in size 3 and up only), though caution should be taken to avoid damaging the epiglottis.[45,46] Fiberoptic examination can confirm the correct positioning of the intubating LMA and the use of the Classic or Proseal LMA during fiberoptic intubation is useful to easily achieve ventilation.[47] (Trying to thread the ETT through the Classic LMA can be challenging and tube dislodgement often occurs). The passage of the LMA is a good conduit for the flexible bronchoscope.

Other supraglottic devices may be useful in children. The Cobra Perilaryngeal Airway (CobraPLA; see Chap. 6 for details) may be inserted easily and efficiently, although reports of high rates (77%) of epiglottic folding,[48] causing laryngeal obstruction, and gastric insufflation can occur and this device offers no protection from regurgitation or aspiration. The i-gel and LMA Supreme are not currently available (fall 2009) in pediatric sizes, although this is expected to change. Benefits of the LMA Supreme are that it can be inserted without any introducer and has the ability to achieve high seal pressures. The reader is referred to the discussion of the Difficult Pediatric Airway in this section for more on the LMA.

T-Piece

To avoid confusion, we will consider only one anesthesia circuit, the T-piece. The T-piece is a valved mechanical device designed to control flow and limit pressure. Introduced in 1937 by Ayre, this device can deliver oxygen or anesthetic gases to an infant or child in such a way that carbon dioxide retention is virtually eliminated. There have been a number of modifications, the most notable being the addition of a bag (the Jackson-Rees modification).[49,50] The T-piece is quite versatile in that it can be used to administer anesthesia to an infant or child in the operating room or during transport to the ward or ICU, for neonatal resuscitation, or whenever the patient needs respiratory assistance for any reason. In resuscitation, T-piece devices consistently achieve target inflation pressures and long inspiratory times.[28] To prevent rebreathing of carbon dioxide, a flow 2.5 times the minute volume should be used. Therefore, from a practical and economic standpoint, the system should not be applied to children weighing more than 20 kg (44 lb).

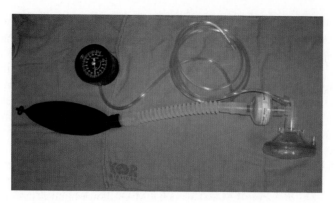

Fig. 10.6 The Jackson-Rees modification of an Ayre T-piece

The modified Ayre T-piece (Mapleson F) consists of a small piece of corrugated tubing about 18 in. long to which a 1-l reservoir bag is attached (Fig. 10.6). The volume of this tube should be at least 75% of the predicted tidal volume. A valve may be placed at the distal end of the tube, or, alternatively, a deliberate leak may be left in the bag to vent any excessive buildup of gases in the system. A right-angle outlet or plastic adapter is attached to the corrugated tubing at its proximal end. Gas enters the right-angle connector via a hollow adapter. The proximal end of the right-angle adapter fits onto any 15-mm connector (mask or endotracheal) tube. The right-angle connector should also have a fitting that allows the attachment of a manometer for monitoring airway pressures. The T-piece, with minor variations, is one of the most common circuits used for manual ventilation of pediatric patients.

Intubation Equipment

The equipment required for intubation in infants is basically the same as that for children and adults, except that a greater variety of ETT sizes and laryngoscope blades should be available when dealing with children. An ETT that fits too tightly can result in decreased mucosal perfusion and subsequent edema.[37] Three ETTs should always be immediately available – the predicted size, one size larger, and one size smaller. When difficulties arise, crucial time may be lost searching for the correct-sized tube, and technical difficulties often do arise from selecting the inappropriate equipment.

Blade Selection

Two working laryngoscopes should always be available for routine anesthesia. The infant's large occiput, the low concavity of their skull (to the age of 6 years), and their relatively large tongue, make the use of curved blades largely unsuitable.[4] They may obscure the view of the larynx. Straight blades are preferred in young children. Since the larynx is located more superiorly and the epiglottis lies at an angle of 45°, these blades directly lift the epiglottis and improve visualization of the vocal cords. The blade should be small enough to enable tracheal tube insertion. The Miller or Wisconsin straight blade is generally the most commonly used blade, although other blades including the Seward, the Cardiff (combining curved and straight blade features), the McCoy (incorporating a lever system) are available and may be useful.[51]

ETT Selection

Tube site (internal diameter in mm) is usually selected on the basis of the child's age in years. The size of tube selected should not be the largest possible, but rather the smallest which will form a good seal. Following is a useful formula to determine the correct size when using uncuffed ETTs for children:

$$(\text{Age in years}/4) + 4 = \text{Inner diameter in mm}$$

When using cuffed tubes, select a tube of 1–2 sizes smaller than that calculated for the uncuffed tube. It can be challenging to determine which size to use for newborns; generally a size 2.5 is used for < 1 kg, size 3 for 1–2 kg, and 3.5 for 2–3 kg. Two other formulas are used to determine how far the tube should be advanced into the trachea:

$$Oral: 12 + \frac{\text{Age}}{2} = \text{tube length (in cm)} \quad Nasal: 15 + \frac{\text{Age}}{2} = \text{tube length (in cm)}$$

Until recently, cuffed tubes were not recommended for use in children less than 8 years of age. This was due to the need for smaller (1–2 sizes) tube sizes enabling the passage of the cuff through the larynx (thus increasing flow resistance in the spontaneously breathing patient), and reports of laryngeal and tracheal mucosal injury caused by overinflation of high-pressure/low-volume cuffs during prolonged intubation in ICU settings. The times are changing and the use of cuffed tubes is becoming more common.[52] Advantages that cuffed tubes might provide include: a reduction in the number of intubation attempts via use of smaller diameter tubes (inflation can accommodate for leaks); the option of providing low or minimal-flow anesthesia or high-pressure ventilation and respective monitoring in certain cases; and the reduction in risk for perioperative tracheal aspiration.[37] They can offer a sealed airway without the use of oversized uncuffed tracheal tubes and reduce the discharge of anesthetic gases.[53] If using cuffed tubes, the intracuff inflation pressure should be monitored continuously. Some authors suggest that these tubes will be preferable when the patient is expected to remain intubated in the postoperative period, such that ventilation and extubation may become easier via the ability to progressively increase the leak around the tube.[16] A new ETT (Microcuff GmbH, Weinheim, Germany) with an ultrathin high-volume, low-pressure polyurethane cuff has shown to provide tracheal sealing with cuff pressures considerably lower than usually accepted.[54]

Flexible Fiberoptic Bronchoscope

Fiberoptic bronchoscopes are available in sizes appropriate for infants and older children, although those small enough to fit infants (size 3.0 or lower) generally do not have a channel for suctioning, application of topical anesthesia, or continuous oxygen flow. The placement of small tubes (e.g., 25 mm ID) may require modified technique, such as using one small bronchoscope to carry the ETT while the biopsy channel of another is used for application of topical anesthesia and oxygen flow.[55] More discussion of technique is included later in this chapter's discussion of Difficult Airways and in Section B.

Rigid Bronchoscopes

Rigid bronchoscopes are not used frequently in children and there are few devices available. These may be beneficial to view difficult anatomy, especially for the experienced operator who finds them easy to use. The lateral illumination provides excellent viewing of the larynx, with superior resolution to the frontal view provided by the flexible fiberscope. Since the technique will require general anesthesia, it is imperative to ensure the patient's airway has been fully evaluated. The small rigid bronchoscopes can mount an ETT and be used for cases of difficulty especially with upper airway pathology. The Bonfils intubation fiberscope has been used with poor success, although the additional use of a laryngoscope may greatly improve the outcome.[56] Section B of this chapter discusses some cases where rigid bronchoscopy may be utilized.

Light Wand

Although proper alignment of the airway axes may improve success when using light wands for intubation, using a light wand can circumvent the need for alignment of the airway in patients with limited movement of the cervical spine or limited mouth opening.[57] This fiberoptic stylet with its lighted tip uses transillumination as a guide for intubation – a bright, well circumscribed glow indicates tracheal placement, whereas a diffuse glow indicates esophageal placement. Several variations are available, although rigid ones are easier to manipulate into correct shape than those that are more malleable. The ETT is carried by a lubricated light wand (keeping the wand short of the tube length by a few millimeters), which is bent to the shape of a hockey stick (90–120°) and advance in the midline while remaining anterior.[3,57] A railroad technique is used for advancing the tube off the light wand. A benefit of the light wand over the fiberoptic intubation is the ability to intubate in the presence of secretions or blood. However, its use does require dimmed room lights and midline laryngeal structures. An anterior jaw lift to elevate the epiglottis may improve success.[57] Smaller ETTs are easier to place than larger ones.

Other Devices for Intubation

Many devices which facilitate or enable direct or indirect visualization of the larynx are available. There are many adapted laryngoscopes developed for use in difficult airways that may be useful in children, with one example being the McCoy laryngoscope. The Belscope may be particularly useful in older children for performing intubation in the presence of a large and occluding tongue. The Shikani Seeing/Optical Stylet is available in pediatric sizes. Fiberoptic and video laryngoscopes (e.g., Bullard and GlideScope) are also available. The reader is referred to Chap. 6 for discussion, including that of pediatric use, of these advanced devices for airway management.

Techniques For Bag-Valve-Mask Ventilation

Bag-valve-mask ventilation (BMV) is the method of choice for children who require ventilatory support in out-of-hospital settings where transport times are short.[28] Self-inflating bags of suitably reduced size are used in infants and children, although bags with at least 450–500 mL capacity are required to deliver an effective tidal volume and longer inspiratory times required by full-term neonates or infants. To the novice, mask ventilation in a child can be quite challenging. The best results are obtained by placing the head in a neutral position (i.e., neither flexion nor extension of the neck) and using one hand to maintain the airway. Excessive pressure should not be exerted in the submental area, because this tends to force the tongue backward toward the posterior pharyngeal wall and creates additional obstruction. Occasionally, both hands will be required to pull the mandible forward. In this situation an assistant may be necessary, especially if the child is apneic. Using the right size mask is imperative and should be individualized to the patient. Masks such as the Rendell-Baker, which have been designed to fit the facial contours of children, will eliminate mechanical dead space.[36] Specially designed clear plastic face masks are recommended for fiberoptic intubation.[37] A summary of the steps to take in a situation of failed mask ventilation is included in Difficult Pediatric Airways of this section.

Techniques of Routine Endotracheal Intubation in Infants and Children

The indications and techniques of endotracheal intubation in children are much the same as those already discussed in adults. Good intubating conditions can result without the use of muscle relaxants, and there should be an evaluation of the risks and benefits of muscle relaxation during intubation, especially in infants.[37,58] Awake intubation was frequently used in infants up to about 6 weeks who presented with pyloric stenosis or intestinal obstruction. Most pediatric anesthesiologists prefer to administer general anesthesia in these cases today. Adolescents may agree to, and be suitable for, awake techniques. Sufficient sedation (e.g., IV ketamine) will be a necessity if awake intubations are attempted. Blind nasotracheal intubation is not recommended in children less than 8–10 years of age, due to anatomic variations: one being the presence of enlarged adenoidal tissue in the nasopharynx, and the other being the acute glottic opening.[59] Fiberoptic intubation is discussed in Difficult Pediatric Airway, found in this section.

Premedication and Induction of Anesthesia

- Premedication is required for awake intubations, although may also be valuable if used prior to induction of anesthesia, especially if there is separation from the child's parents.
- Oral or intravenous midazolam is commonly used for sedation.
- Obtaining an adequate plane of anesthesia while maintaining spontaneous ventilation will be most likely when using inhalation induction. During anesthesia, upper airway obstruction may occur due to relaxation of the airway muscles. Jaw thrusts and proper head positioning should relieve the obstruction, although oral or nasal airways may be required for some cases.

Position

- Place the infant supine with the head resting on a donut-shaped foam pad.
- Before proceeding, deliver oxygen for 1–2 min.
- The infant's neck is then slightly extended by an assistant. Overextension may lead to airway obstruction by flattening the trachea. To further stabilize the head, the assistant should hold it between the palms of both hands. The shoulders can be stabilized by having the assistant press down on them with the ulnar borders of both hands.

Exposure

- Open the infant's mouth using the fingers of the right hand and extend the atlantooccipital joint.
- Using a jaw thrust may help improve visualization of the airway structures.

Visualization

- Hold the laryngoscope in the left hand and introduce the chosen blade (often straight) at the right side of the mouth and advance slowly.

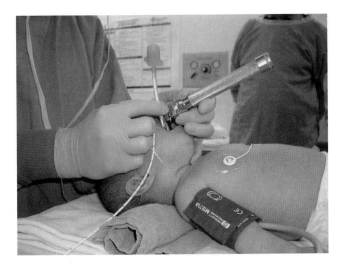

Fig. 10.7 Manual pressure with the little finger may improve visualization of the airway

- Make an effort to recognize anatomic structures as the laryngoscope blade is advanced.
- When the epiglottis is seen, advance the blade beyond the inferior surface and pull the blade forward to slowly withdraw it. The arytenoids first come into view and then the glottis becomes visible. Occasionally, the epiglottis will drop down beneath the tip of the blade. If this happens, advance the blade again, applying slight manual pressure over the hyoid bone with the little finger of the left hand (Fig. 10.7).

Tube Placement

- Insert the ETT and advance it to the midtracheal region.
- An assistant can pull on the right corner of the mouth to allow more room to maneuver the tube.
- Proper depth of ETT can be estimated by multiplying the size of the tube by three (e.g., 4 mm tube should be placed at 12 cm at the tip).

Confirmation

- Clinical assessment and capnography should be used together to confirm tube placement.
- Listen for breath sounds over the stomach and the thorax. Gurgling sounds over the stomach indicate esophageal intubation. Reduced breath sounds over the left, as compared to right, hemithorax may indicate the tube is placed too deep.[1]

If using cuffed tubes, the correctly placed ETT cuff should be felt within the suprasternal notch.[3] The tip of the ETT can move as much as 2 cm during flexion and extension of the head, making it important to auscultate the lung fields every time the head is moved.[2]

- A pediatric end-tidal CO_2 detector should be used if the child is ≤15 kg.

Stabilization and Monitoring

- The tube should be carefully stabilized as previously described.
- The DOPE mnemonic–dislodgement, obstruction, pneumothorax, and equipment– can be recalled to suggest potential ventilation problems. Hand ventilation with 100% oxygen can rule out ventilator issues; auscultation can assess for tube dislodgement; tube kinking or secretions can obstruct the tube and tube suctioning should be performed.

Summary

Tracheal intubation is usually quite an easy procedure in infants and children. Difficult intubation is not as prevalent as in adults. It is important to conduct a proper evaluation and to have all of the necessary and appropriate-sized equipment available. Infants and children desaturate more quickly than adults, so it is important to be well prepared and to have a contingency plan for encountering difficulties with mask ventilation or intubation.

Laryngospasm

Many difficulties can arise in the context of tracheal intubation, many of which are described in detail in Chap. 15. Laryngospasm is included here because of its onerous consequences for younger individuals, especially those between 1 and 3 months of age who desaturate very quickly. Moreover, upper respiratory infections are highly associated (95.8/1,000) with the development of laryngospasm. Although several mechanisms have been described for laryngospasm, the resulting implication is that either the true vocal cords or both the true and false cords have become approximated in the midline to close the glottis and prevent air flow.[2] Laryngospasm often occurs after stimulation of the airway during ventilation or intubation attempts in a lightly anesthetized patient (via sensitizing laryngeal reflexes); although other stimuli that may trigger laryngospasm include chemical irritation of the mucosa by blood secretions or vomitus, visceral pain reflexes, or premature extubation. The higher incidence of laryngospasm in infants 1–3 months of age may be reflective of

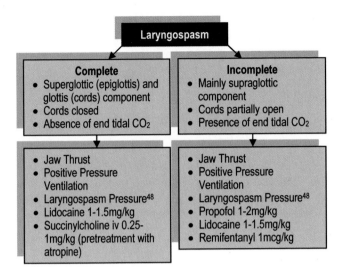

Fig. 10.8 Classification and treatment options of laryngospasm

the tendency for palato-laryngeal engagement (see the earlier section in this Chapter on Distinct Relationship between the Tongue, Pharynx and Larynx in the Infant).[60,61] It is important to distinguish between incomplete and complete laryngospasm, since treatment options may be different (Fig. 10.8). It usually manifests rapidly with desaturation and strenuous respiratory efforts and is ineffectively treated with PPV (regardless of the failure of PPV, many anesthesiologists will apply this technique since on cessation of laryngospasm, oxygen will be delivered immediately).

The best treatment is prevention. There are many pharmacological techniques such as administering IV lidocaine or magnesium prior to extubation, but success with these techniques is limited.[62-64] Nonpharmacological techniques include the "no touch" technique, which is very effective. This technique involves turning patients to the lateral (recovery) position at the end of their procedure, while they are still under adequate anesthetic depth.[65] Inhalation anesthetics are then discontinued and positive ventilation with 100% oxygen is maintained until spontaneous ventilation returns. No further stimulation, besides continuous oximetry monitoring, is allowed until the patients spontaneously wakes up. Tracheal extubation is performed when patients are able to open their eyes.

If laryngospasm does occur, treatment for complete laryngospasm usually includes jaw thrust at the angle of the mandible during PPV with 100% oxygen by BMV and administration of a neuromuscular blocking drug with an anticholinergic pretreatment (atropine before succinylcholine 0.25–1 mg/kg IV) and lidocaine (1–1.5 mg/kg). One technique which is considered by Larson[66] as the best treatment of laryngospasm is the application of a jaw thrust while applying firm bilateral pressure with middle fingers at the cephalad portion of the laryngospasm notch (located behind the lobule of the pinna of each ear), directed inward toward the base of the skull. Oxygen should be administered during the technique. When properly performed, laryngospasm is converted to laryngeal stridor and then to unobstructed respirations. It is believed that this technique works, possibly because of the painful stimulus to the ramus of the mandible, the facial nerve, and perhaps the deep lobe of the parotid gland.

Intubation Trauma

A recent review of airway trauma cases noted that the cause is almost always iatrogenic in nature.[67] Physical evidence of intubation trauma, not always accompanied by clinical signs such as stridor or voice change, includes: stenosis, inflammation and ulceration of the mucosa, submucosal hematoma, necrotic mucosa, granulation tissue which may cause tissue bridging between the vocal chords, and/or complete airway obstructing scar-formation. Intubation injury is mostly due to poor tube selection (oversized and/or overly stiff), and inadequate placement of tubes, as well as, by inappropriate intubation technique and tube dislocation. Solutions lie in a thorough understanding of the pediatric airway and how it differs from the adult airway, as well as, more training for anesthesiologists on endoscopic practices so that they can use simple rigid endoscopes for diagnosis of difficult intubation and airway injury.

The functional significance of the airway comes into play again when considering the etiology of intubation trauma. Until recently, it was thought that the cricoid ring was the smallest point within the pediatric larynx (Eckenhoff's classic article is commonly cited for this although the work of Bayeux in 1897 was the original study).[14] These measurements were based on plasters and anatomical sections of cadavers, the preparation of which may have stretched the laryngeal structures superior to the rigid cricoid cartilage. Moreover, mortuary specimens in neonates may poorly represent thriving infants, since a small cricoid ring size has been correlated to early infant death.[68] Recent investigations in both paralyzed (using video bronchoscopic imaging) and spontaneously breathing (using MRI) patients have found conflicting results, with the joint conclusion that the larynx is in fact not funnel-shaped (with no changes in shape during development) and the level of the glottis measures smallest in both sets of patients.[69, 70] The cricoid "ring" is, in fact, elliptically-shaped. Ultimately, though, the level of most concern will still be that of the cricoid cartilage due to its unyielding, rigid nature, whereas the vocal cords can be distended. This level is "functionally the narrowest portion of the larynx".[70] This will be most critical during prolonged intubation in the intensive care setting where spontaneous breathing is maintained and there will be continual movements around the tube. Besides the above discussed functional anatomy of the epiglottis during infancy, this is another good example of how the functional, in addition to the structural, anatomy is important to consider when evaluating the effects of developmental anatomy on anesthetic practices.

If intubation trauma is suspected, early endoscopic examination of the airway should take place, as early treatment improves outcomes. Newly developed granulation tissue can be reversed with local injection of corticoid crystals, while more solidly developed scar tissue (9–12 months of development) requires time consuming surgical intervention such as tracheolaryngeal resection and stenting. Holzki et al.[67] also note that the cuffed vs. uncuffed pediatric tube debate is not completely solved and that more evidence based, controlled, photo-documented studies are needed to support the correct use and design of cuffed tubes.

Difficult Pediatric Airway

Definition and Classifications

The definition of the difficult airway for children will be the same as for adults: a clinical situation in which a conventionally trained anesthesiologist experiences difficulty with face-mask ventilation of the upper airway, difficulty with tracheal intubation, or both.[71] There are numerous airway problems which will be faced in pediatrics, and although progressive or sudden airway obstruction from causes such as infectious diseases and foreign body aspiration, respectively, will often be considered within the difficult airway category, this text will describe the difficult airway as one in which the main issues are anatomical abnormalities, often associated with congenital or acquired syndromes, which lead to difficult ventilation by face mask or difficult direct laryngoscopy. While these patients may certainly present with chronic obstruction, those patients with progressive or sudden obstruction will be considered in the discussion on Upper Airway Obstruction in the Child, later in this section.

The difficult pediatric airway is rare; usually the airway is just different than the adult airway. Despite this, there is an age distribution seen, with difficult intubation in infants less than 1 year of age reported as 5.3 times greater than in children above this age.[72] The main classifications presented here will be related to whether the difficulty is anticipated or not; regardless, it is imperative to consider planning and preparation for both. Anticipation of a difficult airway in the child will come from a careful history of past anesthesia, targeted physical examination, and identification of patient history as it relates to airway obstruction (e.g., snoring, apnea, daytime somnolence). Many of the factors that are associated with adult difficult airways are not typically present in the child, a few examples being beards, edentulousness, and kyphosis.[16] Anticipation of difficultly with face-mask ventilation will result from the confirmation of a history of snoring, previous anesthetic problems, apnea, daytime somnolence, stridor, hoarse voice, and sleep position. Intubation difficulty expectations will be more related to the physical examination.

Physical examination includes evaluation of:

- Size and shape of head
- Gross facial features
- Size and symmetry of mandible

- Size of tongue
- Prominence of upper incisors
- Range of motion in the jaw, head, and neck

Protruding teeth, limited mouth opening and micrognathia are highly suggestive of difficult laryngoscopy.[73]

Congenital or Acquired Abnormalities Associated with Airway Difficulty

There are several congenital syndromes which are associated with head, neck and cervical spine anomalies and that can complicate the pediatric airway (Table 10.3).[3, 15] Some of the abnormalities can also be acquired, examples include temporomandibular joint dysfunction from trauma (e.g., forceps delivery) or inflammation or microstomia from burns and caustic lesions.

There are also many congenital and acquired causes of airway obstruction, but this will be addressed later in this section of the chapter. Below is a summary of several issues that may arise when attempting mask ventilation or intubation in patients with these malformations. Some approaches to overcome difficulties will be outlined. Otherwise, basic strategies for failed mask ventilation and tracheal intubation are presented under Clinical Scenarios and Strategies. The reader is referred to Marraro's[74] summary of congenital and acquired malformations contributing to the difficult airway in pediatrics.

- Children with craniofacial dysostosis have high arched palates and small nasal passages, leading them to primarily rely on mouth breathing. Occlusion of their oral airway occurs with mouth closure; obstructive apnea can occur due to the high resistance to airflow via the small nares. Preservation of spontaneous ventilation will be paramount.
- Face mask ventilation will be challenging in patients with hemifacial hypoplasia or other distortions in facial features. In this situation the use of an alternative ventilation device (e.g., LMA) may be very beneficial.
- Any condition where there is limited anterior mandibular space (e.g., Pierre-Robin and Treacher-Collins syndromes), relative to the size of the tongue, will make laryngoscopy and tracheal intubation difficult. Intubation through an intubating LMA or with fiberoptics may be necessary.
- Tongue hyperplasia and/or mandibular/maxillary hypoplasia (either will limit the mass ratio of tongue to space), can increase the chance of airway obstruction. Curved blades may assist and allow direct laryngoscopy in patients with large tongues (macroglossia), although direct laryngoscopy may be nearly impossible in some patients with mandibular hypoplasia. Mask ventilation should not be attempted in patients with macroglossia. Oral airways may be effective to maintain airway patency. The use of an alternative device (e.g., LMA) or tracheal intubation may be necessary. The Bullard rigid, fiberoptic laryngoscope may be useful and will usually require the use a stylet or bougie.

Table 10.3 Features of congenital syndromes associated with difficult airways

Anomaly	Syndrome
Ankylosis (temporomandibular joint)	Anthrogryposis, Cocayane
Atlanto-occipital instability	Trisomy 21
Cleft lip and palate	Pierre-Robin, Treacher-Collins
Craniofacial dysostosis (midface hypoplasia, proptosis, high and arched palate and small nasal passages)	Apert, Crouzon, Pfeiffer's
Glossoptosis	Pierre-Robin
Hyperplasia of jaw	Ramon or cherubism
Limited cervical mobility (due to fused or hemivertebrae, neck contractures, joint instabilities)	Klippel–Feil, Juvenile-onset rheumatoid arthritis, Goldenhar's, Freeman–Sheldon, Trisomy 21 (antlanto-axial instability)
Macrocephaly	Hydrocephalus
Macroglossia	Trisomy 21, Beckwith–Wiedemann, Hurler (congenital mucopolysaccharidosis), hypothyroidism, heme- and lymphangiomas of the tongue
Mandibular hypoplasia (often associated with reduced nose–pharynx space) and micrognathia (or retrognathia)	Pierre-Robin, Carpenter, Goldenhar, Crouzon, Freeman–Sheldon, Treacher-Collins (mandibulofacial dysostosis), Stickler's
Maxillary hypoplasia	Apert's, Treacher-Collins
Microsomia	Goldenhar's
Microstomia (reduced mouth opening)	Freeman–Sheldon (whistling face syndrome), Hallermann–Streiff, oto-palatodigital syndromes
Obstructed airway from masses	Neurofibromatosis, Sturge–Weber
Palatoschisis	Pierre-Robin, Treacher-Collins, Goldenhar, Klippel–Feil
Protruding incisors	Cocayane Syndrome
Pharyngomalacia	Trisomy 21
Vocal cord paralysis	Arnold–Chiari, hydrocephalus, encephalocele
Zygomatic hypoplasia	Treacher-Collins

Source: Data from Infosino,[3] Kundra,[15] Brambrink,[37] and Marraro[74]

- It may be difficult to ventilate patients with microsomia (Goldenhar's) using a face mask. Likewise, laryngoscopy may be difficult especially if there is restriction in mouth opening via contractures after past surgery. Ventilation with an LMA or nasal fiberoptic intubation are options.
- Microstomia (reduced opening of the mouth) makes laryngoscopy and endotracheal intubation difficult. Various devices may be considered for ventilation (e.g., nasopharyngeal airways) or intubation (i.e., those which will facilitate intubation with reduced mouth opening; see Chap. 6).
- Any limitation to cervical spine or temporomandibular joint movement can make visualization of the larynx challenging. Intubating patients who have had previous reconstructive surgery may be limited by contractures which limit neck movement. Intubation using a nasal fiberoptic bronchoscope or light wand is a good option. Other intubation devices which minimize cervical movement (e.g., some fiberoptic or video laryngoscopes) may also be considered.

- Glossopexy (tongue sutured to lip) may be necessary in patients with glossoptosis, where the tongue is displaced rostrally to lie at the roof of the mouth.
- Hurler's syndrome (congenital mucopolysaccharidosis) leads to tongue enlargement, soft tissue thickening, and blockage of nasal passages. There is often a history of snoring. Primary goals for these patients are to preserve spontaneous breathing and, when necessary, to intubate via fiberoptic intubation. The intubating LMA will be an option for use during fiberoptic intubation. Unfortunately, progressive airway obstruction can lead to severe respiratory distress which can be untreatable.

The use of the LMA may be an effective method for maintaining patency of the airway, although there may be risks associated with their use. Particularly noteworthy for many of these patients who may also be susceptible to airway obstruction, adequate anesthesia must be provided to avoid laryngospasm which would greatly worsen the scenario.

Anesthetic Management and Induction Technique

Planning is the most important process for managing the difficult airway patient. The anesthetic plan will be largely influenced by the patient physical examination and history, although will also be guided by the surgical procedure and several factors related to the anesthesiologist's experience and familiarity with the available equipment. The speed with which the pediatric patient can desaturate during challenging situations should prompt the anesthesiologist to carefully evaluate each patient to accurately anticipate whether difficulties will arise and generally plan for unforeseen issues regardless of their likelihood. Experience with the normal airway prior to any attempt to deal with a difficult one is paramount and oftentimes additional expertise will be called upon when the difficult airway is suspected. Apart from preparing equipment in a manner to deal with both difficult ventilation and intubation, and preparing the patient in a manner to best facilitate the anesthetic procedures (i.e., careful positioning with props including shoulder rolls/bolster and a pillow to maintain some cervical flexion and atlanto-occipital extension), the induction technique will need to be tailored to the specific needs of the patient. The anesthetic plan should be thoroughly discussed with both the patient (and their parents) as well as the entire surgical team; it should also be well documented. The benefit of the planned surgery should always be weighed against the possible risks of the anesthetic management.[75]

Induction Technique

The main objectives for induction in the difficult airway situation are maintaining spontaneous ventilation and achieving a plane of anesthesia that will enable laryngoscopy. Adequate time for visualization of the structures and performing intubation is essential. Some key considerations are:

- Induction should be smooth and gradual, with the ability to safely abort if alternative plans fail.
- Sedative agents are well known to cause loss of airway muscle tone and to increase airway resistance. In some cases, a smooth induction will be impossible without a small sedative regime, such as oral midazolam 0.3–0.5 mg/kg.
- Atropine (oral 30–40 μg/kg or IM 20 μg/kg) or glycopyrronium are often used to dry secretions and support heart rate during induction.
- While inhalation induction is often the technique of choice due to the ease of maintenance of spontaneous ventilation and avoidance of sedation, there are disadvantages including risks of apnea, laryngospasm, and airway loss.[16] This technique will not be suitable if the face mask does not fit the patient.
- Sevoflurane allows for spontaneous ventilation and easy reversal of anesthetic effects,[76] although propofol and remifentanil can preserve spontaneous ventilation (90% or more of patients will breathe spontaneously with remifentanil 0.05 μg/kg/min) and this drug offers an ultrashort half-life and easy titration.[77] Carefully titrated ketamine 1–2 mg/kg will also work. Often IV induction will commence and sevoflurane will be added to deepen the plane of anesthesia.
- Regardless of whether induction is performed via the inhalation or intravenous route, an intravenous line should be in place prior to airway instrumentation to ensure access for medication to manage the plane of anesthesia.
- Careful consideration should be given to proper mask ventilation technique to ensure the patient's airway does not become obstructed (e.g., covering the nose can be very stressful for the infant).
- In the case of airway obstruction, the patient can be moved to a lateral position and a jaw thrust applied.

Clinical Strategies for Difficult Ventilation and Intubation

Strategies to Overcome Difficulties with Failed Mask Ventilation

- Generally, if mask ventilation has failed on first attempt, the *mask position and seal* should be evaluated.
- Usually, repositioning of the mask or fingers, a change of mask size or type, and ensuring the circuit is continuous will be sufficient, although *additions steps including chin lift jaw thrust or CPAP* may be required.

  – The chin lift reverses the posterior displacement of the epiglottis due to gravity and widens the pharyngeal cavity. One hand is used to lift the inferior border of the mental protuberance to connect the teeth without protruding the mandible. The thumb and first finger form a C-shape to hold the mask while the ring finger performs the lift. Large adenoids and tonsils may limit the efficacy of this maneuver in opening the airway.[78]

- – The mouth can be forced open with a jaw thrust, which requires two hands pulling the mandibular angles upward and anterior. This technique is recommended when the chin lift is not successful.[22] It can also be used to confirm an adequate depth of anesthesia for LMA insertion. LMAs should be avoided in patients with upper airway masses, which will be pushed into the pharynx.
- – CPAP (e.g., 10 cm H_2O) increases the volume and area of the airways. High pressures should be avoided because of the related increase work of breathing, decrease in respiratory compliance and impaired venous return to the heart.

- If adequate gas exchange maintenance is not possible despite these maneuvers, an *oral or nasal airway should be inserted* to hold the tongue forward and relieve obstruction by the lips, teeth, and nose. If the oral airway is too large, however, it may actually cause obstruction (by forcing the epiglottis down over the glottis) or obstruct venous or lymphatic drainage (leading to swelling); and if too small, it may cause obstruction by pushing the tongue backward. The distance between the mouth and the angle of the mandible is a rough guide to the size of airway which will be suitable.[37] Furthermore, a poorly positioned airway can induce pressure necrosis of the tongue.
- If oral airway insertion fails, either *treatment of laryngospasm or bronchospasm* will be necessary, or a *two-person technique* will be warranted.
- The use of an *LMA or other supraglottic airway (e.g., I-gel, SLIPA, COPA)* may be a good choice if the above strategies are not successful.

Strategies to Overcome Difficulties with Tracheal Intubation

Either conventional direct laryngoscopy or an alternative management strategy may be attempted for children with an anticipated difficult airway. An attempt to maintain an extraglottic airway is suitable if the surgery does not require endotracheal intubation. Upon failure of the extraglottic airway, laryngoscopy may be attempted, usually with a straight blade. Prediction of poor viewing during direct laryngoscopy by way of Mallampati classification and anatomical measurements has been shown inaccurate.[15] Performing the intubation in an awake patient (e.g., via fiberoptic intubation) is preferable, although oftentimes anesthesia is needed to be induced and attempting direct laryngoscopy will be reasonable so long as alternative approaches are sought before trauma to the upper airway ensues.[3] In some cases, techniques such as retrograde intubation or cricothyrotomy may be required. A significant number of patients requiring tracheostomies are those with craniofacial anomalies.[79]

In those patients where there is unexpected difficulty, the following steps are suggested[3,16,75]:

1. *Obtain help.*
2. *Maintain ventilation* – if ventilation is not adequate refer to the above strategies. Proceeding with general anesthesia using an LMA may be suitable, depending on the situation.

3. *Reattempt to intubate* with direct laryngoscopy – *optimize patient position* ("sniffing position" with cervical spine flexion, atlanto-occipital extension and chin above sternum), if inadequate consider using *a different blade* (perhaps a McCoy levering or a video laryngoscope such as the GlideScope) or *technique* (a paraglossal[80] or retromolar/right molar[81] approaches may help in infants with their large tongue to space ratio, and involves advancing the blade from the lateral pharyngeal wall), *a stylet or BURP.*
4. *Place LMA* and /or;
5. Proceed to (a) *light wand intubation,* (b) *fiberoptic intubation,* or (c) *intubation through LMA* or other supraglottic device.
6. Limit the number of attempts at intubation to four in order to minimize morbidity.
7. Failed intubation – wake patient up or place a surgical airway (in emergency).

Airway equipment preparations for those cases where there is anticipation of some difficulty should include:

- Various face masks and oropharyngeal airways.
- Two laryngoscopes with straight blades of varying lengths and widths (the McCoy levering may be suitable).
- Multiple ETTs with lubricated intubating stylets preloaded and prepared.
- LMAs of number 1 and 2.
- Appropriate intubating devices (e.g., Fastrach LMA (intubating), lightwand (Trachlight) pediatric Bullard laryngoscope, Glidescope, and infant fiberoptic intubation scope) – all loaded, tested, and lubricated (where appropriate).
- Surgical tracheostomy tray and uncuffed cricothyrotomy set for percutaneous cricothyrotomy.

The application of various alternate laryngoscope blades or modified laryngoscopes (e.g., McCoy, Bullard) may improve intubation success with the difficult airway. An LMA has been used successfully in children as a conduit for endoscopic intubation. In fact, an LMA should be available in all cases of pediatric airway management, particularly when anticipating a difficulty. Flexible or rigid fiberscopes may be used for performing fiberoptic intubation. Lastly, a light wand may be used when direct laryngoscopy or even the fiberoptic bronchoscope has failed. See the equipment section of this chapter for details on devices and their techniques.

Fiberoptic Intubation Techniques

Fiberoptic intubation is viable in infants and neonates due to the development of ultrathin flexible bronchoscopes (2.2–2.5 mm). Adequate time is required for obtaining optimal visibility, thus good oxygenation and deep inhalation anesthesia should be maintained. Adequate topical anesthesia of the airway, especially the larynx, should be provided and all equipment should be available. Nasal or oral routes can be used. Nasal will not only generally be reserved for patients with limited mouth opening or temporomandibular joint rigidity, but also when the surgical access will be optimized. Vasoconstriction will be necessary to limit bleeding and further failure with intubation. A nasal airway placed in the opposite nostril can be used to maintain anesthesia.[4] The ETT should fit snuggly on the fiberscope, and a cuffed ETT may be the best choice for a "tube over scope technique." The smaller fiberscopes, which do not have a suction channel, are often used with this approach. Using the oral route will be more common due to the reduced chance of bleeding, but the technique can be more challenging due to the acute angle of the larynx.

The LMA is a good choice to both maintain anesthesia, and to act as a conduit for intubation.

Various methods of fiberoptic intubation through an LMA have been described. After introducing the bronchoscope through the LMA, lidocaine is sprayed onto the larynx, the bronchoscope is advanced into the trachea and visualization of the carina is obtained. Beyond this the ETT can be railroaded over the bronchoscope or an exchange catheter can be used with or without prior insertion of a guidewire. Despite various strategies to avoid dislodgement of the ETT upon LMA and bronchoscope removal (e.g., joining two ETTs by wedging, taping, or using an adapted female-to-female connectors), the technique can still be awkward and dislodgment may occur.[75]

Another technique involves: inserting a guidewire through the suction channel, removing the fiberscope, railroading an exchange catheter over the guidewire, confirming placement of the exchange catheter (via capnography) after removal of the guidewire, and finally railroading the ETT over the catheter. This technique allows for more flexibility in size of ETT compared to the prior with railroading the ETT over the bronchoscope. This technique will also work when a fiberscope larger than appropriate for the child's trachea is used; the guidewire can be extended beyond the scope prior to ETT insertion. An exchange catheter can be used without a guidewire, with the catheter fitted over an ultrathin fiberoptic bronchoscope. After the catheter is positioned in the trachea, the LMA is removed and the ETT is railroaded over the catheter.

Extubation Considerations for the Difficult Airway

Extubation of the difficult airway can be extremely challenging and both an airway cart and an anesthesiologist should be present. The patient must be fully awake with no residual neuromuscular blockade. There should always be the presence of someone capable of reintubating the patient. If the patient is cooperative, it is advisable to keep an ETT exchanger in place should there be need for reintubation. Patients who have had head or neck surgery should ideally be monitored in the intensive care unit should there be complications such as croup, bleeding, tracheal or esophageal perforation, pneumothorax, trauma, or aspiration. Consideration should also be given to postoperative issues which may compromise respiratory function including significant pain and/or narcotic use or airway edema, as well as other preexisting factors such as restrictive lung disease or neuromuscular weakness. Epidural anesthesia may improve conditions by providing good pain management without large doses of narcotic.

Airway Obstruction in the Child

Infants and children are at a greater risk for airway obstruction than adolescents and adults, due to their small anatomy and reactive physiology. A small decrease in the radius of the airway results in marked increase to the resistance of the airflow (Poiseuille's law) and the work of breathing; the eventual sequelae can include life-threatening hypercapnia and hypoxemia. Unlike the adult patient, there are some considerations in managing pediatric airway obstruction which will complicate both the accurate and efficient diagnosis and treatment, for example, the oftentimes inappropriateness of performing examination or intubation in the awake patient. Some treatments may be most suitable for these patients; an example is the use of heliox (see related section in this chapter). Below is a description of the variable clinical presentation and some of the etiologies and treatments for upper airway obstruction. This Section covers the general clinical presentation, the various etiologies and provides some discussion of clinical management of pediatric upper airway obstruction. The specific considerations for the anesthesiologist and otolaryngologist during endoscopic procedures (many treating obstruction), as presented in Section B, will allow further synthesis of the topic.

Clinical Presentation

Airway obstruction in a child must be taken very seriously. The symptoms and signs are extremely variable and depend upon the etiology and the site of obstruction. Some of the more common symptoms and signs appear in Table 10.4. Obtaining a detailed history is vital for elucidating the cause of upper airway obstruction in children.

The site of an obstruction can, to some degree, be approximated by pinpointing the phase of respiration at which stridor occurs (Table 10.5). Generally, supraglottic lesions (usually of the larynx) cause inspiratory stridor, whereas subglottic lesions cause inspiratory (tracheal) or expiratory (bronchial) stridor. Additional information can be obtained about the nature of the obstruction by studying flow volume loops (which provide a graphic analysis of flow at various lung volumes during continuous inspiration and expiration). These will allow determination of a fixed or variable obstruction and also whether it is intrathoracic or extrathoracic. Although there are exceptions, obstruction that is worse when the patient is asleep is generally pharyngeal (e.g., from tonsils or adenoids), while that which is worse awake (and aggravated by exertion) is laryngeal, tracheal, or bronchial.[82]

The etiology of airway obstruction in a child is usually determined clinically. In less urgent situations the radiologist can provide useful information. If radiological

Table 10.4 Symptoms and signs of airway obstruction.

Symptoms	Signs
Dyspnea	Snoring
Cough	Snorting
Orthopnea	Gurgling
Hoarseness	Stridor
Weakness	Choking
Dysphagia	Chest retraction
Hemoptysis	Nasal flaring
Sore throat	Cyanosis
Exhaustion	Drooling
Nausea	Tachypnea
Vomiting	Unconsciousness

Table 10.5 Stridor: A harsh high-pitched respiratory sound occurring in one or all phases of respiration; usually indicative of upper airway obstruction, the level of obstruction being to some degree determined by the level of the stridor

Level of obstruction	Character
Nose (nasal flaring)	Snoring, snorting
Pharyngeal	Gurgling
Laryngeal, subglottic	Inspiratory
Bronchial	Expiratory

studies are deemed necessary, an individual who is capable of dealing with airway obstruction must remain with the child at all times. Magnetic resonance imaging (MRI) techniques have a new role in diagnosing complicated airway problems in pediatric patients.[83]

Etiology

Congenital

Congenital anomalies are frequently the cause of stridor in infants and children. Laryngeal anomalies are much more frequently the cause of stridor than tracheal anomalies.[82]

Laryngomalacia

Laryngomalacia, with flaccidity of the epiglottis and/or aryepiglottic folds, is responsible for up to 94% of all congenital laryngeal anomalies[82, 84] and is the most common cause of congenital stridor.[85] The onset of symptoms occurs shortly after birth or within the first few months of life. Classically, the infant presents with a high-pitched crowing inspiratory stridor, often associated with feeding problems, respiratory distress, or upper respiratory tract infections. The stridor is caused by loose redundant supraglottic mucosa drawn into the airway during inspiration. Generally one of three abnormalities has occurred:

• Prolapse of redundant arytenoid mucosa into the glottis.
• Short aryepiglottic folds.
• The epiglottis has collapsed posteriorly over the glottis.

Symptoms usually disappear within 18–24 months, and airway intervention is not frequently required. The diagnosis is typically confirmed by flexible transnasal fiberoptic laryngoscopy with the patient anesthetized and spontaneously breathing, while rigid endoscopy may be reserved for inconclusive results or cases where there is suspicion of a synchronous airway lesion.[85] The severity of symptoms rather than the appearance on endoscopy forms the basis for deciding on surgical intervention (e.g., division of aryepiglottic folds or suspension of the prolapsing epiglottis). Unfortunately, underlying neurologic problems may prolong the obstructive symptoms even after surgery.

Congenital Vocal Cord Paralysis

Vocal cord paralysis is the second most common congenital laryngeal anomaly detected in the neonatal period. It may be unilateral or bilateral, although most cases of congenital paralysis are bilateral in nature (acquired paralysis can occur after recurrent laryngeal nerve injury). In most cases, its etiology remains unknown, although increased intracranial pressure may explain it in some cases. Unless there is an obvious precipitating factor, the condition is self-limiting and shows improvement over a period of weeks or months. The diagnosis is confirmed by awake flexible transnasal fiberoptic laryngoscopy and/or bronchoscopy. Radiological assessment is important to diagnose associated central nervous system and cardiovascular abnormalities. Supportive treatment (tube feedings and chest physiotherapy to develop an adequate cough) may be sufficient for unilateral paralysis, although tracheostomy may be necessary in many (approximately 50%) cases of bilateral paralysis.[86] Various types of surgery may be performed, including CO_2 laser treatment for widening the airway, although maintaining the voice and preventing aspiration are the primary aims.[84]

Congenital Subglottic Stenosis

Congenital subglottic stenosis accounts for a third of all congenital laryngeal defects. Thought to be due to failure of the laryngeal lumen to recanalize, it is the second most common cause of upper airway obstruction in infants under 1 year requiring tracheostomy (the most common cause is tracheal stenosis secondary to prolonged endotracheal intubation). The presenting features are stridor, recurrent croup, exertional dyspnea, failure to thrive and recurrent lower respiratory tract infection.[87] The lumen is 4.0 mm in diameter or less at the level of the cricoid and airway obstruction is highly variable (from 0 to 99% depending on grade). Diagnosis is usually by direct laryngotracheal bronchoscopy, and the airway can be sized using increasingly larger ETTs. The "gold standard" treatment for high-severe obstruction (>50%) includes laser excision of the stenosis and laryngotracheal reconstruction (inserting a cartilaginous graft into a vertical laryngotracheal fissure), although better results have recently been found in patients with severe forms after cricotracheal resection.[85, 88]

Miscellaneous

Other congenital anomalies from which there may be airway compromise, include aortic arch defects (leading to vascular compression), hemangiomas, cervical or mediastinum teratomas (embryonal neoplasms), cystic hygroma, laryngeal atresia, web cyst, laryngocele and tracheal anomalies, including posterior laryngeal clefts, tracheomalacia, and complete tracheal rings.

Acquired

Foreign Body Airway Obstruction

Approximately 55% of foreign body airway obstructions (FBAOs) occur in children under 3 years of age.[89] In 2007, 3,700 deaths related to FBAO were reported in the United States (1.2 per 100,000).[90] Food is one of the more common offending agents in children (liquids are the primary cause in infants), particularly hot dogs, peanuts, and spherically shaped candies or fruits. Small plastic toys are also often implicated.[91] FBAO commonly occurs when a child is eating while exercising. Small children (3 years and under) tend to put small objects in their mouth or into their noses that can be swallowed or inhaled during episodes of crying, laughing, or exercise. Furthermore, the lack of molar teeth in young children affects their ability to masticate food. FBAO can be a major cause of morbidity and mortality in children if early treatment is not instigated. Most foreign bodies involving the airway lodge in the main stem bronchi. Life-threatening obstruction occurs when they lodge in the larynx or trachea. Spherical, semirigid, and organic objects are the most hazardous ones, especially if their length is greater than 8 mm.[89, 92]

The approach to FBAO depends upon the degree of obstruction, the state of consciousness, and whether the incident was witnessed or not. The majority of FBAOs (88%) are heralded by a choking episode; therefore, it is important to ask any present witnesses whether choking has occurred.[93] Signs of FBAO may include a sudden onset of respiratory distress with coughing, gagging, stridor, or wheezing,[28] or the patient may be comfortable and in no apparent distress. In fact, physical signs and symptoms have a high sensitivity (they are present) but a very low specificity.[94]

Mild FBAO is characterized by coughing and ability to make sounds; do not interfere with this, although watch for signs of severe obstruction. Severe obstruction should be managed immediately. The diagnosis relies upon bronchoscopy. The treatment of complete and incomplete FBAO is discussed later in this chapter.

Obstructive Sleep Apnea

There is a continuum of childhood obstructive sleep-disordered breathing conditions, including snoring and upper airway resistance syndrome. Obstructive sleep apnea (OSA), the severest of these conditions, is a disorder that is characterized by repeated episodes of partial or complete upper airway obstruction during sleep that results in disruption of normal ventilation and sleep patterns.[95] The prevalence of childhood OSA is upwards of 1–4%.[96] The most common cause is adenotonsillar hypertrophy, although neuromuscular variables likely interact as well. The peak prevalence of OSA occurs in children aged 3–6, a time when the greatest amount of lymphoid tissue is present in the upper airway, relative to its dimensions.[97] A variety of conditions is associated with OSA, including many of those discussed in the difficult airway and upper airway obstruction sections. Obesity may play a role in childhood OSA, although is not the prevalent cause as with adult OSA. Habitual snoring is the most definitive feature of the syndrome, although most children have additional symptoms such as daytime sleepiness and neurocognitive problems.

Treatment of OSA usually consists of tonsillectomy, with adenoidectomy if necessary, although complete cure of the OSA only occurs in 25% of patients and the risk of persistent symptoms is associated with the initial severity of the OBA, family history of OSA and obesity.[98] Weight management is clearly an important postoperative goal. Other treatments include drugs, such as corticosteroids and antibiotics, and continuous positive airway pressure (CPAP).[96]

These patients are at significant risk in the postoperative period for airway obstruction. Problems seen to arise due to an assumption that vigilance is no longer required postoperatively since the obstruction has been relieved. There can be a significantly depressed ventilatory drive due to intra or postoperative narcotic use; additionally, significant postoperative swelling or bleeding may contribute to obstruction. These patients should be monitored postoperatively with pulse oximetry and apnea monitoring.[3]

"Kissing Tonsils" and Sleep Apnea Syndrome

Occasionally, a patient will suffer from the peculiar syndrome of hypertrophied lymphoid tissue associated with sleep apnea. Anesthesiologists and other individuals taking care of these patients should be fully aware of the danger of administering narcotics, which can cause respiratory depression, during the preoperative and postoperative periods.

Subglottic Cysts and Hemangiomas

Previously thought rare, subglottic cysts have been cited as the fourth most common cause of airway obstruction in one recent study.[99] Subglottic cysts are often caused by mucosal damage from endotracheal intubation, with the length of intubation being of little correlation. Many of the children will be ex-premature and intubated in the neonatal period, and the symptoms may be delayed for some time. While the patient is breathing spontaneously, the cysts are treated using laryngeal microinstruments, CO_2 laser, or a microdebrider. Reassessment should be performed 6–8 weeks postprocedure to diagnose recurrence, which may occur in upwards of 50% of cases.[99]

Subglottic hemangiomas result from endothelial hyperplasia and have both a proliferative phase and an involution phase, with gradual resolution of symptoms over a 2–5 year period. During examination, there may be an associated cutaneous hemangioma. During endoscopy, a compressible swelling will be observed, often on the posterior left side. Corticosteroids (systemic or intralesional) may be utilized if surgery is not required (stenosis is not circumferential or >50%), otherwise the abnormal tissue is either excised or bypassed (tracheostomy) until regression. Often multiple strategies are used, the basis for decision often being (like other obstructive conditions) whether the anomaly is unilateral or bilateral and whether there is more or less than 50% obstruction. Bruce and Rothera[85] include their protocol for subglottic hemangioma in their helpful review of upper airway obstruction in children.

Acute or Recurrent Infections

Peritonsillar Infections

Tonsillitis and infectious mononucleosis can both cause airway compromise. Surgical drainage of pus will likely be required to prevent rupture and aspiration complications. Tonsils that have caused airway obstruction may not be surgically removed, due to the risk of excessive bleeding. Conversely, many or most (40–88%) patients who have had airway compromise from infectious mononucleosis require tonsillectomy.

Acute Epiglottitis

Acute epiglottitis is still one of the most feared forms of upper airway obstruction in children. Fortunately, the incidence of *Haemophilus influenzae* type B acute epiglottitis has decreased 100-fold in the United States, Western Europe, Canada, and Australia with the introduction of the conjugate vaccine.[100] However, other organisms cause epiglottitis viz. *H. para-influenzae, Staphylococcus aureus, Streptococcus pneumonia,* and beta-hemolytic streptococci. *H. influenzae* type B disease still occurs in unvaccinated children. Additionally, immune compromised children, for example those with AIDS, or children with hematologic malignancies have been known to suffer from epiglottitis.[101,102] Leukemic infiltration of airway or retropharyngeal tissues or a neutropenic-facilitated focal infectious process may present as a life-threatening upper airway obstruction in acute leukemia.[102] The disease usually occurs in children between ages 2 and 6 and occurs most frequently in the winter and spring months.

The pathological features of acute epiglottitis include fulminant inflammation and swelling of mucous membranes covering the epiglottis, aryepiglottic folds, uvula, and other connective tissue structures and spaces in the supra- and paraglottic regions. The clinical features of acute epiglottis include: "a rapid onset of sore throat and pyrexia; airway obstruction may develop in less than 24 h. Classically, the child appears toxic, adopts a sitting position, has a muffled cough, and experiences difficulty swallowing. As the condition progresses the child appears toxic, develops dysphagia, dysphonia, and drooling." The classic posture of a child in advanced clinical stages of acute epiglottitis is as follows: the child is typically sitting bolt upright, leaning forward with the mouth wide-open, the jaw subluxed, and the head extended. Compared with croup (see below) there is little inspiratory stridor or hoarseness.

The white cell count is usually elevated (>10,000) with marked neutrophilia, but the diagnosis is made on clinical grounds. In less acute cases, lateral neck X-ray may be helpful. A lateral X-ray of the neck reveals the following classic radiologic features of acute epiglottitis: a thickened epiglottis (the "thumb sign") and swollen aryepiglottic folds; and the subglottic region appears normal. Treatment is discussed in a subsequent section.

Acute Laryngotracheitis (Viral Croup)

Viral croup is characterized by progressive inflammation and edema of the entire subglottic tracheobronchial tree. It is characterized by nighttime inspiratory stridor (due to narrowing at the cricoid level) and a barking, hoarse cough and is most commonly seen in children 6 months to 3 years of age. It is often initially associated with inspiratory subcostal and supraclavicular recession, and later by sternal recession and expiratory stridor (via intrathoracic airway obstruction).[103,104]

Parainfluenza virus types 1 and 3 are the most frequent offending agents and this infection has an annual incidence of 1.5 per 100 children under 6 years of age. Croup may also be caused by respiratory syncytial virus, adenovirus, influenza A and B, and occasionally by bacteria (*Mycoplasma pneumoniae*). Croup is characterized by mucosal and submucosal edema of the mucous membranes of the airway in the subglottic region, which are typically loosely attached to the larynx in this region and prone to edema. A 1-mm narrowing of the diameter of the airway in a 2-year-old causes a marked reduction in the cross-sectional area of the trachea (see Fig. 1.26 in Chap. 1).

Viral diseases of the airway are also associated with an increased production of secretions, via disruption of ion transport at the respiratory epithelium, which are often viscous. These factors combine to reduce the cross-sectional area of an already small airway. Children with viral croup usually present with a brief history of an upper respiratory tract infection, with nasal discharge and a "croupy" cough and inspiratory stridor. They will likely complain of a sore throat and have a fever, unlike those patients with spasmodic croup (see next section). A differential diagnosis should be performed and the reader is referred to Bjornson and Johnson.[105] Foreign body aspiration should be ruled out, as should other serious diseases such as bacterial tracheitis and epiglottitis. A–P and lateral neck films may show symmetrical subglottic narrowing ("church steeple" sign) and help to rule out acute epiglottitis. This condition will, though, share some radiological features such as hypopharyngeal dilation and inspiratory tracheal collapse.[103]

The textbook descriptions of acute epiglottitis and croup are not always seen in clinical practice. Quite often there is considerable overlap between the two conditions.[103] When experiencing difficulty distinguishing between acute epiglottitis and croup, information presented in Table 10.6 may be useful. Furthermore, it is important to always include foreign-body airway in the differential diagnosis. Some of the treatment guidelines are included in a subsequent section. Complete details about the controversies surrounding these acute conditions are beyond the scope of this book. For further information, refer to articles by Diaz[103], Barker[106] and Fried.[107]

Acute Bacterial Laryngotracheobronchitis (Bacterial Croup)

The epidemiology of acute infectious upper airway disease has seemed to change due to widespread *Haemophilus influenzae* type B immunization (epiglottitis) and corticosteroid treatment (viral croup), with an increasing contribution from acute laryngotrachobronchitis disease.[108] This form of croup is clinically indistinguishable from the viral form, especially in the early stages, but with progression the secretions become copious, thick, and purulent. It is much more incapacitating than viral croup and these patients often present with high fever and appear quite ill. The disease may develop into sepsis with pneumonia and acute respiratory distress syndrome.

To determine the underlying etiology, cultures from the respiratory tract are needed. The most common organisms cultured are *Streptococcus agalactiae, Streptococcus pneumoniae, Staphylococcus aureus,* and occasionally *Haemophilus influenzae.* A lateral neck X ray may show intraluminal membranes and tracheal wall irregularity.[109] The management is similar in many respects to that of the viral form except more patients will require intubation (94% vs. 17% of patients admitted to the pediatric intensive care unit).[108] Oxygen is administered if necessary. The appropriate antibiotic therapy is commenced. Tracheostomy may be necessary to suction the secretions.

Retropharyngeal Abscess

Retropharyngeal abscesses are usually due to infection of the paramedian chains of lymph nodes, therefore they are contained in the space that lies between the buccopharyngeal fascia and the prevertebral fascia, which extends from the base of the skull down to T1 (see Fig. 1.10 in Chap. 1). Infection in this area may occur from direct trauma, or it may spread from a nasopharyngeal or middle ear infection, or

Table 10.6 Findings and management of croup and epiglottis

Historical findings		Physical findings		Management	
Croup	Epiglottitis	Croup	Epiglottitis	Croup	Epiglottitis
Gradual onset	Abrupt onset	Protective posture absent	Protective posture present	Oxygen essential	Oxygen essential
Sore throat present	Sore throat severe	Low fever	High fever	Antibiotics ineffective	Antibiotics essential
Barking cough	Weak to no cough	Stridor present	Mild to no stridor	Humidification essential	Humidification essential
Mild constitutional symptoms	Severe constitutional symptoms	Cyanosis usually absent	Cyanosis usually present	Aerosolized vasoconstrictors beneficial	Aerosolized vasoconstrictors ineffective
Dysphagia may be present	Dysphagia severe	Retractions initially mild when they occur	Retractions initially marked	Steroids unproven	Steroids unproven
Hoarseness present	Muffled dysphonia progressing to aphonia	Respiratory rate: Tachypnea	Respiratory rate: Tachypnea	No airway intervention if possible, tracheostomy or short-duration nasotracheal intubation	Nasotracheal tube or tracheostomy
Drooling absent	Drooling may be present	Diaphragmatic and abdominal excursions not usually apparent	Diaphragmatic and abdominal excursions marked	Antibiotics ineffective	Antibiotics essential
		Heart rate: Sinus tachycardia, bradycardia with severe hypoxia and preceding cardiac arrest	Sinus tachycardia		
		Nasal flaring may develop/usually present	Nasal flaring may develop/usually present		

Source: Data from Diaz[103]

from hematologic or lymphatic spread. Bacteria responsible for this infection include gram-negative rods, anaerobes, *Staphylococcus aureus, Moraxella,* and group A hemolytic streptococcus. The incidence of retropharyngeal infection appears to be on the rise, with several cases of retropharyngeal infection in one study being methicillin-resistant, and most of these cases leading to mediastinitis and occurring in young infants (6.5 months).[110]

Retropharyngeal abscess usually occurs in children between 2 and 6 years of age (median age in one study was 32.5 months) since the associated lymph nodes often atrophy around the time of puberty.[110] They usually complain of a sore throat and a stiff neck and they are quite often febrile. The diagnosis can be easily confused with acute epiglottitis, but the duration of illness will likely be longer. The symptoms and signs are usually unilateral. A stiff neck and torticollis also help distinguish this condition from acute epiglottitis.

If the clinical signs are confusing, a lateral X ray of the neck taken in extension is recommended. If the width of the retropharyngeal space at the level of C2 is twice that of the diameter of vertebral body, the likelihood of it being a retropharyngeal abscess is very high (sensitivity of approximately 90%).[111]

Airway compromise may occur in these cases, but generally once the diagnosis is made and the appropriate antibiotic prescribed, these children improve quickly. Surgical drainage may be required in some cases. If airway management is required, it may be challenging. The glottis may be difficult to visualize. The airway must be secured without rupturing the abscess; a cuffed ETT will help prevent soiling of the lungs from drainage or potential rupture.

Recurrent Respiratory Papillomatosis

Recurrent respiratory papillomatosis is of viral origin (Human Papilloma Virus types 6 and 11) and is characterized by proliferations of squamous papillomata throughout the entire airway, but predominantly the layrnx.[85,104] Laryngeal involvement will often present as hoarseness and progressive airway obstruction, while that in the tracheobronchial tree will also be obstructive. The current treatment consists of surgical debulking, using CO_2 laser and radiofrequency ablation, and endoscopic microdebridement. The latter may limit the degree of fibrosis and scarring which contribute to poor airway and voice quality.[85] Adjuvant therapies have been used, including interferon, ribavirin, and acyclovir.

Allergic

Laryngeal Edema

Occasionally, a patient will develop an acute allergic reaction following a bee sting or other insect bite that leads to life-threatening laryngeal edema. These children must be treated aggressively with epinephrine, corticosteroids, and antihistamines. And if airway compromise occurs, prompt intubation or tracheostomy may be necessary.

Other

Spasmodic Croup

This condition is characterized by sudden laryngospasm of unknown etiology. Classically, it occurs at night and the child wakes up with a croupy cough. Fever, if present, is usually mild. Occasionally, the parent(s) will bring the child to the hospital and note a marked improvement on arrival due to the moist night air. The airway edema may be caused by an allergic reaction to viral antigens. Patients with spasmodic croup will rarely have radiologic evidence of the disease. The condition responds to epinephrine and steroids may be necessary, because in the early stages the condition is indistinguishable from viral croup. Airway intervention is rarely needed.

Acquired Subglottic Stenosis

Subglottic stenosis may result after intubation, if an incorrect ETT size was used, if there was multiple and/or traumatic intubations, or if the patient was agitated or aggressively moved during intubation. The edema will often subside, although formation of granulation tissue and ulcerations may develop. Management will be required if the child has recurrent respiratory distress or if stridor does not resolve within 7–10 days after extubation.[109]

Neoplasms

Upper airway obstruction can be associated with benign neoplasms or cancer. In the latter case, it may result either from an obstructing tumor or infectious complications (e.g., epiglottitis). Leukemic infiltration (a space-occupying infiltration) of epiglottis or retropharyngeal tissues may have contributed to a life-threatening upper airway obstruction in acute leukemia.[102] Compression of the airway by an anterior mediastinal mass can lead to a critical airway. Lymphoblastic lymphoma or Hodgkin's disease are primary causes of mediastinal masses leading to severe airway compromise.[112]

Trauma, with or without neurologic injury, is another cause of upper airway obstruction in children. Hypotonia caused by neurological disturbances (acquired or congenital) is a fairly frequent cause for tracheostomy in pediatrics.

Inhalation Burn Injury

Airway burns are discussed in Chap. 9, The Difficult Airway, and will present similarly with children as in adults. Severe and rapid swelling can occur and there should be continual monitoring for airway difficulties. Early intubation is essential in many cases, and the use of a cuffed ETT is recommended due to the provision of better sealing should positive end-expiratory pressure be required.[113]

Managing Foreign Body Airway Obstruction (FBAO)

Management in children has many similarities to that in adults, so emphasis will be placed on the differences that pertain to children.

Complete FBAO

In an *infant*, back blows and chest thrusts are recommended to relieve complete airway obstruction, due to possible damage to their relatively large liver. The baby is placed prone, head down, on the rescuer's arm (Fig. 10.9), which in turn rests on the rescuer's thigh. Five back blows (slaps) are delivered. The infant is then turned supine, head down, and five chest thrusts are delivered. The oropharynx should be inspected visually following these maneuvers to see if a foreign body is visible.

When dealing with children older than 1 year, a series of Heimlich maneuvers is performed, in either the upright or supine position. The oropharynx should be inspected in between series. Blind finger sweeps are not recommended at any time. If after two series of age-specific maneuvers in a prehospital setting airway obstruction persists, one should inspect the airway, and if a foreign body is seen, efforts should be made to remove it with Magill forceps. Perform these maneuvers until the foreign body is removed or the patient becomes unresponsive.

If the victim becomes unresponsive, CPR should be started with care to look into the mouth before giving breaths. If the foreign body is in the airway but out of reach, intubation may serve to move the foreign body into one or other main stem bronchi, thereby relieving complete obstruction. If all of these maneuvers fail, a

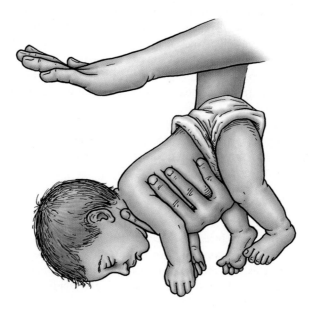

Fig. 10.9 Back blows for infant resuscitation

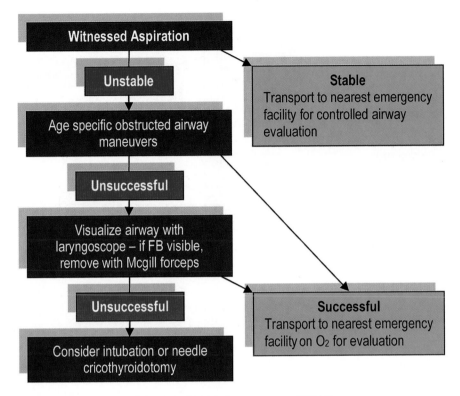

Fig. 10.10 Algorithm outlining out-of-hospital management of FBAO

surgical airway is the only choice. In hospital, a temporary cricothyrotomy can be performed using an 18-gauge needle or catheter to allow oxygen and PPV during transport to the operating room. Microlaryngoscopy and bronchoscopy are performed and the degree of residual injury will determine subsequent steps including short-term intubation or longer-term tracheostomy.[114] See Fig. 10.10 for out-of-hospital management of FBAO. Figure 10.11 presents guidelines for the initial and definitive hospital treatment of this emergency.

Incomplete FBAO

In a child with incomplete airway obstruction, the parent(s) may describe an acute episode of coughing, wheezing, and respiratory distress followed by a symptomless interval; or a history of persistent wheezing may be given. If the problem goes undetected for some time, the child may develop pneumonia, atelectasis, a lung abscess, bronchiectasis, bronchial perforation, or pulmonary hemorrhage. Symptoms include coughing, gagging, cyanosis, and stridor. When they occur in any child, foreign-body aspiration should be high on the list of diagnoses. When organic material (e.g., food) is inhaled, it may go undetected for a time, but it eventually expands due to

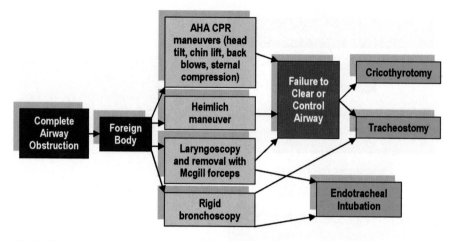

Fig. 10.11 In-hospital management of complete airway obstruction

the absorption of secretions and moisture and an inflammatory reaction occurs in the bronchi. Organic material in the tracheobronchial tree can do one of three things:

- It may be so small as to cause little if any obstruction.
- It may cause complete obstruction during all phases of respiration, resulting in absorption atelectasis.
- It may cause obstructive emphysema secondary to air-trapping during expiration. (Obstruction is mainly expiratory because the increased intrathoracic pressure during expiration narrows the lower airway.)

When a child presents with symptoms of incomplete airway obstruction, the following X-ray views should be obtained:

- Anterior–posterior (AP) and lateral neck
- Inspiratory and expiratory chest
- Barium swallow
- Airway fluoroscopy

If the obstruction is caused by a radiolucent object at the level of the bronchi, the classical picture will be one of obstructive emphysema on the side where the foreign body is located. Although a chest X-ray taken during inspiration may appear relatively normal, one taken during expiration will reveal hyperinflation on the affected side with a mediastinal shift toward the opposite side. It is therefore crucial to take chest X-rays during both inspiration and expiration (Fig. 10.12).

If a radiopaque object is lodged in the larynx, trachea, or a bronchus, radiological findings may be normal or may reveal ipsilateral obstructive emphysema or absorption atelectasis because the object is readily seen. If the object is inhaled, the diagnosis is much easier. Incidentally, even a narrow foreign body accidentally swallowed may be large enough to encroach upon the airway and cause symptoms. For example, ingestion of a jack caused symptoms in the child shown in Fig. 10.13.

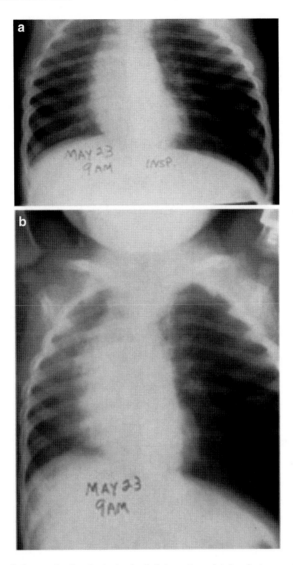

Fig. 10.12 A radiolucent foreign body in the left bronchus. (**a**) Inspiratory and (**b**) expiratory views

Any child with suspected foreign-body aspiration should be brought to a hospital immediately for further investigation.

The gold standard for diagnosing an aspirated foreign body is rigid bronchoscopy under general anesthesia. The procedure for incomplete airway obstruction is as follows:

- Immediate bronchoscopy for severe respiratory distress.
- Urgent bronchoscopy if no distress (wait for stomach to empty).

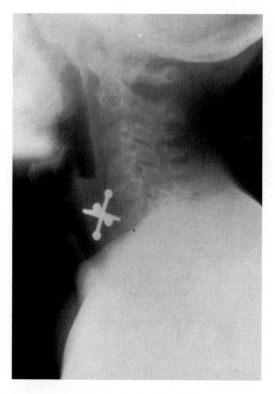

Fig. 10.13 A foreign body (jack) in the esophagus of a child

- Semielective bronchoscopy after workup for suspected aspiration (within 24–48 h).
- Mist tent for 24 h with oxygen enrichment after bronchoscopy.
- Chest physiotherapy after bronchoscopy.

Prior to arrival at the surgical suite, there will likely be placement of a peripheral intravenous catheter. An intramuscular agent, such as ketamine, may be useful when the patient is uncooperative and can be used without significant depression of respiratory drive.[115] Atropine may be useful to dry secretions and to prevent vagal-induced bradycardia from insertion of the bronchoscope. General anesthesia may be induced via inhaled or intravenous agents, with or without maintenance of spontaneous breathing. The routine will depend upon the urgency of the situation and the fasting status of the child. Often total intravenous (TIVA) technique will be used to maintain the source of anesthesia to the patient (e.g., during removal of the bronchoscope) and to reduce exposure of inhalation agents within the operating room.

All patients should receive pulse oximetry and supplemental oxygen may be administered to improve oxygenation. The risks of barotrauma and pneumothorax are too great for jet ventilation. Patients with severe distress may be given heliox (ideally 70% helium, 30% oxygen) to improve gas delivery to the lungs and decrease the work of breathing (by reducing airflow resistance).

The endoscopic identification and foreign body removal can be made more difficult due to local inflammation, including edema and granulation tissue formation which contribute to the obstruction.[116] Furthermore, surgical removal (e.g., thoracotomy) of the foreign body may be necessary if the foreign body is large, sharp and embedded in the tracheal or bronchial wall, or if there is significant difficulty controlling the airway during rigid bronchoscopy.[115] A follow-up bronchoscopy after removal of the foreign body is necessary to rule out additional material and airway injury.[114] Chest X-rays are also performed to monitor for pulmonary compromise. Antibiotic therapy will be necessary if a pneumonic process is active or if mucosal abrasion has occurred.

Treating Epiglottitis and Croup

Epiglottitis

When the diagnosis of acute epiglottitis is suspected, the opinions of the pediatrician, ENT surgeon, radiologist, and anesthesiologist should be sought. If the airway is severely obstructed, radiological studies should be deferred and arrangements made to transport the child to the operating room. An anesthesiologist should remain with the patient at all times and the patient should be treated during examination with high inspired oxygen to prevent hypoxemia and cardiac arrest. If appropriate to perform some investigation prior to intervention, direct inspection of the epiglottis can be indispensable. Otherwise, lateral neck radiographs should be performed and diagnosis will be confirmed in most cases by a "thumb sign," where the vallecula is obliterated by the swollen epiglottis. If the patient has a normal appearing epiglottis, they likely have croup, but one should be warned that normal appearing supraglottic structures do not exclude epiglottitis. This section will mainly focus on the traditional treatment of epiglottitis, being emergency placement of an artificial airway and IV antibiotics. There will also be some comment on more conservative approaches which have been employed with success.

In the past, it was considered a major violation of protocol to examine the airway of a child with suspected acute epiglottitis while the child was awake. Common sense tells us that the diagnostic yield from such an aggressive approach would be low; so therefore, we recommend examination under anesthesia in most circumstances. However, if for some reason the examination is to be carried out in a conscious child, it should be carried out in an operating room and in the presence of airway experts who are prepared to intubate or intervene surgically at any time. Of course, awake intervention may be required without warning if complete airway obstruction occurs at any time or place.

Most experts recommend airway examination under general anesthesia. The most experienced anesthesiologist available should be assigned to the task.

Adequate preoxygenation and an intravenous line should ideally be established prior to induction. Optimally, the child should remain sitting while oxygen (e.g., 100% at 6 L/min) and incremental levels of halothane or sevoflurane are administered by mask to provide slow induction. There is reduced alveolar ventilation and high cardiac output in these patients and it may take as long as 20 min to attain an adequate level of anesthesia to allow airway examination.

Induction may be complicated by complete airway obstruction, laryngospasm, hypotension, cardiac arrhythmias, and cardiac arrest. The vital signs need to be checked frequently throughout the induction, since these patients may be hypovolemic secondary to dehydration; thus, even a low concentration of halothane can cause hypotension. It is a good idea to administer about 10 ml/kg of a salt-rich solution once the intravenous line is established.

After achieving adequate anesthesia, the airway is exposed and an ETT is inserted using direct laryngoscopy (initially) or a rigid bronchoscope. The friable epiglottis should be avoided to prevent trauma, hemorrhage, and laryngospasm. If inflammation is substantial, the tissue will be red and swollen, to the point of obscuring the anatomy. There may be the appearance of a "red cherry" at the base of the tongue: within the center of (not behind) this cherry lies the glottic inlet.[117] It is important to have a wide selection of tubes available. On the initial intubation attempt, a tube at least one full size less than that predicted for the patient's age group should be used. Once the child has been stabilized, it may be preferable to replace the oral tube with a correct-fitting nasal tube, which must be secured with great care. If intubation cannot be achieved after three attempts, one should resort to a surgical tracheostomy or a percutaneous cricothyrotomy tube insertion using Seldinger technique.

Airway equipments which should be available in the operating room include:[117]

- Functional suction device.
- Different sized face masks.
- Two laryngoscope handles and various straight and curved blades of different lengths and widths.
- Sufficient tracheal tubes (4.0, 4.5 and 5.0 mm ID) preloaded with lubricated intubating stylets.
- Two bronchoscopes connected to a light source and suction.
- A tracheostomy tray.
- A cricothyrotomy set.

Once the airway is established, antibiotic therapy (typically for 10 days) should be instituted and must be effective against *Haemophilus influenzae* type B strains and other organisms capable of causing acute epiglottitis; an agent with beta-lactamase resistance is necessary. Blood cultures should be taken before commencing antibiotic therapy.

With the availability of endoscopy, some centers have reported more conservative approaches including management in the ICU without artificial airway placement. The airway is examined in the awake patient (depending on cooperation) using endoscopy (i.e., fiberoptic nasolaryngoscopy or endoscopy with small rigid laryngoscopes) in order to confirm the diagnosis and decide on whether an artificial airway is indicated. If total airway obstruction is not an immediate threat, management with humidified oxygen, inhaled racemic epinephrine, and IV steroids may be successful in preventing complete obstruction. Unlike difficult airway cases, there is little evidence or experience to support the use of alternate intubation devices or fiberoptic intubation.

Croup

One major problem in dealing with croup is deciding whom to admit to the hospital. Fewer than 5% of children with croup are admitted to hospital, but the remainder can usually be managed in the emergency room or at home.[105] Any child who is hypoxic or has symptoms and signs of respiratory failure, tachypnea, dyspnea, cyanosis, lethargy, or retractions should be admitted to hospital.

The first line of treatment in the emergency room has traditionally been humidification, although this treatment is not supported by evidence.[105,118,119] Aerosolized epinephrine is the treatment of choice for children with moderate to severe stridor. The recommended dose of epinephrine is either 0.5 ml of 2.25% racemic epinephrine or 3–5 ml of epinephrine 1:1,000. It is now considered safe to discharge a child from the emergency room after a suitable interval, following an aerosolized epinephrine treatment.[120]

What role do steroids play in the treatment of croup? One metaanalysis showed that the need for endotracheal intubation is significantly reduced in hospitalized children who receive glucocorticoid treatment, while another showed no effect on intubation rates.[121,122] A 12-h reduction in length of stay in the emergency department or hospital and a 50% reduction in return visits and admissions has also been shown.[123] Dexamethasone is the steroid most frequently used and the recommended dose is 0.15–0.6 mg/kg orally or IM. It has been stated that any child who receives an aerosolized racemic epinephrine treatment should also receive steroids.[124] A treatment option should steroids and epinephrine fail is to try administration of the oxygen–helium mixture, Heliox (described in this section of the chapter).

Airway intervention should be avoided if possible. However, if it becomes necessary, the preferred route is oral – at least initially. Approximately 1–3% of children admitted to hospital for croup are intubated.[105] Tracheostomy is rarely necessary and may not be successful since the obstruction occurs at the proximal end of the trachea. To help answer the question of when an artificial airway should be placed, Downes[125] has devised a scoring system that should be used as a guide. Generally, the physical findings of inspiratory and expiratory stridor, barking cough, nasal flaring with retraction, cyanosis in 40% oxygen, and delayed inspiratory sounds are all indications for possible insertion of an artificial airway.

Airway intervention is required when oxygenation and ventilation become compromised. This decision should be made in the operating room with an ENT surgeon, and an anesthesiologist present. During laryngoscopy it is preferable to avoid narcotics, to allow these patients the full benefit of the respiratory drive. To reduce the amount of secretions, anticholinergic drugs should be administered. Many ENT surgeons prefer laryngoscopy under general anesthesia to determine the amount of swelling that remains. A final decision regarding intubation is then based upon these findings. The equipment that should be available is listed above under the section on treating epiglottitis.

Management of the Child with Impending Complete Airway Obstruction

Recognition of impending airway obstruction is crucial because cardiopulmonary arrest is rarely a sudden event; it tends to follow a progressive deterioration in respiratory function.[109] In no area of medicine is closer cooperation required between the anesthesiologist, surgeon, and nursing personnel than when treating a child with upper airway obstruction. Traditionally, in many large centers, children presenting with a critical airway (potentially from acute epiglottitis) were treated by protocol consisting of immediate anesthesia prior to any intervention, and it would be logical if we instituted the same protocol when dealing with any child with upper airway obstruction.

In most instances, the anesthesiologist has time to prepare for the emergency. However, if a child presents *in extremis,* there may be no other option but to secure the airway immediately. The first line of approach should always be ventilation with 100% oxygen; if BMV does not work, insert an LMA or other extraglottic device. (Additionally, any other treatment should commence at this time, for example nebulized epinephrine, antibiotics or steroids.) In many instances, immediate improvement follows. In fact, noninvasive ventilation (e.g., CPAP) may be successful for preventing tracheostomy or optimizing the timing of surgery in patients with congenital syndromes associated with obstruction.[126] If, and when, oxygenation improves, the next step would be to attempt oral endotracheal intubation. Failing that, the only option is a surgical airway. Cricothyrotomy is indicated when the obstruction is at or above the glottic opening. A classic indication is epiglottitis in the older child, after BMV and intubation have failed. Other indications include facial trauma and angioedema.[59] Open cricothyrotomy can only be performed when there is sufficient cricothyroid space (width) and thus is not recommended in children aged 10 and under, as the chances exist of damaging the cricothyroid cartilage or causing laryngeal stenosis and/or permanent damage to speech. Needle cricothyrotomy should only be used as a "last ditch" procedure in children.

The moment the anesthesiologist is alerted that a child has upper airway obstruction, he or she must remain with the patient at all times. Children presenting with upper airway obstruction are often extremely apprehensive, and every effort must be made to calm them. It is often helpful to have one parent remain with the child, at least until the procedure is about to begin. Children suffering from upper airway obstruction usually find the supine position intolerable. Therefore, they should be allowed to remain in the sitting position for as long as possible.

In many situations, proper handling of acute upper airway obstruction in the child requires general anesthesia. Some considerations are listed below:

- With the child in the sitting position, the anesthesiologist should gradually induce anesthesia by delivering a mixture of oxygen and an inhalation agent.
- Firm application of the mask to the patient's face will only frighten the patient and lead to further agitation. The anesthesia circuit, without mask, should be gradually brought closer to the patient's face. Individuals in the operating room should be encouraged to go about their business without making too much noise.
- When unconsciousness occurs, an IV should be established (a tracheostomy set should already be opened).
- Some patients suffering from airway obstruction may be volume-depleted because of fever and the inability to eat or drink; therefore, care should be taken with regards to administering potent inhalation agents, which can cause hypotension. Blood pressure should be carefully monitored.
- If a significant airway problem is suspected, an arterial line should be inserted to obtain subsequent blood samples.
- Sometimes it is quite difficult to judge the depth of anesthesia in these patients. However, with an IV in place, it is reasonable to supplement the inhalation agent by administering propofol, and lidocaine.
- There is considerable controversy about the use of neuromuscular blocking drugs in children with impending upper airway obstruction. Although succinylcholine is used routinely by clinicians in some centers, others shun the use of neuromuscular blockers altogether in this situation. Thus, there are no hard-and-fast rules; however, if a child is paralyzed during the clinician's airway securement process, the *onus rests heavily upon that clinician to maintain adequate oxygenation at all times.*

Intubation Procedure

An array of ETTs and laryngoscope blades should be ready for immediate use. Atropine in a dose of 0.01 mg/kg should be administered intravenously. When an adequate level of anesthesia is achieved, laryngoscopy is performed, and an ETT that is at least one size smaller than normal should be inserted. Laryngeal or tracheal stenoses may need to be dilated using a progression of well lubricated sizes of semirigid tubes.[74] When the airway is secured, the ENT surgeon is likely to perform a laryngoscopy with the ETT in place. If the airway was easy to secure, it may be reasonable to switch to a nasotracheal tube at this time. A soft ETT of ½ caliber less than that reached using dilation is most suitable. The ETT should be securely taped, and the child should be sedated and should have restraints placed on his arms before he awakens. Nursing personnel must be given instructions on how to care for this child postoperatively. In addition to ensuring that the ETT remains in place, the nurse must suction it on a regular basis to prevent it from becoming obstructed. The inspired gases should be humidified (to maintain fluid secretions and facilitate suction) and a minimum amount of CPAP should be applied. A progressive positive end-expiratory pressure level from 5 to 15 cm H_2O should be applied to create an "air pillow" around the tube and promote dilation of the stenotic area.[74] An improvement in stenosis can be confirmed by increasing air leakage. A physician capable of reintubating the trachea should be immediately at hand at all times.

Heliox in Pediatric Airway Management

Heliox decreases the work of breathing and improves gas delivery to the lungs by maximizing laminar airflow and reducing airflow resistance. Since treatment of the obstructive cause or removal of the foreign body may not always be accomplished quickly, heliox can be considered a "therapeutic bridge" until more definite treatment can be instituted.[127] Heliox may be beneficial for both upper and lower (e.g., bronchiolitis) airway obstruction in children. Heliox may improve stridor scores, decrease the work of breathing and improve comfort in the postextubation period; these parameters may help reduce the need for reintubation.[127-129] Heliox may provide benefits similar to racemic epinephrine in patients with moderate to severe croup, and thus could be considered a useful adjunct to standard therapies in the emergency department.[130] Heliox should be administered using a closed system, such that the mask should be held firmly in order to minimize dispersion. The increase in cost between oxygen or room air and the need for specialized equipment will likely limit its use in many centers.

Tracheostomy in the Child

Over the years, the primary indication for pediatric tracheostomy has evolved from acute inflammatory airway obstruction (now relatively rare due to vaccines) to replacing long-term intubation, and its associated chronic laryngotracheal lesions, when ventilatory support is required over many weeks or months.[131] Long-term dependence on ventilatory support may in fact be due to upper airway obstruction (from infection or structural abnormalities), but it is also often associated with trauma (e.g., closed head injuries or basal skull fractures with cerebrospinal fluid leak), bronchopulmonary dysplasia, as well as hypotonia resulting from neurological or neuromuscular disturbances.[132]

Tracheostomy may occasionally be a lifesaving procedure in children, but many have died in the past as a result of immediate or late complications of tracheostomy. In fact, the mortality rate was once quoted as 10% for each year that the tracheostomy remains in place. The fact that more tracheostomies are being performed for chronic illnesses leads to a longer duration of their placement (i.e., lower decannulation rates). Fortunately, overall rates of mortality from tracheostomy complications are decreasing (rates of 1.6–3.6% have been

these diagnostic maneuvers has been disputed in the literature. Biopsies are performed using either optical forceps of varying designs and sizes, or flexible equivalents threaded through the side port of the bronchoscope, allowing simultaneous direct visualization. Both of these procedures can put the patient at risk of injuries to the lips, teeth, and mucosa of the oral cavity, pharynx or tracheo-bronchial tree. Using an atraumatic technique, with appropriate size equipment and depth of anesthesia, is of paramount importance in ensuring safe execution and avoidance of these complications.

Microlaryngoscopy

This is performed using the same position as for bronchoscopy, thus requiring significant extension of the head and neck which poses potential problems to patients with propensity to atlantoaxial subluxation (Down syndrome) or cervical arthrodesis (achondroplastic dwarfs), and arguably some cases of velocardiofacial syndrome. Cases of retro or micrognathia, anteriorly displaced larynges, limited temporomandibular joint range, or microstomia will pose challenges which should be anticipated. An operating laryngoscope is introduced to completely expose the laryngeal inlet, to which a suspension mechanism is attached thereby stabilizing the head and neck. One of the side-ports of the laryngoscope allows the use of an adaptor for connection to the anesthetic circuit. The tip of the laryngoscope should be placed in the apex of the vallecula, lifting the epiglottis out of the field (avoiding traumatizing it), and allowing an unhindered panoramic view of the laryngeal inlet. This allows examination (inspection and palpation) and instrumentation of the larynx, with cold steel conventional instruments, power-assisted debriders, laser beams or fibers, balloon dilation, or application of chemical agents topically or by injection. To provide a clear, dry airway throughout the procedure, appropriately-sized suction (eyeless) aspirators, with thumb controls (occasionally coupled with monopolar diathermy), are used intermittently and atraumatically, in addition to judicious use of topical vasoconstrictors (1:1,000 Adrenaline) applied via small cottonoids.

Anesthetic Considerations for Endoscopic Procedures

Otolaryngological procedures often pose challenges to clinicians, particularly for the otolaryngologist and anesthesiologist, in relation to management of the patient's airway. A distinct feature of any otolaryngologic procedure is that both the anesthesiologist and the surgeon need intimate access to the same anatomical region of the patient. The anesthesiologist is primarily concerned about maintaining a patent airway, oxygenation, and ventilation, with the provision of adequate oxygen and the effective removal of carbon dioxide. The otolaryngologist simultaneously requires both a stable and accessible operative field to optimize the safety and efficacy of the procedure. Occasionally, these goals will conflict and compromise will be required, as reached through joint deliberation and a risk-benefit analysis of the possible anesthetic and surgical techniques. Each case will necessitate an individualized balance of controlled airway reflexes through adequate anesthesia and stable surgical field, both of which must be obtained within the often limited time frame afforded.

A significant consideration in the patient presenting for endoscopy is the presence of coexisting anatomical airway abnormality and compromised respiratory reserve. Perhaps the greatest safety precaution for these cases is choosing anesthetic techniques which provide control of the airway, while ensuring adequate oxygenation and ventilation as needed, all while providing access for the otolaryngologist. There is a wide variety of equipment available for endoscopy procedures as discussed later in this section. Similarly, there are different anesthetic drugs and techniques from which the anesthesiologist can choose. Additionally, the clinician will need to know how to deal with other general pediatric challenges including:

- The uncooperative child
- Rapid desaturation
- Possible difficult venous assess.

When evaluating procedural considerations, the fundamental considerations for the anesthesiologist during otolaryngological procedures are as follows:

- Direct communication between the anesthesiologist and otolaryngological surgeon is vital when developing a sound treatment plan for each patient.
- Planning is essential during pediatric anesthesia in general, but even more critical when considering airway management.

Goals of the Anesthesiologist during Pediatric ENT Procedures

The primary goals for the anesthesiologist during ENT procedures in pediatric patients are to:

- Obtain and maintain adequate oxygenation and ventilation.
- Provide blunted airway reflexes to allow an stable surgical field.
- Minimize hemodynamic responses from manipulation of the airway (bradycardia and increased blood pressure).
- Avoid aspiration and maximize airway protection during perioperative period (i.e., pre and postoperatively).
- Facilitate rapid recovery (i.e., prompt return of consciousness and airway reflexes).
- Ensure amnesia.

General Anesthetic Approaches

A prime determinant of airway safety and success of an otolaryngological procedure in a child relates to the adequacy of anesthesia. There is no one anesthetic technique that can satisfy all of the requirements of every patient: the nature of the airway obstruction, the presence of concomitant lung disease, and the child's level of understanding are all variables that may require a modification of technique. In each case, the skill and experience of the anesthesiologist are crucial to a successful outcome. In the otolaryngology setting, there is often no reasonable time period allowed to ensure an empty stomach. For instance, a patient in whom foreign-body aspiration is suspected should always be assumed to have a full stomach, and appropriate precautions should be taken. The use of agents to reduce the volume and acidity of gastric secretions was outlined when considering Anesthetic Management and Induction Technique of difficult pediatric airways in the previous section of this chapter. Suctioning out stomach contents and the neutralizing gastric acid should be considered. The provision of sedation, route of anesthesia, and use of various options for ventilation will be tailored to each case. In general, but particularly when there is any risk of increased airway obstruction, the author relies upon and prefers to use mask inhalation as the primary route to induce anesthesia. Moreover, in the case of foreign body impaction or obstructive lesion, PPV is avoided.

Planning

Planning is an essential element of the management of the airway. Any infant or child who has airway problems associated with either respiratory infection or feedings will be expected to have the problems in both induction and the emergence phases of anesthesia. Common problems may include a high risk of obstruction, coughing, laryngospasm, and regurgitation. Special attention should be paid to patients with a previous history of difficult anesthesia, and careful preparation for the worst should be carried out. The patient's history may reveal other issues as well, including problems with respiratory infection (suggested by reports of the patient's need to sit up to breathe and problems with feeding) which may lead to severe coughing and cyanosis.

Aside from airway management, keeping neonates and infants warm is extremely important. To avoid a pediatric patient becoming stressed because of cold, the room should be warmed and heating devices (e.g., warming blanket and IV warmers) are necessary. Having adequate help particularly during induction is a must. The anesthesiologist should always request the presence of an assistant skilled in airway and vascular access techniques. Potentially necessary drugs should be available and syringes with premeasured doses of should be prepared.

Managing Uncooperative Children

One of the real challenges for any clinician is to manage an uncooperative child with a difficult airway, particularly on the induction of anesthesia. The nature of the diagnosis, especially that of complete or impending obstruction, may leave the child frightened. Compounding this, poor planning or preparation can easily lead the child to panic. This may not only lead to a very unpleasant induction experience, but may also increase the amount of secretions and otherwise worsen the airway condition. In these situations, the anesthesiologist may elect to vary their technique utilizing several options, some of which are included below.

Induction and Maintenance of General Anesthesia

Generally, mask inhalation induction can only be tolerated well with calm children. In an uncooperative or otherwise agitated child, mask inhalation technique can worsen their response and prove very difficult to perform. Unless exceptional circumstances arise, one should avoid "gorilla inductions" in which the patient is forcefully restrained on the operating table with an anesthetic mask clamped over their face.[135] Many clinicians prefer to administer sedation before induction for an uncooperative child when there are no airway concerns (sedative agents are well known to cause loss of airway muscle tone and to increase airway resistance, making their use in obstruction a serious consideration). The oral route (midazolam 0.5 mg/kg or ketamine 3 mg/kg]), with or without the addition of an anticholinergic (atropine 0.02 mg/kg or glycopyrrolate 0.05 mg/kg) is used to dry secretions and prevent bradycardia, if using inhalational anesthesia. Alternatively, administration of a "stunning" dose of intramuscular (IM) ketamine using 3 mg/kg can provide effective sedation. Moreover, a frightened child who already has an IV catheter in place may be sedated with subanesthetic doses of ketamine; the initial dose is 1 mg/kg followed by titrated doses of 0.5 mg/kg. Following adequate sedation, an inhalation anesthetic can be administered as tolerated.

If not already in place, IV access should be established as soon as possible after the induction to enable speedy medical management of the plane of anesthesia. If the child experiences no intermittent obstruction at the beginning of the induction, it is the author's typical practice to continue the induction slowly. For maintenance, a total intravenous anesthesia (TIVA) infusion of 0.01–0.03 ml/kg/min (using a mixture of 10 mg/ml propofol and 2.5–5.0 µg/ml remifentanil, i.e., 100–300 µg/kg/min of propofol and 0.025–0.075 µg/kg/min remifentanil), is titrated to offer adequate anesthesia while maintaining spontaneous respiration. Younger children (<3 years of age) have been shown to tolerate a higher dose of remifentanil while maintaining spontaneous respiration.[136] If there are concerns over airway obstruction or other compromising situations, a sevoflurane inhalation will be utilized to maintain spontaneous respiration.

The intravenous route, being easily titratable, is used to facilitate control of the airway as much as possible during anesthesia. A high concentration of anesthetic can be achieved in order to depress the protective reflexes and facilitate otolaryngological procedures. Additionally, this mode of anesthesia removes excessive contamination of the room with volatile anesthetics. In those instances when laryngospasm and airway obstruction become irreversible and ventilation of the patient can be impossible despite the mode of anesthesia, serious ventricular bradycardia may occur with high-dose sevoflurane, particularly in combination with remifentanil.

Local Anesthesia of the Airway

Topical anesthesia to the airway can effectively blunt airway reflexes, and is a paramount aspect of the provision of anesthesia for most otolaryngological procedures. Due to its proven efficacy and safety for airway anesthesia, Lidocaine is the most commonly used local anesthetic. While absorption through the pharyngeal and laryngeal mucosa is slow (peak levels 15–20 min), local anesthetic administrated directly into the trachea can be rapidly absorbed. Thus, there is a greater risk for toxicity shortly after delivery. In pediatrics, it is advisable to apply local anesthetic only where needed, using 3–5 mg/kg for regions above the vocal cords and limiting the dose applied below the cords and into the trachea to a limit of 2 mg/kg.

While topical application of local anesthetics in adults is generally easy to accomplish (e.g., via nebulization) in the awake state, in most cases it will be difficult to apply this before induction in children. A nebulizer can be used to deliver lidocaine 4 mg/kg to the airway. When spontaneous respiration is required and inhalation induction is used, there will be the added challenge of deciding upon the timing and route for applying topical anesthesia. One case has been published reporting successful administration of in-circuit nebulized lidocaine simultaneously with sevoflurane induction for the performance of fiberoptic intubation of a difficult pediatric airway (Fig. 10.15).[137] However, further study must be performed to verify the merit of this technique. Otherwise, nasal or laryngeal anesthesia can be achieved after induction while the patient is settled on a face mask, using either xylometazoline 0.05% (Otrivin pediatric nasal drops) via a syringe and atomizer to each nostril, or 2% (4 mg/kg limit) lidocaine using a syringe and nebulizing extension, respectively.[138]

Anesthetic Options During the Airway Procedure (Box 10.2)

Spontaneous vs. Controlled Ventilation

Spontaneous breathing is important especially when there is the presence of intrathoracic obstructive lesions of the large airways. By generating negative intrathoracic

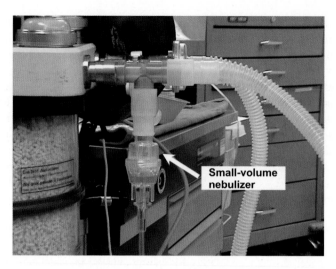

Fig. 10.15 In-circuit nebulized lidocaine setup. A small-volume nebulizer was connected to the inspiratory limb of the circle system via a T-piece adapter

---

Box 10.2   Anesthetic Options for Airway Procedures

Option 1: Spontaneous respiration using total intravenous anesthesia (TIVA) with an infusion of 0.01–0.03 ml/kg/min, using a mixture of 10 mg/ml propofol and 2.5–5 µg/ml remifentanil (i.e., 100–300 µg/kg/min of propofol and 0.025–0.075 µg/kg/min remifentanil).
Option 2: Spontaneous respiration using inhalation agent via insufflations for maintenance and ventilation.
Option 3: Intermittent apnea using inhalation agent or TIVA.
Option 4: Jet ventilation using inhalation agent or TIVA.

---

pressure, spontaneous breaths will often stent open the large airways and also may prevent collapse of the tumor mass onto the large airway. This often permits a certain amount of inspired tidal volume to pass the obstruction. Very limited gas exchange can be achieved with positive controlled ventilation. Moreover, small patients are more prone to barotrauma in the event of restriction in exhalation.

Intubation

Intubation using an ETTETT can allow effective positive ventilation and total control of the airway. However, the presence of the ETT itself within the tight physical space of the pediatric airway limits, makes many airway procedures impossible. In addition, conventional ETTs are contraindicated in laser surgery, as they will easily combust.[138] Tubes with laser resistance are available and include those made of metal (although rigid and having large external diameters) or aluminized plastic (although these are too large for most pediatric patients). Because of this, one technique which has been utilized involves intermittent removal of the tube allowing the operation to proceed for a short period of time, depending on patient tolerance, with reintubation for resumption of oxygenation and ventilation. However, this approach still poses great restriction for many endoscopic procedures and is generally not preferred. Moreover, multiple attempts at intubation may result in varying degrees of trauma to the vocal cords and airway, with the subsequent development of secretions and varying amounts of edema (Fig. 10.16). This, of course, will add to the problems presented by the difficult airway. The use of high-dose steroids in traumatic situations has been utilized. Nasotracheal intubation via flexible fiberoptic endoscopy will be the best choice for intubating the trachea when there are restraints in mouth opening or in head/neck movement. If the oral route is used, various devices may assist with endotracheal intubation of the difficult airway (see Chap. 6).

Another technique which has been described utilizes a nasal tube to maintain inhalation anesthesia, particularly during laser surgery where most ETTs placed in the oral cavity are contraindicated.[138] This author's practice is to cut a polar north ETT short and place it within the nasal cavity, without protrusion beyond the soft palate. A benefit of this method, over gas insufflations through a bronchoscope, is that the anesthesiologist has control over the delivery of gases rather than their administration relating to the surgeon's procedure. As compared to intubation, this technique will enable full access to the larynx. During CO_2 laser surgery, nitrous oxide should not be used as it supports combustion and some of it will be entrained within the operating microscope. During KTP (potassium titanyl phosphate) laser surgery, the anesthetic circuit is removed from the nasal airway and connected to the side-port of the bronchoscope.

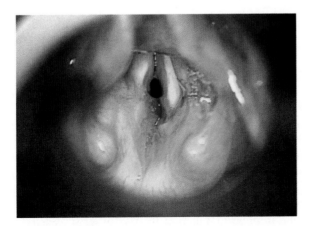

Fig. 10.16 Subglottic edema can result from multiple airway manipulations

Insufflations

A spontaneous ventilation technique using the ventilating bronchoscope can be used.

A standard ETT connector can be modified for attachment to an appropriately-sized nasopharyngeal airway, or the suction channel/side-port of the suspension laryngoscope.

Intermittent Apnea

Intermittent apnea can be beneficial for providing a very short procedure time. This technique is often used in conjunction with intubation, extubation, and reintubation interspersed between the apneic intervals. The duration of apnea is limited by the patient's needs for ventilation and oxygenation. The carbon dioxide pressure will increase 6–7 mmHg within the first minute of apnea and 3–4 mmHg thereafter. This technique is not suitable for use in those patients with limited cardiorespiratory reserve (e.g., congenital heart disease and pulmonary hypertension). The mean length of an apneic episode will be variable within minutes depending on the pulmonary condition of the patients.

Jet Ventilation

Jet ventilation can be accomplished via a cannula connected to the lumen of the laryngoscope. The ventilation can be started with a pressure of 5–10 psi in children and titrated up to provide adequate chest excursions (infant 6–12 psi; children 10–16 psi). However, this technique has not been commonly used in pediatrics, due to its potentially life-threatening complications such as pneumothorax and mediastinal air.[139] Additionally, this ventilatory technique may promote "seeding" of papillomata down the airway during laser surgery.[138]

Emergence and Extubation

Difficulty during induction, and/or airway management, will likely be a good predictor of difficulty during emergence and extubation. These problems may include a low threshold for obstruction, coughing, laryngospasm, and regurgitation. Whenever possible, information from previous anesthetic experiences should be obtained and the anesthesiologist should prepare for the worst. Prevention of aspiration of secretions during emergence and extubation is an important consideration in management of the pediatric airway. Without this prevention, laryngospasm may be precipitated and management of the airway will become much more challenging. Details on techniques to reduce laryngospasm have been included in Section A of this chapter. In order to minimize the risk of airway edema resulting from airway manipulations, the use of 0.1 mg/kg of dexamethasone after or during a difficult intubation is justifiably and commonly used. Patients typically receive humidified oxygen until fully awake to ensure any secretions are easily mobilized.

After the procedure, all patients should be observed in the recovery room or intensive care unit, for as long as any problems of postoperative airway obstruction persist. After extubation the patient's airway may become obstructed and difficult to manage, and if narcotics have been administered, they should be rapidly reversed. The initial dosage of naloxone for this indication is 0.01 mg/kg. If anticholinergic medications were administered prior to the endoscopy, they will provide the dual benefit of decreasing airway secretions and attenuating vagally-mediated bradycardia associated with mechanical stimulation of the airway. Any stridor may be relieved by nebulized adrenaline.

Sedation and analgesia may be required in the intensive care unit, especially after laryngotracheal reconstruction.[140] These patients are often kept intubated for several days to facilitate wound healing, and maintenance of immobility during this period will be important. Sedation is often primarily achieved with benzodiazepines (e.g., midazolam: initial dose 0.05–0.10 mg/kg [6 months to 5 years]; 0.025–0.05 mg/kg [6–12 years]: infusions of 0.025–0.05 mg/kg/h with titrations to effect) and/or propofol (under close monitoring and within limits of 4 mg/kg/h for no more than 48 h), with a variety of adjuvant drugs according to presentation and experience. Opioid analgesic agents and nonsteroidal antiinflammatory drugs (NSAIDS) are commonly used. Alternatively, ketamine or dexmedetomidine may be utilized for their combined sedative-analgesic properties, and the latter for its potential to prevent opioid tolerance when combined infusions are implemented. Paralytic agents are used as a last resort. Regular assessment of sedation and analgesia must be performed to avoid excessive drug doses, or inadequate levels of sedation or analgesia. Sedation scales are commonly used, although BIS scores may be used in some cases (they are inaccurate in children under 5 years of age).

Clinical Scenarios

The following scenarios were selected to illustrate the essence of airway management for endoscopic procedures, as commonly presented to tertiary care facilities, and documented by a retrospective study (unpublished). After obtaining approval of the local Ethical Review Board, a database review was conducted for those patients who required airway endoscopy (laryngoscopy, bronchoscopy), or emergent establishment of a compromised airway at the Stollery Children's Hospital (Edmonton, AB, Canada) since June 2002. The patients were identified from a surgical database (Microsoft Access® 2000) kept prospectively by one of the authors. The database contains demographic data, diagnoses, procedures and other details about urgency, anesthesia, instrumentation, and complications. Figure 10.17 illustrates the data as stratified by diagnoses and urgency.

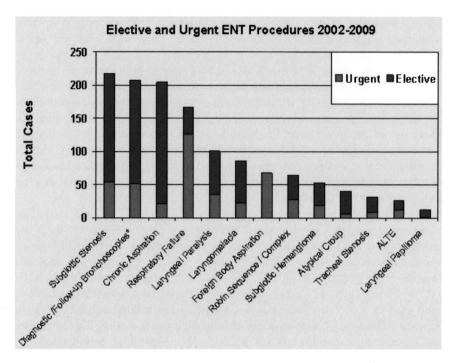

Fig. 10.17 Data from retrospective review of prospectively kept surgical database for ENT cases requiring airway endoscopy (laryngoscopy, bronchoscopy), or emergent establishment of a compromised airway

The following presentations highlight common indications for endoscopy in specific situations encountered by one otolaryngologist. The cases are presented in sequence related to their etiology and level in the laryngo-tracheo-bronchial tree. This classification groups similar presentation modes and challenges with respect to access for securing the airway, and critically compromised pulmonary reserve. While there is some comment on the chosen anesthetic technique, the previous section on Anesthetic Considerations for Endoscopic Procedures can be referred to for more discussion regarding the specific options available for use during each procedure. 10.1 will be referred to at times to consider each option in the context of available choices for anesthetic management.

Upper Airway Pathology

Micro-/Retrognathia

Infants and children with micro-/retrognathia, glossoptosis (Fig. 10.18), upper airway obstruction with or without cleft palate, constitute the range of Robin sequence

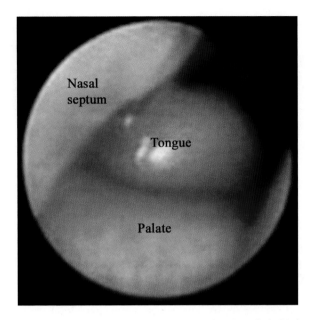

Fig. 10.18 Bronchoscope image demonstrating the tongue riding through the U-shaped cleft palate

and complex.[141] Their presentation mode, acuity and intubation times vary, but their anesthetic management is not commonly an easy affair, even on subsequent visits.

Recently, antenatal diagnosis has offered the alternative of using the EXIT procedure (see related description at the end of the Upper Airway Pathology section) to safeguard the airway, but this has as yet to gain wide acceptance. The more benign, and relatively less common, presentation is with symptoms of sleep disordered breathing, with or without cosmetic concerns. Early warnings should be available to the otolaryngologist or the maxillofacial surgeon in the clinic when assessing the thyromental distance, the Mallampati grade, and level of the cricoid cartilage in relation to the sternum. Any suspicion of difficulties should be supplemented with preoperative sleep studies. Additional signs of decreased respiratory reserve were presented when a barrel-chested adolescent male with Goldenhar syndrome was being investigated for a dental procedure. A useful exercise is to examine such a patient with the flexible fibreoptic laryngoscope while awake in the clinic to determine the utility of nasotracheal intubation over the scope. This technique would be compromised by choanal atresia, stenosis, or severely deviated septa, all of which are prevalent in this group. The endoscopy would also help document the position of the tongue and the larynx, and the feasibility of an awake oral intubation.

Newborn babies may be referred to an anesthesiologist having already been intubated (in essence having decompensated), or with persistent obstruction and varying degree of distress. Neonatal intensive care units will customarily insert a feeding nasogastric or nasojejunal tube to ensure the baby is thriving, and to protect their lower airway. Many patients will improve considerably on that alone, and

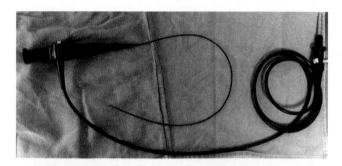

Fig. 10.19 Flexible bronchoscope which can facilitate intubation in the child with a difficult to visualize larynx

others will require maneuvers from semiprone positioning, to insertion of nasopharyngeal airways and, on occasion, continuous positive airway pressure ventilation. Bedside assessment of the phenotype, the vital signs, and the degree of intervention required can help. But the picture can change over time due to more awake hours, increase demand due to sepsis, and concomitant congenital cardiac, metabolic, neurologic and airway conditions.

The most useful, and sometimes the only planned method to secure the airway is intubation over a flexible bronchoscope (Fig. 10.19). It is best performed in the operating room, with available facilities for rigid bronchoscopy and tracheostomy. The procedure is also considered a useful guide to choosing the ultimate long-term method of securing the upper airway – namely a tracheostomy, mandibular distraction, tongue lip adhesion, a nasopharyngeal airway, modification of feeding route or consistency, or indeed none.

Sher et al.[142] described four patterns of obstruction. The first is where the tongue collapses to abut the posterior pharyngeal wall directly; whereas in the second, the soft palate is trapped in between the collapsing tongue and the posterior pharyngeal wall. The third and the fourth is where lateral and circumferential pharyngeal collapse is observed, respectively. The latter two patterns are usually suggestive of the need for a tracheostomy. These patterns could be observed during the awake or the anesthetized status. Rapid onset, short acting agents are the usual choice to give a decent window of time, in addition to topical anesthesia on the larynx. The appropriate size ETT is railed over the bronchoscope, and an assistant is required to introduce the well-lubricated tube through the nose when the endoscopist successfully negotiates the bronchoscope beyond the subglottis.

For an otolaryngologist, adding a bronchoscopy procedure prior to intubation is mandatory, as coexisting airway abnormalities can change the management significantly. The procedure should be performed using the shortest and least traumatic-sized bronchoscope that will do the job. Upon conclusion, if the patient is intubated, the nasotracheal route is preferred to minimize tube-related trauma of the airway. Transfer of the patient to the intensive care unit is usually employed while the patient is breathing spontaneously, and it is highly recommended to attach a label noting a critical airway. Accidental extubation may occur especially in newborns, and the pharmacological balance between sedation and avoidance of muscle relaxation could be elusive.

If a tongue-lip adhesion is required, the intubated baby will not require any special perioperative changes until the surgeon deems the timing suitable for extubation. However, if a bronchoscopy is required as a planned step, or if failure of the operation occurs, the field could become even more challenging. Using the flexible scope in a retrograde fashion to that described could be the best answer to securing an edematous obscure airway.

In those cases where a tracheostomy has been elected, it is of paramount importance to monitor the steps of positioning, as accidental extubation can occur and ensuring correct tube placement is important. After the surgeon has declared that the airway has been entered, and when a tracheostomy tube is to be introduced, the anesthetist should ensure that a reintroduction of the ETT is feasible at any given moment using either a flexible scope or guide wire.

A tracheostomy could obviously, but fortunately not commonly, be the stabilizing technique in an emergency. This situation occurred in the case of one of our patients with near total concomitant subglottic stenosis. The tracheostomy procedure was performed while the anesthetist was providing face mask ventilation. On another occasion in an adolescent with Goldenhar's syndrome, bleeding obscured the field for the endoscopist while attempting an awake endoscopy. A tracheostomy was deemed to require splitting the sternum but instead we elected to perform a cricothyrotomy under local anesthetic coupled with sedation. Intubation was successful through insertion of a Seldinger guide wire, retrieving it from the oral cavity, and then railing the ETT over it, after which the neck wound was closed.

Recurrent Respiratory Papilloma

A 2-year-old girl presented with longstanding dysphonia, and slowly progressive respiratory distress. She was the first born to a white, educated, middle class couple. There was no maternal history of genital human papillomavirus (HPV) infection, and her delivery was by vaginal route and uncomplicated. Owing to the age and the consistent subcostal and suprasternal retraction, no attempt to examine the larynx was made in the outpatient clinic. An urgent hospital admission with a high-dependency bed for postoperative care was requested. The surgeon communicated the high likelihood of recurrent respiratory papilloma with an intention to use the skimmer microdebrider blade. This blade has proven to offer better postoperative comfort, (arguably) less frequent treatment episodes, and superior voice preservation than the CO_2 Laser.[143] The use of this device as opposed to lasers also removes the risk potential for airway fires.

At the first examination, having both the flexible and rigid bronchoscopes afford securing a previously unknown airway, and an opportunity to detect more proximal (nasal and pharyngeal) and distal (tracheal and bronchial) lesions (Fig. 10.20). The latter, in particular, have profound detrimental impact on the long-term prognosis and forewarn a critical airway status. Fortunately in this particular case, the disease was confined to the larynx. A biopsy was obtained for confirming the diagnosis and

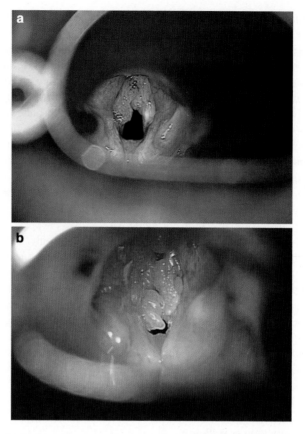

Fig. 10.20 (**a**, **b**) Lesions due to respiratory papilloma. Lesions in the distal airway (trachea, bronchus) can pose serious airway difficulties

subtyping the HPV. The subtype (type 11 vs. 6) along with the disease severity, the clinical complaint (respiratory embarrassment), and a young age at presentation are important pointers to a more aggressive natural history.[144]

After positioning and suspension as previously described, and following the biopsy, the microdebrider is used to debulk the lesion, conserving simultaneously the mucosa of unaffected areas. When a patient's unique natural history is elucidated from prior procedures, one can plan to discharge these patients the same day, with the exception of infants.

Performing the procedure under spontaneous respiration (Box 10.2 Option 1 or 2) is crucial for stabilizing emergently presenting patients, since the observed "bubble" produced during expiration could be the only clue to the whereabouts of the airway lumen. This buys enough time to direct an ETT, or a rigid bronchoscope if necessary, without the risk of total obstruction which may happen while using a muscle relaxant. On the other hand, in previously known patients, the team might choose to perform the procedure using the apneic technique (Box 10.2 Option 3). For some time, jet ventilation has fallen out of favor for fear of distal dissemination of the viral particles, especially during the use of laser evaporation, among other reasons.

This disease is rare (1.7–4.3 per 100,000 incidence in children),[144] but the clinical course has a staggering demand on medical services, with many procedures required per patient, for a very long time. These patients will be a well known group of "frequent fliers" whose information should be shared by the members of the surgical and anesthetic teams.

Subglottic Stenosis/Hemangioma

Subglottic stenosis is probably one of the most common reasons for bronchoscopy in a tertiary referral center (Fig. 10.21). The condition may present at an established

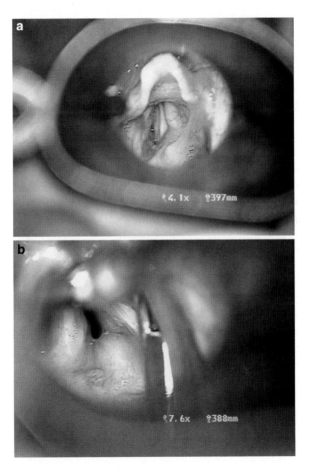

Fig. 10.21 (**a, b**) Subglottic stenosis is one of the most common reasons for bronchoscopy in the pediatric population

stage or "in the making." The latter is usually in an infant or a newborn where repeated attempts to extubate failed in the neonatal (less likely the pediatric) intensive care unit. The common scenario involves a premature baby (severe or moderate), who had been intubated for a prolonged period, and more often than not, had experienced multiple, accidental extubations and hurried reintubations.

Apart from these incidents, it is also customary to elucidate a history of using a larger than age appropriate ETT. The literature supports, to some degree, the incrimination of the larger tube and the prolonged period of ventilation in the pathogenesis of the condition.[145] An older infant or toddler may present with a similar problem or persistent stridor, and variable exertion to breathe upon extubation in pediatric intensive care. These patients are usually those who have undergone major cardiac procedures, and may still have a relatively unstable cardiac status. The observed stenosis in these cases is immature, soft and at a potentially-salvageable stage. The combination of PICU resources, surgeon and anesthesiologist expertise and accurate documentation, allows ample perioperative opportunity to provide an adequate level of care for this situation.

The alternate scenario is that of a toddler with swallowing dysfunction and chronic aspiration, living in the community. In these cases, the patient may harbor a history of prematurity and chronic lung disease and, not uncommonly, ongoing symptoms of esophagitis (either gastro-esophageal reflux disease, or eosinophilic esophagitis). These children will have a less than ideal lung function, and many well be on bronchodilators.

Other children may be undergoing the endoscopy for symptoms of atypical croup. These symptoms usually include episodes of biphasic stridor and barking cough occurring either recurrently, too early in the life-time of the patient (younger than 6 months old), or much later than 4 years of age. A reference to an older hospital chart will usually attest to the story, with documentation of visits to the local emergency departments. Rarely, these children will experience an unusually severe acute "croup" requiring emergency intubation, which will be achieved using a much smaller than appropriate for age tube. In the latter two situations, the stenosis is usually an established one.

The pediatric otolaryngologist's aim is to establish a diagnosis, rank its severity, secure the airway temporarily or definitively, and put forward a plan for later management.

The first step will be to estimate how narrow the airway is. On occasions, the indwelling ETT will give the clue, while in others a prior operative record will determine exactly the grade and state of the stenosis. Generally speaking, the bronchoscopy should be performed with a smaller size instrument than is expected for age and weight, in order to avoid additional trauma. The surgeon may elect initially to inspect, but not to engage the larynx, and proceed only after the subglottis is sized in the fashion described by Cotton and Meyer.[146] These authors consider the appropriate size of ETT to be one that allows an audible air leak around the tube at 20 cm H_2O and, using their standard tables, allocates the stenosis one of four grades. Upon completing that step, an appropriately-sized bronchoscope is chosen and used to inspect the whole of the laryngo-tracheo-bronchial tree. This establishes the length of the stenosis, and whether it is predominantly anterior or posterior. A suspension laryngoscopy confirms the state (soft or mature) of the stenosis, its relation to the level of the glottis, and indeed if another airway problem coexists or not. Also very important, the laryngoscopy discovers whether or not the mobility of the vocal cords is affected (by the same or different pathology).

These steps imply the use of spontaneous respiration at least until all the information regarding dynamic pathologies is gathered (Box 10.2 Options 1 or 2). It has been our experience that "sizing" up the subglottis is better performed while the patient is in a very deep plane of anesthesia, in order to avoid an erroneous impression of stenosis due to laryngospasm. This mode of anesthesia, particularly TIVA, may also allow the surgeon to perform an endoscopic dilation or a debridement using power assisted instruments, or to apply steroids or other pharmacological agents. The latter techniques have recently gained popular support (over lasers and bouginage), hoping that some open subglottic expansion procedures and tracheostomies may be avoided.[147]

If an endoscopic solution is neither feasible nor definitive, the surgeon usually secures the airway with an appropriately-sized tube, simultaneously allowing for easy, uninterrupted, ventilation and lower airway toilet. Cautionary notes regarding the ease of reintubation should be clearly communicated to the relevant unit that will host the patient.

Given the availability of expertise at all levels, and in appropriate facilities, resorting to an immediate tracheostomy is rare. Despite this, it should never be ruled out as a possibility, especially in cases of acute inflammation over and above an existing stenosis. In extreme situations, the operation is performed while the patient is mask ventilated. Preferably still, many centers will stock size 2.0 ETT which will engage most encountered stenoses. Depending on the severity, the general condition (particularly concomitant cardiorespiratory issues), and finally the preferred strategy of the surgeon, either a multiple or single stage reconstruction is chosen if endoscopic means fail.

Many patients will be bronchoscoped while an indwelling tracheostomy is in place, either before or after a repair has been undertaken. This will secure the airway, and ensure enough information is available so that surprises are less likely. The usual aim is to update the grade of the stenosis and the state of the suprastomal region. It is perfectly reasonable to use a muscle relaxant with these patients.

These patients earnestly are another group of the "frequent fliers" for bronchoscopy theaters; their management is multistaged, lengthy, and their share of resources is considerable.

Laryngomalacia (LM)

This is arguably the most common congenital laryngeal anomaly (Fig. 10.22).[148] The presentation is usually within the first 2–3 months of life, in the form of

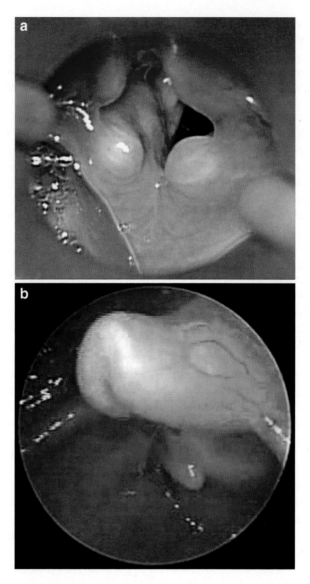

Fig. 10.22 (**a**, **b**) Two examples of laryngomalacia. Laryngomalacia is one of the most common congenital laryngeal abnormalities encountered

inspiratory stridor, associated with variable degree of increased work of breathing.

Later presentations (mean age 6 years) have been recently described with swallowing difficulties, sleep-disordered breathing, and exercise intolerance.[149] A procedure will rarely be performed emergently, but not unusually on an urgent basis. Depending on the severity of airway hindrance, the patient will need either admission to an intensive care admission post endoscopy and surgery, or a high dependency unit. The choice of level of care will be guided by many factors, including (1) prior documentation of the incidence of apparent life threatening episodes (apneic spells, or cyanosis), (2) the average oxygen saturations and respiratory rate, (3) an overnight sleep oximetry or a polysomnography when available, and (4) the requirement of treatment for associated gastro-esophageal reflux disease and/or provision of an alternate route of feeding.

A 6 month-old baby boy, originally from Ghana, presented with a moderately severe picture of LM. In addition to the classical awake symptoms, he also presented with moderate sleep-disordered breathing and required a modified oral diet to minimize the risk of aspiration. The abnormality was detected on flexible endoscopy in the clinic. The parents were counseled for a supraglottoplasty when conservative means evidently did not improve the clinical picture. A high dependency bed was reserved for post surgical care.

The infant was brought into the operating room, and general anesthesia was induced intravenously. The neonatal flexible bronchoscope confirmed the presence of a severe anomaly, permitted evaluation of movement of the larynx, and excluded other upper airway anomalies. Upon rigid bronchoscopy there was no coexistent anomaly in the tracheo-bronchial tree, as cited to occur in between 20 and 60% of patients.[150]

Microlaryngoscopy and supraglottoplasty were subsequently performed, within, as ideal, a free nonintubated airway. This procedure was performed speedily, while accurately dividing the aryepiglottic folds and/or reducing the supraarytenoid tissues, thus allowing for limited edema formation and minimal chances of scar formation. It was performed with the patient breathing spontaneously, and with 50–100% oxygen (plus or minus sevoflurane) insufflated through a designated side port (Box 10.2 Option 1 or 2). While ensuring hemostasis and after administering a dose of dexamethasone (0.1 mg/kg), the patient was transported to the recovery area, breathing spontaneously.

Typically, these patients are prescribed bronchodilators and proton pump inhibitors for a period that varies from 3 to 6 weeks after surgery. Younger babies may require intubation postoperatively, usually for one night.

Laryngeal Paralysis

Movement disorders of the larynx are not uncommon in children. They may present benignly with a voice change (unilateral paralysis, spasmodic dysphonia), or with stridor and aspiration (bilateral paralysis or fixation, vocal cord dysfunction, laryngeal dyskinesia). In the adult patient, many of these disorders could be diagnosed and assessed in the awake state, courtesy of the larger caliber of the available endoscopes and the compliance of the subject. However, in children, anesthesia is used not only because of lack of cooperation and instrument resolution, but also due to the subtle nature of the abnormalities, the critical respiratory embarrassment, and the variation in findings. On these occasions, the aims of the surgeon are to:

document if indeed there is a movement problem (as opposed to simple mucosal lesions causing hoarseness); differentiate mechanical from neurological etiologies; demonstrate and document the variation between awake and sedated status; secure the airway at the conclusion of the procedure; and rule out concomitant airway pathology.

Bilateral laryngeal paralysis, the most pressing of these conditions, is either of central neurological etiology (due to cerebrovascular events or to hydrocephalus), of peripheral neurological etiology (due to iatrogenic postcardiac procedures or to neurotoxicity of vinca alkaloids), or of the idiopathic variety.[151] In our experience, the presentation is more critical the younger the age of onset. Depending on the etiology, concomitant medical conditions may also impact the acuity and urgency of the bronchoscopy.

An initial awake examination in the operating room may be advisable, as the incidence of apparent life-threatening events, or an accompanying compromised cardiac status may preclude an earlier inspection on the ward; in this way, the rapid onset of an unsalvageable situation is preventable. This is followed by an examination using the flexible endoscope, transnasally, while the patient is anesthetized and breathing spontaneously (Box 10.2 Options 1 or 2). While this instrument will allow the examination to take place in as physiological a position as possible, its resolution will be limited, and there will be no opportunity to assess passive mobility. The latter is achieved once a microlaryngoscopy is performed. The challenge for the anesthesiologist here will be to deepen the plane of sedation enough for the patient to tolerate the endoscope placement, while simultaneously allowing inspection of a full range of movement. The surgeon during this stage will also use cold steel instruments to palpate the arytenoids and examine the cricoarytenoid joints for fixation.

An additional examination, which we recently adopted in our institution, is laryngeal electromyography.[152] This is a brief step that offers a permanent record of the neuromuscular integrity governing the two main actions of the larynx. While the larynx is suspended, fine monopolar electrodes are inserted into the laryngeal muscles (namely the thyroarytenoids and posterior cricoarytenoids, bilaterally), while surface electrodes are attached to the chest wall to document synchronous respiratory movement (Fig. 10.23).

The possible patterns found are: normal patterns that are phase-locked to the respiratory cycle, normal patterns that are not locked to the cycle, no tracing at all, or irregular firing. All of the last three patterns can be encountered in laryngeal paralysis. The recording and interpretation requires the presence of a neurophysiologist or a neurologist familiar with the technique. Sources of interference with the recordings include toy bear huggers, intravenous line poles, personnel touching the patient, and nonrespiratory movement. The results can change decisions regarding the management and its timing. There have been no incidents where significant edema or bleeding has occurred.

Our preference for the anesthetic technique is to avoid inhalational agents due to their effect on the mobility and the shorter duration of inspection they afford as opposed to a titratable total intravenous anesthetic (Box 10.2 Option 1).

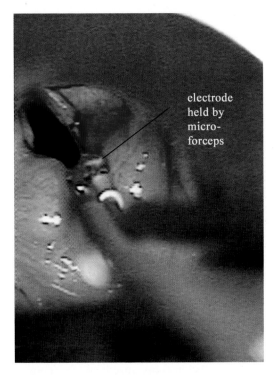

electrode
held by
micro-
forceps

Fig. 10.23 Electromyography allows a permanent record of the neuromuscular integrity of the larynx. The results of this examination must be interpreted by a neurophysiologist or a neurologist familiar with this technique

EXIT Procedure

The Ex-utero intrapartum procedure has been developed to safely deliver a fetus afflicted by a lesion and requiring prolonged maintenance on feto-maternal circulation until another controllable alternative for oxygenation is secured surgically. The arch-example and most common lesion is the cervicofacial lymphatic malformation, which involves the fetal airway (Fig. 10.24). Since the diagnosis is invariably made antenatally (using ultrasound and/or magnetic resonance imaging), it instigates a careful multidisciplinary counseling process (perinatologist, neonatologist, pediatric or fetal surgeon, high risk obstetric surgeon, pediatrician, and anesthetist). Few centers will offer the service, which will be executed on designated sites, by designated teams, and supplanted by various levels of contingency plans.

The EXIT procedure has replaced the Operation on Placental Support (OOPS) procedure as the procedure of choice for fetal airway management. In the OOPS procedure, the fetus is delivered and the uteroplacental circulation is maintained by leaving the umbilical cord intact. There is no attempt to compensate for the loss of uterine volume and unfortunately uteroplacental circulation may not be maintained leading to potential neonatal complications.[153]

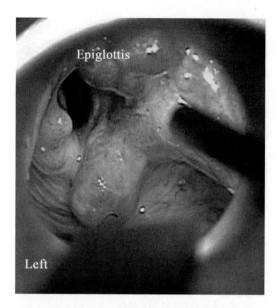

Fig. 10.24 Cervicofacial lymphatic malformation involving the larynx

In contrast, during an EXIT procedure only the fetal head and thorax are delivered; the uteroplacental circulation is optimized; and the uterus is maintained in a state of hypotonia to preserve the uterine volume and prevent placental abruption or maternal hemorrhage (Fig. 10.25).[154]

The EXIT procedure allows for the controlled evaluation of the fetal airway, endotracheal intubation, tracheostomy, or possible neck dissection while avoiding fetal hypoxia, ischemic brain injury or death.[155] The deep maternal anesthesia will also allow for the fetal surgery to be performed without cardiac depression to the fetus while optimizing uterine blood flow.[154] It has been reported that the uteroplacental circulation can be maintained for up to 1 h; however, the average time is 30.3 ± 14.7 min.[154, 156]

The baby whose lesion is depicted in Fig. 10.24 was delivered close to term, and a successful endotracheal intubation was performed. The lymphatic malformation did not affect the airway to a significant degree, and was treated subsequently with sequential sessions of sclerosing agents.

Lower Airway Pathology

Foreign Body Aspiration

The child, usually a toddler, presenting with a potential foreign body aspiration is probably the most common indication for an *emergent* airway endoscopy.

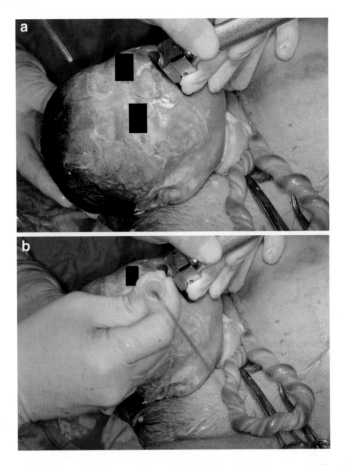

Fig. 10.25 (**a, b**) During an EXIT procedure only the fetal head and thorax are delivered allowing the controlled evaluation and management (including surgical) of the fetal airway

Once a reliable history unfolds that a witnessed choking spell has taken place, the procedure is mandatory, despite the lack of certainty. Time spent in investigations and inaction until signs are evident only serve to complicate the procedure, and possibly turn a safe experience in expert hands to a potentially life-threatening event even in the best of them.[157] Allowing for no more than a handful of hours to pass for a safer induction of anesthesia, the endoscopy should be planned with the team. If the patient is in distress, or a cyanotic spell has been reported, then it is permissible to forgo the empty stomach rule and proceed. Although auscultation and plain chest x-rays can suggest the side maximally affected, the exact location of the foreign body and the degree of affection of the site impacted and the airway distal to it cannot be predicted (Fig. 10.26). And despite the lack of evidence supporting the superiority of employing a spontaneous ventilation technique, vs. using a muscle relaxant, the former allows for

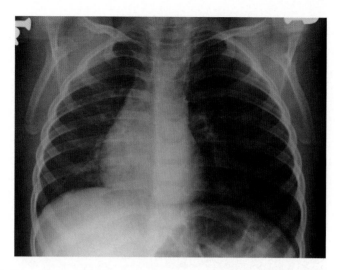

Fig. 10.26 Chest radiograph demonstrating air trapping after accidental inhalation of a foreign body

a preliminary assessment under the safest possible conditions. Examples of the served situations include: bilateral bronchial foreign bodies with partial impaction, tracheal or subglottic foreign bodies, and migrating foreign bodies between the two primary bronchi. Whereas, if the foreign body reaction leads to a small airway spasm, or pulmonary edema coexists, the use of PPV would be greatly facilitated by the use of muscle relaxation. The ancillary use of topical anesthesia in the distal airway, in addition to a vasoconstrictor, can help reduce the reaction to trauma and the concomitant bleeding which are commonly encountered.

The prerequisites for the safe execution of this endoscopy, aside from experience, are an appropriate range of instruments, speedy but not hurried technique, and minimal reinsertions of the endoscope (Fig. 10.27a–c). Constant dialog between the anesthesiologist and the endoscopist on the efficiency of gas exchange is required especially after prolonged scoping in one primary bronchus. Additional instruments such as the Fogarthy balloon catheters, urology stone basket, and fine flexible suction catheter, allow for quicker extraction of some objects (especially blunt and slippery ones), uninterrupted visualization, and more room and time for ventilation through the rigid bronchoscope.

Flexible bronchoscopy is advocated by some publications for initial exploration of the airway, and possibly to enable a less traumatic approach. The availability of fewer and smaller forceps, and the lack of contribution of the instrument to ventilation pose significant drawbacks.

The outcome is usually safe and successful. However, if a respiratory arrest occurs at the primary location, or the foreign body requires an open procedure, the outlook could be significantly more pessimistic.

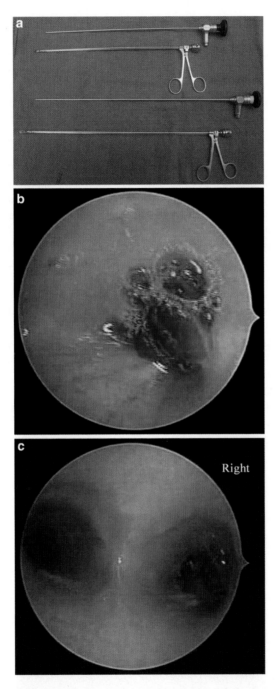

Fig. 10.27 (**a**) Range of instruments in preparation for a rigid bronchoscopy of a patient with a foreign body. (**b**, **c**) Bronchoscope images showing foreign bodies stuck in the bronchus

Tracheal Stenosis

Cases of tracheal stenosis are quite uncommon, and the epidemiology of the congenital (more common) variety and its natural history are poorly documented (Fig. 10.28).[150, 158, 159] However, they pose a substantial challenge during diagnostic and therapeutic procedures. There are two recognized modes of presentation. The first scenario is the infant who, soon after birth or shortly thereafter, presents with respiratory failure, and becomes difficult to ventilate on an intensive care unit; or indeed fails to extubate and requires continuous support.

The second, less common presentation in the authors' institution, is an older child or adolescent with a presumed diagnosis of lifelong asthma and blunted expiratory curves on pulmonary function tests and, occasionally, a highly suggestive plain radiograph of the chest. Concomitant congenital heart and large vessel anomalies are very common, followed by abnormal branching of the tracheobronchial tree. A classically encountered configuration is that of complete tracheal rings,[160] with variable affection of the total length, the cross-sectional area, and the level of maximal stenosis.

Figure 10.28 illustrates a case with more than 50% stenosis, a trachea that allowed negotiation of 2.7 mm rod lens telescope threaded through and beyond an appropriate size ventilating bronchoscope. The maximal stenosis was 1 cm above the carina, and an associated right severe bronchial stenosis was encountered in addition to a pulmonary artery sling (later demonstrated on contrast enhanced computer tomography).

Whereas, to date, the last of three cases never required surgical intervention, the second case was more challenging. In addition to having a longer affected segment,

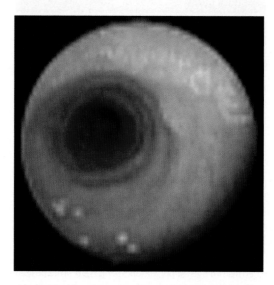

Fig. 10.28 Tracheal Stenosis. An uncommon and relatively poorly understood congenital mal formation

the patient had left-sided pulmonary aplasia and pulmonary hypertension, and continued to exhibit apparent life threatening episodes. He was diagnosed with VACTERL.

The purpose of a full airway endoscopy initially is to establish the diagnosis and to determine the affected site(s), severity and extent of involvement of the airway, and whether associated tracheobronchial anomalies exist. The respiratory status is usually precarious, and avoiding unnecessary instrumentation is crucial to avoid precipitating a crisis mandating emergent establishment of extracorporeal membrane oxygenation (ECHMO). This situation requires prior anticipation by both the surgeon and the anesthesiologist and questions the suitability of the managing center to handle the complexity of the case. In most cases, it must be anticipated that no available ETT or ventilating bronchoscope will be negotiable through the area of maximal stenosis. Upon termination of the procedure, younger children may be returned intubated. Solutions that may irritate the child and again precipitate a respiratory failure should be avoided and, if intubation is the choice, the tube should not engage the stenotic segment to avoid edema or obstruction against the tracheal wall. This arrangement must include the intensivist involved and the on-call pediatric cardiothoracic surgeon.

Notwithstanding the dilemmas posed by availability of surgical talent and of cardiothoracic services, and the general condition of the child addressed, surgical repair has only recently been truly rewarding. The slide tracheoplasty procedure has been well established as a new standard of care, having better results but daunting requirements of ECHMO or cardio-pulmonary bypass and their attending morbidity. Subsequent endoscopies to check the integrity of the repair, possibly dilate or stent stenosed areas, or debride or laser granulations will be required. The myriad of potential findings require the availability of full range of instruments, material, flexibility, and expertise.

Respiratory Failure or Failure to Extubate ICU Children: Children with Known Cardiac, or Neurological Pathology, vs. Virgin Cases

Children and infants may exhibit signs and symptoms of respiratory failure that are hard to ascribe to a specific etiology without examining the large airways. In this section, we would like to attend to a group that is not known to have experienced traumatic or prolonged intubation. Rather, they are residents of intensive care units due to known neurological insults (head injury, hydrocephalus, cervical trauma), have cardiac pathology, or are children presenting with episodic apparent life-threatening episodes. In each situation cardiac and neurological conditions need to be taken into consideration as the anesthetic technique will require modification accordingly, and every effort should be made for appropriate investigation prior to the endoscopy.

Cardiac and large vessel abnormalities are known to be associated with airway pathology, whether congenital or acquired.[161] In fact one could argue that a routine involvement of an airway surgeon in the preoperative investigations and follow-up of these children is well warranted. Most of the pathologies will be dynamic (laryngeal paralysis, and tracheo-bronchomalacia) and require both flexible and rigid endoscopies while spontaneous respiration is maintained. A prime issue with many of these patients is whether the patient is anticoagulated or not, as rigid endoscopy can be relatively hazardous.

Neurological ailments will be mainly associated with issues related to laryngeal competence, respiratory movement, and protection of lower airway. These are more commonly mediated by insults at the brain stem level. Depending on the level of consciousness, bedside examination and reports from neurologists on the presence of gag reflexes, management of salivary secretions, and other accompanying deficits of cranial nerves will provide invaluable information.

Children with apparent life-threatening events require some basic evaluation of neurologic and cardiac function and once these are performed, the usual problems encountered are periodic apnea, gastroesophageal reflux aspiration, laryngeal clefts, or vascular compression syndromes (double aortic arch, innominate artery compression). The question regarding management usually involves whether a tracheostomy is warranted in the first two occasions. Ethical considerations, and issues related to the prognosis of the different scenarios prevail, as does the complexity of whether one etiology vs. the other plays the prime role in promoting the respiratory failure.

Acknowledgments The author would like to thank Jennifer Pillay, Nikki Stalker, and Adam Dryden and Jenkin Tsui for their contribution to this chapter.

References

1. Santillanes G, Gausche-Hill M. Pediatric airway management. *Emerg Med Clin North Am.* 2008;26:961–975, ix.
2. McGoldrick KE. The larynx: normal developmental and congenital anomalies. In: McGoldrick KE, ed. *Anesthesia for Ophthalmic and Otolaryngologic Surgery.* Philadelphia: WB Saunders; 1992:1–14.
3. Infosino A. Pediatric upper airway and congenital anomalies. *Anesthesiol Clin North America.* 2002;20:747–766.
4. Walker RWM. The paediatric airway. In: Calder I, Pearce A, eds. *Core Topics in Airway Management.* Cambridge: Cambridge University Press; 2005:123–129.
5. Crelin ES. Oral cavity and tongue. In: Crelin ES, ed. *Functional Anatomy of the Newborn.* London: Yale University Press; 1973:27–29.
6. Crelin ES. Development of the upper respiratory system. *Clin Symp.* 1976;28:12–13.
7. Laitman JT, Crelin ES, Conlogue GJ. The function of the epiglottis in monkey and man. *Yale J Biol Med.* 1977;50:43–48.
8. Negus VE. *The Comparative Anatomy and Physiology of the Larynx.* London: William Heinemann; 1949.
9. Crelin ES. *The Human Vocal Tract: Anatomy, Function, Development, and Evolution.* New York: Vantage Press; 1987.
10. Polgar G, Kong GP. The nasal resistance of newborn infants. *J Pediatr.* 1965;67:557–567.
11. Williams PL, Warwick R. *Gray's Anatomy.* Philadelphia: W.B. Saunders; 1980.

12. Luten RC, Kissoon N. Approach to the pediatric airway. In: Walls RM, Murphy MF, Luten RC, eds. *Manual of Emergency Airway Management.* 2nd ed. Philadelphia: Lippincott, Williams & Wilkins; 2004:263–281.
13. Godinez RI. Special problems in pediatric anesthesia. *Int Anesthesiol Clin.* 1985;23:88.
14. Eckenhoff JE. Some anatomic considerations of the infant larynx influencing endotracheal anesthesia. *Anesthesiology.* 1951;12:401–410.
15. Kundra P, Krishnan H. Airway management in children. *Indian J Anaesth.* 2005;49: 300–307.
16. Valois T. The pediatric difficult airway. In: Astuto M, ed. *Basics: Anesthesia, Intensive Care and Pain in Neonates and Children.* Italy: Springer; 2009:31–48.
17. Pueschel SM. Atlanto-axial subluxation in Downs syndrome. *Lancet.* 1983;1:980.
18. Bingham RM, Proctor LT. Airway management. *Pediatr Clin North Am.* 2008;55:873–886.
19. Rodenstein DO, Perlmutter N, Stanescu DC. Infants are not obligatory nasal breathers. *Am Rev Respir Dis.* 1985;131:343–347.
20. Litman RS, Wake N, Chan LM, et al. Effect of lateral positioning on upper airway size and morphology in sedated children. *Anesthesiology.* 2005;103:484–488.
21. Arai YC, Fukunaga K, Hirota S, Fujimoto S. The effects of chin lift and jaw thrust while in the lateral position on stridor score in anesthetized children with adenotonsillar hypertrophy. *Anesth Analg.* 2004;99:1638–1641, table.
22. Roth B, Magnusson J, Johansson I, Holmberg S, Westrin P. Jaw lift–a simple and effective method to open the airway in children. *Resuscitation.* 1998;39:171–174.
23. Meier S, Geiduschek J, Paganoni R, Fuehrmeyer F, Reber A. The effect of chin lift, jaw thrust, and continuous positive airway pressure on the size of the glottic opening and on stridor score in anesthetized, spontaneously breathing children. *Anesth Analg.* 2002;94:494–499.
24. Davidovic L, LaCovey D, Pitetti RD. Comparison of 1- versus 2-person bag-valve-mask techniques for manikin ventilation of infants and children. *Ann Emerg Med.* 2005; 46:37–42.
25. Moynihan RJ, Brock-Utne JG, Archer JH, Feld LH, Kreitzman TR. The effect of cricoid pressure on preventing gastric insufflation in infants and children. *Anesthesiology.* 1993;78:652–656.
26. Hunt EA, Fiedor-Hamilton M, Eppich WJ. Resuscitation education: narrowing the gap between evidence-based resuscitation guidelines and performance using best educational practices. *Pediatr Clin North Am.* 2008;55:1025–1050, xii.
27. International Liaison Committee on Resuscitation. 2005 International Consensus on Cardiopulmonary Resuscitation and Emergency Cardiovascular Care Science WithTreatment Recommendations. *Circulation.* 2005;112:III–1–III–136.
28a. American Heart Association. 2005 American heart association guidelines for cardiopulmonary resuscitation (CPR) and emergency cardiovascular care (ECC). *Circulation.* 2005; 112:IV1–IV203.
28b. American Heart Association. 2010 American Heart Association Guidelines for Cardiopulmonary Resuscitation and Emergency Cardiovascular Care. "*Circulation.* 2010;122(suppl 3):S640–S656. Guidelines for Cardiopulmonary Resuscitation and Emergency Cardiovascular Care." *Circulation.* 2010;122(suppl 3):S639–S946.
29. PGAR V. A proposal for a new method of evaluation of the newborn infant. *Curr Res Anesth Analg.* 1953;32:260–267.
30. Roy RN, Betheras FR. The Melbourne Chart–a logical guide to neonatal resuscitation. *Anaesth Intensive Care.* 1990;18:348–357.
31. American Heart Association, American Academy of Pediatrics. 2005 American Heart Association (AHA) Guidelines for Cardiopulmonary Resuscitation (CPR) and Emergency Cardiovascular Care (ECC) of Pediatric and Neonatal Patients: Neonatal Resuscitation Guidelines. *Pediatrics.* 2006;117:e1029–e1038.
32. Halliday HL. Endotracheal intubation at birth for preventing morbidity and mortality in vigorous, meconium-stained infants born at term. *Cochrane Database Syst Rev.* 2001; CD000500.

33. Wiswell TE, Gannon CM, Jacob J, et al. Delivery room management of the apparently vigorous meconium-stained neonate: results of the multicenter, international collaborative trial. *Pediatrics*. 2000;105:1–7.
34. Oca MJ, Nelson M, Donn SM. Randomized trial of normal saline versus 5% albumin for the treatment of neonatal hypotension. *J Perinatol*. 2003;23:473–476.
35. So KW, Fok TF, Ng PC, Wong WW, Cheung KL. Randomised controlled trial of colloid or crystalloid in hypotensive preterm infants. *Arch Dis Child Fetal Neonatal Ed*. 1997;76: F43–F46.
36. Rendell-Baker L. History and evolution of pediatric anesthesia equipment. *Int Anesthesiol Clin*. 1992;30:1–34.
37. Brambrink AM, Braun U. Airway management in infants and children. *Best Pract Res Clin Anaesthesiol*. 2005;19:675–697.
38. White MC, Cook TM, Stoddart PA. A critique of elective pediatric supraglottic airway devices. *Pediatr Anesth*. 2009;19(suppl 1):55–65.
39. Kelly F, Sale S, Bayley G, Cook T, Stoddart P, White M. A cohort evaluation of the pediatric ProSeal laryngeal mask airway in 100 children. *Pediatr Anesth*. 2008;18:947–951.
40. Wheeler M. ProSeal laryngeal mask airway in 120 pediatric surgical patients: a prospective evaluation of characteristics and performance. *Pediatr Anesth*. 2006;16:297–301.
41. Brain AI. The laryngeal mask–a new concept in airway management. *Br J Anaesth*. 1983;55:801–805.
42. Brimacombe JR. *The Laryngeal Mask Anaesthesia: Principles and Practice*. 2nd ed. London: Saunders; 2005.
43. Naguib ML, Streetman DS, Clifton S, Nasr SZ. Use of laryngeal mask airway in flexible bronchoscopy in infants and children. *Pediatr Pulmonol*. 2005;39:56–63.
44. Lopez-Gil M, Brimacombe J, Alvarez M. Safety and efficacy of the laryngeal mask airway. A prospective survey of 1400 children. *Anaesthesia*. 1996;51:969–972.
45. Bagshaw O. The size 1.5 laryngeal mask airway (LMA) in paediatric anaesthetic practice. *Pediatr Anesth*. 2002;12:420–423.
46. Park C, Bahk JH, Ahn WS, Do SH, Lee KH. The laryngeal mask airway in infants and children. *Can J Anesth*. 2001;48:413–417.
47. Walker RW. The laryngeal mask airway in the difficult paediatric airway: an assessment of positioning and use in fibreoptic intubation. *Pediatr Anesth*. 2000;10:53–58.
48. Polaner DM, Ahuja D, Zuk J, Pan Z. Video assessment of supraglottic airway orientation through the perilaryngeal airway in pediatric patients. *Anesth Analg*. 2006;102:1685–1688.
49. Ayre P. Anaesthesia for intracranial operation: new technique. *Lancet*. 1937;1:561.
50. GJ REES. Neonatal anaesthesia. *Br Med Bull*. 1958;14:38–41.
51. Doherty JS, Froom SR, Gildersleve CD. Pediatric laryngoscopes and intubation aids old and new. *Pediatr Anesth*. 2009;19(suppl 1):30–37.
52. Motoyama EK. The shape of the pediatric larynx: cylindrical or funnel shaped? *Anesth Analg*. 2009;108:1379–1381.
53. Weiss M, Dullenkopf A, Bottcher S, et al. Clinical evaluation of cuff and tube tip position in a newly designed paediatric preformed oral cuffed tracheal tube. *Br J Anaesth*. 2006;97: 695–700.
54. Dullenkopf A, Gerber AC, Weiss M. Fit and seal characteristics of a new paediatric tracheal tube with high volume-low pressure polyurethane cuff. *Acta Anaesthesiol Scand*. 2005;49:232–237.
55. Park W, Kim S, Choi H. The two different-sized fibreoptic bronchoscope method in the management of a difficult paediatric airway. *Anaesthesia*. 2001;56:90–91.
56. Bein B, Wortmann F, Meybohm P, Steinfath M, Scholz J, Dorges V. Evaluation of the pediatric Bonfils fiberscope for elective endotracheal intubation. *Pediatr Anesth*. 2008;18:1040–1044.
57. Fisher QA, Tunkel DE. Lightwand intubation of infants and children. *J Clin Anesth*. 1997;9:275–279.

58. Simon L, Boucebci KJ, Orliaguet G, Aubineau JV, Devys JM, Dubousset AM. A survey of practice of tracheal intubation without muscle relaxant in paediatric patients. *Pediatr Anesth.* 2002;12:36–42.
59. Luten RC, Kissoon N, Godwin SA, Murphy MF. Unique airway issues in the pediatric population. In: Hung OR, Murphy MF, eds. *Management of the Difficult and Failed Airway.* New York: McGraw-Hill; 2008:381–388.
60. Roy WL, Lerman J. Laryngospasm in paediatric anaesthesia. *Can J Anesth.* 1988;35:93–98.
61. Kent RD, Vorperian HK. *Development of the Craniofacial-Oral-Laryngeal Anatomy.* San Diego: Singular Publishing Group; 1995.
62. Gulhas N, Durmus M, Demirbilek S, Togal T, Ozturk E, Ersoy MO. The use of magnesium to prevent laryngospasm after tonsillectomy and adenoidectomy: a preliminary study. *Pediatr Anesth.* 2003;13:43–47.
63. Koc C, Kocaman F, Aygenc E, Ozdem C, Cekic A. The use of preoperative lidocaine to prevent stridor and laryngospasm after tonsillectomy and adenoidectomy. *Otolaryngol Head Neck Surg.* 1998;118:880–882.
64. Leicht P, Wisborg T, Chraemmer-Jorgensen B. Does intravenous lidocaine prevent laryngospasm after extubation in children? *Anesth Analg.* 1985;64:1193–1196.
65. Tsui BC, Wagner A, Cave D, Elliott C, El-Hakim H, Malherbe S. The incidence of laryngospasm with a "no touch" extubation technique after tonsillectomy and adenoidectomy. *Anesth Analg.* 2004;98:327–329, table.
66. Larson PC. Laryngospasm – the best treatment. *Anesthesiology.* 1998;89:1293–1294.
67. Holzki J, Laschat M, Puder C. Iatrogenic damage to the pediatric airway. Mechanisms and scar development. *Pediatr Aaesth.* 2009;19 suppl 1:131–146.
68. Sellars I, Keen EN. Laryngeal growth in infancy. *J Laryngol Otol.* 1990;104:622–625.
69. Dalal PG, Murray D, Messner AH, Feng A, McAllister J, Molter D. Pediatric laryngeal dimensions: an age-based analysis. *Anesth Analg.* 2009;108:1475–1479.
70. Litman RS, Weissend EE, Shibata D, Westesson PL. Developmental changes of laryngeal dimensions in unparalyzed, sedated children. *Anesthesiology.* 2003;98:41–45.
71. American Society of Anesthesiologists Task Force on Management of the Difficult Airway. Practice guidelines for management of the difficult airway: an updated report. *Anesthesiology.* 2003;98:1269–1277.
72. Bevilacqua S, Nicolini A, Del SP, et al. [Difficult intubation in paediatric cardiac surgery. Significance of age. Association with Down's syndrome]. *Minerva Anestesiol.* 1996;62:259–264.
73. Frei FJ, Ummenhofer W. Difficult intubation in paediatrics. *Pediatr Anesth.* 1996;6:251–263.
74. Marraro GA. Difficult airway. In: Gullo A, ed. *Anaesthesia, Pain, Intensive Care and Emergency Medicine. Proceedings of the 20th Postgraduate Course in Critical Care Medicine, Trieste Italy 2005.* Milan: Springer; 2006:763–778.
75. Walker RW, Ellwood J. The management of difficult intubation in children. *Pediatr Anesth.* 2009;19(suppl 1):77–87.
76. Kandasamy R, Sivalingam P. Use of sevoflurane in difficult airways. *Acta Anaesthesiol Scand.* 2000;44:627–629.
77. Ansermino JM, Brooks P, Rosen D, Vandebeek CA, Reichert C. Spontaneous ventilation with remifentanil in children. *Pediatr Anesth.* 2005;15:115–121.
78. von Ungern-Sternberg BS, Erb TO, Reber A, Frei FJ. Opening the upper airway–airway maneuvers in pediatric anesthesia. *Pediatr Anesth.* 2005;15:181–189.
79. Tantinikorn W, Alper CM, Bluestone CD, Casselbrant ML. Outcome in pediatric tracheotomy. *Am J Otolaryngol.* 2003;24:131–137.
80. Henderson JJ. The use of paraglossal straight blade laryngoscopy in difficult tracheal intubation. *Anaesthesia.* 1997;52:552–560.
81. Saxena KN, Nischal H, Bhardwaj M, Gaba P, Shastry BV. Right molar approach to tracheal intubation in a child with Pierre Robin syndrome, cleft palate, and tongue tie. *Br J Anaesth.* 2008;100:141–142.

82. Zoumalan R, Maddalozzo J, Holinger LD. Etiology of stridor in infants. *Ann Otol Rhinol Laryngol.* 2007;116:329–334.
83. Donnelly KJ, Bank ER, Parks WJ, et al. Three-dimensional magnetic resonance imaging evaluation of pediatric tracheobronchial tree. *Laryngoscope.* 1994;104:1425–1430.
84. Rutter MJ. Evaluation and management of upper airway disorders in children. *Semin Pediatr Surg.* 2006;15:116–123.
85. Bruce IA, Rothera MP. Upper airway obstruction in children. *Pediatr Anesth.* 2009;19(suppl 1): 88–99.
86. Daya H, Hosni A, Bejar-Solar I, Evans JN, Bailey CM. Pediatric vocal fold paralysis: a long-term retrospective study. *Arch Otolaryngol Head Neck Surg.* 2000;126:21–25.
87. Agrawal N, Black M, Morrison G. Ten-year review of laryngotracheal reconstruction for paediatric airway stenosis. *Int J Pediatr Otorhinolaryngol.* 2007;71:699–703.
88. White DR, Cotton RT, Bean JA, Rutter MJ. Pediatric cricotracheal resection: surgical outcomes and risk factor analysis. *Arch Otolaryngol Head Neck Surg.* 2005;131:896–899.
89. Gregori D, Salerni L, Scarinzi C, et al. Foreign bodies in the upper airways causing complications and requiring hospitalization in children aged 0–14 years: results from the ESFBI study. *Eur Arch Otorhinolaryngol.* 2008;265:971–978.
90. National Safety Council. Injury Facts, 2009 Edition. Internet . 2009. National Safety Council.
91. Harris CS, Baker SP, Smith GA, Harris RM. Childhood asphyxiation by food. A national analysis and overview. *JAMA.* 1984;251:2231–2235.
92. Lima JA. Laryngeal foreign bodies in children: a persistent, life-threatening problem. *Laryngoscope.* 1989;99:415–420.
93. Esclamado RM, Richardson MA. Laryngotracheal foreign bodies in children. A comparison with bronchial foreign bodies. *Am J Dis Child.* 1987;141:259–262.
94. Metrangelo S, Monetti C, Meneghini L, Zadra N, Giusti F. Eight years' experience with foreign-body aspiration in children: what is really important for a timely diagnosis? *J Pediatr Surg.* 1999;34:1229–1231.
95. American Thoracic Society. Standards and indications for cardiopulmonary sleep studies in children. *Am J Respir Crit Care Med.* 1996;153:866–878.
96. Au CT, Li AM. Obstructive sleep breathing disorders. *Pediatr Clin North Am.* 2009;56:243–259, xii.
97. Lerman J. A disquisition on sleep-disordered breathing in children. *Pediatr Anesth.* 2009;19(suppl 1):100–108.
98. Tauman R, Gulliver TE, Krishna J, et al. Persistence of obstructive sleep apnea syndrome in children after adenotonsillectomy. *J Pediatr.* 2006;149:803–808.
99. Watson GJ, Malik TH, Khan NA, Sheehan PZ, Rothera MP. Acquired paediatric subglottic cysts: a series from Manchester. *Int J Pediatr Otorhinolaryngol.* 2007;71:533–538.
100. McEwan J, Giridharan W, Clarke RW, Shears P. Paediatric acute epiglottitis: not a disappearing entity. *Int J Pediatr Otorhinolaryngol.* 2003;67:317–321.
101. Sharma N, Berman DM, Scott GB, Josephson G. Candida epiglottitis in an adolescent with acquired immunodeficiency syndrome. *Pediatr Infect Dis J.* 2005;24:91–92.
102. Singer J, Henry S. Upper airway obstruction as the presenting manifestation of leukemia. *Pediatr Emerg Care.* 2008;24:310–312.
103. Diaz JH. Croup and epiglottitis in children: the anesthesiologist as diagnostician. *Anesth Analg.* 1985;64:621–633.
104. Jenkins IA, Saunders M. Infections of the airway. *Pediatr Anesth.* 2009;19(suppl 1):118–130.
105. Bjornson CL, Johnson DW. Croup. *Lancet.* 2008;371:329–339.
106. Barker GA. Current management of croup and epiglottitis. *Pediatr Clin North Am.* 1979;26:565–579.
107. Fried MP. Controversies in the management of supraglottitis and croup. *Pediatr Clin North Am.* 1979;26:931–942.

108. Hopkins A, Lahiri T, Salerno R, Heath B. Changing epidemiology of life-threatening upper airway infections: the reemergence of bacterial tracheitis. *Pediatrics.* 2006;118:1418–1421.

109. Loftis L. Acute infectious upper airway obstructions in children. *Semin Pediatr Infect Dis.* 2006;17:5–10.

110. Wright CT, Stocks RM, Armstrong DL, Arnold SR, Gould HJ. Pediatric mediastinitis as a complication of methicillin-resistant Staphylococcus aureus retropharyngeal abscess. *Arch Otolaryngol Head Neck Surg.* 2008;134:408–413.

111. Coulthard M, Isaacs D. Retropharyngeal abscess. *Arch Dis Child.* 1991;66:1227–1230.

112. Perger L, Lee EY, Shamberger RC. Management of children and adolescents with a critical airway due to compression by an anterior mediastinal mass. *J Pediatr Surg.* 2008;43: 1990–1997.

113. Fidkowski CW, Fuzaylov G, Sheridan RL, Cote CJ. Inhalation burn injury in children. *Pediatr Anesth.* 2009;19(suppl 1):147–154.

114. Zur KB, Litman RS. Pediatric airway foreign body retrieval: surgical and anesthetic perspectives. *Pediatr Anesth.* 2009;19(suppl 1):109–117.

115. Johnson LB. Management of a 12-year-old child with a foreign body in the bronchus. In: Hung O, Murphy MF, eds. *Management of the Difficult and Failed Airway.* New York: McGraw Hill; 2008:395–399.

116. Ozguner IF, Buyukyavuz BI, Savas C, Yavuz MS, Okutan H. Clinical experience of removing aerodigestive tract foreign bodies with rigid endoscopy in children. *Pediatr Emerg Care.* 2004;20:671–673.

117. Soder CM. Airway management of a child with epiglottitis. In: Hung OR, Murphy MF, eds. *Management of the Difficult and Failed Airway.* New York: McGraw Hill; 2008:389–393.

118. Toward Optimized Practice Program, Edmonton, AB. *Guidelines for the Diagnosis and Management of Croup.* Updated Report. Edmonton, AB: Alberta Medical Association (Canada); 2008.

119. Scolnik D, Coates AL, Stephens D, Da SZ, Lavine E, Schuh S. Controlled delivery of high vs low humidity vs mist therapy for croup in emergency departments: a randomized controlled trial. *JAMA.* 2006;295:1274–1280.

120. Kelley PB, Simon JE. Racemic epinephrine use in croup and disposition. *Am J Emerg Med.* 1992;10:181–183.

121. Cressman WR, Myer CM III. Diagnosis and management of croup and epiglottitis. *Pediatr Clin North Am.* 1994;41:265–276.

122. Ausejo M, Saenz A, Pham B, et al. The effectiveness of glucocorticoids in treating croup: meta-analysis. *West J Med.* 1999;171:227–232.

123. Russell K, Wiebe N, Saenz A, et al. Glucocorticoids for croup. *Cochrane Database Syst Rev.* 2004;CD001955.

124. Bank DE, Krug SE. New approaches to upper airway disease. *Emerg Med Clin North Am.* 1995;13:473–487.

125. Downes JJ, Vidyasagar D, Boggs TR Jr, Morrow GM. Respiratory distress syndrome of newborn infants. I. New clinical scoring system (RDS score) with acid-base and blood - gas correlations. *Clin Pediatr.* 1970;9(6):325–31.

126. Wormald R, Naude A, Rowley H. Non-invasive ventilation in children with upper airway obstruction. *Int J Pediatr Otorhinolaryngol.* 2009;73:551–554.

127. McGarvey JM, Pollack CV. Heliox in airway management. *Emerg Med Clin North Am.* 2008;26:905–920, viii.

128. Kemper KJ, Ritz RH, Benson MS, Bishop MS. Helium-oxygen mixture in the treatment of postextubation stridor in pediatric trauma patients. *Crit Care Med.* 1991;19:356–359.

129. Jaber S, Carlucci A, Boussarsar M, et al. Helium-oxygen in the postextubation period decreases inspiratory effort. *Am J Respir Crit Care Med.* 2001;164:633–637.

130. Smith SW, Biros M. Relief of imminent respiratory failure from upper airway obstruction by use of helium-oxygen: a case series and brief review. *Acad Emerg Med.* 1999;6:953–956.

131. Ozmen S, Ozmen OA, Unal OF. Pediatric tracheotomies: a 37-year experience in 282 children. *Int J Pediatr Otorhinolaryngol*. 2009;73:959–961.
132. Carron JD, Derkay CS, Strope GL, Nosonchuk JE, Darrow DH. Pediatric tracheotomies: changing indications and outcomes. *Laryngoscope*. 2000;110:1099–1104.
133. Mahadeven M, Barber C, Salkeld L, Douglas G, Mills N. Pediatric tracheotomy: 17 year review. *Int J Pediatr Otor*. 2007;71:1829–1835.
134. Carr MM, Poje CP, Kingston L, Kielma D, Heard C. Complications in pediatric tracheostomies. *Laryngoscope*. 2001;111:1925–1928.
135. Berry FA. Anesthesia for the child with a difficult airway. In: Berry FA, ed. *Anesthetic Management of Difficult and Routine Pediatric Patients*. 2nd ed. New York: Churchill Livingstone; 1990:167–198.
136. Barker N, Lim J, Amari E, Malherbe S, Ansermino JM. Relationship between age and spontaneous ventilation during intravenous anesthesia in children. *Pediatr Anesth*. 2007;17:948–955.
137. Tsui BC, Cunningham K. Fiberoptic endotracheal intubation after topicalization with in-circuit nebulized lidocaine in a child with a difficult airway. *Anesth Analg*. 2004;98:1286–1288, table.
138. Best C. Anesthesia for laser surgery of the airway in children. *Pediatr Aaesth*. 2009;19(suppl 1): 155–165.
139. Morris IR. Anesthesia and airway management of laryngoscopy and bronchoscopy. In: Hagberg CA, ed. *Benumof's Airway Management*. 2nd ed. Philadelphia: Elsevier/Mosby; 2007:859–888.
140. Hammer GB. Sedation and analgesia in the pediatric intensive care unit following laryngotracheal reconstruction. *Pediatr Anesth*. 2009;19(suppl 1):166–179.
141. Cohen MM Jr. Robin sequences and complexes: causal heterogeneity and pathogenetic/phenotypic variability. *Am J Med Genet*. 1999;84:311–315.
142. Sher AE, Shprintzen RJ, Thorpy MJ. Endoscopic observations of obstructive sleep apnea in children with anomalous upper airways: predictive and therapeutic value. *Int J Pediatr Otorhinolaryngol*. 1986;11:135–146.
143. Pasquale K, Wiatrak B, Woolley A, Lewis L. Microdebrider versus CO_2 laser removal of recurrent respiratory papillomas: a prospective analysis. *Laryngoscope*. 2003;113:139–143.
144. Gallagher TQ, Derkay CS. Recurrent respiratory papillomatosis: update 2008. *Curr Opin Otolaryngol Head Neck Surg*. 2008;16:536–542.
145. Strong RM, Passy V. Endotracheal intubation. Complications in neonates. *Arch Otolaryngol*. 1977;103:329–335.
146. Meyer CM, O'Connor DM, Cotton RT. Proposed grading system for subglottic stenosis based on endotracheal tube sizes. *Ann Otol Rhinol Laryngol*. 1994;103:319–323.
147. Rutter MJ, Cohen AP, De Alarcon A. Endoscopic airway management in children. *Curr Opin Otolaryngol Head Neck Surg*. 2008;16:525–529.
148. Belmont JR, Grundfast K. Congenital laryngeal stridor (laryngomalacia): etiologic factors and associated disorders. *Ann Otol Rhinol Laryngol*. 1984;93:430–437.
149. Richter GT, Rutter MJ, deAlarcon A, Orvidas LJ, Thompson DM. Late-onset laryngomalacia: a variant of disease. *Arch Otolaryngol Head Neck Surg*. 2008;134:75–80.
150. Yuen HW, Tan HK, Balakrishnan A. Synchronous airway lesions and associated anomalies in children with laryngomalacia evaluated with rigid endoscopy. *Int J Pediatr Otorhinolaryngol*. 2006;70:1779–1784.
151. Chen EY, Inglis AF, Jr. Bilateral vocal cord paralysis in children. *Otolaryngol Clin North Am*. 2008;41:889–901, viii.
152. Jacobs IN, Finkel RS. Laryngeal electromyography in the management of vocal cord mobility problems in children. *Laryngoscope*. 2002;112:1243–1248.
153. Skarsgard ED, Chitkara U, Krane EJ, Riley ET, Halamek LP, Dedo HH. The OOPS procedure (operation on placental support): in utero airway management of the fetus with prenatally diagnosed tracheal obstruction. *J Pediatr Surg*. 1996;31:826–828.

154. Mackenzie TC, Crombleholme TM, Flake AW. The ex-utero intrapartum treatment. *Curr Opin Pediatr.* 2002;14:453–458.
155. Liechty KW, Crombleholme TM, Flake AW, et al. Intrapartum airway management for giant fetal neck masses: the EXIT (ex utero intrapartum treatment) procedure. *Am J Obstet Gynecol.* 1997;177:870–874.
156. Shih GH, Boyd GL, Vincent RD Jr, Long GW, Hauth JC, Georgeson KE. The EXIT procedure facilitates delivery of an infant with a pretracheal teratoma. *Anesthesiology.* 1998;89:1573–1575.
157. Digoy GP. Diagnosis and management of upper aerodigestive tract foreign bodies. *Otolaryngol Clin North Am.* 2008;41:485–496, viii.
158. Fiore AC, Brown JW, Weber TR, Turrentine MW. Surgical treatment of pulmonary artery sling and tracheal stenosis. *Ann Thorac Surg.* 2005;79:38–46.
159. Herrera P, Caldarone C, Forte V, et al. The current state of congenital tracheal stenosis. *Pediatr Surg Int.* 2007;23:1033–1044.
160. Elliott M, Hartley BE, Wallis C, Roebuck D. Slide tracheoplasty. *Curr Opin Otolaryngol Head Neck Surg.* 2008;16:75–82.
161. Guillemaud JP, El-Hakim H, Richards S, Chauhan N. Airway pathologic abnormalities in symptomatic children with congenital cardiac and vascular disease. *Arch Otolaryngol Head Neck Surg.* 2007;133:672–676.

Chapter 11
Fiberoptically Guided Airway Management Techniques

Contents

B.T. Finucane et.al, *Principles of Airway Management*,
DOI 10.1007/978-0-387-09558-5_11, © Springer Science+Business Media, LLC 2010

Introduction

Proficient fiberoptic-guided airway management is the standard of care for advanced practitioners. Mastery of fiberoptic techniques requires training, extensive practice, and an understanding of the equipment. Many medical textbooks describe fiberoptic airway techniques as well as equipment design and function. Most notable is Andranik Ovassapian's *Fiberoptic Endoscopy and the Difficult Airway, 2nd Edition.*[1] Comprehensive and practical review articles on the topic include those by Fulling and Roberts[2] and Dierdorf.[3,4]

Based on its success as an intubating tool for over three decades, it can be argued that the fiberoptic scope is a fundamental piece of airway management equipment. The utility of fiberoptic techniques must not be forgotten or underestimated as new devices like the video laryngoscope gain popularity. Different airway devices offer unique options and all should be included in the airway manager's armamentarium.

The purpose of this chapter is to describe fundamental fiberoptic airway management techniques. Methods to perform tracheal intubation are discussed in detail. Suggestions are made on how to improve one's success in the performance of tracheal intubation using the fiberoptic scope.

Applications

The flexible fiberoptic endoscope has many applications with respect to airway management as summarized on Table 11.1[1,5-7]

One of the major advantages of the fiberoptic endoscope is that it can be used to perform an evaluation of abnormal or traumatized anatomy while the patient is awake, breathing spontaneously, and protecting his own airway. Both the proximal and distal airways can be observed. The practitioner can examine the anatomy, define management options, gather equipment, and summon assistants to help secure the airway.

Table 11.1 Applications of the fiberoptic endoscope in airway management

Diagnostic
  Evaluation of airway anatomy
  Evaluation of equipment placement (endotracheal, endobronchial, nasogastric tubes, LMA)

Therapeutic
  Tracheobronchial lavage
  Removal of foreign bodies
  Oxygenation

Practical
  Endotracheal intubation
  Endobronchial intubation
  Endotracheal tube change
  Special applications (retrograde wire placement, use with new airways, surgical airway
    management, critical care setting)

Sources: From Lefebvre and Stock,[5] Dellinger and Bandi,[6] and Clark et al,[7] Ovassapian[1]

Implementation: Learning the Technique

Over 25 years ago, Dr. Andranik Ovassapian and associates developed a training program based on a series of graduated written learning objectives to teach nasotracheal fiberoptic intubation.[1] Current teaching protocols and formal workshops utilize the graduated approach developed by these pioneers. Models and mannequins are used to teach the manual skills that are required to perform safe and efficient fiberoptic intubations.[1,2]

One can contact the Society for Airway Management,[8] the American Society of Anesthesiologists,[9] or an academic anesthesiology department to ask for information concerning fiberoptic workshops. After attending a workshop, one must refine manual skills by using the fiberoptic endoscope in clinical practice, seeking the guidance of a colleague who is a competent practitioner of fiberoptic techniques. Plan to incorporate fiberoptic techniques into daily practice, using them to manage patients with normal airways. The safe utilization of fiberoptic techniques in no way compromises one's duty to provide the highest quality of professional care to patients. Be assured that fiberoptic intubation performed under the supervision of a competent teacher is safe, comfortable for the patient, and expeditious.[1,10-12] Use the fiberoptic endoscope to perform "routine" intubations instead of using a laryngoscope. Both oral and nasal fiberoptic intubations should be performed. Use the scope to intubate adult and pediatric patients. During this phase of training, learn to protect the fiberoptic endoscope. The instruments are expensive and one can avoid costly repairs by observing a few basic practices that are described in this chapter. After attaining proficiency, continue to use the fiberoptic scope on a routine basis. A comfortable and competent practitioner will be better prepared to deal with patients who have a difficult airway.

In addition to working with a competent colleague, a "fiberoptic cart" that contains all of the equipment necessary to perform fiberoptic intubation must be stocked and readily accessible.[13] (The contents of the cart will be described in detail later in the chapter.) Having the equipment immediately available saves time and encourages one to use the fiberoptic scope in the routine of daily practice.

Many studies have been undertaken to define how many fiberoptic intubations must be performed before one develops reasonable competence. Fulling and Roberts[2] reported that residents required a median of 10 fiberoptic intubation attempts to reach a success rate of 90% on the first try. In clinical practice, variables such as the patient's age, weight, airway anatomy, physical status, mental state (awake, sedated, anesthetized), level of cooperation, as well as the degree of urgency with respect to airway control may affect one's attaining "competence." All of these variables need to be studied in order to establish the number of intubations it takes to attain proficiency. Furthermore, standard goals defining proficiency need to be established.

Indications

Table 11.2[1,14] lists the indications for use of the flexible fiberoptic endoscope as an airway management tool.

Table 11.2 Indications for fiberoptic-guided endotracheal intubation

Routine airway management
Awake Intubation: Any situation where it would be prudent to secure the airway before eliminating the patient's ability to breath and maintain his own airway
Difficult airway management
Known or suspected difficult airway (awake intubations should be method of choice unless the patient is unable to cooperate)
 Trauma
 Tumor
 Burn
 Congenital anomaly
 Infection
 Hematoma
 Obesity
 Arthritis
 History of difficult laryngoscopy or maintenance of mask airway. If the patient has a history of difficult laryngoscopy and easy mask ventilation, the operator may opt to perform the intubation with the patient *asleep*
 High risk of aspiration
Unanticipated difficult airway
 ASA difficult airway algorithm (adjunctive airway tool)[14]
When neurological examination is indicated after tracheal intubation
Cervical spine pathology (unstable or fixed neck)
 Trauma
 Arthritis
Therapeutic
Removal of foreign body from lower airway
Oxygenation
Confirmation of endotracheal tube placement
Bronchopulmonary lavage

One of the most important indications is the performance of an awake intubation on a patient whose airway must be secured without the use of muscle relaxants, deep sedation, or general anesthesia (see Sect. on "Awake Fiberoptic Intubation").

Equipment

In addition to basic airway management supplies, the special equipment needed to perform fiberoptic intubation includes the following items:

1. Intubating airways
2. Masks/adapters
3. Endotracheal tubes
4. Light source
5. Fiberoptic endoscope
6. "Fiberoptic cart," on which all equipment is stored
7. Video equipment if a flexible digital video scope is used

Intubating Airways

Special airways have been designed to facilitate fiberoptic intubation. These airways are used to displace the tongue anteriorly, to help guide the tip of the scope toward the glottis, and to protect the scope from the patient's biting, which could cause expensive damage to the instrument.

Figure 11.1 illustrates an Ovassapian Intubating Airway. Other airways used to facilitate fiberoptic intubation are the Williams Airway Intubator and the Patil-Syracuse airway (Fig. 11.2).

The Ovassapian airway is designed with slotted tube guides that allow the endotracheal tube to be slipped off of the airway after intubation without removal of the 15-mm adapter (Fig. 11.3).

Chung [15] reported modifying of the Williams airway by cutting a 7-mm slot in its anterior wall that would allow the airway to be slipped off the endotracheal tube after successful intubation.

One potentially helpful modification to the Ovassapian airway was reported by Aoyama et al.[16] They suggest placing a black line along the midline of the pharyngeal surface of the airway to help orient the scope's advancement during intubation. The scope is inserted through the Ovassapian airway's slotted tube guides and the black line is followed visually until the scope enters the oropharynx above the glottis. The black line keeps the scope in the midline as it is passed into the patient's airway (Fig. 11.4).

Ravindran [17] suggested that the black line could also help indicate whether the endoscope has been inserted properly along the airway's pharyngeal surface or improperly through a hole in the airway. Goskowicz et al.[18] described the use of a

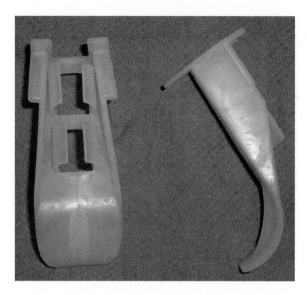

Fig. 11.1 The Ovassapian fiberoptic intubating airway (Manufacturer: Hudson RCI, Research Triangle Park, NC)

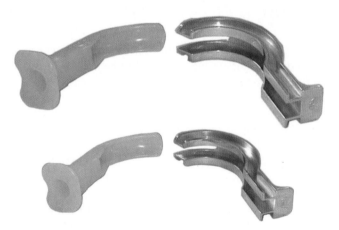

Fig. 11.2 On the *left* is the Williams Airway Intubator (sizes 9 and 10 cm) and, on the *right*, the Patil-Syracuse Oral Airway (sizes 2 and 4) (with permission from Anesthesia Associates, Inc., [AincA], San Marcos, CA)

modified baby bottle nipple as an airway to facilitate intubation in a 7-month-old infant. The nipple had an 8-mm hole cut into its lateral side at its distal end. A mark was placed on the hub of the nipple in line with the distal hole to assure inferior orientation of the hole (Fig. 11.5). Finally, Krensavage [19] suggested that one could use an oral obturator (mouth gag) to open the airway and displace the tongue during fiberoptic intubation.

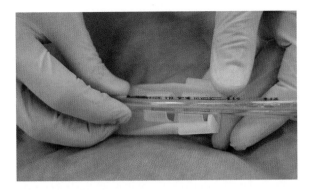

Fig. 11.3 Slotted guides in the Ovassapian airway allow it to be removed easily after the endotracheal tube is in the trachea

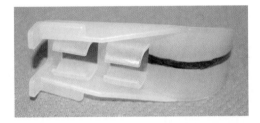

Fig. 11.4 An Ovassapian airway with a *black line* placed along the midline of the pharyngeal surface. When passing the fiberoptic scope into the patient's airway, if the line is followed visually, the scope's tip will stay in the midline and enter the oropharynx superior to the epiglottis and larynx

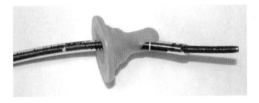

Fig. 11.5 A fiberoptic bronchoscope jacketed with a 4.5-mm internal diameter endotracheal tube placed through a modified baby bottle nipple used as an intubating airway

Masks/Adapters

Specially designed masks and adapters are available that allow mask control of the airway while fiberoptic intubation or airway examination is being performed. A Portex adapter (Smiths Medical, USA) can be fitted onto the mask, or a hole may be drilled through a plastic mask, an adaptation which allows passage of a fiberoptic scope. An airtight diaphragm can be formed over the hole with plastic dressing material through which a small hole is punctured to allow scope passage. Many authors have described creative adaptations and modifications of equipment to augment use during fiberoptic intubation. [20-23] Beware that a number of problems have been reported including fragmentation and separation of mask material and fittings that have endangered patients (Figs. 11.6–11.9).[24-26]

Endotracheal Tubes

Most fiberoptically assisted endotracheal intubations have been performed using standard endotracheal tubes. These tubes are beveled at the tip, though not tapered. Comments concerning tube design and modification will be presented in the Sect. "Success Rate of Fiberoptic Intubation" later in this chapter.

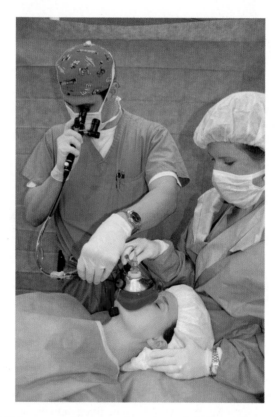

Fig. 11.6 The Patil-Syracuse endoscopy mask can be used to allow delivery of positive pressure ventilation while fiberoptic intubation is undertaken. Endotracheal tubes up to 7.5 mm ID can be passed through the hole in the mask airway

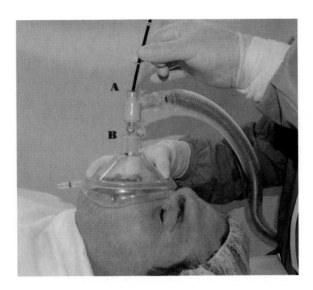

Fig. 11.7 Mask ventilation is maintained while passing the endoscope through the diaphragm of a Portex adapter (Smiths Medical, USA). (*A*) The small aperture of the adapter allows the scope to pass easily for airway examination. An endotracheal tube up to 6.0 mm ID (cuffed) can be passed over the scope if the diaphragm has been removed. Note that a straight connector (*B*) is needed to interface the Portex adapter to the anesthesia mask

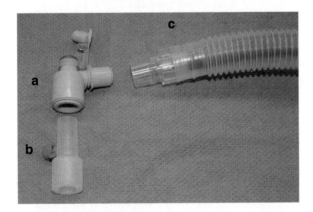

Fig. 11.8 Close up of the Portex adaptor (Smiths Medical, USA) and the other components of the system. (**a**): Portex adapter (**b**): Straight connector (**c**): Anesthesia machine circuit

Light Source

The high intensity light source must be compatible with the fiberoptic scope used to manage the airway (Fig. 11.10). Portable scopes have a small battery-powered light source that attaches to the scope (Fig. 11.11).

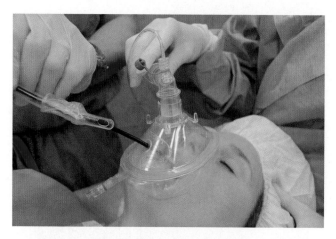

Fig. 11.9 An endoscopy mask can be made by drilling a hole through a standard anesthesia mask and creating a diaphragm with a plastic film dressing. A 0.5-in. hole allows passage of a 7.0-mm ID endotracheal tube. Positive pressure ventilation can be delivered during fiberoptic intubation

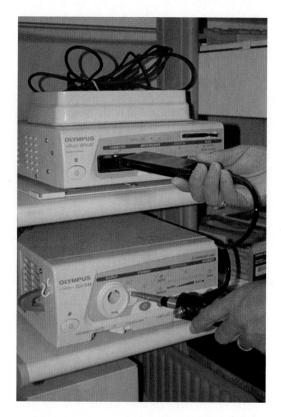

Fig. 11.10 The light cable (*lower*) from the fiberoptic scope is plugged into the light source. Digital systems have a second connection (*upper cable*) for the video connection

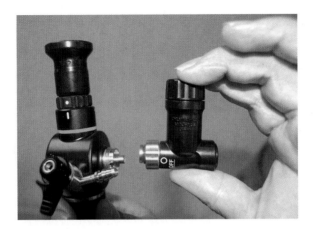

Fig. 11.11 A battery pack – On–Off switch (*right*) is attached to a portable fiberoptic scope

Fiberoptic Endoscope

Many fiberoptic endoscopes are available for use in airway management. When choosing an instrument, consider the following:

1. Cost (most scopes cost more than $8,000, not including video equipment and light source)
2. Size
   (a) Diameter
   (b) Length
3. Angle of tip deflection
4. Field of view
5. Working ports (suction, instrumentation, oxygenation, drug injection)
6. Handle controls
7. Availability of adjunctive equipment
   (a) Teaching attachments
   (b) Video-photographic capability
   (c) Light sources ($5,000, approximate cost)
8. Portability (battery-powered scope)
9. Cleaning protocol
10. Customer service, repair service, and scope loan during the repair period; technical support, educational support by the manufacturer

The basic features of the fiberoptic endoscope are illustrated in Figs. 11.12 and 11.13.

Tables 11.3 and 11.4 summarize design details of scopes that are commercially available from two manufacturers. Bronchoscopes, laryngoscopes, rhinoscopes, intubating laryngoscopes, "mobile" or *portable* scopes that have batteries, and videoscopes are included in the tables. (In general, the depth of field for the listed scopes is 35–50 mm and the light guide cable from the light source is 5–7 ft.)

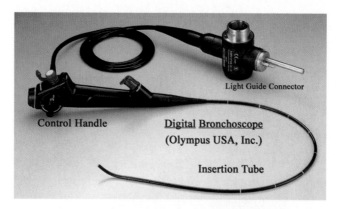

Fig. 11.12 Components of a fiberoptic scope with a cable that attaches to a remote light source (with permission from Olympus America, Inc)

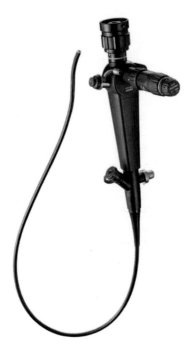

Fig. 11.13 A portable intubating scope manufactured by Pentax. Unlike the digital scope in Fig. 11.12, this scope has an eyepiece and a flexible, coherent light bundle in the insertion tube. The image is transmitted optically to the eyepiece through the coherent fiberoptic bundle. The control handle has an attached battery pack and light source making the scope portable (with permission Pentax Medical Company)

Table 11.3 Olympus endoscopes used for fiberoptic airway management (Olympus USA, Inc.)

Model	Olympus bronchoscopes				
	Insertion tip diameter (mm)	Insertion cord length (mm)	Working port diameter (mm)	Tip deflection (degrees up/down)	Angle of view (degrees)
Bronchoscopes (light source required)					
BF-XP60	2.8	600	1.2	Up/130	180
BF-P60	5.0	600	2.2	180/130	120
BF-3C40	3.6	550	1.2	180/130	120
BF-MP60	4.4	600	2.0	180/130	120
BF-1T60	6.0	600	3.8	180/130	120
BF XT-40	6.2	550	3.2	180/130	120
Portable laryngoscopes					
LF-DP	3.1	600	1.2	120/120	90
LF-TP	5.2	600	2.6	180/130	90
LF-GP	4.1	600	1.5	120/120	90
Video digital bronchoscopes					
BF-Q180	5.5	600	2.0	180/130	120
BF-P180	4.9	600	2.0	180/130	120
BF-XT160	6.3	600	3.2	180/130	120
BF-XP160F	2.8	600	1.2	180/130	90
BF-3C160	3.8	600	1.2	180/130	90
Video processor					
Evis Exera CV-180 video system center					
Light source					
Evis Exera CLV-180 Xenon Light Source					

Portable scopes are extremely utilitarian. They can be used in the intensive care unit (ICU), emergency room, or the operating room. They are lightweight and have excellent optics.

Finally, there are reports of scopes that are custom-made or modified, which have been used to perform fiberoptic intubations. [27,28]

One should contact a sales representative and arrange a demonstration of the scopes that are under consideration for purchase. Most facilities at which fiberoptic intubation is practiced have two scopes, one for adult and one for pediatric use. Serious consideration should be given to the purchase of a portable scope as well. If purchasing a digital video bronchoscope, remember to budget for a video system processor, a special light source, and a viewing monitor.

Fiberoptic Cart

A portable cart should be stocked with all of the equipment needed to perform fiberoptic intubation (Fig. 11.14). This cart should include trays, tubes, or cabinets that protect

Table 11.4 Pentax endoscopes used for fiberoptic airway management (Pentax Medical Company, USA)

Model	Distal tip diameter (mm)	Working cord length (mm)	Working channel diameter (mm)	Tip deflection (degrees up/down)	Angle of view (degrees)
Pentax intubation scopes					
FI-7P	2.4	600	N/A	130/130	95
FI-10P2	3.4	600	1.4	130/130	90
FI-13P	4.2	600	1.8	160/130	95
Portable bedside scopes					
FI-7BS	2.4	600	N/A	130/130	95
FI-9BS	3.0	600	1.2	130/130	90
FI-10BS	3.4	600	1.4	130/130	90
FI-13BS	4.1	600	1.8	160/130	95
FI-16BS	5.1	600	2.6	160/130	95
FI-7RBS	2.4	600	N/A	130/130	95
FI-9RBS	3.0	600	1.2	130/130	90
FI-10RBS	3.4	300	N/A	130/130	95
FI-13RBS	4.1	600	1.8	160/130	95
FI-16RBS	5.1	600	2.8	160/130	95

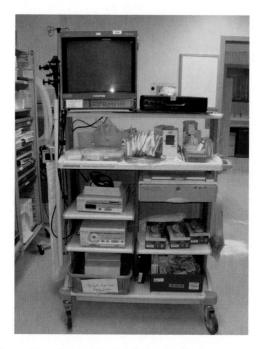

Fig. 11.14 The "fiberoptic cart" stocked with all of the equipment needed to perform fiberoptic intubation

Table 11.5 Contents of the fiberoptic cart

Basic airway management equipment
Various sizes of syringes and needles including Loer Lok tipped syringes
Various sizes of intravenous needles/cannulae
Long cotton swabs, pledgets, forceps, long Q-tips
Gauze
Topical anesthetics
Lidocaine 4%
Lidocaine 1%
Lidocaine 10%
Benzocaine 20%
Viscous lidocaine jelly or ointment 2–2.5%
Local anesthetics for nerve blocks and/or injection through the scope
Lidocaine 1%
Nebulizer for topical application of local anesthetic to the airway
Vasoconstrictor agents
Phenylephrine (Dristan 0.5%)
Oxymetazoline (Afrin 0.05%)
Suctioning equipment
Oxygenation equipment
Tubing
Oxygen source
Masks
Nasal prongs
Fiberoptic intubating airways
Intubating masks/adapters
Fiberoptic light source
Fiberoptic endoscopes (protective trays or tubes for safe storage)
Photographic/video and teaching adapters if desired
"Difficult airway equipment" if so desired, including surgical and percutaneous cricothyroidotomy equipment

the scopes from damage while in storage. *Contaminated equipment must be isolated from clean equipment.* The fiberoptic cart should contain items from Table 11.5.

Techniques of Fiberoptic Intubation

Fiberoptic intubation routed orally or nasally can be performed on:

1. An awake patient
2. An anesthetized patient breathing spontaneously
3. An anesthetized apneic patient

This applies to pediatric as well as adult patients. With the availability of small scopes, very small infants can be intubated using the techniques described in this section. More sophisticated techniques for the intubation of infants are described in detail by Ovassapian.[1]

Awake Fiberoptic Intubation

One of the most important applications of fiberoptic intubation is the performance of an awake intubation on a patient whose airway must be secured *without* the use of general anesthetics, heavy sedation, or muscle relaxants. An awake intubation is performed with the patient breathing spontaneously while he protects his airway. An awake patient maintains muscular support of his neck and can clear saliva and other fluids from his mouth and pharynx.

Writers have long debated the merits of performing fiberoptic intubation on the patient who is "awake" [29] vs. on the patient who is "anesthetized." [30] The consensus now is that the *proficient* practitioner of fiberoptic airway management needs to have mastered *both techniques.* The choice of one technique over the other should be based on clinical demands, not the limited training or experience of the practitioner.

Table 11.2 lists indications to perform *awake* fiberoptic intubation. Fiberoptic intubation of an awake patient may be easier than intubating an anesthetized patient for the following reasons.[1]

1. The awake patient can swallow secretions and help clear the airway.
2. The tongue does not tend to fall back against the pharyngeal wall and obstruct the view of the endoscopist.
3. The awake patient can breathe deeply and phonate, maneuvers that help the endoscopist to visualize the glottis when the anatomy is compromised.
4. Spontaneous ventilation and adequate oxygenation give the endoscopist more time to secure the airway.

Awake fiberoptically assisted intubation can be accomplished quickly and comfortably for the patient. The steps to be taken are listed in Table 11.6.

Selecting the Route of Fiberoptic Intubation

When choosing the route of intubation (nasal or oral), consider pathological and anatomical distortions of the airway, as well as the level of cooperation of the patient. Clinical requirements should also be considered. For example, surgery in the mouth might be an indication for a nasal intubation.

Educate the Patient

A cooperative patient can be intubated much easier than one who is restless or fighting. When faced with the prospect of being intubated awake, most patients are extremely apprehensive. Most, though, cooperate when they understand the reasons behind the decision to intubate awake. One needs to explain the reasons and the plan, assure the patient that his airway will be anesthetized, and remind the patient

Table 11.6 Steps to perform awake fiberoptic intubation

Assess the airway
Decide to perform an awake fiberoptic intubation
Select the route
  Oral
  Nasal
Prepare for contingency interventions
Obtain the equipment: *Fiberoptic cart*
Educate the patient
Educate assistants
Apply appropriate monitors
Administer supplemental oxygen
Administer antisialagogues to decrease airway secretions
Administer vasoconstrictors if nasal route selected
Administer sedation if appropriate
Anesthetize the airway
  Topical anesthetics
  Nerve blocks
  Transtracheal injection
  Through the endoscope
Perform the intubation
Verify correct tube position in the trachea
Further sedation/anesthesia/ventilation

that his cooperation will facilitate the process. When appropriate, administer sedatives, analgesics, and amnestic medications.

Educate Assistants

The person performing the fiberoptic intubation is the airway manager who must ensure that his or her assistants know which monitors to watch, how to provide oxygen and suctioning, how to manipulate the patient's neck and mandible, how to assess the patient's level of consciousness, and how to administer medications. In some cases, a surgeon should be standing by with all of the equipment and assistance necessary to perform an emergency cricothyroidotomy. The airway manager is responsible for maintaining a quiet, organized, and attentive team of assistants.

Monitoring the Patient

The following should be monitored before sedatives are administered and/or the intubation process begins:

1. Oxyhemoglobin saturation.
2. Blood pressure.

3. Electrocardiogram.
4. Ventilation.
5. Patient's level of consciousness: observe and talk to the patient. Sedation may cause hypoventilation, hypoxemia, loss of the airway, and/or unconsciousness.

Oxygen Insufflation Through the Fiberoptic Endoscope

Hershey and Hannenberg [31] reported a case in which a patient who had undergone a fiberoptic intubation suffered gastric rupture. They hypothesized that the rupture was due to oxygen injected through the endoscope into the esophagus. Ovassapian and Mesnick [32] stated that they did not recommend insufflation of oxygen through a scope to assist fiberoptic intubation. If one chooses to insufflate oxygen during the intubation process, whether through the scope or with an independent catheter or airway, one must be advised that the oxygen flow might cause gastric distention, injury, or regurgitation of stomach contents.

Administer Antisialagogues

An antisialagogue drug should be administered before fiberoptic intubation to help minimize airway secretions, thereby improving visualization. [33] Atropine: 0.006 mg/kg IV or IM, or 0.012 mg/kg PO

1. Glycopyrollate: 0.003 mg/kg IV or IM, or 0.006 mg/kg PO
2. Scopolamine: Same as glycopyrollate

If scopolamine is administered, remember that it may cause significant CNS side effects, especially in older patients. These side effects include "motor incoordination, nausea and vomiting, hallucinations, shivering, fever, as well as dry mouth and skin." [34] These effects can be reversed with physostigmine.

Administer Vasoconstrictors

If a nasotracheal intubation is planned, consider administering a topical vasoconstrictor before beginning the intubation. If cocaine is used to provide topical anesthesia, no additional vasoconstrictor is necessary. The vasoconstrictor will serve to open the airway and decrease bleeding, which can obscure visualization. Choose the most patent nasal passage to perform the intubation. To assess patency, ask the patient to breathe through each nostril while obstructing the other and note air movement (Fig. 11.15). Smith and Reid [35] suggest that a more appropriate way to choose the nostril for intubation would be to examine each nasal passage fiberoptically to define preexisting nasal pathology such as septal deviation, and then to select the more patent passage.

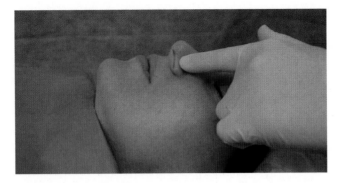

Fig. 11.15 To assess patency of the nasal passage, compress each nostril in turn and choose the more patent side through which to perform a nasal fiberoptic intubation

After choosing the nasal passage, spray a topical vasoconstrictor into the nose.

1. Phenylephrine (Dristan 0.5%): 2–4 sprays
2. Oxymetazoline (Afrin 0.05%): 2–4 sprays

Administer Sedatives and Hypnotics

If safe to do so, a patient should be sedated before an awake intubation is performed. Extreme care should be exercised when sedating a patient with a difficult or tenuous airway. If the patient stops breathing spontaneously, the situation may become critical if mask ventilation proves difficult or impossible. Furthermore, fiberoptic intubation may be more difficult if the patient is not breathing spontaneously.

Sedate the patient *incrementally and slowly*. Set a firm sedation endpoint, such as the following:

> Attempt to establish a level of sedation at which the patient appears comfortable and relaxed while still cooperative, responsive to verbal commands, and breathing spontaneously.

The following intravenous drugs may be used to "sedate" the patient:

1. Midazolam (Versed): 0.01–0.03 mg/kg
2. Diazepam (Valium): 0.01–0.04 mg/kg
3. Fentanyl: 0.4–2.0 μg/kg
4. Morphine: 0.01–0.15 mg/kg
5. Propofol: carefully titrate to the desired effect

The benzodiazepines are also excellent amnestics. After their use, patients often do not remember the intubation process.

Administer Topical Anesthetics (Upper Airway Anesthesia)

For nasal intubations, the nasal passage, nasopharynx, oropharynx, and supraglottic structures must be anesthetized. For oral intubations, the tongue, oropharynx, and supraglottic structures must be anesthetized.

Nebulized (Aerosolized) Lidocaine

Various techniques have been described to apply aerosolized lidocaine to the airway.[36,37] Given time, the entire airway can be anesthetized with this method. One technique (Fig. 11.16) is illustrated using a simple nebulizer containing 4–6 ml of lidocaine 4%.

Topical Anesthetic Sprays and Ointments

The upper airway can be anesthetized with various combinations of local anesthetic sprays and ointments. Topical anesthetics are more effective when applied to a dry mucosal surface.

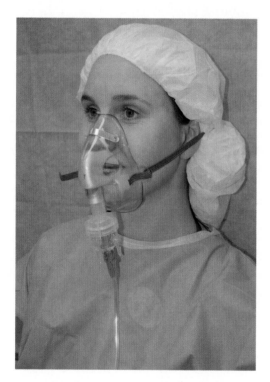

Fig. 11.16 A nebulizer/mask system can be used to administer lidocaine to the entire airway to provide topical anesthesia

Commonly used local anesthetics include the following:

1. Viscous lidocaine jelly or ointment: 2–5%
2. Lidocaine 2%
3. Lidocaine 4%
4. Lidocaine 10%
5. Cocaine 4%
6. Benzocaine 20%
7. Dyclonine 1%

To avoid systemic effects of these local anesthetics, do not exceed the recommended safe doses:

1. Lidocaine: 4–7 mg/kg
2. Cocaine: 1.5–3 mg/kg
3. Benzocaine: 10 mg/kg

Blood concentrations of cocaine after topical or intratracheal[38] administration may remain elevated for a prolonged period of time.

Khorasani et al.[39] documented that the dose of benzocaine that was administered from the commercially supplied canister was modulated by its orientation and residual volume. Ellis et al.[40] reported a case of *methemoglobinemia* after an unknown amount of benzocaine was used to anesthetize the airway in a 76-year-old woman who underwent fiberoptic intubation. In this case, the pulse oximeter reading dropped to 83% saturation and "cyanosis" was observed. A blood gas analyzed at that time revealed a PaO_2 of 502 mmHg and a methemoglobin level of 24% (normal: 0.4–1.5%).

Always monitor the patient for signs of local anesthetic toxicity!

Applying Topical Anesthetics

Many practical and effective methods have been described to apply topical anesthetics to the airway. A few are listed below:

1. Lidocaine gargle[41]: Two aliquots of 5 ml lidocaine 2% (gargle) and 20 ml of lidocaine 1.5% slowly instilled over the posterior tongue.
2. Lidocaine "toothpaste method"[42]: A "line" of lidocaine 5% ointment is placed down the middle of the patient's tongue while he is supine. He is instructed to oppose the tongue to the roof of his mouth, allowing the lidocaine to melt over the mucosal surfaces. A second "line" may be applied.
3. The lidocaine can be injected through the fiberoptic scope[43,44] directly onto the vocal cords and down the trachea (2–4% lidocaine solutions).
4. Dyclonine gargle[45]: Two aliquots of dyclonine 1%, each 12.5 ml, for gargle. (Consider using dyclonine if the patient is "allergic" to common local anesthetics.)

Local anesthetics may cause gagging or nausea and vomiting if swallowed. This can be prevented by suctioning excessive anesthetic solutions that bother the patient.[46]

Administration of Superior Laryngeal Nerve Blocks

The internal branch of the superior laryngeal nerve provides sensory innervation to the epiglottis and larynx above the vocal cords. The nerve can be blocked to provide anesthesia to the glottic structures by one of two methods.

The *internal* method involves placing local anesthetic-soaked pledgets in the piriform fossae bilaterally using a curved Jackson forceps. This method is often not practical because of pathology, secretions, or lack of cooperation in the awake patient.

The *external* method is to inject 2–4 ml of lidocaine 1% through a 23-gauge needle to block the superior laryngeal nerve bilaterally as it passes through the thyrohyoid ligament. Do this by palpating the tip of the thyroid cornu and then run a finger medially 1–1.5 cm and inject at this point. Direct the needle over the thyroid cartilage and aim it toward the thyrohyoid ligament (below the hyoid bone). Insert the needle 1–1.5 cm into the tissue or until it is immediately external to the thyrohyoid ligament (Fig. 11.17). If done correctly, this block will provide sensory anesthesia in 2–5 min.

Tracheal Anesthesia

The trachea and larynx below the vocal cords can be anesthetized by one of three methods:

1. Aerosol nebulizer: lidocaine 2–4% (4–6 ml)
2. Transtracheal injection of local anesthetic: lidocaine 2–4% (4–6 ml)
3. Injection of lidocaine onto the vocal cords and into the trachea through the fiberoptic scope: lidocaine 2–4% (4–6 ml)

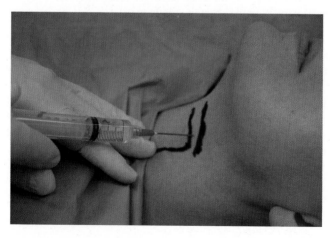

Fig. 11.17 Superior laryngeal nerve block

Transtracheal Injection

The trachea can be anesthetized by injecting 4–6 ml of lidocaine 2–4% through the cricothyroid ligament. The ligament is identified by placing one finger on the thyroid cartilage and the other on the cricoid cartilage. Inject the lidocaine through a small (23-gauge) needle, or a 22-gauge intravenous catheter inserted in the midline. *Aspirate air before injecting.* Remove the needle quickly as the patient will probably cough during local anesthetic injection. The trachea will be anesthetized very quickly (Fig. 11.18).

Care should be taken when performing the superior laryngeal nerve block or the transtracheal injection. Intravascular injection could cause a seizure. Misdirected injection of local anesthetic could cause phrenic nerve block or spinal or epidural anesthesia. Surrounding structures, such as the esophagus, could be damaged. A case of subcutaneous emphysema has been reported after transtracheal injection of local anesthetic.[47] *To avoid these complications, learn to inject local anesthetics through the scope onto the vocal cords and into the trachea.*

Author's Method

The author's method to apply topical anesthetics to the airway is one of many that is efficacious. It will take about 10 min to achieve a good level of anesthesia with the method described. After the antisialagogue has had time to dry the mucous

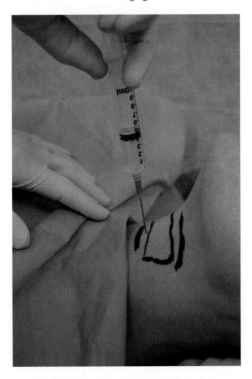

Fig. 11.18 Transtracheal injection of local anesthetic. Aspirate air before injecting the anesthetic solution

membranes, start by applying more dilute solutions of local anesthetics, as the more concentrated solutions tend to irritate the patient's mucosa. The steps to apply topical anesthesia to the airway for fiberoptic intubation are illustrated in Figs. 11.19–24.

Author's method to provide topical anesthesia to the airway for fiberoptic intubation

1. Nebulizer/mask lidocaine: 4–6 ml of 4% lidocaine.
2. Lidocaine 2% dripped onto the nasal and nasopharyngeal mucosa (4–6 ml).
3. Viscous lidocaine 2% applied deeper into the nasal passage with long Q-tip swabs.
4. Lidocaine 10% (or benzocaine 20%) applied to the nasal and nasopharyngeal mucosa with spray and long Q-tip swabs.
5. Lidocaine 10% (or benzocaine 20%) applied to the tongue and oropharyngeal mucosa with sprays.
6. Supplement with lidocaine 2–2.5% ointment on the tongue and in the nose. One can apply 5% ointment to a tongue blade and place it on the patient's tongue. This maneuver can be repeated. The author calls this technique "application of a *lidocaine lollipop*".
7. *Test the level of anesthesia with a tongue blade and a long Q-tip before inserting the fiberoptic scope or the endotracheal tube!* (Fig. 11.24).

One may skip steps 2–4 if an oral intubation is planned.

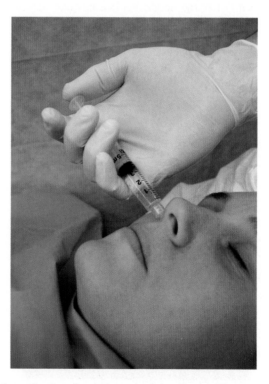

Fig. 11.19 Begin the application of topical anesthesia by dripping lidocaine 2% into the patient's nose

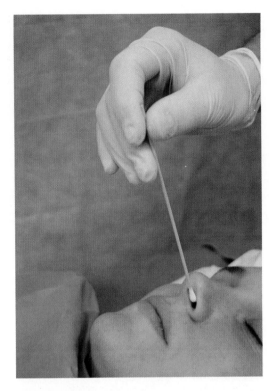

Fig. 11.20 Viscous lidocaine (2–2.5%) can be applied to the deeper mucosal surfaces by means of a long Q-Tip swab

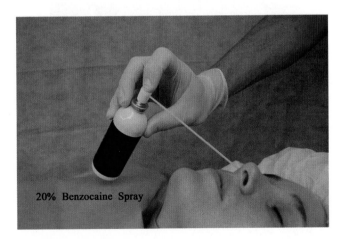

Fig. 11.21 More concentrated anesthetics such as lidocaine 10% and benzocaine 20% can be sprayed into the nose and applied to deeper mucosal surfaces with long Q-tip swabs soaked with the anesthetic solutions

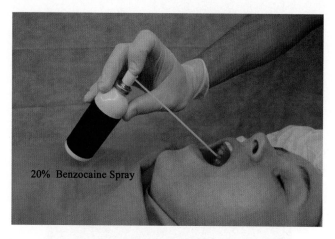

Fig. 11.22 Concentrated anesthetics can be sprayed on the tongue and into the oropharynx

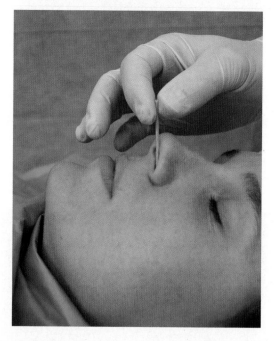

Fig. 11.23 Test the level of the nasal topical anesthesia by stimulating the nasal and nasopharyngeal surfaces with a long Q-tip. The patient should feel no discomfort

Awake Intubation Techniques

Whether one performs a nasal or oral intubation, oxygen should be administered to the patient. Figures 11.25 and 11.26 illustrate two oxygen delivery systems.

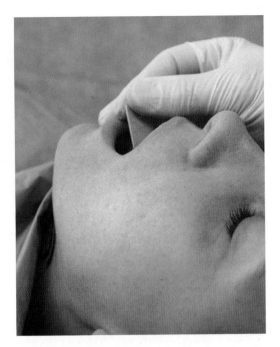

Fig. 11.24 Test the level of the oral and oropharyngeal anesthesia by touching the tongue and the pharyngeal wall with a tongue blade. The patient should experience no discomfort or gag reflex

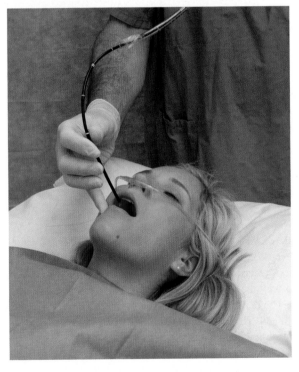

Fig. 11.25 Nasal prongs can be used to supplement oxygen during oral fiberoptic intubation

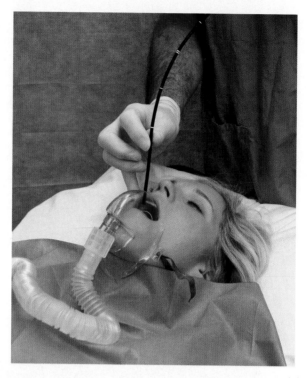

Fig. 11.26 A modified face mask can be used to supplement oxygen during nasal fiberoptic intubation

Manipulating the Scope

One can stand at the patient's side or at his head to perform fiberoptic intubation. The techniques described refer to an operator standing at the patient's head, facing the patient. The controls of the scope are operated by the nondominant hand. The fine movements involved with fiberoptic intubations are made with the dominant hand, moving the scope forward and back and guiding it in right and left turns. The dominant hand may gently contact the patient's face to sense depth of scope insertion and movement of the patient during endoscopy (Fig. 11.27).

The handle of the scope should be held so that the black reference marker, seen through the eyepiece, is oriented at the 12 o'clock position. The black reference marker orients the scope anteriorly and in the midline. The tip of the scope can be curved upward or downward with the hand controls. The operator can also activate suctioning with a hand control. The depth to which the scope is inserted into the airway is controlled by the dominant hand. The operator should look through the scope as it is inserted and try to recognize anatomic landmarks as soon as possible. To turn the scope to the right, the operator curves the tip upward, then turns the handle to the right, leaning one's body into the turn. To turn the scope to the left, the operator curves the tip upward, then turns the handle to the left, leaning to the left. *Do not try to turn the scope by twisting the fiberoptic*

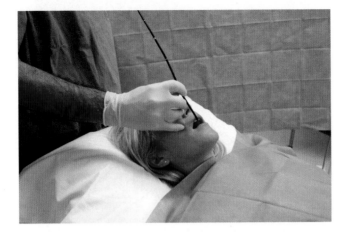

Fig. 11.27 The endoscopist stands at the patient's head and directs the scope's fine movements with his dominant hand which should come into gentle contact with the patient's face

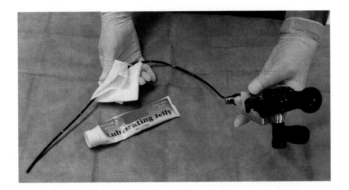

Fig. 11.28 The endoscope should be well lubricated with lubricating-Jelly or viscous anesthetic gel

bundle! This maneuver will damage the scope! Direct the scope with short, controlled movements. Finally, be careful to hold the scope with the fiberoptic bundle fully extended so that the glass fibers are not broken by coiling or angulation.

Prepare the Scope and Endotracheal Tube

One should lubricate both the endoscope and the endotracheal tube to decrease friction and ease insertion. The tube and scope can be lubricated with a water-soluble gel (Fig. 11.28). Lubricate the inside of the tube as well by passing a flexible catheter covered with gel through the tube (Fig. 11.29).

Before lubricating the tube, soften it by placing it in some warm, sterile water or saline (Fig. 11.30). This is especially important if a nasal intubation is planned.

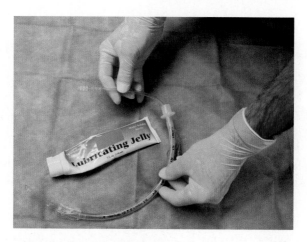

Fig. 11.29 To facilitate passage of the endoscope, the inside of the endotracheal tube should be lubricated. A flexible suction catheter covered with lubricating-Jelly or viscous anesthetic gel can be run through the tube to deposit lubricant inside

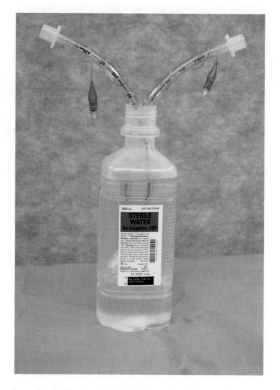

Fig. 11.30 The endotracheal tube can be softened in warm water or saline. A softer tube will curve more easily and cause less trauma to the nasal passage

Immediately before starting the intubation, be sure to focus the scope and clean the viewing channel. The scope's tip can be warmed by running the tip under warm water or by placing it near the outflow of a forced air warming device.[48] This strategy will help prevent fogging when the scope is placed into the patient's airway.

Awake Nasotracheal Fiberoptic Intubation

With the operator standing at the patient's head, initiate the intubation with the tip of the endotracheal tube in the patient's nasal passage or with the tube pulled proximally onto the endoscope (Fig. 11.31).

If starting with the tip of the tube in the nasal passage, *do not pass the tube as far as the pharynx or the tube will direct the scope toward the esophagus.* One advantage of starting with the tube pulled onto the endoscope is that the tube will not impede the scope's movement or tip deflection, making maneuvering of the scope and tip easier.

With the patient's head in a neutral or slightly extended position (if safe),[49] insert the tip of the scope into the nose. *Begin viewing through the scope immediately.* If the tip of the endotracheal tube is already in the nose, observe the endotracheal

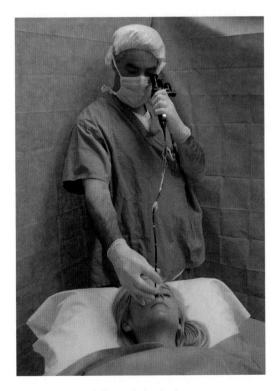

Fig. 11.31 Performing a nasotracheal fiberoptic intubation

tube through the scope and watch the endoscope pass out of the tube. Next, watch the scope move through the nasal passage and enter the pharynx. At this point, deflect the tip of the scope *upward*. The epiglottis and glottic opening should come into view in the midline. If the laryngeal structures are not seen, move the tip of the scope to the right and left by rotating the handle and leaning into the turn. Ask the patient to take a deep breath or vocalize. Movement of the larynx may make it easier to visualize the epiglottis or glottis. Once the glottis is visualized, move the scope toward the opening. Spray local anesthetic through the working channel of the scope to anesthetize the vocal cords and trachea. Anticipate coughing at this point. Once the patient is calm, pass the endoscope into the trachea and observe the tracheal rings and the carina.

When the scope is in the trachea, slide the tube over the scope into the trachea. This maneuver should be easy. However, one may find that the endotracheal tube encounters resistance to passage. *Do not force the endotracheal tube.* One may try various rotational maneuvers to help the tip of the tube to pass into the trachea.[50-52] Start by turning the tube 90° clockwise before passage (for nasal intubation). If this maneuver does not work, try turning the tube 90° counterclockwise. If the tube still does not pass, consider using a tube with a different tip, an anode tube, or a smaller endotracheal tube. If the tube feels like it is "stuck" to the endoscope, *do not force the tube off the scope! Doing so can cause an expensive tear to the scope's outer sheath.* Instead, try to inject a few ml of saline into the distal end of the tube. This maneuver may lubricate the scope and allow the tube to be passed over the scope.[53] If the tube remains "stuck" to the scope, remove the scope and tube as one unit and start again. See subsequent sections of this chapter on improving success of fiberoptic intubation.

Once the tube has successfully been passed into the trachea, note its depth, verify that the tube is in the trachea by observing the carina, inflate the cuff, and remove the scope. Confirm tube placement. (See Sect. on "Confirming Tube Placement" later in the chapter.)

One common problem encountered by the novice is poor visualization or observing the notorious "red out" when looking through the scope. Use the suction liberally. Take the scope out and clean the tip as often as is necessary. Do not deflect the tip of the scope onto a mucosal surface. Be careful not to pass the scope quickly into the esophagus. The vocal cords usually come into view when the scope is passed only 5–10 cm into the airway.

Awake Orotracheal Fiberoptic Intubation

With the operator standing at the patient's head, have the patient place his head in a neutral or slightly extended (sniff) position if safe to do so. Have an assistant lift the mandible.

The mandibular lift maneuver is very important. The epiglottis will be lifted off the pharyngeal wall and the operator will be able to visualize the glottis

Rotation of the Endotracheal Tube

For an oral intubation, rotation of the endotracheal tube 90° counterclockwise before advancing it into the trachea is one solution that is commonly suggested by fiberoptic endoscopists.[64-67] Cossham[68] reported this rotational maneuver in 1985. The reason the maneuver may be successful is that it positions the beveled side of the tube's tip posteriorly so that the pointed tip of the tube is not directed toward either arytenoids or the epiglottis. Wheeler and Dsida[69] suggest that the endotracheal tube be preloaded onto the endoscope with a 90° counterclockwise rotation. For a nasal intubation, Wheeler et al.[70] suggested that a 90° clockwise rotation be applied so the bevel is in the anterior position.

Alternate Endotracheal Tube Tip Designs

Many authors reported that endotracheal tubes with different tip designs may facilitate passage of the tube through the glottic opening. Three articles[71-73] report that the silicone-tipped, beveled tube that is supplied with the Intubating Laryngeal Mask Airway (Laryngeal Mask Company, UK) (Fig. 11.33) is easier to pass into the trachea than are standard endotracheal tubes. In Europe, this tube is referred to as an Intavent Tube. In the United States, the intubating LMA system is called the Fastrach (LMA, North America) and the tube is called the Fastrach Endotracheal Tube. Jones et al.[74] described the Moore tapered-tip endotracheal tube that was demonstrated to facilitate fiberoptic intubation. Another tube with a tapered, flexible tip, the Parker Flex-Tip (Parker Medical, Englewood, CO) (Fig. 11.34), was demonstrated to be easier and quicker to pass over a scope than an endotracheal tube with a standard tip, when no rotational maneuvers were applied to facilitate intubation.[75] Critics of the study commented that 90° counterclockwise rotation of the tube did increase ease of

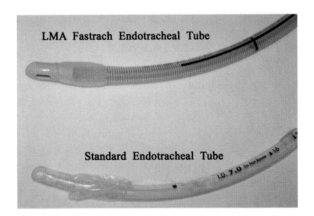

Fig. 11.33 The tube from an Intubating LMA Kit has a soft silicone beveled tip

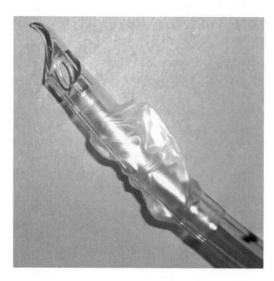

Fig. 11.34 The Parker Tube has a tapered tip. Its tip facilitates passage into the trachea when the tube is passed over the fiberoptic scope

intubation and they suggested that the standard intubating protocol should include the rotational maneuver.[76] *On a personal note, the author of this chapter endorses the use of the Parker tube, especially during awake fiberoptic intubation when the laryngeal structures may still be mobile and sensitive to tactile stimulation.*

Brull et al.[77] conducted a study comparing the flexometallic (anode) tube with a standard endotracheal tube and found that the flexible tube was easier to pass over a bronchoscope. In contrast, Hakala et al.[78] found that the anode tube was harder to pass. Suffice it to say, one should not force a tube into the trachea. If it is difficult to pass the tube, in spite of applying rotational maneuvers, consider selecting a tube with a different tip configuration.

Tube Size and Fiberoptic Scope Diameter

One common observation concerning arytenoid cartilage impingement is that if the endotracheal tube's internal diameter is much larger than the fiberoptic endoscope, the tube will lose track during passage into the trachea and impinge on the cartilage. Many suggestions have been made to remedy this problem. Rosenblatt[79] tested the efficacy of the "double setup endotracheal tube," described by Marsh[80] to facilitate fiberoptic intubation (Fig. 11.35). The conclusion was that the tapered configuration to the intubating system, created by passing the tip of a 5.0-mm endotracheal tube through a 7.5-mm endotracheal tube, facilitated fiberoptic intubation. Note that a small diameter endoscope must be used with this technique, (3.5-mm outside diameter (OD) or smaller). Jackson et al.[81] supported this conclusion in a subsequent study of the double setup.

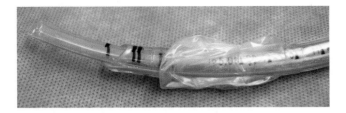

Fig. 11.35 The double setup endotracheal tube configuration forms a "taper" by passing a 5.0-mm endotracheal tube through the tip of a 7.5-mm endotracheal tube

Others have postulated using sleeves[82] and airway exchange catheters[83,84] to direct the tube into the trachea. There are as many critics as proponents of these techniques. Each practitioner should experiment with modified devices and practice on mannequins before applying a new technique to a patient.

Conclusions

All of the suggestions to make passage of the endotracheal tube easier have not been compared and tested against one another. However, the following comments summarize the literature reviewed for this chapter.

How to make passage of the endotracheal tube from the fiberoptic scope easier

1. Make sure the patient is in the proper position (jaw thrust).
2. Make sure the airway is anesthetized (topical or general anesthesia).
3. Use familiar equipment (airways, masks, scopes, tubes, etc.).
4. Use a scope that is nearly the same size as the internal diameter of the endotracheal tube. Make sure the scope is lubricated and moves freely within the tube.
5. Consider using a taper-tipped endotracheal tube (Parker tube[Parker Medical, Englewood, CO] or an ILMA tube).
6. When passing the tube orally, rotate the tube 90° counterclockwise to facilitate passage through the glottis.
7. When passing the tube nasally, rotate the tube 90° clockwise.
8. If passage is difficult, try releasing the jaw thrust, flexing the neck, or removing the intubating airway.

Complications of Fiberoptic Intubation

The complications associated with fiberoptic intubation are rare. Table 11.9 lists a variety of complications that are associated with the technique.

A study by Heidegger et al.[85] found that the incidence of vocal cord sequellae was 8.5% in fiberoptically intubated patients vs. 9.3% in patients intubated with a laryngoscope. None of the injuries were persistent. Postoperative hoarseness was reported

Table 11.9 Complications of fiberoptic intubation

Laryngospasm
Bronchospasm
Gagging
Vomiting (aspiration)
Hematoma (at the sight of transtracheal injection of local anesthetic)
Nerve block and transtracheal injection-related problems
  Seizures
  Injury to surrounding structures
  Epidural or spinal injection of local anesthetic
  Nerve injury
  Barotrauma (subcutaneous emphysema)
Over sedation
  Loss of the airway
  Hypoventilation/hypoxemia
Barotrauma, gastric distension/rupture, if oxygen is insufflated through the endoscope
Cardiovascular problems
  Hypertension
  Tachycardia
  Vagal reflexes
Damage to the scope or other equipment
Unpleasant recall by the patient
Trauma to teeth or structures in the mouth, pharynx, larynx, or the trachea

Source: Data from Ovassapian[1]

to be 4% in both groups. The injuries included hematoma, erythema, and edema of glottic structures including the vocal cords, the arytenoids, and the vestibular ligament. More serious injuries, such as avulsion of the right arytenoid cartilage, have been reported.[86] All manipulations undertaken during fiberoptic intubation should be appropriate, gentle, and precise. *Never force the scope or tube into the airway!*

Special Uses of the Fiberoptic Endoscope

The fiberoptic endoscope has many applications other than intubation of the trachea. A few of these will be discussed in more detail. They include the following:

1. Endobronchial tube placement
2. Retrograde wire-guided intubation
3. Endotracheal tube change
4. Use in the ICU
5. Pediatric use
6. Use with other airway equipment: Combitube, COPA, LMA, I-Gel, LT-S supraglottic airway, modified nasal airway
7. Video fiberoptic systems
8. Use of the fiberoptic endoscope as a conduit for jet ventilation

  9. Intubation of a prone patient[87,88]
 10. Use of the fiberoptic endoscope in the "difficult airway" scenario

Cautionary Note: All of the techniques described above should be practiced on models and mannequins before being attempted on a patient! Learn under the guidance of a skilled endoscopist.

Endobronchial Tube Placement

The fiberoptic scope can be used to verify that a double-lumen endotracheal tube has been placed correctly. To confirm proper tube placement, the operator looks down the *tracheal lumen* of the double-lumen tube and visually verifies the following:

1. That the tip of the endobronchial tube has entered the correct mainstem bronchus.
2. That the cuff on the distal or bronchial end of the tube can *barely* be seen at the carina when the cuff is inflated. This will verify that the distal tip of the tube is not too far into the mainstem bronchus.

Retrograde Wire-Guided Intubation

The fiberoptic endoscope may be used to assist retrograde wire-directed intubation. (See Chap. 12.) The technique has been described by many authors and used to intubate adult[89] and pediatric[90] patients. The steps of the technique follow:

1. Check equipment. Make sure the wire to be passed is at least 6–10 in. longer than the fiberoptic endoscope and that it passes through the working port of the scope.
2. Place a lubricated endotracheal tube over the fiberoptic bundle and run it back to the handle of the scope.
3. Pass the retrograde wire through the cricothyroid ligament and direct it out through the mouth or nose as described in Chap. 12.
4. Pass the wire through the distal end of the fiberoptic scope and feed it all the way through the scope so that it comes out of the proximal end of the working port. Have an assistant grasp or clamp the wire to keep it from being lost in the scope.
5. Pass the scope along the wire into the airway. View its passage through the airway. Watch as it passes into the trachea.
6. Pass the tube into the trachea, positioning it above the carina. The tube and scope can be moved together. Provide slack in the wire by feeding more wire through the cricothyroid ligament. If the wire kinks or prohibits insertion of the scope and tube, it can be cut off at the skin and pulled back through the scope. Do not cut the wire until the scope is definitely in the trachea.
7. Remove the wire.
8. Inflate the cuff and verify placement of the tube in the trachea.
9. Remove the endoscope.

Endotracheal Tube Change

A patient's endotracheal tube may need to be changed because of cuff failure or tube damage. Executing a tube change with the fiberoptic endoscope requires *expert skill* with the instrument. Equipment for and personnel competent to perform an emergency cricothyroidotomy should be standing by if the technique is attempted on a patient with a very tenuous or abnormal airway *since loss of the airway during tube changing could be a life-threatening event.*

1. Apply appropriate monitors.
2. Allow the patient to continue breathing spontaneously if he is doing so.
3. Denitrogenate the lungs by placing the patient on 100% oxygen for at least 5 min.
4. Judiciously consider the appropriateness of sedation, topical anesthesia, and nerve blocks. Apply topical anesthesia to the trachea by injecting 2–4 ml of lidocaine 4% into the endotracheal tube.
5. Consider the risks and benefits of nasal vs. oral intubation.
6. Pass a lubricated endotracheal tube onto the fiberoptic bundle and slide it back to the handle.
7. Gently insert the endoscope nasally and advance it until the existing tube can be seen passing into the glottis. Carefully examine the anatomy and review contingency plans.
8. At this point, one has two options:
   (a) One may pass the fiberoptic scope into the trachea alongside the existing tube before removing the tube. The scope may have to pass *anterior to the existing tube as it enters the anterior commissure of the glottic opening.*[1] Deflate the cuff of the existing tube to allow passage of the scope. After the scope is in the trachea, remove the existing tube and pass the new tube into the trachea. Confirm tube placement.
   (b) Sometimes the scope will not pass into the trachea with the existing tube in place. In this case, pass the new tube down to the end of the scope and position the scope close to the glottic opening. Remove the existing tube and insert the scope into the trachea. Advance the new tube over the scope. One can make this option safer by passing a flexible tube changer or a bougie through the damaged tube before removing it. If the new tube or scope cannot be passed into the trachea, one can attempt to pass a tube over the airway exchange catheter into the trachea.

Case Report

The author was consulted to "change an oral endotracheal tube because the patient had bitten into the tube" causing a leak. The pulmonologist stated that the "cuff of the tube could not be inflated," and hypothesized that the air channel to the cuff had been bitten through. The patient was observed to be morbidly obese with a swollen tongue, a short fat neck, a small mouth, and limited neck mobility. The patient was obtunded after suffering a stroke and was orally intubated and mechanically ventilated. Normal blood gases on an FiO_2 of 0.4 were maintained.

On examination of the patient's endotracheal tube, it was noted that the tube was taped at 17 cm at the teeth. The respiratory therapist reported that "at least 30 cc of air was put into the cuff," but the leak remained. Review of the chest X-ray revealed that the tip of the endotracheal tube was at the level of the larynx.

In this case, the patient did not need a tube change, but needed to have the tube inserted into the trachea. However, because of morbid obesity and inability to cooperate, simply advancing the tube into the trachea blindly could pose a problem. What if the tip of the tube were to slip off of the larynx and go into the esophagus?

The author ordered that the patient be placed on 100% oxygen for 5 min. Viscous lidocaine was applied to the patient's tongue. Then 2 mg of midazolam was given. All of the equipment needed to reintubate the patient was on hand and verified to be functional. The patient's trachea was instilled with 2% lidocaine via the endotracheal tube. The author inserted the fiberoptic scope into the patient's mouth to the right of the oral airway. The cuff of the endotracheal tube was observed to be herniated out of the glottis. An assistant was asked to place a tube changer through the endotracheal tube into the trachea. The respiratory therapist was asked to slowly deflate the cuff of the endotracheal tube while it was under fiberoptic observation. Once the cuff was observed to deflate (after nearly 30 cc of air was removed!), the therapist was asked to advance the tube into the trachea. The author watched the tube slide into the trachea. After the cuff passed the vocal cords, the tube was advanced 2–3 cm. The tube changer was removed, breath sounds were auscultated on positive pressure ventilation, carbon dioxide was detected by the therapist, and the author confirmed that the endotracheal tube was in place. The fiberoptic scope was removed and chest X-ray verified proper tube position.

This *case report* documents how the fiberoptic scope was used to diagnose and to treat a potentially dangerous airway problem. No other instrument would be as useful.

Techniques to use in the ICU

All of the techniques that have been described can be used in the ICU. In addition, other specific uses in this setting include the following:

1. Endotracheal and endobronchial lavage and suctioning
2. Evaluation of airway anatomy for trauma, foreign bodies, or pathology at any level
3. Verifying the position of other equipment (NG tube)
4. Obtain samples for bacterial/cytological examination

Pediatric Use

Every use described for adults can be applied to pediatric patients. The fiberoptic endoscope has been used: to evaluate the airways of very young awake patients,[91,92] to intubate pediatric surgical patients who were anesthetized and difficult to intubate with standard instruments,[93] or predicted to be difficult.[94] As well, it can be used to manage the airways of pediatric patients with known bronchial pathology.[95] The airway manager must master fiberoptic airway management techniques that are applicable to pediatric as well as to adult patients.

Fiberoptic Endoscopy and Adjunctive Airway Devices

Gaitini et al.[96] described a nasal fiberoptically guided intubation in an anesthetized patient who had a Combitube in place. The fiberoptic scope was advanced until the pharyngeal section of the Combitube was seen positioned superolaterally to the larynx. The pharyngeal cuff was partially deflated and the bronchoscope was passed into the trachea. After the patient was intubated, the Combitube was removed. A similar technique was described by Ovassapian et al.[97]

Gaitini et al.[98] also published a study comparing 20 anesthetized, nonparalyzed, spontaneously breathing patients with 20 anesthetized, paralyzed, and mechanically ventilated patients who had a Combitube placed after induction of anesthesia. The patients were intubated using a nasotracheal fiberoptic technique. An armored endotracheal tube was used in the study. The pharyngeal cuff was partially deflated during the intubation. The rates of successful intubations were 90% in the spontaneously breathing group of patients and 75% for the paralyzed patients.

Kraft et al.[99] described a modified Combitube that allowed passage of the fiberoptic scope through the airway. The technique described by Kraft et al. also required use of a guide wire over which the endotracheal tube was placed.

These reports document that fiberoptic intubation directed outside a Combitube, which is already in place, is a reasonable option to consider if one deems it necessary to exchange the Combitube with an endotracheal tube.

COPA (Cuffed Oropharyngeal Airway)

Hawkins et al.[100] described a fiberoptic intubation technique in which a scope, covered with an Aintree intubation catheter, was passed through a COPA airway into the trachea of 20 anesthetized, paralyzed patients. The scope and COPA were then removed, leaving the Aintree catheter in the trachea. A standard endotracheal tube was then "railroaded" over the catheter into the trachea. The authors reported that all patients were successfully intubated. The only difficulty arose when the operator failed to lubricate the Aintree catheter.

Greenberg and Kay[101] reported a study of 40 anesthetized patients who were intubated either nasally or orally with a COPA in situ. The fiberoptic endoscope was passed outside of the COPA and the cuff was not deflated. After the scope was passed into the trachea, the COPA was removed and an endotracheal tube was passed into the trachea over the scope. The authors reported one episode of coughing causing transient hypoxemia, and one patient being withdrawn from the study because of "secretions." The authors concluded that the COPA should be considered as a useful adjunct to fiberoptic intubation, especially since the device allows ventilation during the intubation process to continue.

LMA (Laryngeal Mask Airway)

Fiberoptic intubations have been performed for years through the LMA.[102,103] The LMA has proven to be a useful guide through which to perform neonatal and pediatric laryngoscopy and bronchoscopy.[104] Fiberoptic intubation techniques utilizing the LMA have been described for pediatric surgical patients, some with preexisting difficult airway anatomy.[105,106]

The manufacturers of the LMA promote the *Fastrach-LMA* (LMA North America), which is designed to facilitate "blind" intubations through the mask and to be used as an intubating LMA with the fiberoptic endoscope. The *Fastrach* is packaged with three reusable *Fastrach Endotracheal Tubes* that have silicone tapered tips. The *Fastrach-LMA* has a modified diaphragm (epiglottic elevator) through which an endoscope and a tube can be passed.

In practice, the LMA is used most often to facilitate fiberoptic intubation in an anesthetized patient. However, an LMA may be placed in an awake patient who is topically anesthetized and/or sedated. To use the *Fastrach* to facilitate fiberoptic intubation, start by placing it in proper pharyngeal position and then inflate the cuff. The patient can be ventilated or he may breathe spontaneously. Next, place an endotracheal tube (without the 15-mm adapter) onto the fiberoptic bundle of the scope. Pass the scope through the *Fastrach* into the trachea. Pass the tube over the scope into the trachea. Remove the scope. Next, place a "stabilizer bar or device" on the end of the endotracheal tube. The "stabilizer device" holds the endotracheal tube in place as the *Fastrach* is withdrawn from the mouth. Place a standard airway into the patient's mouth, replace the 15-mm adapter on the distal end of the tube, inflate the cuff, and verify tube position. One may not wish to remove the *Fastrach;* however, the patient may damage it by biting (Figs. 11.36–38).

Other Devices

Successful fiberoptic intubation through an I-Gel supraglottic airway (Intersurgical Ltd., Wokingham, UK) was reported in two cases of patients with suspected difficult airways.[107]

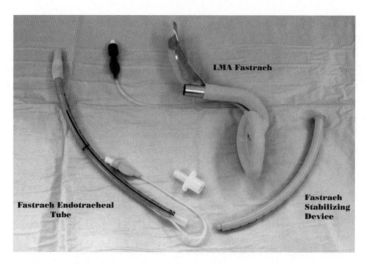

Fig. 11.36 The Fastrach LMA, Fastrach Endotracheal Tube, and the "stabilizing device" used to hold an endotracheal tube in place if the Fastrach is removed after fiberoptic intubation (LMA North America Inc., with permission)

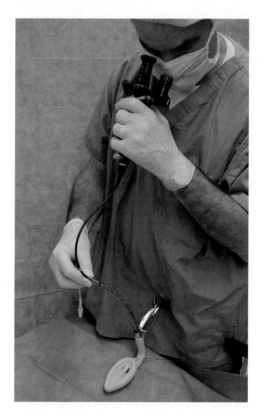

Fig. 11.37 Fiberoptic intubation through a Fastrach LMA (LMA North America Inc., with permission)

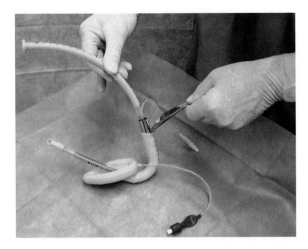

Fig. 11.38 Use the "stabilizing device" to hold the endotracheal tube in place as the Fastrach is withdrawn from the mouth (LMA North America Inc., with permission)

Another author reported intubating an infant with Boring-Oritz Syndrome with a supraglottic LT-S in situ.[108] Finally, Metz and Beattie[109] described modification of a nasal trumpet by inserting the 15-mm adaptor from a 7.0 to 8.0 endotracheal tube into the trumpet end of the airway. Once the nasal airway was in place, an assistant could administer oxygen through a standard circuit while the primary operator performed an oral fiberoptic intubation. Many other creative modifications have been reported and can be devised by the practitioner. Test the modified equipment before using it on a patient. Insure that no parts can come loose and be lost in the airway or the esophagus.

Fiberoptic Endoscope and Jet Ventilation

The fiberoptic endoscope has been used as a conduit to apply jet ventilation. One example describing its use was published by David et al.[110] They applied low-frequency jet ventilation through the suction channel of an endoscope that had been passed through the tracheal anastomosis of a patient who required aggressive pulmonary toilet. The technique, as described, was both simple and efficacious. If the fiberoptic scope is used to deliver jet ventilation, the patient should be monitored for signs of barotrauma.

Fiberoptic Endoscopy in the Difficult/Emergent Airway Scenario

What is the place of the fiberoptic endoscope in the difficult/emergent airway scenario?

In the recent past, severe criticism had been leveled by some towards practitioners who reported using a fiberoptic scope to manage an "emergent" airway.[111] However, fiberoptic intubation is offered as one choice on the ASA's Difficult Airway Algorithm. It is an option listed on the "nonemergency pathway."[14] A quote from Dr. Ovassapian, commenting on the use of the fiberoptic scope in difficult situations, puts the argument into proper perspective.[112]

> The only thing hindering the routine use of (the) fiberscope (endoscope) in failed intubation, is lack of experience, skill, and confidence.

As training has improved, and experience has been gained with the fiberoptic scope to manage all types of airway contingencies, harsh opinions of the past are no longer credible. In fact, a survey of Canadian anesthesiologists reported that "Direct laryngoscopy and fiberoptic bronchoscopy were the preferred technique(s) for intubation…" in a variety of difficult airway scenarios.[113]

The ASA Difficult Airway Algorithm suggests one way to think about managing the difficult airway. One must weigh one's airway management skills, strengths, and weaknesses when dealing with the emergency airway. Roberts[114] offered many thoughtful observations and suggestions concerning various options. *In the final analysis, one must decide how aggressively to apply fiberoptic airway management skills when faced with a difficult or emergent airway. The proficient fiberoptic endoscopist is entitled to include fiberoptic techniques on any arm of his difficult airway algorithm.*

Optical Intubating Stylets

The optical stylet is another class of optical intubating devices. Clinical studies and case reports have documented their efficacy. For one reason or another, they have not yet achieved the overwhelming popularity of the fiberoptic scope. Table 11.10 lists a few examples of optical intubating stylets.

Before purchasing an intubating scope or stylet, have the salesperson present a formal demonstration of its use on models, provide training material including videos, and arrange to borrow a scope to test it clinically.

Table 11.10 Optical and digital intubating stylets

Shikani (optical): (Clarus Medical, Minneapolis, MN)
Levitan (optical): (Clarus Medical)
Claris video system (digital): (Clarus Medical)
WuScope(optical): (Achi Corp, San Jose, CA)

Summary

The refinement of fiberoptic airway management techniques and the proliferation of teaching workshops are testimonies to the utility of this unique and versatile airway intervention. To gain *proficiency* using the fiberoptic scope, one should:

1. Attend a workshop presented by a recognized authority in the field of fiberoptic airway management.
2. Develop an organized and efficient training protocol.
3. Practice as many different fiberoptic airway techniques as possible under the guidance of a competent colleague.
4. Use the fiberoptic endoscope on a *routine* basis.
5. Apply the techniques to pediatric as well as adult patients.

Finally, one must honestly evaluate and trust one's level of competence using the fiberoptic scope. The fiberoptic scope can be used for routine, difficult, or emergent airway management depending on one's level of training and confidence.

References

1. Ovassapian A. *Fiberoptic Endoscopy and the Difficult Airway.* 2nd ed. Philadelphia: Lippincott-Raven; 1996.
2. Fulling PD, Roberts JT. Fiberoptic intubation. *Inter Anesth Clin.* 2000;38(3):189-217.
3. Dierdorf SF. The physics of fiberoptic endoscopy. *Mt Sinai J Med.* 1995;62(1):3-9.
4. Dierdorf SF. Use of the flexible fiberoptic laryngoscope. *Mt Sinai J Med.* 1995;62(1):21-26.
5. Lefebvre DL, Stock MC. Fiberoptic glottic examination to promote safe prolonged tracheal intubation. *Anesthesiology.* 1988;69:A177.
6. Dellinger RP, Bandi V. Fiberoptic bronchoscopy in the intensive care unit. *Crit Care Clin.* 1992;8:755.
7. Clark PT et al. Removal of proximal and peripheral endobronchial foreign bodies with the flexible fiberoptic bronchoscope. *Anaesth Intensive Care.* 1989;17:205-208.
8. Society for Airway Management. PO Box A 3982, Chicago, IL 60690-3982; Tel: (773) 834-3171; http://www.samhq.org.
9. American Society of Anesthesiologists. 520 N. Northwest Highway, Park Ridge, IL 60068-2573; Tel: (847) 825-5586; http://www.asahq.org.
10. Erb T, Hampl KF, Schurch M, Kern CG, Marsch SC. Teaching the use of fiberoptic intubation in anesthetized, spontaneously breathing patients. *Anesth Analg.* 1999;89:1292-1295.
11. Erb T, Marsch SCU, Hampl KF, Frei FJ. Teaching the use of fiberoptic intubation for children older than two years of age. *Anesth Analg.* 1997;85:1037-1041.
12. Schaefer HG, Marsch SC, Keller HL, et al. Teaching fiberoptic intubation in anaesthetized patients. *Anaesthesia.* 1994;49(4):331-334.
13. Mallios C, de Quelerij M, Gerritsen P, Medici G, Poorten FV, et al. Fiberoptic cart for intubation and teaching. *Can J Anaesth.* 1998;45(12):1220-1221.
14. ASA Difficult Airway Algorithm. 2001. Available at: http://www.asahq.org; 2001. Accessed 29.11.09.

15. Chung D. A modified Williams airway intubator to assist fiberoptic intubation. *Can J Anaesth.* 1998;45(1):95.
16. Aoyama K, Seto A, Takenaka I. Simple modification of the Ovassapian fiberoptic intubating airway. *Anesthesiology.* 1999;91(3):897.
17. Ravindran RS. Another advantage of marking Ovassapian fiber-optic intubating airway. *Anesthesiology.* 2000;92(6):1843.
18. Goskowicz R et al. Fiberoptic tracheal intubation using a nipple guide. *Anesthesiology.* 1996;85(5):1210.
19. Krensavage TJ. Oral obturator a useful adjunct for fiberoptic tracheal intubation. *Anesthesiology.* 1996;85(4):942.
20. Higgins MS, Marco AP. An aid in oral fiberoptic intubation. *Anesthesiology.* 1992;77:1236.
21. Frei FJ, Ummenhofer W. A special mask for teaching fiber-optic intubation in pediatric patients. *Anesth Analg.* 1993;76:458.
22. Okuda M, Hirano K, Utsunomiya H, Konishi K, Muneyuki M, Matsumoto J. A new device for fiberoptic endotracheal intubation under general anesthesia. *Anesthesiology.* 1988;69:637.
23. Nagaro T, Hamami G, Takasaki Y, Arai T. Ventilation via a mouth mask facilitates fiberoptic nasal tracheal intubation in anesthetized patients. *Anesthesiology.* 1993;78:603.
24. Waring PH, Vinik HR. A potential complication of the Patil-Syracuse endoscopy mask. *Anesth Analg.* 1991;73:668.
25. Williams L, Teague PD, Nagia AH. Foreign body from a Patil-Syracuse mask for fiberoptic intubation. *Anesth Analg.* 1991;73:359.
26. Davis K. Alterations to the Patil-Syracuse mask for fiberoptic intubation. *Anesth Analg.* 1992;74:472.
27. Guzman JL. Use of a short flexible fiberoptic endoscope for difficult intubations. *Anesthesiology.* 1997;87(6):1563-1564.
28. Saruki N, Saito S, Sato J, Kon N, Tozawa R. Swift conversion from laryngoscopic to fiberoptic intubation with a new, handy fiberoptic stylet. *Anesth Analg.* 1999;89:526-528.
29. Morris IR. Fibreoptic intubation. *Can J Anaesth.* 1994;41(10):996-1008.
30. Cole AR, Mallon JS, Rolbin SH, Morris IR. Fibreoptic intubation. *Can J Anaesth.* 1995;42(9):840.
31. Hershey MD, Hannenberg AA. Gastric distention and rupture from oxygen insufflation during fiberoptic intubation. *Anesthesiology.* 1996;85(6):1479-1480.
32. Ovassapian A, Mesnick PS. Oxygen insufflation through the fiberscope to assist intubation is not recommended. *Anesthesiology.* 1997;87(1):183.
33. Brookman CA, Teh HP, Morrison LM. Anticholinergics improve fiberoptic intubating conditions during general anaesthesia. *Can J Anaesth.* 1997;44(2):165-167.
34. Ezri T, Szmuk P, Konichezky S, Abramson D, Geva D. Central anticholinergic syndrome complicating management of a difficult airway. *Can J Anaesth.* 1996;43(10):1079.
35. Smith JE, Reid AP. Selecting the safest nostril for nasotracheal intubation with the fibreoptic laryngoscope. *Br J Anaesthesia.* 1999;82(suppl 1):26.
36. Balatbat JT, Stocking JE, Rigor BM. Controlled intermittent aerosolization of lidocaine for airway anesthesia. *Anesthesiology.* 1999;91(2):596.
37. Smith T. Jetting lidocaine through the atomizer. *Anesthesiology.* 1999;90(2):634.
38. Barclay PM, O'Sullivan E. Systemic absorption of cocaine during fibreoptic bronchoscopy. *Br J Anaesth.* 1999;83:518P-519P.
39. Khorasani A, Candido KD, Ghaleb AH, Saatee S, Appavu SK. Canister tip orientation and residual volume have significant impact on the dose of benzocaine delivered by Hurricane spray. *Anesth Analg.* 2001;92:379-383.
40. Ellis FD, Seiler JG III, Palmore MM Jr. Methemoglobinemia: a complication after fiberoptic orotracheal intubation with benzocaine spray. *J Bone Joint Surg Am.* 1995;77(6):937-939.
41. Chung DC, Mainland PA, Kong AS. Anesthesia of the airway by aspiration of lidocaine. *Can J Anaesth.* 1999;46(3):215-219.
42. Drummond JC. Airway anesthesia: the toothpaste method. *Can J Anaesth.* 2000;47(1):94.

43. Jones JM, Bramhall J. Airway anaesthesia during fibreoptic endoscopy. *Can J Anaesth.* 1997;44(7):785.
44. Vloka J, Hadzic A, Kitain E. A simple adaptation to the Olympus LF1 and LF2 flexible fiberoptic bronchoscopes for instillation of local anesthetic. *Anesthesiology.* 1995;82(3):792.
45. Bacon GS, Lyons TR, Wood SH. Dyclonine hydrochloride for airway anesthesia: awake endotracheal intubation in a patient with suspected local anesthetic allergy. *Anesthesiology.* 1997;86(5):1206-1207.
46. Benumof JL. Upper airway obstruction. *Can J Anaesth.* 1999;46(9):906.
47. Wong D, McGuire GP. Subcutaneous emphysema following trans-cricothyroid membrane injection of local anesthetic. *Can J Anaesth.* 2000;47(2):165-168.
48. Dunn SM, Pulai I. Forced air warming can facilitate fiberoptic intubations. *Anesthesiology.* 1998;88(1):282.
49. Roberts JT et al. Why cervical flexion facilitates laryngoscopy with a Macintosh laryngoscope, but hinders it with a flexible fiberscope. *Anesthesiology.* 1990;73:A1012.
50. Katsnelson T, Frost EA, Farcon E, Goldiner PL. When the endotracheal tube will not pass over the flexible fiberoptic bronchoscope. *Anesthesiology.* 1992;76:151.
51. Cossham PS. Fibreoptic orotracheal intubation. *Br J Anaesth.* 1999;83(4):683-684.
52. Randell T. Response to Cossham. *Br J Anaesth.* 1999;83(4):683-684.
53. Krensavage TJ. Saline solution as lubrication to manipulate a stuck fiberoptic bronchoscope. *Anesth Analg.* 1999;88:965.
54. Aoyama K, Takenaka I, Nagaoka E, Kadoya T, et al. Jaw thrust maneuver for endotracheal intubation using a fiberoptic stylet. *Anesth Analg.* 2000;90(6):1457-1458.
55. Aoyama K, Yamamoto T, Takenaka I, Sata T, Shigematsu A. The jaw support device facilitates laryngeal exposure and ventilation during fiberoptic intubation. *Anesth Analg.* 1998;86(5):432-434.
56. Aoyama K, Nagaoka E, Takenaka I, Kadoya T. New jaw support device and awake fiberoptic intubation. *Anesth Analg.* 2000;91(5):1309-1310.
57. Johnson C, Hunter J, Ho E, Bruff C. Fiberoptic intubation facilitated by a rigid laryngoscope. *Anesth Analg.* 1991;72:714.
58. Dennehy KC, Dupuis JY. Fibreoptic intubation in the anaesthetized patient. *Can J Anaesth.* 1996;43(2):197.
59. Archdeacon J, Brimacombe J. Anterior traction of the tongue – a forgotten aid to awake fiberoptic intubation. *Anaesth Intensive Care.* 1995;23(6):750-757.
60. Slots P, Reinstrup P. One way to ventilate patients during fibreoptic intubation. *Acta Anaesthesiol Scand.* 2001;45:507-509.
61. Chen L, Sher SA, Aukburg SJ. Continuous ventilation during transnasal fiberoptic bronchoscope-aided tracheal intubation. *Anesth Analg.* 1996;82(3):674.
62. Cavdarski A. Continuous ventilation during transnasal fiberoptic intubation. *Anesth Analg.* 1996;83:1133.
63. Reed AP. Predictable problems with flexible fiberoptic laryngoscopy. *Mt Sinai J Med.* 1995;62(1):31-35.
64. Asai T, Shingu K. Difficulty in advancing a tracheal tube over a fibreoptic bronchoscope: incidence, causes and solutions. *Br J Anaesth.* 2004;92(6):870-881.
65. Johnson DM, From AM, Smith RB, From RP, Maktabi MA. Endoscopic study of mechanisms of failure of endotracheal tube advancement into the trachea during awake fiberoptic orotracheal intubation. *Anesthesiology.* 2005;102(5):910-914.
66. El-Orbany MI, Salem MR, Joseph NJ. Letter to editor; Tracheal tube advancement over the fiberoptic bronchoscope: size does matter. *Anesth Analg.* 2003;97:301.
67. Schwartz D, Connelly NR, Dunn SM. Letter to editor; Fiberoptic intubation. *Anesthesiology.* 2006;104:377.
68. Ho AM, Karmaker MB. Letter to the Editor; Facilitating endotracheal tube advancement during fiberscope-assisted intubation: giving due credit. *Anesthesiology.* 2006;104:376.

69. Wheeler M, Dsida RM. Letter to editor; Undo your troubles with the tube: how to improve your success with endotracheal tube passage during fiberoptic intubation. *Anesthesiology.* 2006;104:378.
70. Wheeler M, Dsida RM, Kristensen MS. Letter to editor; Fiberoptic intubation: troubles with the tube. *Anesthesiology.* 2003;99(5):1236.
71. Barker KF, Bolton T, Cole S, Coe PA. Ease of laryngeal passage during fiberoptic intubation: a comparison of three endotracheal tubes. *Acta Anaesthesiol Scand.* 2001;45:624-626.
72. Greer JR, Smith SP, Strang T. A comparison of tracheal tube tip design on the passage of an endotracheal tube during oral fiberoptic intubation. *Anesthesiology.* 2001;94(5):729-731.
73. Greer R et al. Comparison of two tracheal tube tip designs for oral fiberoptic intubation. *Br J Anaesth.* 2000;84(2):281.
74. Jones HE, Pearce AC, Moore P, et al. Fiberoptic intubation: influence of tracheal tube tip design. *Anaesthesia.* 1993;48:672-674.
75. Kristensen MS. The parker flex-tip tube versus a standard tube for fiberoptic orotracheal intubation. A randomized double-blind study. *Anesthesiology.* 2003;98(2):354-358.
76. Ho AM, Chung DC, Karmakar MK. Letter to editor; Is the parker flex-tip tube really superior to the standard tube for fiberoptic orotracheal intubation? *Anesthesiology.* 2003;99(5):1236.
77. Brull SJ, Wiklund R, Ferris C, Connelly NR, Ehrenwerth J, Silverman DG. Facilitation of fiberoptic orotracheal intubation with a flexible tracheal tube. *Anesth Analg.* 1994;78:746-748.
78. Hakala P, Randell T, Valli H. Comparison between tracheal tubes for orotracheal fiberoptic intubation. *Br J Anaesth.* 1999;82(1):135-136.
79. Rosenblatt WH. Overcoming obstruction during bronchoscope-guided intubation of the trachea with the double setup endotracheal tube. *Anesth Analg.* 1996;83:175-177.
80. Marsh NJ. Easier fiberoptic intubations. *Anesthesiology.* 1992;76:860-861.
81. Jackson AH, Wong P, Orr B. Randomized, controlled trial of the double setup tracheal tube during fibreoptic orotracheal intubation under general anaesthesia. *Br J Anaesth.* 2004;92(4):536-540.
82. Ayoub CM, Rizk MS, Yaacoub CI, Baraka AS, Lteif AM. Advancing the tracheal tube over a flexible fiberoptic bronchoscope by a sleeve mounted on the insertion cord. *Anesth Analg.* 2003;96(1):290-292.
83. Mohammad I, Katarzyna K, Salem MR. Letter to editor; Use of cook airway exchange catheter® to facilitate fiberoptic intubation: are we trying to solve a problem that we created? *Anesthesiology.* 2003;98:1293.
84. Roth R, Neustein S. Letter to editor; Dueling fiberoptic bronchoscope techniques. *Anesth Analg.* 2004;98(1):276.
85. Heidegger T, Lukas S, Villiger CR. Fiberoptic intubation and laryngeal morbidity: a randomized controlled trial. *Anesthesiology.* 2007;107:585-590.
86. Aoyama K, Takenaka I. Letter to editor; Markedly displaced arytenoids cartilage during fiberoptic orotracheal intubation. *Anesthesiology.* 2006;104:378-379.
87. Hung M, Fan S, Lin C, Hsu Y, Shih PY, Lee TS. Emergency airway management with fiberoptic intubation in the prone position with a fixed flexed neck. *Anesth Analg.* 2008;107:1704-1706.
88. Kramer DC, Lo JC, Gilad R, Jenkins A. Letter to editor; Fiberoptic scope as a rescue device in an anesthetized patient in the prone position. *Anesth Analg.* 2007;105(3):890.
89. Gupta B, McDonald J, Brooks J, Mendenhall J. Oral fiberoptic intubation over retrograde guidewire. *Anesth Analg.* 1989;68:517.
90. Audenaert SM, Montgomery CL, Stone B, Akins RE, Lock RL. Retrograde-assisted fiberoptic tracheal intubation in children with difficult airways. *Anesth Analg.* 1991;73:660.
91. Downing GJ, Kibride HW. Evaluation of airway complications in high-risk preterm infants: application of flexible fiberoptic airway endoscopy. *Pediatrics.* 1995;95(4):567-572.
92. Berkowitz RG. Neonatal upper airway assessment by awake flexible laryngoscopy. *Ann Otol Rhinol Laryngol.* 1998;107:75-80.

93. Blanco G et al. Fibreoptic nasal intubation in children with anticipated and unanticipated difficult intubation. *Paediatr Anaesth.* 2000;111:49-53.
94. Hakala P, Randell T, Meretoja OA, Rintala R. Orotracheal fibreoptic intubation in children under general anaesthesia. *Paediatr Anaesth.* 1997;7:371-374.
95. Monrigal JP, Granry JC. Excision of bronchogenic cysts in children using an ultra-thin fibreoptic bronchoscope. *Can J Anaesth.* 1996;43(7):694-696.
96. Gaitini LA, Vaida SJ, Fradis M, Somri M, Yanovski B, Kalderon N. Replacing the combitube by an endotracheal tube using a fibre-optic bronchoscope during spontaneous ventilation. *J Laryngol Otol.* 1998;112:786-787.
97. Ovassapian A, Liu S, Krejcie T. Fiberoptic tracheal intubation with combitube in place. *Anesth Analg.* 1993;76:S315.
98. Gaitini LA, Vaida SJ, Somri M, Fradis M, Ben-David B. Fiberoptic-guided airway exchange of the esophageal-tracheal combitube in spontaneously breathing versus mechanically ventilated patients. *Anesth Analg.* 1999;88:193-196.
99. Kraft P, Röggla M, Fridrich P, Locker GJ, Frass M, Benumof JL. Bronchoscopy via a redesigned combitube in the esophageal position: a clinical evaluation. *Anesthesiology.* 1997;86:1041-1045.
100. Hawkins M, Osullivan EO, Charters P. Fibreoptic intubation using the cuffed oropharyngeal airway and Aintree intubation catheter. *Anaesthesia.* 1998;53:891-894.
101. Greenberg RS, Kay NH. Cuffed oropharyngeal airway (COPA) as an adjunct to fiberoptic tracheal intubation. *Br J Anaesth.* 1999;82:395-398.
102. Chen L. Continuous ventilation during trans-laryngeal mask airway fiberoptic bronchoscope-aided tracheal intubation. *Anesth Analg.* 1996;82:891-892.
103. Barnett RA, Ochroch EA. Augmented fiberoptic intubation. *Crit Care Clinics.* 2000; 16(3):453-462.
104. Hinton AE, O'Connell JM, van Besouw JP, Wyatt ME. Neonatal and paediatric fibre-optic laryngoscopy and bronchoscopy using the LMA. *J Laryngol Otol.* 1997;111:349-353.
105. Holmstrom A, Akeson J. Fibreoptic laryngotracheoscopy via the LMA in children. *Acta Anaesth Scand.* 1997;41:239-241.
106. Walker RWM, Allen DL, Rothera MR. A fibreoptic intubation technique for children with mucopolysaccharidoses using the LMA. *Paediatric Anaesth.* 1997;7:421-426.
107. Michalek P, Hodgkinson P, Donaldson W. Fiberoptic intubation through an I-gel suproglottic airway in two patients with predicted difficult airway and intellectual disability. *Anesthesia and Analgesia.* 2008;106:1501-1504.
108. Lotz G, Schalk R, Byhahn C. Letter to editor; Laryngeao tube s-II to facilitate fiberoptic endotracheal intubation in an infant with boring-opiz syndrome. *Anesth Analg.* 2007;105(5):1516-1517.
109. Metz S, Beattie C. A modified nasal trumpet to facilitate fibreoptic intubation. *Br J Anaesth.* 2003;90(3):388-391.
110. David I et al. Jet ventilation for fiberoptic bronchoscopy. *Anesthesiology.* 2001;94(5):930-932.
111. Deam R, McCutcheon C, Wong D, McGuire G. Letter to editor; Management choices for the difficult airway. *Can J Anesth.* 2003;50(6):623.
112. Ovassapian A. Fibreoptic bronchoscope and unexpected failed intubation. *Can J Anaesth.* 1999;46:806-807.
113. Jenkins K, Wong D, Correa R. Management choices for the difficult airway by anesthesiologists in Canada. *Can J Anesth.* 2002;49(8):850-856.
114. Roberts J. Fiberoptic intubation and alternative techniques for managing the difficult airway. *ASA Refresher Course.* 1999;136.

Chapter 12
Surgical Options in Airway Management

Contents

B.T. Finucane et al., *Principles of Airway Management*,
DOI 10.1007/978-0-387-09558-5_12, © Springer Science+Business Media, LLC 2011

Introduction

The airway manager faces no challenge greater than that of dealing with an apneic patient whom he "cannot intubate, [and] cannot ventilate."[1] Before the patient suffers irreversible hypoxic injury, the airway manager must be prepared to establish a surgical airway. The purpose of this chapter is to describe surgical airway management options for those not trained to perform a surgical tracheostomy.

Oxygenation vs. Ventilation

The prime objective of managing the critical airway is to establish a route for oxygen delivery to the patient's lungs. Although ventilation may be desirable, oxygenation is lifesaving. The surgical airway creates a route for oxygen delivery when standard airway management techniques fail.

Airway Algorithms

Algorithms designed to deal with difficult airway scenarios have been described in previous chapters of this book. Algorithms and protocols are structured courses of action proposed to lead to a predefined outcome. Algorithms offer specific directions to deal with the difficult airway. The practitioner can study these suggestions at his leisure, then he can prepare by learning techniques and procuring equipment that he will need to treat the patient with a critical airway. Preparation must be made in advance. One's course of action should be logical, methodical, and nonredundant. At some point, the algorithm will lead to surgical options in airway management. This chapter addresses these options.

Preparing to Manage the Surgical Airway

Managing the surgical airway demands *psychological*, *logistical*, and *clinical* preparation.

1. *Psychological preparation:* The airway manager must be prepared to abandon standard and familiar airway management techniques in the critical situation and to undertake more invasive surgical interventions.
2. *Logistical preparation:* All surgical airway management equipment must be immediately available and functional.
3. *Clinical preparation:* The airway manager must establish a protocol or algorithm to deal with the difficult airway, including surgical options. Potential problems must be anticipated and critical events recognized. Finally, the practitioner must be trained and proficient in the use of all equipment specified in the protocol.
4. *Psychological preparation:* Few situations are more challenging than the one faced by the airway manager who recognizes that the patient is not breathing and cannot be ventilated or intubated. One is often reluctant to admit that familiar and standard techniques have failed. To be psychologically prepared to establish a surgical airway consider the following points:

   (a) Admit that a patient *will* present with a life-threatening airway problem that cannot be rectified with standard techniques.
   (b) Admit that standard techniques can and do fail.
   (c) Establish, learn, and trust protocols and algorithms dealing with surgical airway intervention.
   (d) Once it is recognized that standard techniques have failed, be prepared to institute the protocol *immediately.*
   (e) Recognize that *time* is the most critical variable in the protocol. Do not waste it! If one technique is unsuccessful, proceed to the next step on the protocol.
   (f) Expect to assume total responsibility for managing the airway.
   (g) Accept help from those more proficient and immediately available to help.
   (h) Realize that some patients will experience a poor outcome or death *despite* one's best efforts.

5. *Logistical preparation:* All of the equipment necessary to establish a surgical airway must be functional and immediately available. The equipment should be stored on a cart or tray that can be transported to the site where it is needed. The equipment should be inspected at regular intervals and documented to be in working order. One should practice retrieving, setting up, and using emergency airway equipment to retain proficiency.

6. *Clinical preparation:* To be clinically prepared, one should adopt a protocol or algorithm designed to guide one's actions in managing the surgical airway. The algorithm may be one that is already published (ASA Difficult Airway Algorithm), one that is modified, or one that is uniquely designed for a given practice. The protocol should be logical, practical, and thorough. The practitioner should know, trust, and modify the protocol as indicated by new knowledge and experience. Proficiency in the use of all equipment specified in the protocol is required.

The most difficult aspect of clinical preparation involves recognizing the critical events that dictate the need to establish a surgical airway. At some point, one must admit that standard techniques have failed and that the patient cannot be ventilated or intubated. Worse, the patient is likely to experience hypoxic injury or death *unless* a surgical airway is established. The timing of the decision is critical and depends on experience, skill, and knowledge. If one is *psychologically, logistically,* and *clinically* prepared to establish a surgical airway, valuable time can be saved. Even with the equipment on hand, it will take a few minutes to establish and confirm that a satisfactory surgical airway has been established.

Surgical Options in Airway Management

The techniques described in this chapter proceed from the most simple to the more complex. When confronted with a difficult airway one must weigh the risks and benefits of each technique and choose the one with the highest probability of success. This decision is often difficult to make. One needs to be *taught* by an experienced person and must *practice* surgical techniques to maintain *proficiency*.

Techniques

The terms *cricothyrotomy* and *cricothyroidotomy* are used interchangeably in this chapter.
The techniques to be described in this chapter include the following:

1. Needle/catheter cricothyroidotomy
2. Retrograde catheter-guided intubation

3. Minitracheostomy
4. Percutaneous dilatational tracheostomy (PDT)
5. Adjunctive equipment and techniques
6. Emergency surgical cricothyrotomy
7. Formal tracheostomy

Needle/Catheter Cricothyroidotomy

Objective of the Technique

The objective is to insert a catheter(s) into the trachea through which oxygen can be inspired or injected with low-pressure or high-pressure systems. This technique is considered to be a temporary intervention utilized until a more formal airway can be established.

Needles and catheters inserted percutaneously into the trachea through the cricothyroid or another tracheal membrane have been used to provide oxygenation and sometimes ventilation in both pediatric and adult patients.[2] Anecdotal reports have appeared in the literature for years. Utility of the technique has been documented in animal[3] and human subjects. Variables such as catheter design, material, diameter, driving pressures,[4,5] lung compliance, ventilatory rates, I:E ratios, and delivery systems have been studied. Many authors[1,6-10] have proposed systems utilizing the needle/catheter, jet injectors,[11] jet stylets,[12,13] jet cannulae,[14] and modified tube changers.[15] Airway experts endorse the technique.[16] Needle/catheter cricothyroidotomy is the *first step* in many other surgical airway maneuvers – for example, retrograde catheter-guided intubation, minitracheostomy, and percutaneous dilatational cricothyrotomy.

Equipment

The following equipment is needed to perform a needle/catheter cricothyroidotomy:

1. 14-gauge or 16-gauge intravenous needle/catheter.
2. Nonkinking "dilator"-type catheter.
3. Guide wire that passes through the 14-g or 16-g catheter and over which the dilator can be passed (size: 0.025–0.035 in.).
4. Skin prep solution.
5. Lidocaine 1%.
6. 3-ml syringe with 25-g needle.
7. 20-ml syringe.
8. Sterile saline solution.
9. Scalpel blade (#11).
10. *All inclusive kit*: Emergency Transtracheal Airway Catheter®(Cook Medical, Bloomington, IN) (Figs. 12.1 and 12.2).

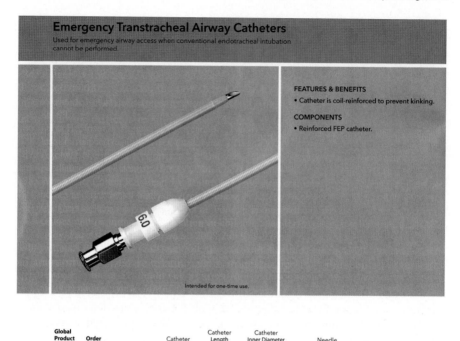

Emergency Transtracheal Airway Catheters
Used for emergency airway access when conventional endotracheal intubation cannot be performed.

FEATURES & BENEFITS
• Catheter is coil-reinforced to prevent kinking.

COMPONENTS
• Reinforced FEP catheter.

Intended for one-time use.

Global Product Number	Order Number	Catheter Fr	Catheter Length cm	Catheter Inner Diameter mm	Needle Gage
G10338	C-DTJV-6.0-5.0-BTT	6.0	5.0	2	15
G09413	C-DTJV-6.0-7.5-BTT	6.0	7.5	2	15

Fig. 12.1 Emergency transtracheal airway catheter® (Cook Medical, Bloomington, IN, with permission)

Technique

Proceed as follows:

1. Administer 100% oxygen to the patient with a face mask (if breathing spontaneously) or with a resuscitation bag-mask system.
2. Extend the neck (if safe to do so).
3. Prepare the skin with disinfectant solution (if time permits).
4. Palpate the thyroid and cricoid cartilages in the midline. The cricothyroid membrane lies between these structures. (*Note:* To reduce the likelihood of vascular injury or glottic damage one author[17] suggests using a subcricoid approach [through the cricotracheal ligament], one level down.)
5. Inject lidocaine intradermally and submucosally down to the trachea (if time permits).
6. Put 5–10 ml of saline in the 20-ml syringe.
7. Put the needle/catheter device on the 20-ml syringe.
8. Insert the needle through the tracheal membrane with a slight caudal angle. Aspirate on the 20-ml syringe. Air will be aspirated into the syringe when the needle enters the trachea. Advance the device a few millimeters and slide the catheter into the trachea, removing the needle.

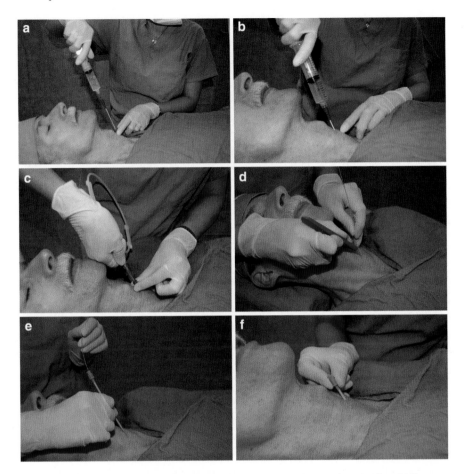

Fig. 12.2 Steps in the needle/catheter cricothyroidotomy. (**a**) Locate the cricothyroid ligament between the thyroid and cricoid cartilages. (**b**) Insert a needle through the ligament, pointing it slightly caudally. Suction with the syringe. Once the needle/catheter is in the trachea, air will flow into the syringe. Insert the catheter into the trachea and remove the needle. At this point, you may try to oxygenate the patient through the catheter. If desired, a more rigid cannula can be used to replace the catheter (which may kink). (**c**) Merely pass a guide wire through the cannula. Remove the cannula leaving the wire in the trachea. (**d**) Make an incision along the wire into the trachea and, (**e**) Pass a nonkinking dilator over the wire. (**f**) Insert the cannula and remove the wire. To avoid trauma or a mainstem cannulation, do not pass the cannula more than a few inches into the trachea. Secure it by hand or with a suture

9. Aspirate air through the catheter to insure that it is still in the trachea.
10. At this point, one may try to deliver oxygen into the trachea (see below).
11. Exchange the thin-walled catheter with a rigid dilator to prevent kinking. To do this, pass the guide wire through the catheter, remove the catheter, make a small incision into the trachea by sliding the scalpel blade along the wire, and place the dilator (or rigid catheter) into the trachea. Remove the wire and aspirate air through the rigid dilator to insure tracheal placement.

12. Using the Cook Emergency Transtracheal Airway Catheter (Cook Critical
    Care, Bloomington, IN) eliminates the need to switch to a more rigid catheter.
    The needle-catheter of this kit is inserted as described in Steps 1–9. Since the
    catheter is of rigid design Steps 10 and 11 are eliminated.

Comments on Catheter Insertion and Function

Sdrales and Benumof[18] suggested that one may ease insertion of the catheter and
lessen the likelihood of kinking if the needle were bent 15°, about 2.5 cm from the
distal tip, and if the needle were inserted at a 15° angle to the skin. Southwick[19]
reported that at least one manufacturer had already marked a "precurved" transtracheal catheter (VBM Medizintechnik, Germany). Soto and Mesa[20] pointed out that
newer needle/catheter systems designed to prevent accidental needle sticks, such as
the BD InSyte Autogard catheter (BD, Franklin Lakes, NJ), cannot be attached to
a syringe to be used as described above. Finally, Ames and Venn[21] reported a case
where the catheter was lacerated near its hub. Although the tip of the catheter was
in the trachea, enough oxygen leaked through the laceration to cause subcutaneous
emphysema.

At this stage of the needle/cricothyroidotomy technique, a large bore rigid catheter or cannula has been inserted into the trachea. The next step is to *oxygenate* and/
or *ventilate* the patient.

Oxygenation Through the Catheter

Two methods may be used to oxygenate the patient through a tracheal catheter.
A *low-pressure* system may be the only option available and it may provide oxygenation but not ventilation. A *high-pressure* system has been demonstrated to
provide oxygenation and, in some cases, ventilation, and it is the preferred option.

Expiration of Gases

When using any system observe for expiration of gas from the lungs. This is especially true when using a *high-pressure* oxygenation system. If the glottis is not
totally obstructed, gas can escape through the nose or mouth. If the glottis or upper
airway is obstructed, a second cannula or a valve (stopcock or other device) will
have to be added to the system to allow for expiration.

Low-Pressure Oxygenation Systems

Some authors think that low-pressure oxygenation systems "should not be considered."[22] The author of this chapter disagrees. A low-pressure system may be the only

system available. These systems may be lifesaving until a formal cricothyroidotomy has been performed or a high-pressure system is substituted. Five low-pressure systems will be described. These include:

1. Spontaneous ventilation
2. Apneic oxygenation
3. Resuscitation bag
4. Anesthesia machine circuit
5. ENK oxygen flow modulator set© (Cook Critical Care, Bloomington, IN)

Spontaneous Ventilation

Successful ventilation and oxygenation through one or two large-bore (12-gauge) intravenous catheters inserted into the trachea of a spontaneously ventilating patient has been documented.[23] However, research on models[24,25] has demonstrated that the work of breathing through 12-gauge to 14-gauge catheters dramatically increased from 250 to 12,000% depending on flow. Two 12-gauge catheters inserted into the trachea of a spontaneously breathing patient may be lifesaving. Oxygen can be supplied to the catheters as shown in Fig. 12.3a. Oxygen should also be administered with a face mask–resuscitation bag system, since some gas exchange through the upper airway may occur.

Apneic Oxygenation

Even if the patient were apneic, oxygen may be delivered through a tracheal catheter at relatively low flows (5–10 L/min) and low pressures. The oxygen supply hose will have to be fitted with a male Luer-Lok fastener on the distal end to connect to the tracheal catheter. Animal studies have documented the efficacy of the technique[26,27]. One should look for signs of overdistension of the lungs and listen for expiration of gas through the mouth.

Resuscitation Bag and Circle System Bag on an Anesthesia Machine

A manual resuscitation bag or the low-pressure component of an *anesthesia machine circuit (bag)* may be interfaced with the tracheal catheter to supply oxygen. Use the highest flow of oxygen that is available when using these systems. Neither system will provide ventilation though either may be used in an attempt to deliver oxygen to the patient until a more effective airway is established.

For either system to be used a 15-mm adapter interface has to be established. Three methods can be used. The following equipment is needed:

1. 3-ml Luer-Lok syringe with plunger removed
2. 10-ml Luer-Lok syringe with plunger removed

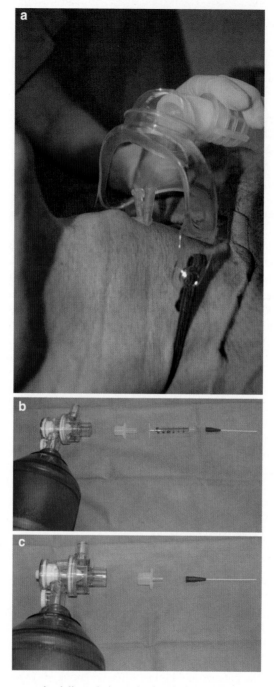

Fig. 12.3 (**a**) Oxygen can be delivered via tracheal collar to a patient breathing spontaneously through two large-bore (12-gauge) tracheal catheters. (**b**) An interface may be created between a resuscitation bag and the tracheal catheter using a 3-ml syringe and the 15-mm adapter from a 7.5-mm ID endotracheal tube. (**c**) An interface may be created between a resuscitation bag and the tracheal catheter using a 15-mm adapter from a 3.0-mm ID endotracheal tube.

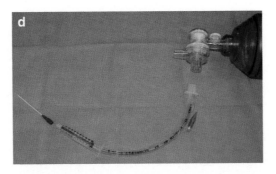

Fig. 12.3 (continued) (**d**) An interface may be created between a resuscitation bag and the tracheal catheter using a 10-ml syringe and a 7.0-mm ID endotracheal tube with the cuff inflated to create a tight seal

3. 15-mm adapter from a 7.5-mm ID endotracheal tube
4. 15-mm adapter from a 3.0-mm ID endotracheal tube
5. 7.0-mm endotracheal tube with a 10-ml syringe attached to the pilot balloon port
6. Resuscitation bag or anesthesia machine circuit
7. Oxygen source and tubing

Three interfaces can be established:

1. Connect the 3-ml syringe to the tracheal catheter. Insert the adapter from the 7.5-mm ID endotracheal tube into the open end of the syringe (Fig. 12.3b).
2. Alternatively, one could insert the adapter from a 3.0-mm ID endotracheal tube directly into the tracheal catheter (Fig. 12.3c).
3. The third option is to connect a 10-ml syringe to the tracheal catheter. Insert a 7.0-mm endotracheal tube into the syringe and blow up the cuff until tight (Fig. 12.3d).

After establishing the 15-mm adapter interface, the resuscitation bag or the bag of the anesthesia machine may be used to deliver oxygen to the patient. The bag should be compressed vigorously and the flow of oxygen to the bag should be high. Pressure in the bag will be high due to resistance. The mouth and nose of the patient may be held closed if gas escapes during inspiration.

Figure 12.4 shows the contents of the Enk Kit marketed by Cook Critical Care. The Enk catheter is attached to the nipple of an oxygen flow meter. Positive pressure is generated when the operator occludes the holes in the Enk Modulator Set. The kit can be used in any setting where standard oxygen flow meters are in use. *Remember:* Low-pressure systems will not ventilate the patient. Convert to a high-pressure system or a more formal airway *as soon as possible!*

High-Pressure Systems

The use of high-pressure (50 psi) "jet" ventilation has been advocated as the optimal modality for oxygenating and ventilating a patient whose trachea has been

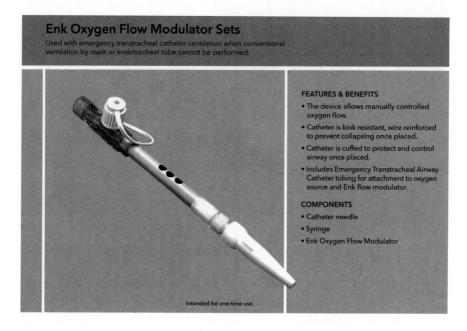

Enk Oxygen Flow Modulator Sets

Used with emergency transtracheal catheter ventilation when conventional ventilation by mask or endotracheal tube cannot be performed.

FEATURES & BENEFITS

• The device allows manually controlled oxygen flow.

• Catheter is kink resistant, wire reinforced to prevent collapsing once placed.

• Catheter is cuffed to protect and control airway once placed.

• Includes Emergency Transtracheal Airway Catheter tubing for attachment to oxygen source and Enk flow modulator.

COMPONENTS

• Catheter needle

• Syringe

• Enk Oxygen Flow Modulator

Intended for one-time use.

Global Product Number	Order Number	Catheter Fr	Catheter Length cm	Catheter Inner Diameter mm	Needle Gage
G12398	C-EFMS-100	6.0	7.5	2	15
G13145	C-EFMS-101	6.0	5.0	2	15

Fig. 12.4 Enk oxygen flow modulator set© (Cook Medical, Bloomington, IN, with permission)

cannulated.[1] Although true jet ventilation may or may not occur depending on many factors (e.g., glottic closure above the catheter), a high-pressure ventilating device does deliver large volumes of oxygen (500 ml/s) to the trachea even through a small catheter (14- or 16-gauge). Two high-pressure systems will be described.

Anesthesia Machine Flush Valve

Anesthesia machines deliver oxygen at pressures less than 10 psi[5] when the flush valve is activated. However, if a high-pressure jet ventilating system (50 psi) is not immediately available, the anesthesia flush valve system is a convenient substitute and is available in every operating room. Morley and Thorpe[28] reported that a 1-second press of the flush valve delivered 628 ml of oxygen to their test analyzer through a system made of IV tubing.

Equipment Needed

To connect the anesthesia machine to the tracheal catheter, the following equipment is needed:

1. An anesthesia machine.
2. 5–6-foot length of noncompliant tubing with a 15-mm adapter bonded to its proximal end and a male Luer-Lok needle attachment bonded to its distal end.
3. High-flow stopcock bonded in line into the noncompliant tubing.

Attach the equipment as follows: .

1. Plug the 15-mm adapter into the fresh-gas outlet of the anesthesia machine. (*Note:* A plastic adapter fits more firmly than a metal adapter.)
2. Attach the Luer-Lok to the tracheal catheter.
3. Activate the system by pushing the flush valve of the anesthesia machine. Hold inspiration for 1 s. Observe the patient for chest movement, both inspiration and expiration. If expiration does not occur, relieve pressure by opening the system with the stopcock.
4. Repeat inspirations 8–10 times per minute (Fig. 12.5).

High-Pressure "Jet" Ventilation

To apply high-pressure "jet" ventilation through the tracheal cannula, the following equipment is required:

1. A high-pressure oxygen source, 50 psi (wall or portable).
2. A formal "jet" ventilator with appropriate connector to interface with the oxygen source.
3. A male Luer-Lok bonded to the distal end of the system with a high-flow stop-cock bonded in line is used to relieve pressure if the lungs do not deflate through the glottis.

To use this equipment, proceed as follows:

1. Attach the "jet" ventilator to the oxygen source.
2. Connect the distal end of the tubing via the Luer-Lok fitting to the tracheal cannula.
3. Activate the jet ventilator for 0.5–1 second and observe the patient for chest movement or signs of barotrauma (Fig. 12.6).
4. Repeat the activation 6–10 times per minute.
5. If the lungs do not deflate, open the stopcock to relieve pressure.

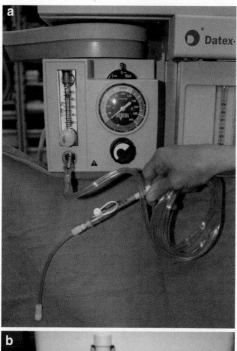

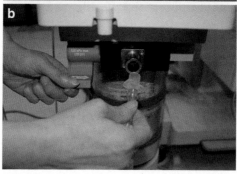

Fig. 12.5 (a) An ENK oxygen flow modelator can be used as a "jet" ventilator with the device attached to the O₂ Flow meter. (b) A "jet" ventilator can be made of rigid tubing with a male Luer-Lok interface bonded to its distal end. The proximal end of the system is a 15-mm plastic adapter from an endotracheal tube bonded to the tubing. The 15-mm adapter is inserted into the fresh-gas outlet of an anesthesia machine. The system is activated by pressing the flush valve of the machine

Cautionary Note: Barotrauma is a significant complication of this technique. Observe the patient carefully to detect whether or not the cannula remains in the trachea and insure that the patient has time to exhale by observing the chest and listening for gas to escape either through the glottis or the stopcock.

Efficacy of the Technique

Patel[29] documented that percutaneous transtracheal jet ventilation instituted in the *emergency setting* provided safe and effective oxygenation to patients whose

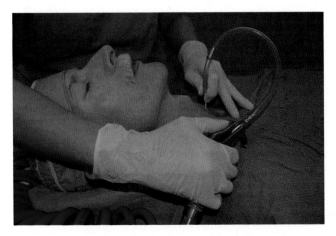

Fig. 12.6 A formal "jet" ventilator driven by a high-pressure oxygen source

oxygenation could not be maintained with bag-mask systems and who had proven to be difficult to intubate. In 23 of 29 patients (79.3%), tracheal cannulation and jet oxygenation were successful. Failure occurred in 6 patients for the following reasons:

1. Poor landmarks because of obesity and short neck ($n=2$)
2. Poor landmarks because of previous tracheostomy ($n=1$)
3. Catheter kinking ($n=2$)
4. Catheter misplacement because of improper technique ($n=1$)

Two of these six patients were intubated over an airway exchange catheter, while four of the patients were subsequently intubated after several attempts. Many anecdotal reports support the technique's clinical efficacy.

Obtaining a Formal Airway

All of the systems described thus far should be considered to be temporary interventions to provide oxygen. After the patient has stabilized, one must proceed to the next step: that is to *establish a formal airway*. At this point, the following options should be considered.

1. If drugs were used to facilitate intubation, the patient may be allowed to wake up with the tracheal catheter left in place until he is able to spontaneously ventilate and to protect his airway. (This option implies that there is no airway pathology that would obstruct spontaneous breathing.)
2. Further attempts to intubate with adjunctive equipment (e.g., fiberoptic bronchoscope, video laryngoscope, or retrograde catheter) may be undertaken with the tracheal catheter in place.
3. Emergency cricothyroidotomy may be performed.

The algorithm or protocol should outline all of the steps necessary to establish a formal airway.

Complications of Needle/Catheter Cricothyroidotomy[1,2,30]

There are many complications associated with needle/catheter cricothyroidotomy techniques. These include the following:

1. *Barotrauma* (subcutaneous emphysema, pneumothorax, pneumomediastinum, pneumopericardium)
2. Breakage or bending of the needle
3. Kinking, dislodgement, or breakage of the catheter
4. Perforation of the esophagus or other structures in the neck or thorax
5. Bleeding at the insertion site or into the trachea, causing obstruction
6. Expiratory obstruction
7. Hypoventilation with hypercapnia and acidosis
8. Sore throat
9. Infection

The complication rate can be expected to be higher in pediatric patients, patients with abnormal anatomy, or patients with coagulopathies. Use of the technique for infants and very small children has been questioned.

Be Prepared to Perform a Needle/Catheter Cricothyroidotomy

Needle/catheter cricothyroidotomy techniques have been included in many difficult airway algorithms and protocols. However, the question remains, *who is ready to perform a needle cricothyroidotomy?* Davies[31] asked this question to physicians in 184 accident and emergency departments treating more than 30,000 patients per year in Great Britain. He reported that "47% of the departments had made provision for immediate use of needle cricothyroidotomy. Forty-five percent of the doctors interviewed were fully conversant in the use of needle cricothyroidotomy." He concluded that provisions to use the technique immediately were generally inadequate. He recommended that all departments should provide the necessary equipment and training to their physicians so they could use the equipment properly. If one includes needle/catheter cricothyroidotomy techniques in his algorithm, *make sure the equipment is available and functional, and practice the technique on a regular basis! This can be done with commercially available airway models.*

Retrograde Catheter-Assisted Intubation

Objective of the Technique

A retrograde wire or catheter passed from the trachea, through the glottis into the upper airway may be used to guide an endotracheal tube between the vocal cords into the trachea.[17,30,32,33]

This technique may be planned from the onset or used as a rescue option if attempts to intubate a patient fail and the glottic opening is not completely obstructed.

The retrograde wire technique has been used in a variety of patients including infants,[34] adults receiving a double-lumen endobronchial tube,[35] and in those undergoing cardiac surgery.[36] Many suggestions have been made concerning its application.[37–40] A training model using patients scheduled for elective tracheostomy has been described.[41] Transtracheal injection of lidocaine and laryngeal nerve blocks have made retrograde intubation more comfortable for the awake patient.[42]

Equipment

1. Oxygen source and insufflation device
2. Skin prep cleaning solution
3. Lidocaine 1%
4. 3-ml syringe with 25-gauge needle
5. 10-ml syringe
6. Saline
7. Laryngoscope
8. Magill forceps
9. 12–14 gauge intravenous needle/catheter
10. 10–14 gauge rigid transtracheal catheter or dilator
11. A plastic (e.g., epidural or angiographic) catheter at least 20 in. long
12. Guide wire (at least 20 in. long), 0.035-in. diameter
13. Suture needle with 1-0 silk suture attached
14. Various sizes of endotracheal tubes
15. Suction apparatus
16. *All Inclusive Kit*: Cook® Retrograde Intubation Sets (Cook Medical, Bloomington, IN)

Methods

Three methods to perform a retrograde wire or catheter-assisted intubation are presented:

Method 1: Using a plastic catheter or guide wire (Fig. 12.7).

1. Administer oxygen to the patient with oral insufflation and/or nasal prongs.
2. Extend the patient's neck.
3. Palpate the cricothyroid ligament (or the next lower tracheal membrane).
4. Inject local anesthetic into the skin overlying the ligament.
5. Attach the 10-ml syringe containing 5-ml of saline to the 12–14 gauge needle/catheter, puncture the cricothyroid membrane or the second tracheal membrane, aspirate air, advance 2–3 mm, then thread the catheter into the trachea. If a rigid dilator is available, substitute it with the standard intravenous needle/catheter. A wire can be passed through the rigid catheter.

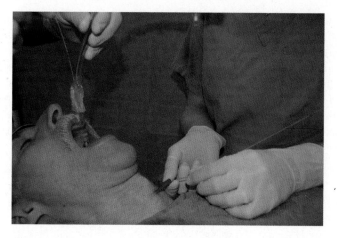

Fig. 12.7 A retrograde wire passed out of the mouth extends through the side port of an endotracheal tube. The tube passes over the wire into the trachea. When the tip of the tube gets to the glottis, passage into the trachea may be facilitated by twisting the tube to the left or right

6. Remove the needle, aspirate air again.
7. Thread the plastic retrograde catheter or the guide wire through the catheter into the pharynx.
8. Visualize the pharynx with a laryngoscope.
9. With the Magill forceps, direct the catheter or wire out of the mouth, or toward the nasal passage, while gently advancing from below.
10. Gain control of the catheter or wire as it exits the mouth or nose.
11. Option One (Retrograde catheter or wire): Thread an endotracheal tube over the catheter or wire into the trachea. The wire may pass through the Murphy eye of the endotracheal tube or through the tube's central lumen.[33]

   (a) Remove the catheter or guide wire from below while advancing the endotracheal tube once the tip of the tube has entered the trachea.
   (b) Inflate the cuff of the tube and ventilate the patient.

12. Option two: If using a Cook Retrograde Intubation Set© (Cook Critical Care, Bloomington, IN), one can pass an intubating catheter into the trachea. A Rapi-fit© adaptor can be attached to the catheter to transform the catheter into an oxygenation conduit. The contents of the Cook kit are shown in Fig. 12.8. Lenfant et al[43] reported an improved success rate if the operator threaded the endotracheal tube over the guide wire, passed the tube into the trachea, passed the intubating catheter through the endotracheal tube, and then removed the wire while passing the endotracheal tube over the intubating catheter that had been left in the trachea as a guide stent.

Method 2: Using a silk suture to guide the tube into the trachea

1. Pass the retrograde plastic catheter out through the mouth as described in Method 1.
2. Suture a silk tie onto the end of the catheter.

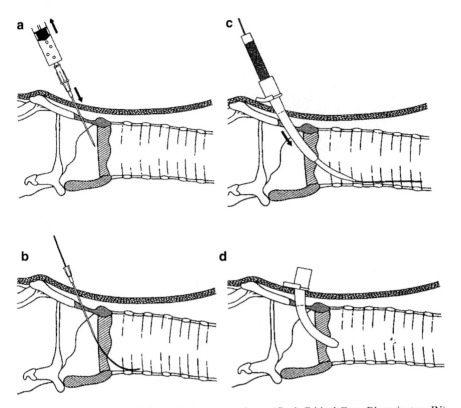

Fig. 12.12 Insertion of a Melker cricothyrotomy airway (Cook Critical Care, Bloomington, IN) (From Chan et al.,[52] with permission)

Complications and Problems with Minitracheostomies

Minitracheostomy kits used under controlled conditions appear to be safe and efficacious. Complication rates were reported to range from 10 to 17% (mostly minor and nonfatal).[53–55] Reported complications are listed below:

1. Difficult insertion[56–59]
2. Misleading signs of tracheal positioning[56]
3. Pneumothorax[60]
4. Surgical emphysema[61]
5. Bleeding[49,62,63]
6. Respiratory difficulty – insufficient respiratory support after placement[64]
7. Loss of the introducer into the pleural space[65]
8. Esophageal perforation[66–68]
9. Neck extension during insertion – may be contraindicated if underlying cervical spine injury is suspected[69]

a

ARNDT EMERGENCY CRICOTHYROTOMY CATHETER SET

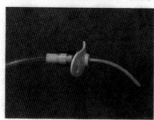

Used for emergency airway access when conventional endotracheal intubation and ventilation cannot be performed.

• Airway access is achieved utilizing percutaneous entry (Seldinger) technique via the cricothyroid membrane.

• Subsequent dilation of the tract and tracheal entrance site permits passage of the emergency airway.

Supplied sterile in peel-open packages. Intended for one-time use.

| | SYRINGE | | | INTRODUCER NEEDLE 18 gage appropriate length | | TFE CATHETER INTRODUCER NEEDLE 18 gage appropriate length |

AMPLATZ EXTRA STIFF WIRE GUIDE
.038 inch diameter stainless steel appropriate length with flexible tip

Female Luer Lock Connector

Airway Catheter

Dilator

15 mm Connector

AIRWAY CATHETER ASSEMBLY
Reinforced FEP catheter and radiopaque dilator

15 mm Connector

CONNECTING TUBE
For use with ventilatory device

Male Luer Lock Connector

Sets consist of items shown above, sterile water, scalpel and cloth tracheostomy tape strip for fixation of airway catheter.

SET ORDER NUMBER	AIRWAY CATHETER		NEEDLE	Global Product Number
	Inner Diameter	Length	Gage	
C-DTJV-9.0-6.0-ARNDT	3 mm	6 cm	18	G08251

Fig. 12.13 (**a**) Arndt Emergency Cricothyrotomy Catheter Set (Cook Medical, Bloomington, IN, with permission). (**b**) Inserting the needle and guide wire of an Arndt kit. Air is aspirated through the side port as the needle enters the trachea. The guide wire is left in the trachea. (**c**) Inserting the minitrach of an Arndt kit. (**d**) The Arndt cricothyroidotomy catheter in place

10. Cricothyroid ligament ossification[70]
11. Upper airway CPAP during and after minitracheostomy placement – predisposing to barotrauma[71]
12. Stenosis
13. Laryngeal damage
14. Placement of the catheter into the pretracheal or paratracheal space[53]

Contraindications for Use of Minitracheostomy Techniques

Although the minitracheostomy has been used on pediatric patients,[72] its role in managing the emergency airway in small children needs further study. Historically, the contraindications to its use have been the following:

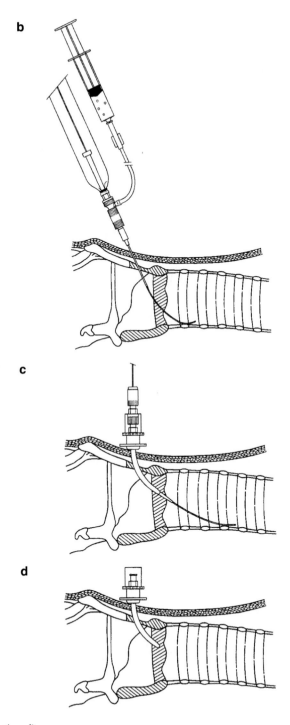

b

c

d

Fig 12.13 (continued)

1. Pediatric patients
2. Obesity or obscure airway anatomy
3. Coagulopathies
4. Platelet count less than 100,000
5. Calcified larynx

Percutaneous Dilational Tracheostomy (PDT)

Objective of the Technique

The objective of PDT is to establish a large-bore percutaneous tracheal airway utilizing techniques that require minimal surgical incision and/or dissection. Although originally intended for use in emergency or elective settings, PDT is currently recommended for elective use only.

Powell et al[73] published a review of the literature on PDT and offered the following historical perspective of the subject:

1. *1969*: Toye and Weinstein described a technique that was based on a single tapered dilator that was advanced into the airway over a guide catheter. The dilator had a recessed blade that was designed to cut tissue as the dilator was forced into the trachea.
2. *1985*: Ciaglia et al described a technique that was based on the Seldinger technique of passing dilators of increasing diameter over a guide wire that had been inserted into the trachea. A formal tracheostomy tube is passed into the trachea over an *appropriately sized* dilator.
3. *1989*: The Rapitrac (Fresenius, Runcorn, Cheshire, UK), developed by Schachner et al, utilized a cutting-edged dilating forceps device, which was passed under force into the trachea over a guide wire.
4. *1990*: Griggs et al reported a guide wire dilating forceps (GWDF) that did not have a cutting edge like the Rapitrach, which were passed under force into the trachea over a guide wire.

In *1995*: Fantoni described a technique involving a single percutaneous dilatational device that was passed through the trachea and skin from an internal approach. By the end of the 1990s many authors were strong proponents of the technique when used to establish an elective tracheostomy in critically ill, long-term ventilator-dependent patients.[75] Others showed no great advantage of the technique when compared to traditional surgical tracheostomy.

The following aspects of PDT will be addressed in more detail:

1. Cost considerations
2. Complications
3. Comparison of the PDT with surgical tracheostomy
4. Comparison of different PDT techniques

5. Current patterns of PDT utilization
6. Training considerations
7. Examples of PDT techniques and kits

General Comments

1. The vast majority of articles discussing PDT deal with patients who require *elective* tracheostomy.
2. Few writers advocate the use of PDT to establish an *emergency airway.* Surgical cricothyroidotomy is considered the preferred interventional method in the emergency setting.
3. PDT should be used *only* when immediate surgical backup is available to perform an open tracheostomy should PDT insertion fail.
4. Fiberoptic guidance of PDT insertion is the standard of care

Cost Considerations

PDT performed in the ICU offered a cost/charge savings as compared to open tracheostomy performed in the operating room in most of the studies on cost.[73,76–80] However, one study documented that the cost/charge savings was greatest when open tracheostomy was performed in the ICU. One should be careful when analyzing cost and charge data as cost sensitive variables are not well-controlled.

Complications Associated with PDT

In 1998, Powell et al[73] published a review of the literature up to 1995 that dealt with complications associated with PDT. Their investigation identified 40 studies containing 1,684 patients. Various PDT techniques were compared. Tables 12.1–12.3 summarize their findings. For comparison, they reported data from two studies of the standard tracheostomy.
Important conclusions from this paper were the following:

1. The Rapitrac had a high perioperative complication rate.
2. Most of the complications associated with PDT occurred earlier in the process of learning the technique. Precautions should be undertaken to prevent complications resulting from inexperience.
3. The Toye and Griggs methods utilizing dilational forceps, were not studied by investigators who had not invented the techniques.
4. More follow-up studies were needed to define complications associated with PDT.

Table 12.1 Postoperative complications for four percutaneous tracheostomy methods and standard tracheostomy

Complication (%)	Toye	GWDF	Rapitrac	PDT	Standard tracheostomy
Bleeding	–	2.0	1.1	2.1	(1–37)
Tube occlusion	–	–	0.4	0.3	2.7
Tube displacement	–	–	1.5	0.6	1.5 (0–7)
Emphysema	4.0	–	2.7	0.9	0.9 (0–9)
Subcutaneous or mediastinal					
Wound infection	1.0	–	0.4	1.5	1.0
Tracheoinnominate fistula	–	–	–	0.2	0.4–4.5
Tracheoesophageal fistula	–	–	0.4	–	0.2
Vocal cord paralysis	–	–	–	0.1	0.0
Overall	5.0	2.0	6.5	5.5	
	(5/100)	(5/248)	(17/262)	(59/1074)	

Source: Powell[73] with permission

Table 12.2 Late and/or postdecannulation complications for four percutaneous tracheostomy methods and standard tracheostomy

Complication (%)	Toye	GWDF	Rapitrac	PDT	Standard tracheostomy
Tracheal stenosis	–	–	0.8	1.0	0.5
Disfiguring scar	–	–	0.8	0.1	–
Residual stoma	–	–	–	0.2	0.2
Granulation of stoma	–	–	0.4	0.6	0.4
Overall	0.0	–	1.9	1.9	
	(0/100)	(NR)	(5/262)	(20/1074)	

NR not reported
Source: Powell[73] with permission

In 1999, Moe et al[81] published another literature review in which over 1,500 cases involving various PDT techniques were identified. They also presented a prospective series of 130 cases that they performed using Ciaglia's PDT technique. Tabulation of their findings are presented in (Table 12.3)

The methods of PDT utilized were the following:

Method 1: Toye
Method 2: Rapitrac
Method 3: Ciaglia Kit
Method 4: Griggs (dilating forceps)
Method 5: Hazard, modified Ciaglia technique
Method 6: Wang (Shiley Kit)

USZ University of Zurich Hospital series of 130 patients utilizing Ciaglia, Cook kit
AVE Average of the seven methods listed above
OT Open Tracheostomy (five references listed by Moe et al) (Table 12.4)

Table 12.3 Complications of tracheostomy by type and method

	1	2	3	4	5	6	USZ	AVE	OT
No. of procedures	94	150	428	228	79	7	130	1,116	
Total complications (%)	16	19	8	3	16	71	7	10	6–66
Type of complication									
Death	1	0.7	0.2			14		0.4	0–80
Major hemorrhage		0.7	0.2	0.8	4			0.6	0–36
Pneumothorax	1	1.3			3	14	0.7	0.6	0.5–4
Paratracheal insertion	6					14	2	0.8	0.5
Accidental de cannulation	1	2	0.5					0.5	3–4
Tracheal perforation					1	14		0.2	
Trach tube occlusion			0.7					0.3	1–11
Inability to complete procedure		4.7	0.2			14	2	1	
Cardiac dysrhythmia		1.3	0.2					0.3	1–4
Wound infection	1		1		3		0.7	0.8	1–36
Tracheal stenosis			0.2		3			0.3	0.4–60
Trach cartilage damage		2						0.3	
Tracheoesoph fistula		0.7						0.09	0.5–2
Tracheomalacia		0.7						0.09	
Subcutaneous. emphysema	4	2	0.7		3		0.7	1.1	1–3
Mild hemorrhage		1.3	3	2			2	2	
Hematoma	1							0.09	
Stomal granulation		2.7	0.7					0.6	
Change of voice			0.7					0.3	
Poor cosmetic result		1.3			1			0.3	

Source: Modified from Moe[81] with permission

Table 12.4 Complication and mortality rates

Method	Complication rate (%)	Mortality rate (%)
PDT	11.7	0.3
Traditional tracheostomy	15.8	1.6

Source: Billy and Bradrick[82] with permission

Moe et al also listed the following *contraindications to percutaneous tracheostomy:*

1. Pediatric or other small airway
2. Scarring in operative field
3. Obesity obscuring landmarks of palpation
4. Edema in pretracheal region
5. Mass or tumor in or near operative field

6. Patients difficult to intubate for any reason
7. Diseases of urgent or emergent nature
8. Nonintubated patients
9. Any case expected to be technically difficult

Important conclusions from this paper include the following:

1. Techniques using sharp instrumentation such as the Toye, Griggs, and Rapitrac have "poor performance records" when compared to the Ciaglia PDT.
2. Modification to the Ciaglia PDT did not decrease complications.
3. In the emergency setting, cricothyroidotomy is more effective than PDT to *establish a definitive airway*.
4. In their institution, the cost for PDT was slightly higher than that of open tracheostomy.
5. PDT "should be performed only by physicians with detailed knowledge of the anatomy and physiology of the upper airway, with skills in emergent tracheostomy, and preferably by surgeons with extensive experience in airway management and intubation."
6. The Ciaglia Kit (Cook Critical Care, Bloomington, IN) set a "new gold standard for tracheostomy" performed electively in the prospective study portion of the paper.

Billy and Bradrick[82] reviewed 19 studies including 1,012 patients who had undergone PDT. They compared PDT complication and mortality rates with those of 1,925 patients who had undergone traditional tracheostomy (Table 12.4).

These authors also warned against the use of PDT in the emergency setting, or for patients with potentially unstable airways.

Bobo and McKenna[83] reported the overall complication rates compiled from 18 studies (some of which were reviewed in previous papers) and concluded that PDT appeared to be safe and efficient. They warned against using the technique in the emergency setting.

Muhammand et al[84] published a retrospective study of 497 patients who had undergone PDT. Significant hemorrhage occurred in 4.8% of their patients. They concluded that the risk of hemorrhage could be reduced if the PDT were placed above the fourth tracheal ring, that fiberoptic endoscopy should be used to confirm correct placement, that the neck should not be fully extended, and that if one suspects abnormal anatomy, diagnostic tests such as ultrasound could define vascular anatomy in the neck.

Vigliaroli et al[85] presented the results of 304 PDTs with the Ciaglia Kit. Table 12.5 summarizes their findings.

The investigators examined the larynx and trachea of 41 patients up to 1,115 days after extubation. Mucosal findings were similar to those found after standard tracheostomy.

Finally, Gaukroger and Allt-Graham[86] reported the complications associated with the use of the Ciaglia PDT in 50 patients. One patient (who was anticoagulated when the PDT was placed) had a clot in the trachea 4 h after placement. Another patient dislodged her tracheostomy tube after 3 days and it could not be replaced.

Table 12.5 Complications of PDT ($n = 304$ patients)

Complication	Incidence (%)
Pneumothorax	0.3
Tube displacement	1.0
Peritracheal insertion improper	0.7
Tracheoesophageal fistula	0.3
Tracheocutaneous fistula	0.7
Tube occlusion	0.7
Endoluminal tube displacement	1.0
Wound infection	1.7

Source: Vigliaroli et al[85] with permission

She subsequently had a formal surgical tracheostomy. In 3 patients, the guide wire kinked in the final stages of the procedure resulting in pretracheal placement of the tracheostomy tube. In all 3 patients, the complication was recognized immediately and all patients were successfully percutaneously intubated over a guide wire that had been repositioned.

Prospective Studies and PDT Complication Rates

The largest single-center prospective study reporting experience with PDT was that of Kearney et al.[75] Over an 8-year period, experienced surgeons performed 827 PDTs on 824 patients using the Ciaglia technique exclusively. For the first half of the study (1990–1996), the investigators used the Ciaglia Percutaneous Tracheostomy Introducer Set (Cook Intensive Care, Bloomington, IN). After 1996, they used the Sims Per-Fit Kit (Sims Inc., Keene, NH), which had a "tracheostomy tube specifically designed for percutaneous placement." They found no differences between kits with respect to outcome. The overall results of the study are summarized in Table 12.7. Tables 12.6–12.9 summarize the specific complications reported by Kearney et al.

These investigators did not advocate the use of PDT in the emergency setting. They noted that Cook had introduced a simplified PDT kit with "a better tracheostomy tube-dilator interface."

Kearney et al concluded that "PDT is a technical improvement over the open surgical technique. On the basis of our study, we believe that PDT is the preferred method for intubated critically ill patients who require elective tracheostomy."

Other prospective studies published between 1996 and 2000, in which the Ciaglia technique was used documented similar low mortality rates associated with PDT insertion.[87–93] In these studies, the majority of PDTs were inserted by surgeons or surgical residents. In a few, internists and an anesthesiologist inserted the PDT. The fiberoptic bronchoscope was used to facilitate PDT and to confirm correct tube

Table 12.6 Single-center 8-year experience with percutaneous dilational tracheostomy

Type of study: prospective
Personnel performing PDT: trained surgeons
Number of patients: 824
Number of PDTs: 827
Mean procedure time: 15 min
Intraoperative complication rate: 6%
Procedure-related death rate: 0.6%
(Immediate) postoperative complications: 5%
Mean follow-up more than 1 year, tracheal stenosis rate: 1.6%

Source: Kearney et al[75] with permission

Table 12.7 Surgical complications (827 procedures)

Complication	Number	%
No complication	778	94.0
Premature extubation	9	1.0
Bleeding/no transfusion	7	0.9
False passage	6	0.7
Tracheostomy tube size	5	0.6
Pneumothorax	4	0.5
Guidewire displacement	4	0.5
Unable to complete procedure	2	0.2
Subcutaneous emphysema	2	0.2
Transient hypotension	2	0.2
Difficult tube placement	2	0.2
Tracheal laceration	2	0.2
Tracheoesophageal fistula	2	0.2
Other[a]	4	0.5

[a] Puncture of endotracheal tube balloon, needle insertion at wrong level, puncture of tracheal ring, and bleeding with transfusion

Source: Kearney et al[75] with permission

Table 12.8 Postoperative complications (827 procedures)

Complication	Number	%
No complication	781	95.0
Bleeding without transfusion	13	1.6
Airway obstruction with decannulation	8	1.0
Bleeding with transfusion	5	0.9
Premature extubation	4	0.5
Stomal infection	4	0.5
Excessive granulation tissue	5	0.6
Other[a]		

[a] Dysphagia, hoarseness, aspiration, balloon rupture, and subcutaneous emphysema

Source: Kearney et al,[75] with permission

Table 12.9 Postdischarge complications

Complication	Number[a]	%
No complications	522	95.4
Dysphagia	10	1.8
Tracheal stenosis or malacia	5	0.9
Airway obstruction with decannulation	4	0.7
Hoarseness	3	0.5
Other[b]	4	0.7

[a] Of 548 (80 of the 628 patients discharged were lost to follow-up)
[b] Aspiration, excessive granulation tissue, subglottic web, and stomal infection
Source: Kearney et al[75] with permission

placement by most investigators, though not all. In all of the studies, the PDT was deemed to be safe and efficacious. Many studies also claimed a "cost" savings when PDT was used. *None of the authors advocated use of the PDT in the emergency setting.*

Since publication of the last edition of this book, new PDT devices have been introduced to the market. Some devices are no longer available or have been modified. Complications have been reported with each device. For example, the PercuTwist™ Tracheostomy Dilator Set (Rusch, Kernen, Germany) received favorable comment from Sengupta et al[94] and Westphal et al[95]. However, Scherrer et al[96] reported a double fracture of the second tracheal ring with avulsion and migration of the fractured cartilage. As new PDT devices are more thoroughly tested, other complications and the frequency with which they occur will be reported.

Conclusions Regarding PDT-Related Complications

Many studies documented that the Ciaglia PDT technique is safe, efficacious, and cost-effective. The technique is not advocated for emergency use. It should be used by *experienced physicians. Immediate surgical backup should be available.* Fiberoptic bronchoscopic guidance is suggested to minimize complications associated with PDT insertion.

Comparisons Between the Ciaglia PDT and Open Tracheostomy

In 1909, Jackson standardized the open tracheostomy technique used by surgeons today. Many studies over the past decade have compared this "gold standard" to various percutaneous dilational tracheostomy methods (primarily the Ciaglia technique). While some studies endorse open tracheostomy as the technique of choice to establish an elective surgical airway,[97–99] others found that PDT was also safe and efficacious when performed by a trained surgeon.[100–102] PDT has gained considerable popularity in some areas[103] and has proven superior to open tracheostomy in prospective studies.[53,104] A more recent metaanalysis of a systematic literature review[105] supported the proposition "…that PDT, performed electively in the ICU, should be the method of choice for performing tracheostomies in critically ill adult patients."

Debate over the Best Method to Establish an Elective Surgical Airway Continues

Investigators have used tests including bronchoscopy, MRI, radiographic studies, pulmonary function testing, and physical examination to define and evaluate long-term complications of PDT vs. open tracheostomy. Using endoscopy to evaluate the airway, one investigator noted a very high incidence of asymptomatic "airway abnormalities" after PDT in 36 of 41 survivors.[106] Other studies showed much lower rates of long-term PDT-related sequellae.[107–110] The reasons for this discrepancy remains unresolved due to the unfortunate number of patients lost to follow-up. Norwood et al[111] evaluated long-term complications in 100 of 422 patients who had undergone PDT. Of these 100 patients, 38 agreed to computerized tomography (CT) and fiberoptic airway endoscopy, 10 patients had CT only, while 52 were evaluated by interview alone. The most common complications that were reported were voice change (27%), mild tracheal stenosis (21%), and vocal cord abnormalities (11%)

Disagreement continues as to the preference of PDT vs. open tracheostomy used to establish an elective surgical airway. To read more on this topic, consider the debate between Bernard and Kenady,[112] proponents of conventional surgical tracheostomy, and Griffen and Kearney,[113] proponents of PDT. Excellent reviews by Barba[114] and Pryor et al[115] summarized various surgical techniques commonly undertaken in the ICU setting, including PDT, tracheostomy, and cricothyroidotomy.

Comparisons of Different PDT Techniques

Recent publications documented clinical comparisons of various PDT techniques. Most studies are prospective, though the methodology utilized to collect the data varied.

Byhahn et al[116] compared the Ciaglia Blue Rhino (CBR) (Cook Critical Care, Bloomington, IN) to the standard Ciaglia PDT in 50 patients. The mean procedure time for the Blue Rhino was 165 s vs. 386 s for the standard Ciaglia PDT. Tracheal cartilage rupture occurred in 9 of 25 patients in the Blue Rhino group vs. 2 of 25 in the standard PDT group. The authors noted that the long-term sequellae of tracheal ring fracture needs further study. Other complications with the standard PDT included posterior tracheal wall injury (2/25), pneumothorax (1/25), and bleeding during tracheostomy tube change (1/25). No life-threatening complications were associated with use of the Blue Rhino. The authors concluded that the "new CBR is more practicable than PDT."

Westphal et al[117] compared the standard Ciaglia PDT and the Fantoni translaryngeal technique (TLT) in 90 patients. They reported that the mean procedure time for the TLT was slightly shorter than for PDT, 9.8 vs. 10.4 min. Complications for PDT included severe bleeding (1/45), aspiration of blood (4/45), and lower postoperative PaO_2/FiO_2. The main complications of the TLT technique were difficult retrograde wire placement (14/45) and higher $PaCO_2$ intraoperatively. The authors concluded that both techniques were "safe and attractive" to establish long-term airway access in critically ill patients.

In a study by Byhahn et al,[118] the Griggs Guide Wire Dilating Forceps (GWDF) and Fantoni TLT techniques were compared in 100 patients. The mean procedural time was shorter for the GWDF technique, 4.8 vs. 9.2 min. The overall complication rates for both groups were 4%. Complications of the GWDF included moderate to severe bleeding in 2 of 50 patients. Complications of the TLT included tracheal wall rupture in 1 of 50 patients and pretracheal tube placement in 1 of 50 patients. They rated both techniques safe when performed by experienced physicians.

Three studies compared the GWDF technique and the standard Ciaglia PDT. Nates et al,[119] in a study of 100 patients, documented a slightly shorter mean procedural time for PDT than for GWDF, 9.3 vs. 10 min. They preferred standard PDT to GWDF because of a lower overall complication rate (2% vs. 25%). The major complication with GWDF was bleeding Van Heerden et al[120] studied 54 patients and reported equal rates of bleeding between GWDF and PDT patients. The major difference between groups was reported to be more difficult tracheostomy tube change at day 7 with the Ciaglia group (4/29) due to a smaller stoma size. The authors regarded both techniques to be safe. Finally, Ambesh and Kaushik[121] compared the techniques in a study that included 80 patients. The mean procedural time was shorter for the GWDF group, 6.5 vs. 14 min. The complication rates were similar for both groups with two exceptions. Stomal dilation was more difficult with the PDT technique, while tracheal cannulation was more difficult with the GWDF group. No clinical tracheal stenosis at 9 months postdecannulation was reported in patients from either group. The authors reported that both techniques were safe and easy to use.

Two studies compared the Portex PCK™ (Portex Cricothyroidotomy Kit, Smiths Medical International, Hythe, Kent, UK) with the Melker cricothyroidotomy (Cook Medical, Bloomington, IN). One study was conducted on mannequins[122] and the other on human cadavers[123]. The PCK™ has an indicator "flag" that helps guide its tube-over-needle insertion. The authors of both studies concluded that PCK™ insertion times were slightly shorter than times recorded for the Melker kit. Statistically, complication and success rates were similar for the two techniques. However, the types of complications and/or injuries produced by the PCK™ kits were deemed to be more significant. The participants in the mannequin study "chose to use the wire-guided (Melker) device in a clinical emergency situation." Both kits are acceptable for emergency airway management use. The clinician will reduce complications and assure proficiency if he practices insertion on teaching models with the kit of his choice.

In conclusion, the studies reported that the PDT techniques analyzed were safe and efficacious when used by experienced physicians. Fiberoptic bronchoscopic guidance was recommended by all authors. It was reported that TLT could be used with pediatric patients, a claim not made for standard Ciaglia PDT. Finally, no authors endorsed any technique for use in the emergency setting.

Percutaneous Dilatational Tracheostomy Devices

Many PDT devices are available. The six PDT's listed below are examples of devices that have different design characteristics. Specific details of each can be viewed on the manufacturers' websites. A few of the more popular devices are discussed in more detail.

1. Ciaglia Blue Rhino® Percutaneous Introducer (Cook Medical, Bloomington, IN)
2. Ciaglia Blue Dolphin™ Balloon Percutaneous Tracheostomy Introducer (Cook Medical, Bloomington, IN)
3. Portex® Griggs Forceps Technique Kits [not for use in the USA] (Portex®, Smiths Medical Intenational [UK])
4. Fantoni Translaryngeal Tracheostomy Kit (Mallinckrodt, Europe)
5. Portex® ULTRAperc Percutaneous® Single Dilator Technique Kits® (Smiths Medical, USA)
6. PercuTwist™ (Rusch)

Ciaglia Blue Rhino® Percutaneous Introducer (Cook Medical, Bloomington, IN)
The Ciaglia Blue Rhino® (Cook Medical, Bloomington, IN) is a very popular PDT device.

The following figure shows the components of the set as marketed by Cook Medical, Bloomington, IN (Fig. 12.14).
Instructions for use of the Blue Rhino®

1. The PDT is inserted through the first or preferably the second tracheal membrane.
2. After identifying the proper level, locally inject lidocaine with epinephrine and make a vertical 1.5-cm incision in the midline from the lower edge of the cricoid cartilage. One may gently dissect the incision with a curved mosquito clamp down to the anterior tracheal wall. Next, use a finger to dissect the front of the trachea and to displace thyroid tissue downward.
3. After deflating the endotracheal tube cuff, pull the tube back 1 cm. (A fiberoptic bronchoscope can verify that the tip of the tube is still in the trachea and guide the operator with the next four steps.)
4. Direct the introducer needle in a posterior/caudad direction into the trachea observing air aspiration to verify that the tip of the needle has entered the trachea. Inject 1.0 cc of lidocaine into the trachea and remove the needle Attach a syringe half filled with lidocaine to the needle/catheter and reinsert the tip into the trachea. Aspirate on the needle to make sure that the tip is still in the trachea by

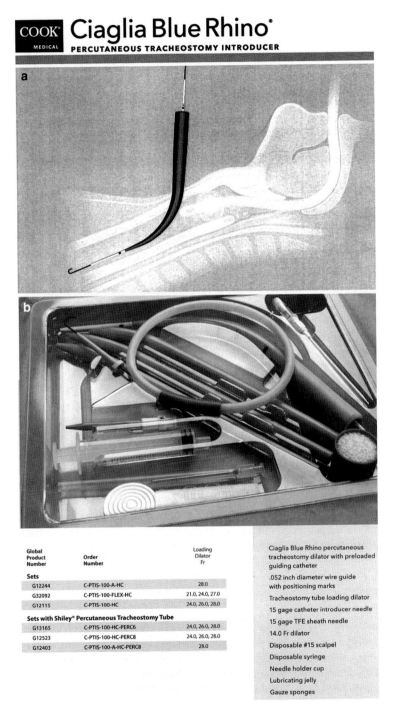

Global Product Number	Order Number	Loading Dilator Fr
Sets		
G12244	C-PTIS-100-A-HC	28.0
G32092	C-PTIS-100-FLEX-HC	21.0, 24.0, 27.0
G12115	C-PTIS-100-HC	24.0, 26.0, 28.0
Sets with Shiley® Percutaneous Tracheostomy Tube		
G13165	C-PTIS-100-HC-PERC6	24.0, 26.0, 28.0
G12523	C-PTIS-100-HC-PERC8	24.0, 26.0, 28.0
G12403	C-PTIS-100-A-HC-PERC8	28.0

Ciaglia Blue Rhino percutaneous tracheostomy dilator with preloaded guiding catheter

.052 inch diameter wire guide with positioning marks

Tracheostomy tube loading dilator

15 gage catheter introducer needle

15 gage TFE sheath needle

14.0 Fr dilator

Disposable #15 scalpel

Disposable syringe

Needle holder cup

Lubricating jelly

Gauze sponges

Fig. 12.14 (**a**) Ciaglia Blue Rhino® Percutaneous Introducer. (**b**) Contents of the Blue Rhino® introducer kit (Cook Medical, Bloomington, IN, with permission)

observing for air. Move the endotracheal tube to make sure that the needle has not impaled the tube or cuff (the needle will move if it has impaled the endotracheal tube).

5. When the needle's position is verified, remove the needle and advance the catheter into the trachea; aspirate for air. Remove the syringe and insert the 0.052-in. "J" wire into the trachea.

6. Following the direction of the arrow on the guiding catheter, advance the guiding catheter over the wire guide to the skin-level mark on the wire guide. Insert the guiding catheter and wire guide *as a unit* into the trachea until the safety ridge on the guiding catheter is to the skin level. *The end of the guiding catheter with the safety ridge should be introduced toward the patient.* Align the proximal end of the Teflon guiding catheter at the mark on the proximal portion of the wire guide. This will assure that the distal end of the guiding catheter is properly positioned back on the wire guide, preventing possible trauma to the posterior tracheal wall during subsequent manipulations. Position the guiding catheter and wire guide *as a unit* so that the safety ridge on the guiding catheter is at the skin level.

7. Activate the EZ-Pass hydrophilic coating by immersing the distal end of the Ciaglia Blue Rhino® dilator in sterile water or saline.

8. Advance the Ciaglia Blue Rhino® dilator and the guiding catheter as a unit over the wire guide while maintaining the wire guide position. Align the proximal end of the guiding catheter at the mark on the proximal portion of the wire guide. This will assure that the distal end of the guiding catheter is properly positioned back on the wire guide, preventing possible trauma to the posterior tracheal wall during subsequent manipulations.

9. Begin to dilate the access site by advancing the guiding catheter and Ciaglia Blue Rhino® dilator as a unit over the wire guide into the trachea. *To properly align the dilator on the wire guide/guiding catheter assembly, position the proximal end of the dilator at the single positioning mark on the guiding catheter. This will assure that the distal tip of the dilator is properly positioned at the safety ridge on the guiding catheter to prevent possible trauma to the posterior tracheal wall during introduction.* While maintaining the visual reference points and positioning relationships of the wire guide, guiding catheter, and dilator, advance them *as a unit* to the skin-level mark on the Ciaglia Blue Rhino® dilator. Care *must* be taken not to advance the Blue Rhino® dilator beyond the black skin-level mark. Advance and pull back the dilating assembly several times to perform effective dilation of the tracheal entrance site.

10. Remove the Ciaglia Blue Rhino® dilator, leaving the wire guide/guiding catheter assembly in position. *Note:* The wire guide must always lead the dilator and the guiding catheter assembly to prevent possible trauma to the posterior tracheal wall during dilation. Care must be taken to keep the guiding catheter assembly properly aligned with the mark on the proximal portion of the wire guide.

11. Slightly overdilate the tracheal entrance site to a size appropriate for passage of the tracheostomy tube of choice; overdilate to allow easy passage of the balloon portion of the tracheostomy tube into the trachea.

12. Preload the flexible tracheostomy tube to be inserted on the appropriate-size blue dilator by first generously lubricating the surface of the dilator. Position the tracheostomy tube onto the dilator so that its tip is approximately 2 cm back from the distal tip of the dilator. Make sure the balloon is totally deflated. Thoroughly lubricate the tracheostomy tube assembly prior to insertion. The sizing chart below should be used as a guide to assure correct fit.

Note: Dual cannula tracheostomy tubes may also be placed using this technique. The inner cannula must be removed for introduction. Always check fit of dilator to tracheostomy tube prior to insertion. *Follow tracheostomy tube manufacturer's instructions for testing of balloon cuff and inflation system prior to insertion.*

13. Advance the preloaded tracheostomy tube over wire guide/guiding catheter assembly to the safety ridge and then advance as a unit into the trachea. As soon as the deflated balloon enters the trachea, withdraw the blue dilator, guiding catheter, and wire guide.
14. Advance the tracheostomy tube to its flange. *Note:* If using a dual cannula tracheostomy tube, insert the inner cannula at this point.
15. Connect the tracheostomy tube to the ventilator, inflate the balloon cuff, and remove the endotracheal tube. *Note:* Prior to complete removal of the endotracheal tube, test ventilation through the tracheostomy tube.
16. Perform suction to determine if any significant bleeding or possible obstruction exists that has not been noted to this point.
17. If necessary, one suture may be placed at the bottom of the initial incision.

After placement apply Neosporin dressing to the stoma site 3 times per day (TID) for 3 days. Elevate the head of the patient's bed 30–40° for 1 h after insertion (Figs. 12.15–12.22).

Precautions

1. Always confirm access into trachea by air bubble aspiration.
2. Maintain safety positioning marks of wire guide, guiding catheter, and dilators during dilating procedure to prevent trauma to posterior wall of the trachea.
3. Tracheostomy tube should fit snugly to dilator for insertion. Generous lubrication to the surface of the dilator will enhance fit and placement of the tracheostomy tube.
4. Use the fiberoptic bronchoscope to guide insertion of the PDT.

Clinical use of the Ciaglia Blue Rhino® kit has been described by Byhahn et al and Bewsher et al.[124,125] (Fig. 12.23).

The *Ciaglia Blue Dolphin*™ (Cook Medical, Bloomington, IN) is the first PDT that combines balloon dilation and tracheal tube insertion. The balloon minimized airway leakage during insertion. A video of the device's insertion can be viewed on www.cookmedical.com.

Portex® Griggs Forceps Technique Kits (GWDF) (Smiths Medical, International [UK])

The GWDF Tracheostomy Kit is not available in the United States. However, it has been used extensively in other countries.[118,120,126–128] The principal instrument in

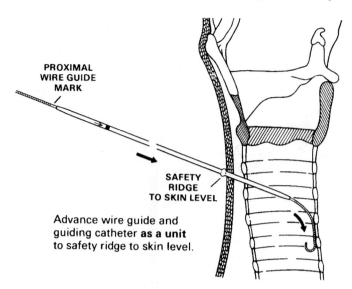

Fig. 12.19 Advance wire guide and guiding catheter *as a unit* to safety ridge to skin (Cook Critical Care, Bloomington, IN, with permission)

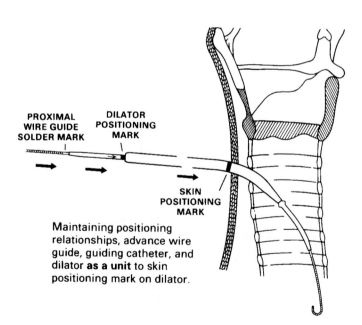

Fig. 12.20 Maintaining positioning relationships, advance wire guide, guiding catheter, and dilator *as a unit* to skin positioning mark on dilator (Cook Critical Care, Bloomington, IN, with permission)

TRACHEOSTOMY TUBE

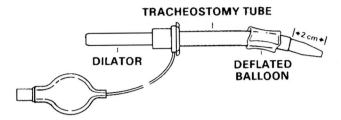

Fig. 12.21 Tracheostomy Tube Used with Cook Pot Kit (Cook Critical Care, Bloomington, IN, with permission).

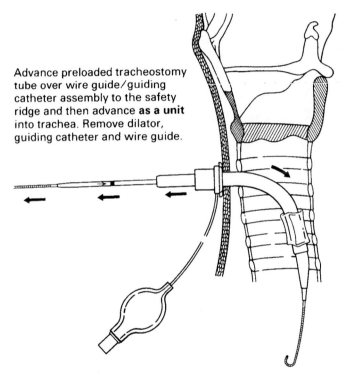

Advance preloaded tracheostomy tube over wire guide/guiding catheter assembly to the safety ridge and then advance **as a unit** into trachea. Remove dilator, guiding catheter and wire guide.

Fig. 12.22 Advance preloaded tracheostomy tube over wire guide. Guiding catheter assembly to the safety ridge and then advance *as a unit* into trachea. Remove dilator, guiding catheter and wire guide (Cook Critical Care, Bloomington, IN, with permission)

the kit is a modified Howard Kelly forceps with a curved tip. The blades of the tip have a guide wire groove that, when the forceps is closed, will allow the wire to pass through the forceps' blades (Fig. 12.24).

To perform the GWDF technique, the following steps are undertaken.[118,120,129]

1. A 2-cm horizontal incision is made through the skin at the desired tracheal level (between the second and third tracheal ring).

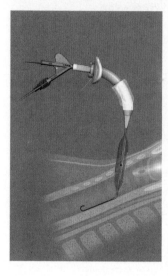

Ciaglia Blue Dolphin
Balloon Percutaneous Tracheostomy Introducer

Sets:	Loading Dilator French Size
C-PTBS-2400	24
C-PTBS-2600	26
C-PTBS-2700	27
C-PTBS-2800	28
C-PTBS-3000	30
Trays:	
C-PTBSY-2400	24
C-PTBSY-2600	26
C-PTBSY-2700	27
C-PTBSY-2800	28
C-PTBSY-3000	30

The set consists of a balloon-tipped catheter loading dilator assembly; Cook inflation device; wire guide; 18-gage introducer needle; 18-gage TFE sheath needle; needle holder cup; 14 French dilator; large full body drape with clear plastic window; gauze pads, disposable syringe; measuring tape; disposable safety scalpel; and lubricating jelly. A separate, sterile tracheostomy tube is also included in an optional set. (Described below)

The tray contains the set components and other items necessary for a bedside procedure including lidocaine; 22-, 25- and 18-gage needles; double swivel connector; Chlorhexidine/alcohol prep solution; suture with needle; CSR wrap; and prep tray. A separate, sterile tracheostomy tube is also included in an optional tray. (Described below)

Ciaglia Blue Dolphin
Balloon Percutaneous Tracheostomy Introducer
Including Percutaneous Cuffed Tracheostomy Tubes

Sets:	Loading Dilator French Size
C-PTBS-2600-PERC6	26
C-PTBS-2800-PERC8	28
Trays:	
C-PTBSY-2600-PERC6	26
C-PTBSY-2800-PERC8	28

Fig. 12.23 Ciaglia Blue Dolphin™ balloon percutaneous tracheostomy introducer (Cook Medical, Bloomington, IN, with permission)

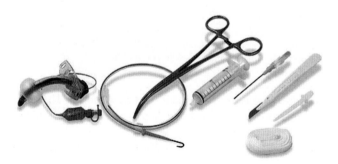

Fig. 12.24 Portex® Griggs™ percutaneous dilation blue line ultra® tracheostomy kits (Smiths Medical, International [UK], with permission)

2. A guide wire is inserted as described in the Ciaglia PDT technique. Fiberoptic guidance is recommended to insure that the wire is placed in the midline.
3. The GWDF is closed over the wire and passed through the dilated tract to the pretracheal wall. The forceps can be opened to dilate the tract.
4. The GWDF is then passed into the trachea (with fiberoptic guidance).
5. The forceps are then opened (using both hands) to the diameter desired (the diameter of the stoma tract).
6. The forceps are removed with the blades "open" to dilate the tract.[120]
7. An appropriately sized tracheostomy tube with obturator is inserted over the wire.
8. The wire and obturator are removed, the cuff inflated, and ventilation begun.

Clinicians using the Griggs GWDF warn that the procedure is not for emergency tracheostomy use and should be performed with fiberoptic guidance.

Fantoni Translaryngeal Tracheostomy Kit (Mallinckrodt, Europe)

Translaryngeal tracheostomy (TLT) was described by Fantoni and Ripamonti in 1995.[74] Since then, the technique has been used in Europe, Canada, and Australia. A clinical kit is not yet available in the United States. The technique is unique in that the tracheostomy tube is passed from within the trachea outward through the skin. The technique has been studied by many authors[130-133] and is deemed to be an acceptable percutaneous tracheostomy technique. Westphal et al[133] used TLT to perform 120 elective percutaneous tracheostomies. They concluded that the technique, as performed in the intensive care unit, was "safe and cost-effective."

The first step in performing the Fantoni technique for PDT is to insert a guidewire through the cricothyroid membrane using the components contained in the kit. Cricothyroid puncture and guidewire insertion are performed under fiberoptic guidance with the scope placed to the end of the endotracheal tube. The wire is passed in retrograde fashion parallel to the endotracheal tube through the glottis and out of the mouth. The remaining steps of the technique are illustrated in Figs. 12.25–12.28.

The reader can contact the manufacturer of other PDT devices to obtain insertion instructions and other product information.

Adjunctive Equipment and Techniques Used to Facilitate PDT Placement and other Surgical Airway Management Options

Many authors have published letters and studies suggesting that various percutaneous tracheostomy procedures could be more safely or efficiently performed if a variety of adjunctive equipment and techniques were used by the airway manager. This section of the chapter will review some of these suggestions.

Fiberoptic Bronchoscope

Many investigators and clinicians advocate using the fiberoptic bronchoscope when performing most elective percutaneous tracheostomy interventions. The fiberoptic

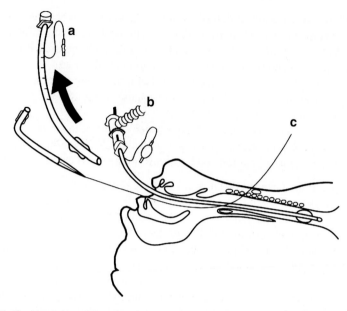

Fig. 12.25 The Fantoni translaryngeal tracheostomy (TLT). The endotracheal tube, (**a**) was replaced under direct laryngoscopy with the thin tube of the set (**b**), the tracheostomy tube is connected to the guide wire and, (**c**), by pulling the wire's distal end, is advanced to the trachea (from Westphal et al,[133] with permission)

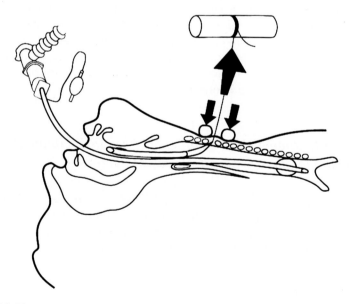

Fig. 12.26 The Fantoni TLT. By pulling the wire and by using digital counterpressure, the tracheostomy tube is advanced through the anterior tracheal wall and the soft tissues of the neck (from Westphal et al,[133] with permission)

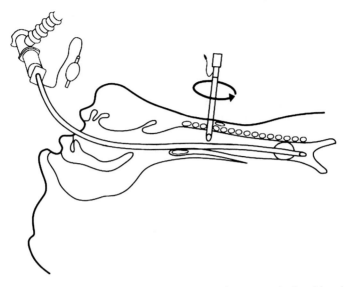

Fig. 12.27 The Fantoni TLT. Correct placement of the tracheostomy tube is achieved with 180° rotation by means of an obturator. Intratracheal rotation of the tracheal cannula can be done either with the thin endotracheal tube in place or after removal (from Westphal et al,[133] with permission)

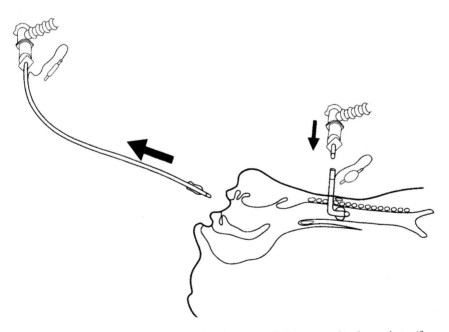

Fig. 12.28 The Fantoni TLT. The cuff is inflated, and the tube is connected to the respirator (from Westphal et al,[133] with permission)

scope is used to visually guide the operator when the following maneuvers are undertaken:

1. To verify that the tip of the endotracheal tube is below the cords and above the level of proposed tracheostomy site after the tube has been pulled back.
2. To confirm that the level of the proposed tracheostomy is correct (usually the first or second tracheal membrane) and in the midline.
3. To guide initial needle-thyroidotomy to help prevent posterior tracheal wall or endotracheal tube perforation.
4. To direct and confirm proper placement and direction of the catheter, guide wire, and/or guiding cannula into the distal trachea.
5. To monitor formal tracheostomy tube placement.
6. To inspect and/or suction the trachea and bronchi after formal tracheostomy tube placement.

Bouvette and Fuhrman[134] commented that use of the fiberoptic bronchoscope "does not guarantee 100% success of elimination of all complications" associated with PDT. Furthermore, Mphanza and Jacobs[135] remark that use of the fiberoptic bronchoscope may not improve safety, and in some cases may make ventilation more difficult while performing PDT. This could cause an increase in $PaCO_2$ that could lead to deleterious consequences if the patient had increased intracranial pressure. Perhaps the use of end-tidal CO_2 monitoring in selected patients could be used to guide the operator's adjustment of ventilator parameters during PDT placement.

At the present time, most, though not all clinicians and investigators advocate the routine use of the fiberoptic bronchoscope while performing a variety of elective percutaneous tracheostomy techniques.

Video-Assisted Endoscopy

Ciaglia[136] suggested that a video-assisted bronchoscope could be used when a PDT is performed. The advantage of this technique is that the video picture is viewed by the clinician who is performing the PDT, allowing "the operator [to] see the field and be guided in management." Ciaglia wrote that "in this way, PDT could become a minimally invasive procedure with maximally increased visibility." The equipment to perform video-assisted endoscopy is marketed by many manufacturers of fiberoptic equipment. Video-assisted endoscopy equipment can be moved easily into the ICU or operating room for routine use during elective PDT.

Laryngeal Mask Airway (LMA)

Dexter[137] first reported performing PDT in patients ventilated with an LMA in 1994. He used a fiberoptic bronchoscope to guide PDT placement. Others have reported performing PDT using the LMA as an adjunctive aid.[138–141]Quinio et al[142] published a case report of Fantoni TLT placement in a patient whose airway was managed with an LMA. These authors claimed that the technique's main advantages included easier and safer fiberoptic bronchoscopic manipulation, since they did not have to pass the scope through an endotracheal tube. They further pointed out that there was no risk of endo-tracheal tube displacement or cuff or tube perforation with the tracheostomy needle. They warned, though, that the technique involved a risk of aspiration and that it might be contraindicated if the patient had upper airway pathology or "stiff" lungs.

Lightwand (Trachlight, Laerdal Medical Inc., Wappingers Falls, NY)

Addas et al[143] published a case series of 11 patients in which they used a Trachlight as an adjunctive aid for performing Ciaglia PDT. All of the patients studied were intubated at the time of PDT. Following is a summary of their methods.

1. Mark a reference point on the patient's neck (the level of the first and second tracheal ring or between the cricoid cartilage and the first tracheal ring).
2. Cut the endotracheal tube so the lightwand's tip is at the end of the tube when the lightwand is inserted. (The lightwand has centimeter markings along its shaft.)
3. Remove the stiff retractable stylet from the lightwand.
4. Place the lightwand in the endotracheal tube.
5. Deflate the endotracheal tube's cuff.
6. Withdraw the endotracheal tube and lightwand as a unit until the transillumination of the wand can be seen 1 cm above the marked site of insertion of the needle.
7. Secure the tube.
8. Remove the lightwand.
9. Reinflate the cuff and ventilate the patient
10. Proceed with the Ciaglia PDT technique. The authors dissected down to the trachea, displacing the soft tissue and thyroid gland, and punctured the trachea between the second and third tracheal ring.

The authors reported that PDT was successful in all of their patients. The mean time to perform the technique was 17.8 min. They reported no complications caused by the Trachlight.

The authors commented that the technique described was "blind" and that it should be used cautiously in patients with a coagulopathy. They also warned that the technique should be avoided in patients in which transillumination might be com-promised, such as those who have a short or "thick" neck or those who are obese.

It is postulated that the Trachlight might be an inexpensive adjunctive aid to those who routinely perform PDT "blindly".

Endotracheal Tube Exchangers

Hollow endotracheal tube exchangers have been used as adjunctive aids during PDT. Cooper et al[144] described the use of a tube exchanger (Endotracheal

Ventilation Catheter; CardioMed Supplies, Inc.; Gormley, Ontario, Canada) and a manually cycled jet ventilator during PDT placement. The tube exchanger was placed in the trachea with its end at the same level as the end of the endotracheal tube. Ventilation and oxygenation was provided via jet ventilation during PDT placement. Deblieux et al[145] published a case series in which they placed a 4.7-mm O.D., perforated disposable tube exchanger (C-CAE-14.0-83, Cook Critical Care, Bloomington, IN) through the endotracheal tube and advanced it blindly 5–8 cm into the trachea past the endotracheal tube's tip. These authors did not ventilate their patients through the tube exchanger. The exchanger was left in place during PDT. They implied that the tube exchanger could have been used to jet-ventilate the patient or as a guide for reintubation if the endotracheal tube was inadvertently pulled out during PDT placement. While both techniques have merit, neither was reported to be routinely used in the clinical studies reported earlier in this chapter. Further research is needed to define potential complications that could result from use of either technique.

Ultrasound Guidance of PDT

In 1999, Muhammad et al[146] used diagnostic ultrasound to assess the suitability of four patients to undergo PDT in the ICU. They postulated that ultrasonic evaluation of the pretracheal region could identify patients in whom aberrant anatomy would make PDT more difficult. Anatomic anomalies such as an aberrant blood vessel, deviated trachea, or a very short neck could be identified and evaluated by ultrasonic examination. The findings of the examination could then direct the operators to modify the PDT technique or choose to perform a formal operative tracheostomy. They presented two patients, one with a large pretracheal vein crossing anterior to the thyroid isthmus and one with a very short cricoid-sternal distance in whom they opted to perform operative tracheostomy. In the other two patients, both exhibiting short cricoid-sternal distances, the ultrasound was used to guide correct needle placement for the PDT. The authors did not specify details of the ultrasonic "guidance." They also discussed technical limitations of the ultrasonic equipment at their disposal. They predicted that technological developments would make ultrasonic guidance of PDT more practicable in the future.

Rigid Bronchoscope

Brimacombe and Clarke[147] published a case report and the findings from a series of six additional patients in whom a rigid bronchoscope was used to assist PDT. They found that the view through the rigid scope was excellent and that suctioning a large clot from the distal airway was easily accomplished.

Ventilation and oxygenation could also be maintained through the rigid scope. They reported that the scope's position was easy to maintain. They felt that the two main limitations of the technique were the risk of aspiration during performance of PDT and lack of training in rigid bronchoscopic techniques for most nonsurgical clinicians who perform PDT in the ICU. They concluded that use of the rigid bronchoscope as an adjunct to performing PDT merited further research.

Chest Radiographs After PDT

Many clinicians who perform PDT obtain routine, *immediate* (within 1 h) postprocedural chest radiographs to document the presence or absence of complications. The cost-benefit aspects of this practice have come under scrutiny. Donaldson et al[148] published a prospective case series of 54 patients who underwent PDT, 18 of whom received *immediate* (less than 1 h) postprocedural chest radiographs, while 35 received a *delayed* (2–12 h) postprocedural chest radiograph. One patient died immediately after PDT and was not included in the study. They found "no incidents of pneumothorax, pneumomediastinum, or tracheostomy tube malposition in any patient." They concluded that obtaining a routine, *immediate* post-PDT chest radiograph was not cost-effective. They recommended that an *immediate* post-PDT should be obtained if the procedure was difficult, if the PDT was performed for urgent or emergency indications, if the anatomy was abnormal or altered, or if the patient required high levels of positive-pressure ventilation. They opined that significant pneumothorax, the most critical post-PDT radiographic finding, could be diagnosed clinically. Whether or not a chest radiograph should be obtained routinely after uneventful PDT placement has been challenged by other clinicians concerned with cost containment.

Capnography During Transtracheal Needle Cricothyrotomy

Tobias and Higgins[149] studied capnography traces obtained during needle cricothyrotomy in dogs. They documented that the capnograph rapidly detected CO_2 when the needle entered the trachea. They also documented that the CO_2 trace was lost when the tip of the needle was passed through the posterior tracheal wall. They recorded capnographic traces of dogs breathing spontaneously and of dogs that were apneic. Finally, they demonstrated that the plunger of the syringe to which the needle was attached did not need to be pulled back for CO_2 to be detected by the capnograph. They concluded by writing, "Regardless of the reason for the needle cricothyrotomy, the monitoring of CO_2 from the needle during advancement serves as an additional safety measure to ensure the intratracheal location of the needle or catheter."

Fiberoptic Bronchoscope to Aid Retrograde Wire–Directed Intubation

The placement of a retrograde wire from the trachea through the upper airway (mouth or nose) used to direct endotracheal tube placement has already been discussed. Several authors have suggested modifying the technique by using the fiberoptic bronchoscope to facilitate intubation. Bissinger et al[150] reported passing a bronchoscope (loaded with a reinforced 6.5–8.5-mm I.D. endotracheal tube) over a retrograde wire that had been passed through the cricothyroid membrane. They successfully intubated 89 of 93 patients. They reported a problem with "hanging up" of the endotracheal tube as it was passed over the scope through the glottis in 5 of 93 patients, a phenomenon that was overcome by simple maneuvers such as jaw thrust or rotation of the endotracheal tube. The technique was abandoned in four patients who were fiberoptically intubated with conventional techniques. Commenting on this article, Eidelman and Pizov[151] suggested that the technique be modified – first, by placing a rigid plastic guide over the retrograde wire; second, by passing an endotracheal tube (with a pediatric bronchoscope in its lumen but not over the wire) into the trachea as far as the guide wire entry point; third, at this point, passing the bronchoscope into the distal trachea; fourth, removing the guide wire; and finally, passing the endotracheal tube into the trachea over the bronchoscope. In response, Bissinger et al[152] stated that the Eidelman-Pizov modifications did not necessarily prevent "hanging up" of the endotracheal tube. They suggested that the retrograde wire could be passed through the side hole of the endotracheal tube so it could be passed further into the trachea before the guide wire is removed. Roberts and Solgonik[153] reported a successful retrograde intubation with a technique similar to that described by Eidelman and Pizov.[151] Finally, Rosenblatt et al[154] reported a case in which a fiberoptic bronchoscope was passed in retrograde fashion through a surgical cricothyroidotomy into the upper airway of a patient with severe upper airway edema. Attempts to intubate the patient with a laryngoscope and conventional fiberoptic techniques had been unsuccessful. Before passing the retrograde bronchoscope, the patient had already been intubated with a 6.0-mm I.D. tube that had been surgically placed through the cricothyroid membrane. A guide wire was passed through the scope and then a 7.5/5.0-mm double endotracheal tube setup was advanced over the scope and wire until its tip could be seen through the tracheal stoma. The scope was removed, as was the 5.0-mm extender tube, leaving the 7.5-mm endotracheal tube in the trachea, over the wire. The bronchoscope was then passed through the endotracheal tube, alongside of the wire, and positioned in the distal trachea. The wire was removed and the endotracheal tube was passed into the trachea using the bronchoscope as a stylet.

If one considers using the fiberoptic bronchoscope to assist retrograde wire–directed intubation, the practitioner has the option of choosing a technique in which the wire is passed through the scope or a technique in which the scope is passed alongside the wire. Both techniques have been used successfully to intubate patients with difficult airway anatomy.

Learning Percutaneous Tracheostomy

It is logical to assume that a learning curve would be associated with the adoption of any new surgical procedure. As experience is gained, the complication rate would be expected to drop. Donaldson et al[155] cited references pertaining to this phenomenon by earlier investigators (before 1995). In their study, resident otolaryngologists were taught to perform elective Ciaglia PDT under the supervision of "an attending otolaryngologist experienced in PDT" who was present throughout the procedure. Bronchoscopic guidance was utilized in all cases. They concluded that no learning curve was demonstrated and that PDT could be taught safely to resident physicians who were appropriately supervised.

In another study, Massick et al[156] demonstrated that when a single operator was learning Ciaglia PDT, in their case the senior attending surgeon involved with the study, a "steep" learning curve was demonstrated. Their prospective cohort study of 100 patients, 20 patients in each group, revealed that the perioperative and postoperative complication rate was higher in the first group than in any other group. They also noted that the late complication rate was higher in the last 50 patients as compared to the first 50. They did not use bronchoscopic guidance to aid the PDT. They noted also that patients with abnormal cervical anatomy had a higher complication rate when compared to patients with normal anatomy. The late complication rate did not depend on the operator's experience level. Future studies will establish the learning curve for practitioners of other specialities (general surgery, intensive care physicians, anesthesiologists) who learn various PDT techniques.

Clinical Patterns of PDT Utilization

A survey of 100 adult critical care units in the UK[157] revealed the following information concerning PDT use:

1. Used PDT for elective tracheostomy: 93%
2. Used fiberoptic guidance of PDT placement: 73%

This study confirmed the widespread use of PDT in responding British ICU's in 2003. A publication in 2008 concluded that "Percutaneous dilatational tracheostomy is the procedure of choice for tracheostomy in critically ill patients in Germany."[158] PDT was used routinely in 86.1% of the ICU's while only 13.9% used surgical tracheostomy only. The most common percutaneous device used in German ICU's was the Ciaglia Blue Rhino® (69%) (Personal communication from Kluge, S).

The investigators documented 98% utilization of the fiberoptic bronchoscope to guide and verify PDT placement in German ICU's. The authors reported that

PDT devices were used routinely in ICU's in the UK (97% with 83% fiberoptic guidance), Spain (72% with 16% fiberoptic guidance), the Netherlands (62% with 36% fiberoptic guidance), and in Switzerland (57% with no data on fiberoptic guidance).

Teaching Surgical Airway Techniques

Two ways to teach surgical airway techniques are to use anatomical models, either synthetic or animal,[159] and to develop protocols allowing students (at any level) to use interventional airway equipment in the course of daily practice.[160] One study demonstrated that anesthesiologists who were shown a 3-min training film could perform a cricothyroidotomy using the Melker Emergency Percutaneous Dilational Set (Cook Medical, Bloomington, IN) within 40 s after five insertion attempts utilizing a mannequin model.[161] Professional organizations such as the American Society of Anesthesiologists, Society for Airway Management, and the Difficult Airway Society (UK) sponsor or present difficult and surgical airway training programs.

Contraindications to Performing Percutaneous Tracheostomy

The contraindications to performing percutaneous tracheostomy vary depending on technique. Contraindications are relative or absolute depending on many factors such as the experience of the operator, institutional standards, availability of ancillary help, time constraints, and the stage of technical development and knowledge concerning a particular intervention. The following list includes conditions and situations constituting traditional contraindications to performing percutaneous tracheostomy techniques:

1. Emergency situations
2. Inability to establish a surgical airway immediately should the technique fail
3. Abnormal cervical or pretracheal anatomy

   (a) Morbid obesity
   (b) Thyroid tissue at the level of proposed tracheostomy
   (c) Aberrant blood vessels
   (d) Short neck
   (e) Previous neck/tracheal surgery

4. Infection at the proposed tracheostomy site
5. Burns
6. Pregnancy
7. Cervical spine instability
8. Uncontrolled coagulopathy

9. Nonintubated patient
10. Pediatric patient
11. Previous sternotomy

Emergency Percutaneous Tracheostomy

Unfortunately, there is a paucity of scientific information concerning the application of percutaneous tracheostomy techniques in the setting of emergency airway management. Eisenburger et al[162] reported that in a simulated "emergency" setting, the success rate for performing a surgical cricothyrotomy was 70% as compared to a success rate of 60% for percutaneous dilational cricothyrotomy (Arndt Emergency Cricothyrotomy Catheter Set, Cook Critical Care, Bloomington, IN) for a group of inexperienced clinicians. More studies need to be conducted to compare various techniques under controlled conditions. The authors of studies concerning PDT almost unanimously caution against use of the technique in the emergency setting.

Emergency Surgical Cricothyrotomy

An emergency surgical cricothyrotomy is undertaken if an apneic or obstructed patient faces imminent hypoxic injury and airway management techniques, both conventional and surgical, have failed or are deemed to fail within a critical time framework. The critical triggers in this scenario are "Cannot intubate, cannot ventilate!" and cannot establish a percutaneous cannula for oxygenation.

Anatomy of the Cricothyroid Space

The cricothyroid membrane is located in the anterior midline between the lower border of the thyroid cartilage and the upper border of the cricoid cartilage (Fig. 12.29).

The average size of the cricothyroid membrane is 9×30 mm. To perform a cricothyrotomy, a midline approach is used. Bleeding is a major complication of the procedure. Goumas et al[163] performed an autopsy study of 107 cadavers to define the vascular anatomy of the cricothyroid space. They considered veins greater than 2 mm in diameter to be "important," implying that this size vein had the potential to cause significant perioperative bleeding. The findings of their anatomic investigation are summarized in Table 12.10.

Since the fewest vascular structures were found in the midline, these investigators recommended that the midline of the cricothyroid space be identified "every time" a cricothyrotomy is performed.

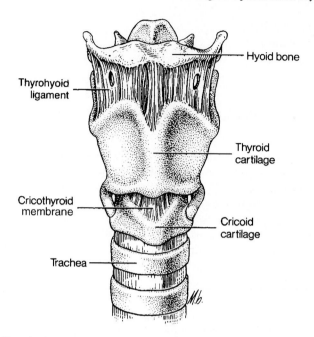

Hyoid bone

Thyrohyoid
ligament

Thyroid
cartilage

Cricothyroid
membrane

Cricoid
cartilage

Trachea

Fig. 12.29 The cricothyroid membrane lies between the thyroid and cricoid cartilages. The *cricothyroid space,* which lies between the membrane and the skin, contains many anatomic structures as defined by Goumas et al.[163]

Table 12.10 Anatomy of the cricothyroid space (107 cadavers studied)

Structure	Located in the midline	Located within 1 cm of the midline
Veins greater than 2 mm diameter (all veins were superficial)	11 (10.2%)	30 (30.8%)
Artery (1 mm)	4 (3.7%)	
Network of small veins		27 (25%)
Dense network of veins		1 (1%)
Lymph node	1 (1%)	
Pyramidal lobe of thyroid		7 (6.5%)
Two pyramidal lobes		1 (1%)

Source: Goumas et al[163] with permission

General Comments

Schroeder[164], reviewing the topic of cricothyroidotomy from the otolaryngologist's point of view, cited evidence that in the emergency situation, airway intervention at the cricothyroid level should be considered as reasonable an option as tracheostomy at a lower level. The advantages of the cricothyroidotomy over a lower tracheostomy were reported to be: (1) similar complication rates; (2) landmarks are easier to identify; (3) cricothyroidotomy is faster to perform, especially in the hands of a nonsurgeon; (4) less risk of pneumothorax; (5) less bleeding; (6) less risk of tracheoinnominate artery fistula; (7) less risk of tracheoesophageal fistula; (8) less cervical hyperextension is required; (9) a dislodged tube is easier to reinsert; (10) the surgical site is higher, perhaps of importance if lower neck surgery or a sternotomy had been or will be performed after the cricothyroidotomy. In more *elective* situations, the author cited references that favored a lower tracheostomy level, such as with: (1) pediatric patients; (2) patients who had been previously intubated; (3) patients with laryngeal infection or trauma; (4) patients who used their voices professionally (perhaps to lessen the incidence of vocal changes posttracheostomy). Three other important comments made by the author are the following: in order to avoid vocal cord damage, as the cords lie 0.5–2 cm above the cricothyroid membrane, the scalpel blade should incise the membrane with its tip pointed inferiorly. The author warned against damaging the thyroid or cricoid cartilages to lessen the incidence of postoperative stenotic complications. Finally, because the average size of the cricothyroid membrane was 9×30 mm, the author recommended use of a tracheostomy tube with an 8.5-mm O.D.

Outcome Studies

The results of retrospective outcome studies published in the 1990s are summarized in Tables 12.11[165,166] and 12.12[167]. In most cases, a trained surgeon performed the cricothyroidotomy or tracheostomy. In 28 of 29 cases, in which the surgical airway was established outside of the emergency room or operating room, the speciality of the operator was not specified.

   These studies indicate that trained medical personnel have a high rate of success performing emergency cricothyroidotomy. The importance of training programs

Table 12.11 Cricothyroidotomy outcome studies

Study	No. of patients	Success rate	No. of prehospital patients	No. of in-hospital patients	Complication rate
Hawkins et al.[165]	66	98.5%	8	58	3%
Isaacs[166]	65	95.4	20	45	Early: 15.4% Late: 7.4% (2/27)
Literature review[163]	320	96%			Early: 14.3%

Table 12.12 Emergency cricothyroidotomy vs. tracheostomy

Number of patients		Success rate		Complications	
Crico	Tracheo	Crico	Tracheo	Crico	Tracheo
20	14	87%	100%	20%	21%

Two patients were successfully converted from cricothyroidotomy to tracheotomy
All patients were managed surgically except 1, who had a successful orotracheal intubation
Needle cricothyroidotomy–jet ventilation was attempted in three patients. The technique failed in all three cases secondary to misplacement of catheter placement
Source: Gillespie and Eisele[167] with permission

such as the Advanced Trauma Life Support program outlined by the American College of Surgeons was noted.

Prehospital Airway Management Including Cricothyroidotomy

There are many reports of emergency responders using cricothyrotomy to establish a definitive airway in the prehospital setting. Most papers describe retrospective series. Some emergency response teams had physicians trained in airway management attending to all patients. Some did not. Some intubation protocols called for the use of paralytic agents, others did not. Different drugs were used to "sedate" patients prior to intubation, some of which may not have been administered prudently. Blind nasotracheal intubation was used by some responders, others did not utilize the technique. The indications to perform emergency cricothyrotomy in the field are not uniform. The level of training and proficiency to perform cricothyrotomy is not the same for all emergency personnel.

Despite these variables, the published reports offer interesting findings. Leibovici et al[168] reported on 29 cricothyroidotomies performed in the field in Israel, a country in which all cases were reported to a national trauma registry. Teams of responders always contained a physician. Group 1 teams included physicians who were surgeons, anesthesiologists, otolaryngologists, thoracic surgeons, plastic surgeons, obstetricians, or intensive care specialists. Group 2 teams included physicians who were general practitioners, internists, cardiologists, and pediatricians. All of the physicians in both groups had ATLS training, while only 3 had prior experience with cricothyroidotomy. The primary indication to perform an emergency cricothyroidotomy was failure to intubate despite no apparent anatomic distortion ($n=13$) and trauma to the anatomic landmarks of the pharynx and larynx ($n=12$). The results of the study indicate an overall success rate of 89.6%. Two of thirteen cricothyroidotomies using the Seldinger method (Cook Cricothyroidotomy Set, Cook Critical Care, Bloomington, IN) and 1 of 16 standard surgical cricothyroidotomies failed. All three patients made it to the hospital. The investigators found no statistical differences between groups, although all failures were reported by Group 2 teams. The only significant acute complication reported was failure to establish an airway.

Gerich et al,[169] in a prospective study designed to evaluate the efficacy of a rapid sequence intubation protocol, analyzed the findings reported on 383 acutely injured patients in the field who required airway control. The response team included a physician surgical resident and a paramedic with more than 10 years experience. The resident had at least 3 years of postgraduate training, 6 months training in intensive or critical care medicine, and 24 months in general or trauma surgery. The teams successfully intubated 373 of 383 patients (97%). Cricothyroidotomy was performed successfully in all eight cases in which it was attempted. The indications for cricothyroidotomy included failure to intubate ($n=2$), patient trapped in the vehicle ($n=2$), facial fractures or trauma ($n=3$), and clenched teeth ($n=1$). This group accounted for approximately 2% of the trauma patients. All but one of these patients subsequently died from their injuries. The authors concluded that trained EMS personnel should be able to successfully intubate patients in the field and that the rate of emergency cricothyroidotomy can be kept low. In response to this report, Brohi et al[170] reported that their EMS protocol called for use of suxamethonium. They reported that only 3 of 37 patients who received a cricothyroidotomy did so after failed intubation (0.2%). Their cricothyroidotomy rate was 2.5%.

Jacobson et al[171] reported that over a 5-year period, nonphysician ambulance teams under study in Indianapolis, Indiana, established 509 "definitive" airways. The majority of patients were intubated, while 50 surgical cricothyroidotomies were performed (9.8%). Indications to perform cricothyroidotomy were masseter spasm ($n=23$), upper airway visualization problems from blood or vomit despite suctioning ($n=18$), facial fractures that posed a contraindication to nasal intubation ($n=16$), and entrapment of the patient in the vehicle ($n=5$). Fifteen patients had more than one indication. The paramedics performed successful emergency cricothyroidotomy 94% of the time. The authors cited four other references in which nonphysician EMS teams performed emergency cricothyroidotomy, reporting success rates ranging from 88 to 99%.

In conclusion, trained physicians and nonphysicians report very good success rates with the technique, generally about 95%. Large-scale, prospective studies are needed to define optimal protocols regarding use of emergency cricothyroidotomy in the prehospital setting.

Emergency Cricothyroidotomy Techniques

Three cricothyroidotomy techniques will be presented. The first two techniques are described in a paper by Holmes et al.[172] In this paper, two groups were randomly selected from 27 emergency medicine interns, 1 junior medicine resident, and 4 senior medical students. None of the subjects had experience with surgical cricothyroidotomy. One group was taught the *standard technique* and the other was taught the *rapid 4-step technique* in a 15-min training session. Each subject then performed a cricothyroidotomy on an adult cadaver and was allowed one attempt to insert a No. 6 Shiley tracheostomy tube. The groups were then taught the alternative technique and were tested on their performance of that technique. The necks of the cadavers were dissected and complications were noted.

Standard Technique

Instruments

Scalpel with no. 11 blade
Trousseau dilator
Hemostats
Tracheal hook
No. 6 Shiley tracheostomy tube

Position: Standing at the patient's right side.
Steps

1. Midline vertical incision, 4 cm long, over the cricoid membrane.
2. Identification of the cricothyroid membrane by means of blunt dissection.
3. Short horizontal stab incision in the lower part of the cricothyroid membrane.
4. Stabilization of the larynx with a tracheal hook at the inferior aspect of the thyroid cartilage.
5. Dilatation of the ostomy with curved hemostats.
6. Placement of the Trousseau dilator in the incision, with dilatation of the ostomy.
7. Placement of the Shiley tube in the trachea.

Rapid 4-Step Technique[173]

Instruments

> Scalpel with no. 20 blade
> Tracheal hook
> No. 6 Shiley tracheostomy tube

Position: Standing at the patient's left side.
Steps

1. Identification of the cricothyroid membrane by palpation (a vertical incision through the skin to allow palpation of the cricothyroid membrane is recommended if the cricothyroid membrane cannot be initially identified on palpation).
2. Horizontal stab incision through the skin and cricothyroid membrane with the scalpel.
3. Stabilization of the larynx with the tracheal hook at the inferior aspect of the ostomy (on the cricoid cartilage), providing caudal traction.
4. Placement of the Shiley tube in the trachea.

The results of the study are summarized in Table 12.13.

Major complications included complete transection of the cricoid cartilage and posterior tracheal/esophageal perforation.

Table 12.13 Comparison of two cricothyroidotomy techniques

Parameters	4-Step technique	Standard technique
Successful airway (%)	28/32 (88%)	30/32 (94%)
Complications (%)		
Inadvertent tracheotomy	4/32 (13%)	7/32 (22%)
Other complications	8/32 (25%)	5/32 (16%)
Major complications	3/32 (9%)	1/32 (3%)
Time (seconds)		
Mean ± SD	43.2±44.6	138.8±93.4
Median (25th–75th percentiles)	32 (24–42)	114 (74–154)

Source: Holmes et al,[172] with permission

Alternative Techniques

Wong and Bradrick,[16] (p206) in Hagberg's *Handbook of Difficult Airway Management,* described two modifications to the techniques described above. They state that a horizontal, rather than a vertical, incision at the level of the cricothyroid

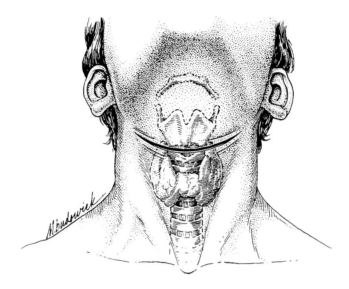

Fig. 12.30 The cricothyroidotomy incision

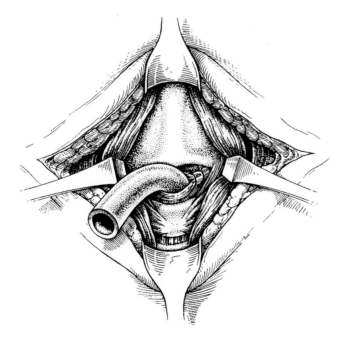

Fig. 12.31 Inserting the tube into a tracheostomy

membrane is acceptable (Figs. 12.30 and 12.31). They also comment that the surgical opening can be dilated with the handle of the scalpel by inserting it into the stoma and rotating it.

Complications of Emergency Cricothyroidotomy[16,174]

1. Failure to obtain an airway
2. Tracheostomy tube displacement or misplacement
3. Injury to laryngeal structures
4. Pneumothorax, pneumomediastinum
5. Damage to other structures in the neck (esophagus, blood vessels)
6. Vocal cord damage
7. Voice changes (hoarseness, change of pitch)
8. Subglottic stenosis, especially in children
9. Eating/swallowing problems
10. Posterior/lateral tracheal damage
11. Cellulitis
12. Aspiration
13. Shortness of breath
14. Unsightly scar

Most of the late-term complications associated with emergency cricothyroidotomy were considered to be minor. In fact, some of the reported complications could have been caused by the primary trauma and not the cricothyroidotomy.

Contraindications to Emergency Cricothyrotomy

In the setting of the emergency airway, the contraindications to performing a cricothyroidotomy are few. Most authors, though, warn that the technique is not suitable for "young children" or infants.

Cricothyrotomy and the Unstable Cervical Spine

Cricothyrotomy has been advocated by some authors to be the method of choice to establish an emergency airway in a patient with known or suspected unstable cervical spine. Gerling et al[174] studied the magnitude of cervical movement associated with the performance of cricothyrotomy on 13 surgically induced unstable cervical spine cadaveric preparations. They reported that the cervical movement associated with the procedure was "less than the threshold for clinical significance." Anterior–posterior displacement was 1–2 mm, while less than 1 mm of axial compression was demonstrated. They concluded by stating that "these results support the safety of cricothyrotomy in the presence of an unstable c-spine." Management of the airway in patients with unstable cervical spine is dealt with in other sections of the book.

Seldinger Technique Emergency Cricothyroidotomy vs. Standard Surgical Cricothyroidotomy

Schaumann et al[175] published a study comparing the Seldinger technique based Arndt Emergency Cricothyroidotomy Catheter Set (Cook Medical, Bloomington, IN) vs. the standard surgical cricothyroidotomy technique in human cadavers. Twenty emergency physicians were given verbal instructions on the two techniques for cricothyroidotomy tube insertion. The authors reported that the tube was placed properly in 88.2% of the Seldinger technique insertions vs. 84% of the surgical insertions. They also reported that the time to first ventilation was statistically significantly shorter for the Seldinger technique insertions vs. the surgical insertions: 108.6 ± 59.5 s vs. 136.6 ± 66.3 s. Finally, no injuries were reported for the Seldinger group vs. six punctures of thyroid vessels in the surgical group. While criticisms of the study's methodology have been published[176,177], the authors maintain that implications of their findings are clinically relevant. Future investigations may compare the efficacy of the devices used in the clinical setting.

Formal Tracheostomy

The technique of formal tracheostomy is not described in this book since it should be performed only by a trained surgeon. The indications for and complications of the technique are presented below.

Most tracheostomies are performed on ventilator-dependent patients or on patients with impaired airway defensive reflexes. When to perform the tracheostomy is controversial. An endotracheal tube may cause upper airway, laryngeal, or tracheal damage that could lead to long-term complications. However, tracheostomy is not without risk. The indications and advantages to performing a tracheostomy include the following:

Indications and Advantages of Tracheostomy[178]

1. Long-term secure airway
2. Enhances patient comfort
3. Might make pulmonary suctioning easier
4. Allows the patient to speak
5. Patients can take oral nutrition
6. Might decrease the likelihood of long-term swallowing dysfunction

7. Diminishes the likelihood of laryngeal injury
8. May be needed to establish an airway for head/neck surgical procedures

Complications of Tracheostomy

Goldenberg et al[179] reported the incidence of tracheostomy-related complications in a retrospective study of 1,130 consecutive patients.

1. Tracheal stenosis (1.85%)
2. Hemorrhage (0.8%)
3. Tracheocutaneous fistula (0.53%)
4. Infection (0.44%)
5. Tube decannulation/obstruction (0.35%)
6. Subcutaneous emphysema (0.08%)
7. Pneumothorax (0.26%)
8. Tracheoesophageal fistula (0.08%)

Other complications[178,180]

  9. Laryngeal nerve damage
10. Mediastinal sepsis
11. Air embolism during operation
12. Laryngeal incoordination (phonation or breathing difficulty)
13. Unsightly scar

The complications associated with tracheostomy are similar for adult and pediatric patient populations. Tracheostomy-related mortality is reportedly 0.5–5%[181] in the pediatric population.

Rigid Bronchoscopy

A rigid bronchoscope may be inserted to provide an airway during surgery involving the trachea, mediastinum, vascular rings, aberrant innominate artery, or the removal of foreign bodies. In most circumstances an experienced surgeon will insert the bronchoscope. The airway operator must be ready to assist the surgeon and to connect the bronchoscope to the anesthesia circuit to provide oxygen, ventilation, and/or anesthesia gases to the patient.

Summary

This chapter has presented a description of surgical equipment and techniques used to manage the difficult airway. Time is the limiting factor if the patient faces imminent hypoxic injury. It is difficult to decide which techniques are most applicable in the emergency situation. If one decides to include any of the equipment or techniques described in this chapter on his *difficult airway algorithm,* he must familiarize himself with the equipment, learn the techniques, and practice the techniques to maintain proficiency.

Percutaneous tracheostomy techniques were discussed in detail in the chapter. *These techniques should be used only in the elective setting.*

Unfortunately, the literature does not offer convincing evidence that one surgical airway management technique is better than another in the *emergency setting.* Since most clinicians are familiar with the Seldinger technique to insert intravenous catheters, surgical airway options based on the technique have been developed. *The emergency airway practitioner should select and master one needle/rigid catheter technique (be prepared to deliver high-pressure oxygen via jet ventilator) and one minitracheostomy technique. In addition, one must be prepared to perform an emergency cricothyrotomy before the patient experiences hypoxic injury.* These recommendations are not scientifically supported. They represent the opinion of the author of this chapter.

Many educational courses offer useful instruction in surgical airway management. Contact the American Society of Anesthesiologists (Park Ridge, IL) or the Society for Airway Management (Chicago, IL) for information concerning their educational programs and publications. Finally, the websites of the manufacturers of the equipment described in this chapter, for example Cook Medical Products (Bloomington, IN) at www.cookmedical.com offer on-line educational material that illustrate use of their emergency airway equipment.

References

1. Benumof JL, Scheller MS. The importance of transtracheal jet ventilation in the management of the difficult airway. *Anesthesiology.* 1989;71:769.
2. Smith RB, Schaer WB, Pfaeftle H. Percutaneous transtracheal ventilation for anesthesia and resuscitation: a review and report of complications. *Can J Anaesth.* 1975;22:607.
3. Zornow MH, Thomas TC, Scheller MS. The efficacy of three different methods of transtracheal ventilation. *Can J Anaesth.* 1989;36:624.
4. Gaughan SD, Ozaki GT, Benumof JL. A comparison in a lung model of low- and high-flow regulators for transtracheal jet ventilation. *Anesthesiology.* 1992;77:189.
5. Gaughan SD, Benumof JL, Ozaki GT. Can an anesthesia machine flush valve provide for effective jet ventilation? *Anesth Analg.* 1993;76:800.
6. Klein DS, Lees DE. Emergency cricothyroidotomy: a flexible device in the operating room. *South Med J.* 1989;82:661.
7. Kross J, Zupan JT, Benumof JL. A contingency plan for tracheal intubation. *Anesthesiology.* 1990;72:577.
8. Delaney WA, Kaiser RE. Percutaneous transtracheal jet ventilation made easy. *Anesthesiology.* 1991;74:952.
9. Ho AM. A simple anesthesia machine-driven transtracheal jet ventilation system [letter]. *Anesth Analg.* 1994;78:405.
10. Meyer PD. Emergency transtracheal jet ventilation system. *Anesthesiology.* 1990;73:787.

11. Benumof JL, Gaughan S. Connecting a jet stylet to a jet injector. *Anesthesiology.* 1991;74: 963.
12. Gaughan SD, Benumof JL, Ozaki GT. Quantification of the jet function of a jet stylet. *Anesth Analg.* 1992;74:580.
13. Schapera A, Bainton CR, Kraemer R, Lee K. A pressurized injection/suction system for ventilation in the presence of complete airway obstruction. *Crit Care Med.* 1994;22:326.
14. McLellan I, Gordon P, Khawaja S, Thomas A. Percutaneous transtracheal high frequency jet ventilation as an aid to difficult intubation. *Can J Anaesth.* 1988;35:404.
15. Chipley PS, Castresana M, Bridges MT, Catchings TT. Prolonged use of an endotracheal tube changer in a pediatric patient with a potentially compromised airway. *Chest.* 1994; 105:961.
16. Hagberg CA. *Handbook of Difficult Airway Management.* Philadelphia: Churchill Livingstone; 2000:194.
17. Shantha TR. Retrograde intubation using the subcricoid region. *Br J Anaesth.* 1992;68:109.
18. Sdrales L, Benumof JL. Prevention of kinking of a percutaneous transtracheal intravenous catheter. *Anesthesiology.* 1995;82:288.
19. Southwick JP. Precurved transtracheal catheters [letter]. *Anesthesiology.* 1995;82(5):1302.
20. Soto R, Mesa A. New intravenous catheter not suitable for trans-tracheal jet ventilation [letter]. *Anesth Analg.* 2001;92:1074.
21. Ames W, Venn P. Complication of the transtracheal catheter [letter]. *Br J Anaesth.* 1998; 81(5):825.
22. Peak DA, Roy S. Needle cricothyroidotomy revisited. *Ped Emerg Care.* 1999;15(3):224.
23. Dallen LT, Wine R, Benumof JL. Spontaneous ventilation via transtracheal large-bore intravenous catheters is possible. *Anesthesiology.* 1991;75:531.
24. Fawcett W, Ooi R, Riley B. The work of breathing through large-bore intravascular catheters. *Anesthesiology.* 1992;76:323.
25. Banner MJ et al. Excessive work imposed during spontaneous breathing through transtracheal catheters. *Anesthesiology.* 1992;77:A1231.
26. Mingus ML et al. Transtracheal oxygenation using simple equipment and low pressure oxygen delivery. *Anesthesiology.* 1988;69:A835.
27. Mackenzie CF, Barnas G, Nesbitt S. Tracheal insufflation of oxygen at low flow: capabilities and limitations. *Anesth Analg.* 1990;71:684.
28. Morley D, Thorpe CM. Apparatus for emergency transtracheal ventilation. *Anaesth Intensive Care.* 1997;25:675.
29. Patel RG. Percutaneous transtracheal jet ventilation. *Chest.* 1999;116(6):1689.
30. Poon YK. Case history number 89: a life-threatening complication of cricothyroid membrane puncture. *Anesth Analg.* 1976;55:298.
31. Davies P. A stab in the dark! Are you ready to perform needle cricothyroidotomy? *Injury.* 1999;30:659.
32. Hwa-Kou K. Translaryngeal guided intubation using a sheath stylet. *Anesthesiology.* 1985;63:567.
33. Bourke D, Levesque PR. Modification of retrograde guide for endotracheal intubation. *Anesth Analg.* 1974;53:1013.
34. Schwartz D, Singh J. Retrograde wire-guided direct laryngoscopy in a 1-month-old infant. *Anesthesiology.* 1992;77:607.
35. Alfrey DD. Double-lumen endobronchial tube intubation using a retrograde wire technique. *Anesth Analg.* 1993;76:1374.
36. Nicholson SC, Black AE, Kraras CM. Management of a difficult airway in a patient with Hurler-Scheie syndrome during cardiac surgery. *Anesth Analg.* 1992;75:830.
37. Abou-Madi MN, Trop D. Pulling vs. guiding: a modification of retrograde guided intubation. *Can J Anaesth.* 1989;6:336.
38. King HK, Long-Fong W, Ahsanul KK, Daniel JW. Soft and firm introducers for translaryngeal guided intubation. *Anesth Analg.* 1989;68:826.

39. Dhara SS. Retrograde intubation: a facilitated approach. *Br J Anaesth*. 1992;69:631.
40. Sanchez AF, Morrison DE. In: Hagberg CA, ed. *Handbook of Difficult Airway Management*. Philadelphia: Churchill Livingstone; 2000 [chapter 6].
41. Guggenberger J, Lenz G. Training in retrograde intubation. *Anesthesiology*. 1988;69:292.
42. Mahiou P, Korach JM, Emplier FT, Ecoffey C, Pasteyer J. Retrograde tracheal intubation combined with laryngeal nerve block in conscious trauma patients. *Anesthesiology*. 1988;71: A199.
43. Lenfant F, Benkhadra M, Trouilloud P, Freysz M. Comparison of two techniques for retrograde tracheal intubation in human fresh cadavers. *Anesthesiology*. 2006;104:48–51.
44. Parmet JL, Metz S. Retrograde endotracheal intubation: an underutilized tool for management of the difficult airway. *Contemp Surg*. 1996;49(5):300–306.
45. Bhattacharya P, Biswas BK, Baniwal S. Retrieval of a retrograde catheter using suction, in patients who cannot open their mouths. *Br J Anaesth*. 2004;92:888.
46. Hatton K, Price S, Craig L, Grider JS. Educating anesthesiology residents to perform percutaneous cricothyrotomy, retrograde intubation, and fiberoptic bronchoscopy using preserved cadavers. *Anesth Analg*. 2006;103:1205–8.
47. Marciniak D, Smith CE. Emergent retrograde tracheal intubation with a gum-elastic bougie in a trauma patient. *Anesth Analg*. 2007;105:1720–1721.
48. Mathews HR, Hopkinson RB. Treatment of sputum retention by minitracheostomy. *Br J Surg*. 1984;71:147.
49. Hutchinson J, Hopkinson RB. How to insert a minitrach. *Br J Hosp Med*. 1989;42:112.
50. Ala-Kokko TI, Kyllonen M, Nuutinen L. Management of upper airway obstruction using a Seldinger minitracheostomy kit. *Acta Anaesth Scand*. 1996;40:385.
51. Corke C, Cranswick P. A Seldinger technique for minitracheostomy insertion. *Anaesth Intensive Care*. 1988;16:206.
52. Chan TC, Vilke GM, Bramwell KJ, Davis DP, Hamilton RS, Rosen P. Comparison of wire-guided cricothyrotomy versus standard surgical cricothyrotomy technique. *J Emerg Med*. 1999;17(6):957.
53. Van Heurn LWE, van Geffen GJ, Brink PRG. Percutaneous subcricoid minitracheostomy: report of 50 procedures. *Ann Thorac Surg*. 1995;59:707.
54. Wain JC, Wilson DJ, Mathisen DJ. Clinical experience with minitracheostomy. *Ann Thorac Surg*. 1990;49:881.
55. Pedersen J et al. Is minitracheostomy a simple and safe procedure? A prospective investigation in the ICU. *Intensive Care Med*. 1991;177:333.
56. Randell T et al. Minitracheostomy: complications and follow-up with fiberoptic tracheoscopy. *Anaesthesia*. 1990;45:875.
57. Randell T, Lindgren L. Inadvertent submucosal penetration with a minitracheostomy cannula inserted by the Seldinger technique. *Anaesthesia*. 1991;46:801.
58. Hammond J, Bray B. A serious complication of minitracheostomy. *Anaesthesia*. 1992;47: 538.
59. Combes P et al. Minitracheostomy: impossible cannulation. *Br J Anaesth*. 1991;66:275.
60. Silk JM, Marsh AM. Pneumothorax caused by minitracheostomy. *Anaesthesia*. 1989;44:663.
61. Fisher JB. Surgical emphysema, minitracheostomy, and HFJV. *Intensive Care Med*. 1992;18: 317.
62. Campbell AM, O'Leary A. Acute airway obstruction as a result of minitracheostomy. *Anaesthesia*. 1991;46:854.
63. Daborn AK, Harris NE. Minitracheostomy: a life-threatening complication. *Anaesthesia*. 1989;44:839.
64. Russell WC. Complications and inappropriate use of minitracheostomy. *Anaesth Intensive Care*. 1989;17:513.
65. McEwan A et al. A serious complication of minitracheostomy. *Anaesthesia*. 1991;46:1041.
66. Allen PW, Thornton M. Oesophageal perforation with minitracheostomy. *Intensive Care Med*. 1989;15:543.

67. Claffey LP, Phelan DM. A complication of cricothyroid "minitracheostomy": oesophageal perforation. *Intensive Care Med.* 1989;15:140.
68. Ryan DW, Dark JH, Misra U, Pridie AK. Intra-oesophageal placement of minitracheostomy tube. *Intensive Care Med.* 1989;15:538.
69. Brathwaite CEM. Rapid percutaneous tracheostomy. *Chest.* 1991;100:1475.
70. Pedersen J, Lou H, Schurizek BA, Melsen NC, Juhl B, et al. Ossification of the cricothyroid membrane following minitracheostomy. *Intensive Care Med.* 1989;15:272.
71. Woodcock T. Mask CPAP and minitracheostomy: a cautionary tale. *Intensive Care Med.* 1991;17:436.
72. Allen PW, Hart SM. Minitracheostomy in children. *Anaesthesia.* 1988;43:760.
73. Powell DM, Price PD, Forrest LA. Review of percutaneous tracheostomy. *Laryngoscope.* 1998;108:170.
74. Fantoni A, Ripamonti D. A breakthrough in tracheostomy techniques: translaryngeal tracheostomy. *8th European Congress of Intensive Care Medicine.* Athens, Greece; 1995: 1031–1034.
75. Kearney PA, Griffen MM, Ochoa JB, Boulanger BR, Tseui BJ, Mentzer RM. A single-center 8-year experience with percutaneous dilational tracheostomy. *Ann Surg.* 2000;231(5):701.
76. Schwann NM. Percutaneous dilational tracheostomy: anesthetic consideration for a growing trend. *Anesth Analg.* 1997;84(4):907.
77. Fernandez L, Norwood S, Roettger R, Gass D, Wilkins H III. Bedside percutaneous tracheostomy with bronchoscopic guidance in critically ill patients. *Arch Surg.* 1996;131:129.
78. Cobean R, Beals M, Moss C, Bredenberg CE. Percutaneous dilational tracheostomy: a safe, cost-effective bedside procedure. *Arch Surg.* 1966;131:265.
79. Chendrasekhar A et al. Percutaneous dilatational tracheostomy: an alternative approach to surgical tracheostomy. *Southern Med J.* 1995;88(10):1062.
80. McHenry CR, Raeburn CD, Lange RL, Priebe PP. Percutaneous tracheostomy: a cost-effective alternative to standard open tracheostomy. *Am Surg.* 1997;63:646.
81. Moe KS, Schmid S, Stoecki SJ, Weymuller EA. Percutaneous tracheostomy: a comprehensive evaluation. *Ann Otol Rhinol Laryngol.* 1999;108:384.
82. Billy ML, Bradrick JP. Percutaneous dilatational subcricoid tracheostomy. *J Oral Maxillofac Surg.* 1997;55:981.
83. Bobo ML, McKenna SJ. The current status of percutaneous dilational tracheostomy: an alternative to open tracheostomy. *J Oral Maxillofac Surg.* 1998;56:681.
84. Muhammad JK, Major E, Wood A, Patton DW. Percutaneous dilatational tracheostomy: haemorrhagic complications and the vascular anatomy of the anterior neck: a review based on 497 cases. *Int J Oral Maxillofac Surg.* 2000;29:217.
85. Vigliaroli L, DeVivo P, Mione C, Pretto G. Clinical experience with Ciaglia's percutaneous tracheostomy. *Eur Arch Otorhinolaryngol.* 1999;256:426.
86. Gaukroger MC, Allt-Graham JA. Percutaneous dilatational tracheostomy. *Br J Oral Maxillofac Surg.* 1994;32(6):375.
87. Barrachina F, Guardiola JJ, Ano T, Ochagavia A, Marine J. Percutaneous dilatational cricothyroidotomy: outcome with 44 consecutive patients. *Intensive Care Med.* 1996;22:937.
88. Petros S, Engelmann L. Percutaneous dilatational tracheostomy in a medical ICU. *Intensive Care Med.* 1997;23:630.
89. Carrillo EH, Spain DA, Bumpous JM, Schmieg RE, Miller FB, Richardson JD. Percutaneous dilational tracheostomy for airway control. *Am J Surg.* 1997;174:469.
90. Suh RH, Margulies RH, Hope ML, Ault M, Shabot MM, et al. Percutaneous dilatational tracheostomy: still a surgical procedure. *Am Surg.* 1999;65:928.
91. Velmahos GC, Gomez H, Boicey CM, Demetriades D. Bedside percutaneous tracheostomy: prospective evaluation of a modification of the current technique in 100 patients. *World J Surg.* 2000;24:1109.
92. Marx WH, Ciaglia P, Graniero KD. Some important details in the technique of percutaneous dilatational tracheostomy via the modified Seldinger technique. *Chest.* 1996;110(3):762.

93. Walz MK, Peitgen K, Thurauf N, et al. Percutaneous dilatational tracheostomy – early results and long-term outcome of 326 critically ill patients. *Intensive Care Med.* 1998;24:685.
94. Sengupta N, Ang KL, Prakash D, Ng V, George SJ. Twenty months'routine use of a new percutaneous tracheostomy set using controlled rotating dilation. *Anesth Analg.* 2004;99: 188–192.
95. Westphal K, Maeser D, Scheifler G, Lischke V, Byhahn C. PercuTwist: a new single-dilator technique for percutaneous tracheostomy. *Anesth Analg.* 2003;96:229–232.
96. Scherrer E, Tual L, Dhonneur G. Tracheal ring fracture during a percutwist tracheostomy procedure. *Anesth Analg.* 2004;98:1451–1453.
97. Porter JM, Ivatury RR. Preferred route of tracheostomy – percutaneous versus open at the bedside: a randomized, prospective study in the surgical intensive care unit. *Am Surg.* 1999;65:142.
98. Massick DD, Yao S, Powell DM. Bedside tracheostomy in the ICU: a prospective randomized trial comparing open surgical tracheostomy with endoscopically guided percutaneous dilational tracheostomy. *Laryngoscope.* 2001;111:494.
99. Grover A, Robbins J, Bendick P, Gibson M, Villalba M. Open versus percutaneous dilatational tracheostomy: efficacy and cost analysis. *Am Surg.* 2001;67:297.
100. Lim JW, Friedman M, Tanyeri H, Lazar A, Caldarelli DD. Experience with percutaneous dilatational tracheostomy. *Ann Otol Rhinol Laryngol.* 2000;109:791.
101. Gysin C, Dulguerov P, Guyot JP, Perneger T, Abajo B. Chev- rolet JC. Percutaneous versus surgical tracheostomy: a double-blind randomized trial. *Ann Surg.* 1999;230(5):708.
102. Stoeckli SJ, Breitbach T, Schmid S. A clinical and histologic comparison of percutaneous dilatational versus conventional surgical tracheostomy. *Laryngoscope.* 1997;107:1643.
103. Street MK, Boyd O. Tracheostomy: the change in practice in a region over a decade. *Br J Anaesth.* 2000;84(5):689P.
104. Friedman Y et al. Comparison of percutaneous and surgical tracheostomies. *Chest.* 1996; 110(2):480.
105. Delaney A, Bradshaw S, Nalos M. Percutaneous dilational tracheostomy versus surgical tracheostomy in critically ill patients: a systematic review and meta-analysis. *Critical Care.* 2006;10:R55.
106. Carney AS. The use of MRI to assess tracheal stenosis following percutaneous dilatational tracheostomy [letter]. *J Laryngol Otol.* 1998;112:599.
107. Fischler MP, Kuhn M, Cantieni R, Frutiger A. Late outcome of percutaneous dilatational tracheostomy in intensive care patients. *Intensive Care Med.* 1995;21:475.
108. Callanan V, Gillmore K, Field S, Beaumont A. The use of MRI to assess tracheal stenosis following percutaneous dilatational tracheostomy. *J Laryngol Otol.* 1997;111:953.
109. Rosenbower TJ, Morris JA Jr, Eddy VA, Ries WR. The long-term complications of percutaneous dilatational tracheostomy. *Am Surg.* 1998;64:82.
110. Leonard RC, Lewis RH, Singh B, Van Heerden PV. Late outcome from percutaneous tracheostomy using the Portex kit. *Chest.* 1999;115(4):1070.
111. Norwood S, Vallina VL, Short K, Saigusa M, Fernandez LG, McLarty JW. Incidence if tracheal stenosis and other late complications after percutaneous tracheostomy. *Ann Surg.* 2000;232(2):233.
112. Bernard AC, Kenady DE. Conventional surgical tracheostomy as the preferred method of airway management. *J Oral Maxillofac Surg.* 1999;57:310.
113. Griffen MM, Kearney PA. Percutaneous dilational tracheostomy as the preferred method of airway management. *J Oral Maxillofac Surg.* 1999;57:316.
114. Barba CA. The intensive care unit as an operating room. *Surg Clin North Am.* 2000; 80(3):957.
115. Pryor JP, Reilly PM, Shapiro MB. Surgical airway management in the ICU. *Crit Care Clin.* 2000;16(3):473.
116. Byhahn C, Wilke HJ, Halbig S, Lischke V, Westphal K. Percutaneous tracheostomy: Ciaglia blue rhino versus the basic Ciaglia technique of percutaneous dilatational tracheostomy. *Anesth Analg.* 2000;91:882.

117. Westphal K, Byhahn C, Wilke HJ, Lischke V. Percutaneous tracheostomy: a clinical comparison of dilatational (Ciaglia) and translaryngeal (Fantoni) techniques. *Anesth Analg.* 1999;89:938.
118. Byhahn C, Wilke HJ, Halbig S, Lische V, Westphal K. Bedside percutaneous tracheostomy: clinical comparison of Griggs and Fantoni techniques. *World J Surg.* 2001;25:296.
119. Nates NL, Cooper DJ, Myles PS, Scheinkestel CD, Tuxen DV. Percutaneous tracheostomy in critically ill patients: a prospective, randomized comparison of two techniques. *Crit Care Med.* 2000;28(11):3734.
120. Van Heerden PV, Webb SAR, Power BM, Thompson WR. Percutaneous dilational tracheostomy – a clinical study evaluating two systems. *Anaesth Intensive Care.* 1996;24:56.
121. Ambesh SP, Kaushik S. Percutaneous dilational tracheostomy: the Ciaglia method versus the Rapitrach method. *Anesth Analg.* 1998;87:556.
122. Assmann N, Wong D, Morales E. A comparison of a new indicator-guided with a conventional wire-guided percutaneous cricothyroidotomy device in mannequins. *Anesth Analg.* 2007;105:148–154.
123. Benkhadra M, Lenfant F, Nemetz W, Anderhuber F, Feigl G, Fasel J. A comparison of two emergency cricothyroidotomy kits in human cadavers. *Anesth Analg.* 2008;106:182–185.
124. Byhahn C, et al. Percutaneous tracheostomy "Ciaglia blue rhino": experiences in 120 critically ill adults [Poster presentation B16]. *Anesthesiology.* 2001;October(suppl).
125. Bewsher MS, Adams AM, Clarke CWM, Mcconachie J, Kelly DR. Evaluation of a new percutaneous dilatational tracheostomy set. *Anaesthesia.* 2001;56:859.
126. Steele APH, Evans HW, Afaq MA, et al. Long-term follow-up of Griggs percutaneous tracheostomy with spiral CT and questionnaire. *Chest.* 2000;117(5):1430.
127. Raine RI et al. Late outcome after guide-wire forceps percutaneous tracheostomy – a prospective, randomized comparison with open surgical tracheostomy. *Br J Anaesth.* 1999;82(suppl 1):168.
128. Watters MPR et al. Tracheal rupture during percutaneous tracheostomy: safety aspects of the Griggs method. *Br J Anaesth.* 2000;84(5):671P.
129. Bliznikas D. Percutaneous tracheostomy, *eMed J.* 2001;2(11). www.emedicine.com.
130. MacCallum PL, Parnes LS, Sharpe MD, Harris C. Comparison of open, percutaneous, and translaryngeal tracheostomies. *Otolaryngol Head Neck Surg.* 2000;122(5):686.
131. Karnik A, Freeman JW. Translaryngeal tracheostomy technique (TLT): prospective evaluation of 164 cases. *Br J Anaesth.* 1999;82(suppl 1):169.
132. Vecchiarelli P et al. Fantoni's trans-laryngeal tracheostomy: two years of experience. *Br J Anaesth.* 1999;82(suppl 1):167.
133. Westphal K et al. Tracheostomy in cardiosurgical patients: surgical tracheostomy versus Ciaglia and Fantoni methods. *Ann Thor Surg.* 1999;68:486.
134. Bouvette M, Fuhrman TM. Preventing complications during percutaneous tracheostomy [letter]. *Anesthesiology.* 1999;90(3):918.
135. Mphanza T, Jacobs S. Letter in reply to reference 142. *Anesthesiology.* 1999;90(3):918.
136. Ciaglia P. Video-assisted endoscopy, not just endoscopy, for percutaneous dilatational tracheostomy. *Chest.* 1999;115(4):915.
137. Dexter T. The laryngeal mask airway: a method to improve visualization of the trachea and larynx during fiberoptic assisted percutaneous tracheostomy. *Anaesth Intensive Care.* 1994;22:35.
138. Lyons BJ et al. The LMA simplifies airway management during percutaneous dilational tracheostomy. *Acta Anaesthesiol Scand.* 1995;39:414.
139. Brimacombe J. Letter. *Anaesthesia.* 1994;49:358.
140. Verghese C, Rangasami J, Kapila A, Parke T. Airway control during percutaneous dilatational tracheostomy: pilot study with the intubating LMA. *Br J Anaesth.* 1998;81(4):608.
141. Zuleika M, Jacobs S, Mphanza T, Brohi F. The use of the LMA in suitable ICU patients undergoing percutaneous dilational tracheostomy. *Intensive Care Med.* 1997;23(1):129.

142. Quinio P et al. Translaryngeal tracheostomy through the intubating LMA in a patient with difficult tracheal intubation. *Intensive Care Med.* 2000;26(6):820.

143. Addas BM, Howes WJ, Hung OR. Light-guided tracheal puncture for percutaneous tracheostomy. *Can J Anesth.* 2000;47(9):919.

144. Cooper RM et al. Facilitation of percutaneous dilational tracheostomy by use of a perforated endotracheal tube exchanger. *Chest.* 1996;109(4):1131.

145. Deblieux P, Wadell C, McClarity Z, DeBoisblanc BP. Facilitation of percutaneous dilational tracheostomy by use of a perforated endotracheal tube exchanger. *Chest.* 1995;108(2):572.

146. Muhammad JK, Patton DW, Evans RM, Major E. Percutaneous dilatational tracheostomy under ultrasound guidance. *Br J Oral Maxillofacial Surg.* 1999;37(4):309.

147. Brimacombe J, Clarke G. Rigid bronchoscope: a possible new option for percutaneous dilational tracheostomy. *Anesthesiology.* 1995;83(3):646.

148. Donaldson DR, Emami AJ, Wax MK. Chest radiographs after dilatational percutaneous tracheostomy: are they necessary? *Otolaryngol Head Neck Surg.* 2000;123(3):236.

149. Tobias JD, Higgins M. Capnography during transtracheal needle cricothyrotomy. *Anesth Analg.* 1995;81:1077.

150. Bissinger U, Buggenberger H, Lenz H. Retrograde-guided fiberoptic intubation in patients with laryngeal carcinoma. *Anesth Analg.* 1995;81:408.

151. Eidelman LA, Pizov R. A safer approach to retrograde-guided fiberoptic intubation [letter]. *Anesth Analg.* 1996;82:1107.

152. Bissinger U et al. Letter in reply to reference 159. *Anesth Analg.* 1996;82:1108.

153. Roberts KW, Solgonick RM. A modification of retrograde wire-guided, fiberoptic-assisted endotracheal intubation in a patient with ankylosing spondylitis. *Anesth Analg.* 1996;82: 1290.

154. Rosenblatt WH, Angood PB, Maranets I, Kaklamanos IG, Garwood S. Retrograde fiberoptic intubation. *Anesth Analg.* 1997;84:1142.

155. Donaldson DR, Emami AJ, Wax MK. Endoscopically monitored percutaneous dilational tracheostomy in a residency program. *Laryngoscope.* 2000;110:1142.

156. Massick DD et al. Quantification of the learning curve for percutaneous dilatational tracheostomy. *Laryngoscope.* 2000;110:222.

157. Russon K, Clark J, Hutchinson S. Variations in tracheostomy practive in uk critical care units. *Br J Anaesth.* 2004;92:621P.

158. Kluge S, Brumann HJ, Maier C, Klose H, Meyer A, et al. Tracheostomy in intensive care unit: a nationwide survey. *Anesth Analg.* 2008;107:1639–1643.

159. Gardiner Q, White PS, Carson D, Shearer A, Frizelle F, Dunkley P. Technique training: endoscopic percutaneous tracheostomy. *Br J Anaesth.* 1998;81(3):401.

160. Gerig HJ, Heidegger T, Ulrich B, Grossenbacher R, Kreienbühl G. Fiberoptically-guided insertion of transtracheal catheters. *Anesth Analg.* 2001;93:663.

161. Wong D, Prabhu Atul J, Coloma M, Imasogie Ngozi, Chung F. What is the minimum training required for successful cricothyroidotomy? A study in mannequins. *Anesthesiology.* 2003;98:349–53.

162. Eisenburger P, Laczika K, List M, Wilfing A, Losert H, et al. Comparison of conventional surgical versus Seldinger technique emergency cricothyrotomy performed by inexperienced clinicians. *Anesthesiology.* 2000;92(3):687.

163. Goumas P, Kokkinis K, Petrocheilos J, Naxakis JS, MocHLouust G. Cricothyroidotomy and the anatomy of the cricothyroid space: An autopsy study. *J Laryngol Otol.* 1997;111:354–356.

164. Schroeder AA. Cricothroidotomy: when, why, and why not? *Am J Otolaryngol.* 2000; 21(3):195.

165. Hawkins ML et al. Emergency cricothyrotomy: a reassessment. *Am Surg.* 1995;61:52.

166. Isaacs JH Jr. Emergency cricothyrotomy: long-term results. *Ann Surg.* 2001;67:346–349.

167. Gillespie MB, Eisele DW. Outcomes of emergency surgical airway procedures in a hospital-wide setting. *Laryngoscope.* 1999;109:1766.

168. Liebovici D et al. Prehospital cricothyroidotomy by physicians. *Am J Emerg Med.* 1997;15(1):91.
169. Gerich TG, Schmidt U, Hubrich V, Lobenhoffer HP. Prehospital airway management in the acutely injured patient: the role of surgical cricothyrotomy revisited. *J Trauma.* 1998;45(2):312.
170. Brohi K et al. Letter to editor. *J Trauma.* 1999;46(4):745.
171. Jacobson LE, Gomez GA, Sobieray RJ, Rodman GH, Solotkin KC, Misinski ME. Surgical cricothyroidotomy in trauma patients: analysis of its use by paramedics in the field. *J Trauma.* 1996;41(1):15.
172. Holmes JF, Panacek EA, Sakles JC, Brofeldt BT. Comparison of 2 cricothyrotomy techniques: standard method versus rapid 4-step technique. *Ann Emerg Med.* 1998;32(4):442.
173. Brofeldt BT, Holmes JF, Panacek EA, Sakles JC. An easy cricothyrotomy approach: the rapid four-step technique. *Acad Emerg Med.* 1996;3:1060.
174. Gerling MC et al. Effect of surgical cricothyrotomy on the unstable cervical spine in a cadaver model of intubation. *J Emerg Med.* 2001;20(1):1.
175. Schaumann N, Lorenz V, Schellongowski P, Staudinger T, Locker GJ, et al. Evaluation of Seldinger technique emergency cricothyroidotomy versus standard surgical cricothyroidotomy in 200 cadavers. *Anesthesiology.* 2005;102:7–11.
176. Dulguerov D, Gysin C. Letter to the editor. *Anesthesiology.* 2005;103:667.
177. Price R. Letter to the editor. *Anesthesiology.* 2005;103:667–668.
178. Spaite DW, Joseph M. Prehospital cricothyrotomy. *Ann Emerg Med.* 1990;19:279.
179. Goldenberg D, Ari EG, Golz A, Danino J, Netzer A, Joachims HZ. Tracheostomy complications: a retrospective study of 1130 cases. *Otolaryngol Head Neck Surg.* 2000;123(4):495.
180. Johnson DR et al. Cricothyrotomy performed by prehospital personnel: a comparison of two techniques in a human cadaver model. *Am J Emerg Med.* 1993;19:207.
181. Wetmore RF et al. Pediatric tracheostomy: a changing procedure? *Ann Otol Rhinol Laryngol.* 1999;108:695.

Chapter 13
Mechanical Ventilation and Respiratory Care

Contents

B.T. Finucane et al., *Principles of Airway Management*,
DOI 10.1007/978-0-387-09558-5_13, © Springer Science+Business Media, LLC 2011

Introduction

Mechanical ventilation (MV) and respiratory care provide support to the patient who cannot maintain viable oxygenation, ventilation, and/or protective airway reflexes. Support is initiated when the patient cannot maintain a safe level of homeostasis. Support is withdrawn when the patient is able to breathe without artificial assistance. The level and duration of support depend on the cause of the respiratory system's failure and the patient's response to therapy.

There are many conditions that cause respiratory system decompensation. Common causes include the following:

Infection
1. Bacterial
2. Viral
3. Other microbes

Obstructive airway disease
1. Asthma
2. Bronchitis
3. COPD
4. Emphysema

Trauma
1. Lung contusion and chest wall injury
2. Burn pathology
3. Chemical exposure

Pharmacologic causes
1. Depressant drug overdose
2. Neuromuscular relaxants

Neuromuscular disease
1. Coma, stroke, altered mental status impairing protective airway reflexes
2. Neuromuscular diseases causing weakness
3. Inability to metabolize muscle relaxant drugs

Cardiovascular/renal diseases
1. Heart failure
2. Pulmonary edema
3. Renal failure

Metabolic causes
1. Malnutrition
2. Metabolic acidosis

Many of these conditions cause similar pathology. This includes the loss of lung volume (decreased functional residual capacity (FRC)), lower lung compliance,

Ventilatory Orders (Adult)

1. FiO_2
   Hundred percent until the first blood gas result has been obtained (FiO_2 may be decreased as the disease state permits, but oxyhemoglobin saturation should remain at or above 90%).

2. Tidal volume
   6–10 cc/kg body weight (see discussion of acute respiratory distress syndrome (ARDS) later in this chapter)

3. Frequency
   Eight to twelve breaths per minute (IMV = 8–12/min)

4. Distending airway pressure
   The amount of CPAP or PEEP to be applied depends on the degree of shunt (venous admixture), the patient's lung compliance, and FRC (5 cm H_2O is considered "physiologic PEEP" and should be applied if ventilatory support is extended beyond a few minutes.)

5. Modality of ventilation
   The modality of ventilation depends on patient variables such as strength, depth of sedation, mental and nutritional status, and type and magnitude of pathology or injury. Weaning expectations and clinical preference also play roles in the modality of ventilation that is selected. Currently PSV, IMV, and PRVC (pressure-regulated volume-controlled ventilation) with appropriate levels of PEEP and CPAP are popular modalities of ventilation.

Comments on the Modality of Ventilation

No single modality of ventilation has proven to be superior to others. Some modalities decrease the work of breathing while others allegedly increase a patient's comfort. Some modalities are more likely to produce barotrauma, at least theoretically. Others demand patient participation. The clinical experience of the physician often dictates the modality of ventilation that is selected. One should consider the expected duration of ventilatory support, the type and degree of pathology, as well as the weaning strategy when selecting the modality of ventilation. Table 13.2 presents a few salient comments on various modalities of ventilation summarized from an excellent review article on the subject.[1]

Pediatric and Neonatal Ventilation

Historically, neonates and premature infants were ventilated with IPPV (intermittent positive-pressure ventilation) and CPAP.[5] Over the past two decades, a better understanding of the pathogenesis of hyaline membrane disease (HMD), bron-

Table 13.2 Modalities of ventilation

Target	Mode	Breath trigger	Comments
Volume	CMV (VCV)	Mechanical	No spontaneous patient breath
			Eliminates work of breathing
			Pressure limit set at 60 cm H_2O
			Patients often heavily sedated, anesthetized, paralyzed
Volume	VAV	Patient	Assisted breaths delivered at full volume
			May induce respiratory alkalosis, hypokalemia, arrhythmias
Volume	VACV	Mechanical and patient	Machine delivers backup
			May induce respiratory alkalosis
Volume	IMV	Mechanical and patient	Useful weaning modality
			Preset IMV rate
			No assisted breaths; therefore, hemodynamics may be improved with less likelihood of developing respiratory alkalosis
			Higher work of breathing than with PSV
Pressure	PSV	Patient	High degree of patient-ventilator interaction
			Possibly improves patient comfort
			Decreased work of breathing
			Lower peak airway pressures
			If PS level high, may induce respiratory alkalosis
Pressure	PCV and IRV	Mechanical	I:E ratio greater than 1:2 for IRV
			May evoke patient discomfort
			May adversely affect hemodynamics
			May produce intrinsic PEEP
Pressure	PACV	Mechanical and patient	May be weaned to PSV as patient's condition improves and mean airway pressure decreases to 15 cm H_2O and inspiratory time < 0.8 s

chopulmonary dysplasia (BPD), and retrolental fibroplasia have led clinicians to introduce many new therapeutic agents and techniques (surfactant, steroids, lower FiO_2) and to utilize newer monitors such as transcutaneous oxygen, carbon dioxide analyzers, and oxyhemoglobin saturation monitors. Many of the current modalities of ventilation have been used to support neonatal and pediatric patients, such as PSV,[6] proportional-assist ventilation,[7] and various assisted modalities.[5] Ventilators such as the Siemens 300 are designed for neonatal and pediatric use. It is beyond the scope of this book to discuss, in detail, the merits of each of these modalities. However, if the patient does not have severe lung disease, the following ventilator orders can be written for the typical patient under 10 kg.

Ventilator Orders for the Infant Under 10 kg

FiO_2	Start with 100%, but wean to keep oxyhemoglobin saturation greater than 90%
Frequency	18–20 Breaths per minute
Airway pressures	Inspiratory: limit to 18–20 cm H_2O
	Expiratory: 2 cm H_2O
PEEP or CPAP	As clinically indicated
Arterial blood gases	As indicated

Larger children may be ventilated with the same targets and goals as an adult. If a neonatal or premature patient presents with *severe* pulmonary dysfunction, a neonatologist or pediatrician must be consulted to manage ventilatory support.

Weaning the Patient from Mechanical Ventilation

As the patient's condition improves, the pathology resolves, his alertness approaches his normal level, and paralytic agents are discontinued and fully reversed, mechanical support can be weaned toward eventual discontinuation and extubation. The rapidity of weaning depends primarily on resolution of the disease or condition that necessitated the initiation of ventilatory support. The five parameters delineated in the initial orders may be weaned in the following fashion:

1. FiO_2
   The FiO_2 should be weaned as quickly as possible to below 40%. The oxyhemoglobin saturation should remain at 90% or greater and the PaO_2 at or above 60 mmHg.

2. Tidal volume
   The volume delivered by the ventilator remains constant.

3. Frequency
   The ventilator's rate can be weaned when the patient starts breathing spontaneously. Wean the rate to keep the arterial pH in the normal range (7.35–7.45).

4. PEEP or CPAP level
   The level of distending airway pressure may be weaned by titrating it against the patient's PaO_2, the FiO_2 needed to maintain oxygenation goals, and clinical signs that the patient's work of breathing is improving such as a decrease in the spontaneous respiratory rate and increase in tidal volume. If high levels of PEEP or CPAP are required (above 15 cm H_2O) a pulmonary artery catheter can be inserted to measure mixed venous oxyhemoglobin saturation, a value needed to

calculate the shunt fraction. Distending airway pressure should be applied to maintain a shunt fraction at or below 18%.

5. Modality of ventilation

IMV: Wean by decreasing the IMV rate

PSV: Wean the "plateau pressure" in 1–2 cm H_2O increments to 10–15 cm H_2O. Do not wean below 8 cm H_2O

CMV: Allow the paralytic agents and sedatives to wean off, then convert to IMV

Assisted modalities: Incrementally decrease the frequency

Finally, the clinician should consider a final *T-tube trial* for an appropriate time interval before discontinuing ventilatory support. With a T-tube the patient receives supplemental oxygen without ventilatory support.

Extubation Criteria

Extubation can be considered when all of the following criteria are met:

- Adequate oxygenation and ventilation can be maintained by the patient. The oxyhemoglobin saturation is at or above 90% with a FiO_2 of 40% or less, and CPAP is less than or equal to 5 cm H_2O. The pH should be above 7.35 while the patient receives 2 or fewer mechanical breaths per minute. The level of pressure support should be in the range of 8–10 cm H_2O.
- The measured vital capacity is at least 15 ml/kg and the negative inspiratory force is less than −20 cm H_2O.
- The patient is alert, cooperative, and oriented. He has active cough, gag and swallow reflexes. (The competence of the cough reflex can be tested when the trachea is stimulated during suctioning. The gag reflex can be tested by stimulating the pharynx with a tongue blade.)
- No airway obstruction after extubation is anticipated.

If all of these criteria are met, a safe extubation should be accomplished. If a patient displays permanent loss of reflexes, such as after a stroke, tracheostomy should be considered.

Troubleshooting Ventilator Problems

Modern ventilators are equipped with many monitors and alarms to assure proper function and patient safety. However, ventilators can fail or become disconnected. Furthermore, the patient may develop a new condition that affects ventilation, often quickly and dramatically. Emergency equipment must be immediately available to assist in these circumstances. This equipment includes an oxygen source, a self-inflating ventilation bag, suctioning equipment, and airway masks and intubation

Table 13.3 Difficulty with ventilation

Patient problems	Equipment problems
Chest wall	Misplacement of tube
Obesity	Endobronchial
Stiff chest syndrome	Esophageal
Pleura	Submucosal
Hemothorax	Laryngeal (cuff between vocal cords)
Hydrothorax	Extubation
Pneumothorax	Obstruction
Tumor	Kinking
Lung parenchyma	Biting
Adult respiratory distress syndrome	Foreign body
Aspiration	Blood/secretions
Atelectasis	Cuff
Chronic obstructive pulmonary disease	Overinflated
Pulmonary edema	Herniation
Tumor	Leaks
Bronchi	Circuit
Obstruction	Valves
Reactive airway disease	Leaks
Larynx and trachea	Soda lime exhaustion
Stenosis	Increased resistance
Tumor	Ventilator
Mouth	Disconnects
Oral hygiene	Loss of power
Loose teeth	O_2 delivery
Nose	Failure
Sinusitis	Crossed gas lines/contamination
Bleeding	Disconnects

equipment. If a ventilator appears to be malfunctioning or the patient develops distress or signs of hypoxemia *hand ventilate the patient with a self-inflating bag and 100% oxygen and call the respiratory therapist to check the machine.*

Table 13.3 lists some common problems and complications that might make ventilation difficult.

Figure 13.1 may help guide your approach to evaluating ventilatory difficulty.

Current Strategies and Practices in Mechanical Ventilation and Respiratory Care

The remainder of the chapter will deal with current strategies and practices in MV and respiratory care. The following topics will be addressed:

1. ALI/ARDS (acute lung injury/acute respiratory distress syndrome)
2. Ventilation strategies

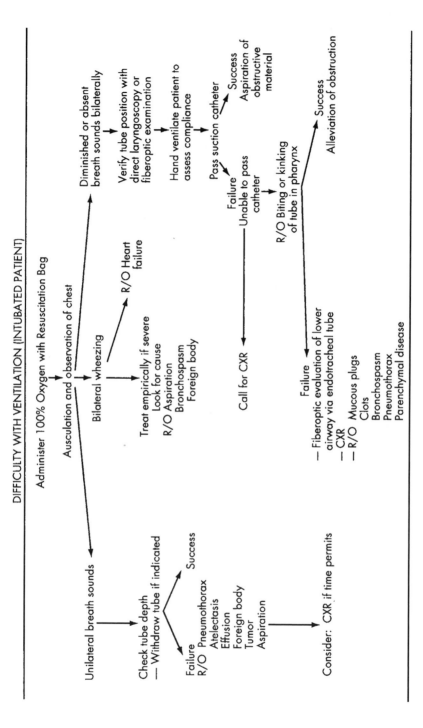

Fig. 13.1 A difficulty-with-ventilation algorithm for the intubated patient

3. Recruitment maneuvers
4. Alternative modalities of ventilation
5. New weaning strategies
6. Complications of mechanical ventilation
7. Ventilator associated pneumonia
8. Closed-circuit suctioning
9. Portable ventilators
10. Hyperbaric oxygenation
11. Ethical considerations of mechanical ventilation
12. Future ALI/ARDS research

The presentations are cursory by design to fit the scope of this textbook. Critical care medicine is a complex subspecialty. Many textbooks are available that deal with all aspects of this discipline to which the reader is directed for more exhaustive study and edification.

ALI/ARDS (Acute Lung Injury/Acute Respiratory Distress Syndrome)

The term *adult respiratory distress* was first used by Ashbaugh et al in 1967 to describe a pulmonary syndrome in adults that resembled respiratory distress in infants.[8] For years, the condition was referred to as *ARDS* (adult respiratory distress syndrome). The syndrome was characterized by acute onset, tachypnea, hypoxemia, poor lung compliance, and bilateral pulmonary infiltrates. The hypoxemia could be treated with PEEP. The mortality rate was reported to be as high as 90%. It was recognized that ARDS was not necessarily a primary disease but rather the pulmonary manifestation of many different pathologic and traumatic processes. ARDS was often associated with multiple organ dysfunction and failure. In 1994, the European-American Consensus Committee on ARDS agreed on the following definitive features of the syndrome.

European-American Consensus Committee on ARDS:
1994[8-10] Definitive features of ALI/ARDS

1. Acute onset
2. Bilateral infiltrates on chest X ray
3. Hypoxemia:

ALI: PaO_2/FiO_2 ratio less than 300 mmHg
ARDS: PaO_2/FiO_2 ratio less than 200 mmHg

4. No evidence of left atrial hypertension:

(Pulmonary artery occlusion pressure [wedge] less than 18 mmHg)

The committee also recommended that the syndrome be called *acute respiratory distress syndrome* rather than *adult respiratory distress syndrome*.

Investigators studied many therapeutic and supportive interventions to improve the outcome of patients with ARDS. With the recognition that the syndrome represented the pulmonary component of many different processes and the introduction of PEEP to improve oxygenation so the patient would not die of hypoxia, the mortality rate has dropped to the 25–50% range. More recently, a better understanding of the pulmonary effects of PPV and PEEP, the hormonal and humeral components of the syndrome, and the early discovery of loss of surfactant with ARDS have led to a multitude of proposals to "treat" ARDS.

McIntyre et al[8] have reviewed the literature in a comprehensive paper published in 2000. They considered the findings of 285 papers dealing with various aspects of ARDS-related clinical trials. They evaluated the "quality of evidence" supporting various conclusions and practices. Furthermore, they rated the conclusions and practices in terms of the level of recommendation.

Rating Systems for Scientific Evidence and Recommendations[8]

Rating System for Quality of Evidence

Level 1: Large, randomized, prospective, controlled investigations
Level 2: Small, randomized, prospective, controlled trials with uncertain results
Level 3: Nonrandomized, concurrent, or historical cohort investigations
Level 4   Peer-reviewed state-of-the-art articles, review articles, editorials, or substantial case series
Level 5: Nonpeer reviewed published opinions, such as textbook statements or official organizational publications

Rating System for Recommendations

(a) Convincingly justifiable on scientific evidence alone (2 Level 1 investigations)
(b) Justifiable by available scientific evidence (1 Level 1 investigation)
(c) Reasonably justifiable by available scientific evidence and strongly supported by expert critical care opinion (Level 2 investigations only)
(d) Adequate scientific evidence is lacking but widely supported by available data and expert critical care opinion (Level 3 data)
(e) No scientific data exists to justify support (Level 4 and 5 publications)

Of all of the therapeutic interventions reviewed, only one, the *lung protective ventilator strategy*, was strongly supported. Lower tidal volumes and airway pressures should be used when ventilating patients with ALI/ARDS. Their suggested strategy utilized a tidal volume 6 ml/kg with driving pressures (PSV plateau and peak inspiratory pressure delivered with IMV or CMV) in the range of 20–25 cm H_2O above PEEP levels. One may have to tolerate "permissive hypercapnia" with this ventilatory strategy.

V_t=tidal volume [liters]). Clinical guidelines to facilitate weaning are being developed and tested.[47]

To facilitate difficult weaning, consider the points listed in Table 13.6.[48-51]

Complications of Mechanical Ventilation

Many of the complications associated with mechanical ventilation such as equipment failure, upper airway trauma and injury, and barotrauma have already been mentioned. More recent investigators are looking into many new and intriguing

Table 13.5 Causes of difficult weaning

Inadequate respiratory center output
   Residual effect of sedative drugs
   CNS damage
   Severe metabolic alkalosis
Increase in respiratory workload
   Increased minute ventilation
      Hyperventilation from pain, anxiety, restlessness
      Increased metabolic rate from excessive feeding or sepsis
      Increased physiologic dead space
   Increased elastic workload
      Low thoracic or lung compliance
      Intrinsic PEEP
   Increased restrictive workload
      Lower airway obstruction
      Thick or copious airway secretions
      Artificial airway (endotracheal tube)
      Ventilator circuitry and demand valve
      Postextubation upper airway obstruction
Respiratory pump failure
   Thoracic wall abnormality or disease
   Peripheral neurologic disorder
      Phrenic nerve injury
      Cervical spine damage
      Critical care neuropathy
      Guillain–Barre syndrome
   Muscular Dysfunction
      Malnutrition, muscular catabolism
      Pulmonary hyperinflation
      Severe electrolyte and metabolic disorders
      Prolonged postneuromuscular blockade effect
Left ventricular failure
   Left ventricular dysfunction
   Coronary artery disease

Source: Lessard and Brochard,[46] with permission

Table 13.6 Things to consider to facilitate difficult weaning

Recognize and correct the causes of weaning failure
Define a patient-specific weaning program
Consider psychological factors (gain patient cooperation, mobilization, sleep at night, oral feeding, TV, radio, newspapers, hypnosis)[48]
Provide adequate nutritional support
Correct metabolic abnormalities
Optimize cardiac function
Reduce the imposed work of breathing (aspirate airway, consider bronchodilators and corticosteroids, replace a partially obstructed endotracheal tube, consider tracheostomy, optimize ventilator settings [inspiratory flow], optimize sensitivity of ventilator triggers, carefully add external PEEP [in patients with intrinsic PEEP and expiratory flow limitation – e.g., COPD], allow permissive hypercarbia)
Improve the patient's respiratory capacity (consider theophylline), consider respiratory muscle training program
Consider deflating the endotracheal tube cuff[49] to improve the patient's ability to handle secretions and to decrease airway flow resistance[50]
Consider alternative ventilatory modalities such as mask ventilation[49,51]
Manage the case with a specialized team

areas of research associated with mechanical ventilation. For example, investigators have begun to define specific lung injury caused by mechanical ventilation itself. Suter[52] summarized biochemical components of lung injury in ventilated subjects. He stated:

> "It has become evident that MV (mechanical ventilation) using large tidal volumes without PEEP and/or causing overdistension of lung units produces significant inflammatory changes in the lung. In experimental and human studies, a marked increase in leukocytes and pro-inflammatory cytokines was noted in bronchoalveolar lavage fluid during the application of more 'aggressive' ventilatory strategies as compared with more 'protective' modes, i.e., lower Vt applied on the steeper part of the pressure-volume curve, thereby avoiding repeated opening and closing, and also overdistension of the lung. It has also been shown that regular stretching of alveolar cells in culture produces release of cytokines when small amounts of lipopolysaccharides are present. These data provide a cellular explanation of the inflammatory changes observed."

Many other investigators are studying the humoral and cellular effects of mechanical ventilation. As a result of this research, as has been noted, clinicians are more prone to use lower tidal volumes and to utilize modalities of ventilation that create lower overall airway pressures.

Ventilator Associated Pneumonia

A critical review by Pneumataikos et al[53] graded the quality of evidence and the strength of recommendations made by authors of research articles that examined various aspects of ventilator associated pneumonia (VAP). They claimed that VAP occurred in 9–27% of all ventilated patients. The two classifications of VAP are early onset (occurring in the first 96 h of intubation) and late onset (occurring after 96 h).

Following is a summary of the review:

1. Selective decontamination of the subglottic space: strongly recommended.
2. Prevention of biofilm formation: weak recommendation.
3. Use of specific antiseptic impregnated endotracheal tubes: weak recommendation.
4. Synchronized mucus aspiration in the distal end of the ETT: clinical studies are required to confirm animal study findings in mechanically ventilated patients.
5. Elimination of the ETT biofilm: clinical studies are needed to define the efficacy of biofilm elimination as a preventive strategy against VAP.
6. Early tracheostomy: no recommendations can be addressed because of insufficient evidence.
7. Noninvasive ventilation: "when feasible and not medically contraindicated, the use of noninvasive ventilation instead of tracheal intubation may result in lower risk for development of VAP."
8. Conclusion: the strongest evidence supports subglottic space suctioning of secretions if the patient is intubated for 72 h or more.

In summary, the authors concluded with the following statement:

> VAP is a nosocomial lung infection more related with the presence of an endotracheal tube in the patient's airway than with the ventilator per se. The term "endotracheal tube-associated pneumonia" could be recommended as describing better the pathogenesis than the term "ventilator-associated pneumonia."

Their evaluation of the literature supports practicing selective decontamination of the subglottic space. This is achieved by using an endotracheal tube such as the Hi-Lo©. Evac endotracheal tube manufactured by Mallinkrodt that is equipped with a suctioning channel used to clear secretions from the subglottic space. Future research will address many other issues related to VAP.

Closed-Circuit Suctioning

Studies support the use of closed-circuit suctioning of the endotracheal tube to decrease the likelihood of cross-contamination between the bronchial system and gastric juices[54] as well as the preservation of oxygenation levels[55] during tracheal lavage. A literature survey by Subirana et al[56] of data to 2006 concluded that closed vs. open suctioning of the trachea had no effect on the risk of VAP or mortality. More study is required in this area.

Portable Ventilators

Portable ventilators can be used when transporting or resuscitating patients. One such ventilator, the Pneupac Ventipac portable gas-powered ventilator, is described by McCluskey and Gwinnutt.[57] Before using any medical device, such as a ventilator, one must receive expert training in its operation.

Hyperbaric Oxygenation

Hyperbaric oxygenation has been reported to reverse both the clinical symptoms and EKG changes of cardiac ischemia in two case reports of patients with profound anemia.[58] The technique requires a hyperbaric chamber and expert operation to avoid complications.

Ethical Considerations of Mechanical Ventilation

Investigators have examined and reported on various ethical considerations associated with mechanical ventilation. One such paper deals with the development of a questionnaire to elicit patient preferences with respect to intubation.[59] Decisions made when treating ventilated patients are often profound, if not life-ending. Patients, families, and physicians need to develop better means to communicate.

Future ALI/ARDS Research

Future research will include studies concerning hormonal and humeral regulation and response to ALI/ARDS, new modalities of ventilation, liquid ventilation, carbon dioxide washout techniques, positioning (prone vs. supine), and the role of nitric oxide to treat ALI/ARDS patients. The effects of alveolar recruitment will be better defined. New and better monitors will be developed. Novel approaches to understand, treat and to moderate the body's response to ARDS and the side effects of mechanical ventilation will be advanced. Two examples of these approaches include the application of vaporized perfluorobexane used to attenuate ventilator-induced lung injury,[60] and the autologous transplantation of endothelial progenitor cells to treat chemically induced ALI.[61] Future ALI/ARDS research will be conducted by basic and clinical scientists in all subspecialties of medicine.

Summary

This chapter has reviewed the basic considerations of mechanical ventilation and respiratory care. Equipment was described. Ventilation and weaning goals and protocols were discussed. Current ventilation strategies were outlined. The concept of a protective ventilation strategy was considered in some detail. The goals of mechanical ventilation and respiratory care are to maintain oxygenation and ventilation while at the same time deliver therapy that is not injurious to the patient. When managing patients, set to specific and realistic goals and utilize the newest monitors to assure patient safety. Finally, remember that *ventilators can fail and a patient's condition may deteriorate quickly*. In these situations, *revert to the basics. Check the endotracheal tube, administer 100% oxygen with a self-inflating resuscitation bag, auscultate the chest for breath sounds, and keep a finger on the pulse and an eye on the patient. Do not hesitate to call for help*!

References

1. Sladen, RN. Current concepts of mechanical ventilation. *IARS Review Course Lectures.* 1999;86–92.
2. Siemens Servo Screen 390 V2.0/3.X operating manual.
3. Siemens Servo Ventilator 300/300A operating manual 8.1/9.1.
4. Ouellet P. *Waveform and Loop Analysis in Mechanical Ventilation.* Solna: Siemens-Elema; 1997.
5. Kossel H, Versmold H. 25 Years of respiratory support of newborn infants. *J Perinat Med.* 1997;25:421–432.
6. Tokioka H, Nagano O, Ohta Y, Hirakawa M. Pressure support ventilation augments spontaneous breathing with improved thoracoabdominal synchrony in neonates with congenital heart disease. *Anesth Analg.* 1997;85:789–793.
7. Schulze A, Gerhardt T, Musante G, et al. Proportional assist ventilation in low birth weight infants with acute respiratory disease: a comparison to assist/control and conventional mechanical ventilation. *J Pediatr.* 1999;135(3):339–344.
8. McIntyre RC, Pulido EJ, Bensard DD, Shames BD, Abraham E. Thirty years of clinical trials in acute respiratory distress syndrome. *Crit Care Med.* 2000;28:3314–3331.
9. Shapiro MB, Anderson HL III, Bartlett RH. Respiratory failure: conventional and high-tech support. *Surg Clin North Am.* 2000;80(3):871–883.
10. Bernard GR, Artigas A, Brigham KL, et al. The American-European Consensus Conference on ARDS: definitions, mechanisms, relevant outcomes, and clinical trial coordination. *Am J Respir Crit Care Med.* 1994;149:818–824.
11. Cereda M. In: 2006 ASA Refresher Course: Lecture 134.
12. Moloney ED, Griffiths MJD. Protective ventilation of patients with acute respiratory distress syndrome. *Br J Anaesth.* 2004;92:261–270.
13. Rouby J, Constantin JM, Girardi CR, Zhang M, Lu Q. Mechanical ventilation in patients with acute respiratory distress syndrome. *Anesthesiology.* 2004;101:228–234.
14. Gropper MA. In: 2007 ASA Refresher Course: Lecture 137.
15. Tung A. In: 2005 ASA Refresher Course: Lecture 211.
16. Schwartz DE. In: 2004 ASA Refresher Course: Lecture 308.
17. Michelet P. Editorial: hypercapnic acidosis: how far? *Anesthesiology.* 2008;109:771–772.
18. Schultz MJ, Haitsma JJ, Slutsky AS, Galjic O. What tidal volumes should be used in patients without acute lung injury? *Anesthesiology.* 2007;106:1226–1231.
19. Putensen C, Wrigge H. Editorial: tidal volumes in patients with normal lungs: one for all or the less, the better? *Anesthesiology.* 2007;106:1085–1087.
20. Licker M, Diaper J, Ellenberger C. Letter: perioperative protective ventilatory strategies in patients without acute lung injuries. *Anesthesiology.* 2008;108:335–336.
21. Rossi A, Ranieri M. Positive endexpiratory pressure. In: Tobin MJ, ed. *Principles and Practice of Mechanical Ventilation.* New York, NY: McGraw-Hill; 1994:259–303.

22. Celebi S, Koner O, Menda F, et al. The pulmonary and hemodynamic effects of two different recruitment maneuvers after cardiac surgery. *Anesth Analg.* 2007;104:384–390.
23. Celebi S, Kiner O, Menda F, et al. Pulmonary effects of noninvasive ventilation combined with the recruitment maneuver after cardiac surgery. *Anesth Analg.* 2008;107:614–619.
24. Oczenski W, Hormann C, Keller C, et al. Recruitment maneuvers after a positive end-expiratory pressure trial do not induce sustained effects in early adult respiratory distress syndrome. *Anesthesiology.* 2004;101:620–625.
25. Rouby JJ. Lung overinflation. The hidden face of alveolar recruitment. *Anesthesiology.* 2003;99:2–4.
26. Wilcox FE, Brower RG, Stewart TE, et al. Recruitment maneuvers for acute lung injury: a systematic review. *Am J Respir Crit Care Med.* 2008;178(11):1156–1163.
27. Meade MO, Cook DJ, Griffith LE, et al. A study of the physiologic responses to a lung recruitment maneuver in acute lung injury and acute respiratory distress syndrome. *Respir Care.* 2008;53:1441–1449.
28. Stapleton RD. Editorial. Recruitment maneuvers in acute lung injury: What do the data tell us? *Respir Care.* 2008;53:1429–1430.
29. Hansen LK, Koefoed-Nielsen J, Nielsen J, Larsson A. Are selective lung recruitment maneuvers hemodynamically safe in severe hypovolemia: an experimental study in hypovolemic pigs with lobar collapse. *Anesth Analg.* 2007;105:729–734.
30. Hansen LK, Sloth E, Nielsen J, et al. Selective recruitment maneuvers for lobar atelectasis: effects on lung function and central hemodynamics: an experimental study in pigs. *Anesth Analg.* 2006;102:1504–1510.
31. MacIntyre NR. High-frequency ventilation. In: Tobin MJ, ed. *Principles and Practice of Mechanical Ventilation.* New York: McGraw-Hill; 1994.
32. Sakuragi T, Shono S, Yasumoto M, Arizono H, Dan K. High-frequency jet ventilation during fiberoptic laser resection of tracheal granuloma in a small child. *Anesth Analg.* 1996;82:889.
33. Meduri GU, Mauldin GL, Wunderink RG, Leeper KV, Jones C, Tolley E. Noninvasive mechanical ventilation via face mask in patients with acute respiratory failure who refused endotracheal intubation. *Crit Care Med.* 1994;22(10):1584–1590.
34. Natalini G, Cavaliere S, Seramondi V, et al. Negative pressure ventilation vs external high-frequency oscillation during rigid bronchoscopy. *Chest.* 2000;118(1):18–23.
35. Neumann P, Hedenstierna G. Ventilatory support by continuous positive airway pressure breathing improves gas exchange as compared with partial ventilatory support with airway pressure release ventilation. *Anesth Analg.* 2001;92:950–958.
36. Smith RPR, Fletcher R. Airway pressure release ventilation in cardiac surgery patients. *Br J Anaesth.* 2000;84(2):272.
37. Branson RD, Hurst JM. Differential lung ventilation. In: Peral A, Stock MC, eds. *Handbook of Mechanical Ventilatory Support.* Baltimore: Williams and Wilkins; 1992:185–193.
38. Smith RB. Continuous flow apneic ventilation. In: Perol A, Stock MC, eds. *Handbook of Mechanical Ventilatory Support.* Baltimore: Williams and Wilkins; 1992:175–184.
39. Okazaki J, Isono S, Tanaka A, Tagaito Y, Schwartz A, Nishino T. Usefulness of continuous oxygen insufflation into trachea for management of upper airway obstruction during anesthesia. *Anesthesiology.* 2000;93(1):62–68.
40. Wolf AR. Blood gas changes during apnoeic oxygenation in infants and children. *Br J Anaesth.* 1997;78(4):473.
41. Liebenberg CS, Raw R, Lipman J, Moyes DG, Cleaton-Jones PE. Small tidal volume ventilation using a zero deadspace tracheal tube. *Br J Anaesth.* 1999;82(2):213–216.
42. Ranieri VM, Grasso S, Mascia L, et al. Effects of proportional assist ventilation on inspiratory muscle effort in patients with chronic obstructive pulmonary disease and acute respiratory failure. *Anesthesiology.* 1997;86:79–91.
43. Bratzke E, Downs J, Smith RA. Intermittent CPAP: a new mode of ventilation during general anesthesia. *Anesthesiology.* 1998;89:334–340.

44. Perel A, Stock MC. *Handbook of Mechanical Ventilatory Support*. Baltimore: Williams and Wilkins; 1992.
45. Tobin MJ. *Principles and Practice of Mechanical Ventilation*. New York: McGraw-Hill; 1994.
46. Lessard MR, Brochard LJ. Weaning from ventilatory support. *Clin Chest Med*. 1996;17(3):475–489.
47. Walsh TS, Dodds S, McArdle F. Evaluation of simple criteria to predict successful weaning from mechanical ventilation in intensive care patients: clinical investigation. *Br J Anaesth*. 2004;92:793–799.
48. Treggiari-Venzi MM, Suter PM, deTonnac N, Romand JA. Successful use of hypnosis as an adjunctive therapy for weaning from mechanical ventilation. *Anesthesiology*. 2000;92:890–892.
49. Shneerson JM. Editorial. Are there new solutions to old problems with weaning? *Br J Anaesth*. 1997;78(3):238–240.
50. Bapat P, Verghese C. Cuff deflation for easier weaning from ventilation. *Br J Anaesth*. 1997;79(1):145.
51. Girault C, Briel A, Hellot MF, et al. Noninvasive ventilation as a systemic extubation and weaning technique in acute-on-chronic respiratory failure. *Am J Respir Crit Care Med*. 1999;160:86–92.
52. Suter PM. Does mechanical ventilation cause lung injury? *IARS Review Course Lectures*. 2001;104–105.
53. Pneumatikos IA, Dragoumanis CK, Bouros DE. Ventilator-associated pneumonia or endotracheal tube-associated pneumonia? *Anesthesiology*. 2009;110:673–680.
54. Rabitsch W, Kostler WJ, Fiebiger W, et al. Closed suctioning system reduces cross-contamination between bronchial system and gastric juices. *Anesth Analg*. 2004;99:886–892.
55. Lasocki S, Lu Q, Sartorius A, Fouillat D, Remerand F, Rouby JJ. Open and closed–circuit endotracheal suctioning in acute lung injury. *Anesthesiology*. 2006;104:39–47.
56. Subirana M, Sola I, Benito S. Closed tracheal suction systems versus open tracheal suction systems for mechanically ventilated adult patients. *Anesth Analg*. 2008;106:1326.
57. McLuskey A, Gwinnutt CL. Evaluation of the pneupac ventipac portable ventilator: comparison of performance in a mechanical lung and anaesthetized patients. *Br J Anaesth*. 1995;75(5):645–650.
58. Greensmith JE. Hyperbaric oxygen reverses organ dysfunction in severe anemia. *Anesthesiology*. 2000;93:1149–1152.
59. Dales RE, O'Connor A, Hebert P, Sullivan K, McKim D, Llewellyn-Thomas H. Intubation and mechanical ventilation for COPD: development of an instrument to elicit patient preferences. *Chest*. 1999;116(3):792–800.
60. Gama de Abreu M, Wilmink B, Hubler M, Koch T. Vaporized perfluorohexane attenuates ventilator-induced lung injury in isolated perfused rabbit lungs. *Anesthesiology*. 2005;102:597–605.
61. Lam C, Liu Y, Hsu J, et al. Autologous transplantation of endothelial progenitor cells attenuates acute lung injury in rabbits. *Anesthesiology*. 2008;108:392–401.

Chapter 14
Extubation Strategies: The Extubation Algorithm

Contents

Introduction

The American Society of Anesthesiologists' difficult airway algorithm was introduced in 1993 and revised in 2003[1]. Hagberg,[2] Wilson,[3] and others have published thoughtful critiques of the algorithm, offering numerous modifications to expand its application. The algorithm has achieved "Gold Standard" status in its current form (see Chap. 9). It represents the definitive schematic approach to "front-end" difficult airway management.

Less has been published addressing a schematic approach to "exit strategies" concerning extubation of the difficult airway. To wit, a new *extubation algorithm* is presented herein.

B.T. Finucane et al., *Principles of Airway Management*,
DOI 10.1007/978-0-387-09558-5_14, © Springer Science+Business Media, LLC 2011

Purpose of an Algorithm

An algorithm is a set of instructions for carrying out a procedure usually with the requirement that the procedure terminates at some point.[4]

To be useful, an algorithm must be easy to understand, based on creditable experience and research, and be simple to follow to a defined endpoint. The validity of the instructions should be subjected to scientific scrutiny. Algorithms may be amended to include new instructions and to eliminate invalid, unnecessary, or redundant steps.

The A.S.A. difficult airway algorithm proposes a set of instructions that, if followed successfully, terminates with the establishment of a secure airway. The usefulness of the algorithm has been validated in clinical practice. It helps anesthesiologists organize their thinking and preparation when dealing with the difficult airway.

Purpose of an Extubation Algorithm

An extubation algorithm summarizes airway strategies in schematic form that would lead to a successful extubation. Before examples of extubation algorithms are presented, a few preliminary comments are offered concerning extubation of the patient in general.

Extubation Criteria[1]

Before a patient is extubated, he must meet the following criteria:
   Routine extubation criteria (assuming the airway is normal)

1. CNS criteria

    (a) The patient should be awake and cooperative.
    (b) Protective reflexes are present (cough, gag, and swallow).

2. Ventilation and oxygenation criteria

    (a) The patient is breathing spontaneously.
    (b) The respiratory rate is less than 25/min.
    (c) The tidal volume is at least 5 ml/kg.
    (d) The vital capacity is at least 15 ml/kg.
    (e) The arterial pH is greater than 7.35.
    (f) The arterial $PaCO_2$ is less than or equal to 50 mmHg.
    (g) The oxyhemaglobin saturation is greater than or equal to 90% when the FiO_2 is less than or equal to 0.4.

3. Neuromuscular criteria

    (a) The patient has unassisted head lift greater than 5 s.
    (b) Full reversal from neuromuscular relaxant drug blockade has been documented by testing with a nerve stimulator.

Extubation Criteria Following a Difficult Intubation

Before extubating a patient following a difficult intubation or an intubation requiring special airway equipment such as a fiberoptic bronchoscope, additional criteria must be met. These include the following:

1. *Type I causes of difficult intubation*: If the difficult intubation was caused by a *reversible* phenomenon, that cause must have been eliminated and the airway returned to its normal anatomical configuration prior to extubation. Examples of such causes include:

   (a) Trauma
   (b) Bleeding
   (c) Laryngeal edema (trauma, burns, angioedema, toxic irritation)
   (d) Airway distorted by a foreign body
   (e) Airway distorted by abscess, infection, hematoma, or tumor

Reversal of transient causes of difficult intubation can be verified by examination of the airway prior to extubation utilizing physical examination, direct laryngoscopy, fiberoptic evaluation, observation made with a video laryngoscope, and a thorough review of appropriate radiographic tests. The criterion to extubate after a Type I cause of difficult intubation is resolution of the pathology or abnormality to normal airway anatomy.

2. *Type II causes*: If the difficult intubation was caused by an *irreversible* phenomenon, the practitioner must define the cause of the difficulty and its exact effect on the patient's airway anatomy, prior to extubation. A detailed plan to deal with all anticipated contingencies must be made and all special airway equipment and personnel must be on hand prior to extubation. *Sometimes the best or only plan to deal with irreversible causes of a difficult intubation is to establish an elective surgical airway prior to extubation.*

Examples of irreversible causes of difficult intubation include:

   (a) Craniofacial abnormalities
   (b) Arthritis affecting neck mobility and positioning and/or the laryngeal anatomy
   (c) Obesity affecting neck mobility as well as oral and pharyngeal anatomy
   (d) Laryngeal pathology such as cricoarytenoid arthritis, laryngomalacia, post-operative surgical changes
   (e) Tracheomalacia
   (f) Contractures after burn injury
   (g) Permanent airway distortion after following trauma, infection, or tumor
   (h) Tumor mass in the airway itself
   (i) Lingual tonsils

The fact that a patient has a permanent condition that makes intubation difficult does not mean that extubation cannot be accomplished with success. Should such a condition exist, special considerations and preparations must be made prior to extubation. The extubation algorithm proposes ways to deal with special case extubations. The criteria to extubate after a Type II cause of difficult intubation are that the patient meets all routine extubation criteria and that the anatomy has not undergone any further deleterious changes since intubation.

In summary, to extubate a patient after difficult intubation, all the *routine extubation criteria* as well as *extubation criteria following difficult intubation* must be met. Should a patient have a permanent condition that makes intubation difficult, a plan to deal with every known contingency, as well as special airway equipment and experienced personnel, must be on hand when extubation is attempted.

Strategies to Extubate a Patient with a Difficult Airway

Thomas Mort[5] wrote an excellent article describing strategies to deal with extubation of the patient with a difficult airway. Earlier chapters of this book deal in detail with many of the topics addressed in his article. Importantly, he warns that intubation, ventilation, respiratory care, and extubation carry inherent risks that can cause additional airway trauma and/or distortion. Iatrogenic pathology must be kept in mind when planning an extubation strategy.

The strategy to extubate a patient with a difficult airway involves the following steps:

1. The patient meets all *routine extubation criteria.*
2. The patient meets all *extubation criteria following a difficult intubation.*
3. A contingency plan to deal with anticipated and unanticipated difficulties is in place.
4. All airway equipment is on hand and in working order. Backup equipment is readily available.
5. Extra assistance is on hand. Each person knows his role in the extubation strategy.
6. Personnel and equipment are on hand, should an emergency surgical airway be required.
7. "Cuff Leak test" confirms airway patency around the endotracheal tube.
8. All visual and radiographic evaluations of the airway predict successful extubation.
9. Follow the extubation algorithm.

American Society of Anesthesiologists Task Force on the Management of the Difficult Airway: Strategy for Extubation of the Difficult Airway

In 2003, the A.S.A. Task Force on the Management of the Difficult Airway[6] published the following comment concerning a strategy for extubation of the difficult airway:

> The literature does not provide a sufficient basis for evaluating the benefits of an extubation strategy for the difficult airway. The Task Force regards the concept of an extubation strategy as a logical extension of the intubation strategy. Consultant opinion strongly supports the use of an extubation strategy.

The Task Force recommends that a "preformulated strategy for extubation of the difficult airway" be in place before extubation. The strategy should include:

1. Consideration of the merits of extubating the patient when he is awake or unconscious (for the anesthetized patient).
2. Evaluation of factors that could have an adverse impact on ventilation after extubation.
3. Formulation of a plan to deal with loss of the airway after extubation.
4. Consideration of the use of a rigid airway guide over which the endotracheal tube is withdrawn. The guide would be left in the trachea to expedite reintubation.

The Task Force's recommendations are prudent and should be included in an extubation algorithm.

Difficult Airway Extubation Algorithms

As of 2009, no extubation algorithm has been proposed by a consortium of airway management experts. None has been endorsed by the American Society of Anesthesiologists. While many writers have addressed the myriad aspects concerning extubation of the difficult airway, only a few have set forth algorithms to deal with the topic. While no algorithm can be failure proof, algorithms are useful teaching tools and guides to clinicians. Algorithms provoke thought and preparation. For an algorithm to be useful, the practitioner must be thoroughly knowledgeable of its contents and purpose before an airway management situation becomes emergent.

Hagberg et al.[2] have published a thoughtful review that presents a set of five new airway algorithms. Combined, the five algorithms propose an expanded and more comprehensive plan to deal with the difficult airway than that presented by the A.S.A. difficult airway algorithm. One of the algorithms deals with extubation of the patient with a difficult airway.

Hagberg et al. Extubation Algorithm (Fig. 14.1)

The five algorithm set proposed by Hagberg et al. is more comprehensive than the A.S.A. algorithm. Because it is more comprehensive, it is more complex and time-consuming to follow than the A.S.A. algorithm. An extubation algorithm should require that assistance be on hand prior to the attempted extubation. That would include a surgeon to perform an emergency cricothyroidotomy if the planned extubation is of a particularly difficult patient. Finally, a more comprehensive extubation algorithm would detail more options utilizing a variety of airway management equipment and techniques.

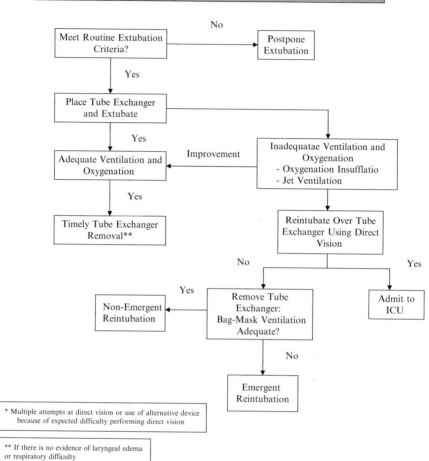

Fig. 14.1 The Hagberg et al. extubation algorithm (with modification) (Hagberg et al.[2] with permission)

For such a modified extubation algorithm, a few prerequisites are stipulated:

1. The extubation algorithm may be applied to any patient who was difficult to intubate or whose airway anatomy changed after intubation rendering extubation predictably difficult.
2. The extubation algorithm will not include strategies applied to the extubation of patients with normal airways.
3. The equipment cited on the extubation algorithm may be substituted with other equipment more familiar to the reader based on his clinical experience.

After the algorithm is presented, the remainder of the chapter will expound on a few of its details.

Extubation Algorithm for Patients with Difficult Airways (Fig. 14.2)

Performing the Leak Test Prior to Extubation

The leak test demonstrates that air can pass between the endotracheal tube and the laryngotracheal mucosal surfaces when the cuff is deflated. The leak documents that an air channel is opened around the tube when marginal airway pressures are exerted on the endotracheal tube – patient airway system. Two tests can be performed. With the cuff deflated, the *positive pressure test* produces an audible gas leak when 20–25 cm H_2O pressure is applied to the endotracheal tube. The *negative pressure test* produces an audible leak when the patient takes a breath with the cuff down and the end of the endotracheal tube blocked. Neither test proves that the airway will remain patent on extubation, but a negative leak test, *no leak demonstrated*, should make the practitioner more cautious. A negative leak test with visual confirmation of severe upper airway edema should persuade the practitioner to delay extubation until resolution of the edema and demonstration of a positive leak test.

Preoxygenation

Preoxygenation or denitrogenation of the lungs should be performed before extubation. The patient's functional residual capacity (FRC) should be fully oxygenated, should extubation fail. A few precious minutes would then be secured, should reintubation be necessary. With an FiO_2 of 1.0 and the patient breathing tidal volume breaths, preoxygenation should be achieved in 3–5 min.[7] To be on the safe side, preoxygenate for at least 5 min before attempting extubation. Keep in mind that the FRC is often diminished in supine or recumbent patients or in those with lung disease.

Airway Anesthesia Prior to Extubation

Many of the options to be discussed require oral, pharyngeal, laryngeal, or tracheal instrumentation. The practitioner should consider administering topical lidocaine, cocaine, or benzocaine to the mucosal surfaces of the airway before instrumentation. Topical anesthesia assures that the patient will better tolerate the instrumentation and be more willing and able to cooperate and to respond to instructions.

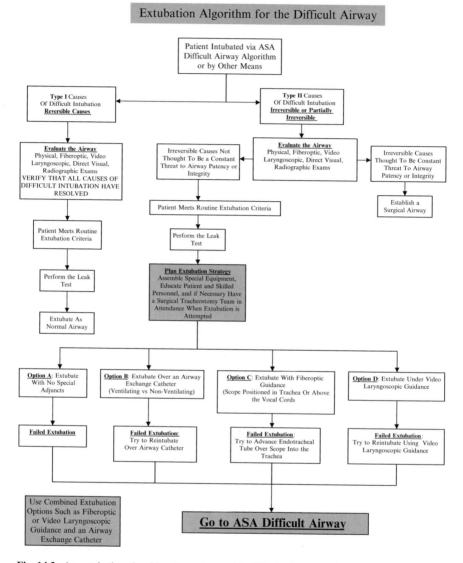

Fig. 14.2 An extubation algorithm for patients with difficult airways. The algorithm incorporates the recommendation of the A.S.A. Task Force on Management of the Difficult Airway

Patient Education Prior to Extubation

Extubation of an awake patient under any circumstances can cause fear, anxiety, and concern in the patient. The patient, the only one with something to lose, is the most important player on the extubation team. Make sure the patient understands the complete extubation plan as well as the role he is expected to play. A cooperative patient is essential to a well-planned extubation strategy.

Option A: Extubation over an Airway Guide

This method of extubation of the difficult airway has received the most attention. This option entails extubating the patient with a guide, stent, or airway exchange catheter (AEC) passed through the endotracheal tube, then leaving the guide in the trachea during the immediate postextubation period. In theory, should the extubation fail, the tube (or a smaller one) could be passed back into the trachea to secure the airway. The literature supports the technique as applied to patients with suspected difficult extubations. Mort[8] cited an 87% first time success rate of reintubation over an AEC after failed extubation with an overall success rate of 92%. He suggested that utilization of an "AEC is an efficient method of maintaining continuous access to the airway after extubation, as it is well tolerated and potentially offers a clinically valuable conduit for reintubation… ." Failure of the technique was attributed to inadvertent withdrawal of the AEC from the glottis and to severe laryngeal edema. An accompanying editorial[9] supported Mort's conclusion. Note that an AEC is included on the Hagberg et al. algorithm. It is referred to as a TE (tube exchanger).

The duration for which an AEC is left in after extubation is variable, depending on the patient's condition, the airway anatomy, and the probability of failed extubation. The AEC is usually left in place for a range of time varying from a few minutes to a few hours. Smaller catheters may be tolerated better than larger ones. However, larger guides may be better conduits for reintubation.[8]

The guide should be left in until the practitioner is satisfied that the patient can maintain airway patency on his own (Figs. 3–9).

Problems associated with the use of an airway extubation guide include:

1. Trauma to airway, oral, pharyngeal, or esophageal anatomy
2. Barotrauma, should a jet ventilator be used with a ventilating guide
3. Inadvertent displacement of the guide into the pharynx or esophagus
4. Breakage of the guide and endotracheal tube dislodgement[10]

Option B: Extubation with Fiberoptic Guidance

The fiberoptic endoscope can be used to evaluate airway anatomy prior to extubating a patient who was difficult to intubate. The scope can also be used during the extubation process. One use of the scope is to use it as the *extubation guide*. After placing the scope through the endotracheal tube and passing it to the carina, the tube is withdrawn from the trachea. The scope is left in place until such time that it is deemed that the extubation has been successful and then the scope is removed. Should reintubation be required, the clinician should try to pass the tube over the scope back into the trachea. Alternatively, the scope can be preloaded with a smaller "rescue" endotracheal tube and then passed into the trachea, above or below the existing endotracheal tube, before the tube is removed. The scope is left in the trachea as described above. Should the patient require reintubation, the smaller

FROVA INTUBATING INTRODUCERS

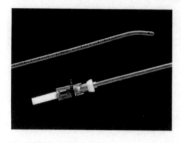

Used to facilitate endotracheal intubation and to allow simple endotracheal tube exchange. Use of removable Rapi-Fit* Adapter permits use of ventilatory device if necessary during exchange procedure. Supplied sterile in peel-open packages. Intended for one-time use.

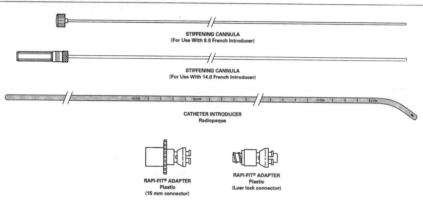

STIFFENING CANNULA
(For Use With 8.0 French Introducer)

STIFFENING CANNULA
(For Use With 14.0 French Introducer)

CATHETER INTRODUCER
Radiopaque

RAPI-FIT® ADAPTER
Plastic
(15 mm connector)

RAPI-FIT® ADAPTER
Plastic
(Luer lock connector)

Global Product Number	Order Number	CATHETER French Size	Length	Inner Diameter	Use in Replacement of Endotracheal Tube with Inner Diameter[1]
G12591	C-CAE-8.0-35-FII	8.0	35 cm	1.6 mm	3 mm or larger
G11915	C-CAE-14.0-65-FII	14.0	65 cm	3 mm	6 mm or larger
Without Stiffening Cannula					
G13307	C-CAE-14.0-65-FI	14.0	65 cm	3 mm	6 mm or larger

[1]Endotracheal tube not included.

Patent Number 5,052,386

Fig. 14.3 The Cook Frova intubating introducer can be used as a ventilating airway exchange catheter (AEC). Note that the introducer can be fitted with a 15 mm Rapi-Fit© adaptor for oxygenation/ventilation using an anesthesia machine circuit or a self-inflating resuscitation bag. The introducer can also be fitted with a Rapi-Fit© Luer lock adapter if high pressure jet ventilation/oxygenation is utilized

"rescue" endotracheal tube can be advanced into the trachea. Another use of the scope is to preload it with a "rescue" tube and position the scope just above the glottic opening. Observe the removal of the existing tube and keep the scope in place until the need for immediate reintubation had passed. This use of the scope is riskier than the first two options and it is not recommended if the anatomy is grossly distorted or the patient was difficult to mask ventilate. Finally, the scope can be used to directly place an endotracheal tube over an A.E.C. if passage of the tube into the trachea is impeded at the glottis. The scope permits the clinician to visualize the glottic opening and the structures surrounding it to help guide an endotracheal

AINTREE INTUBATION CATHETER

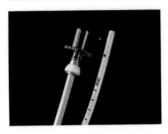

Used for uncomplicated, atraumatic endotracheal tube exchange.

• Use of removable Rapi-Fit® Adapter permits use of ventilatory device if necessary during exchange procedure.

• Catheter has larger 4.7 mm lumen.

• Through-lumen design of catheter with distal sideports ensures adequate air flow.

• Blunt tip of catheter is atraumatic to internal structures.

• Centimeter marks facilitate accurate placement with shortened endotracheal tubes.

Supplied sterile in peel-open packages. Intended for one-time use.

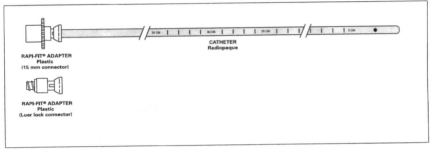

Global Product Number	Order Number	French Size	Length	Inner Diameter	Use in Replacement of Endotracheal Tube with Inner Diameter
G10789	C-CAE-19.0-56-AIC	19.0	56 cm	4.7 mm	7 mm or larger

Patent Number 5,052,386

Fig. 14.4 The Cook Aintree intubation catheter can also be used as an exchange catheter. It has a large inner diameter, which makes oxygenation/ventilation easier. The Aintree catheter comes with both types of Rapi-Fit© adaptors

tube into the trachea. The operator is reminded that topical anesthesia helps the patient tolerate airway instrumentation. Also, appropriate steps must be taken to protect the scope from damage, by either the patient biting it or the operator applying unnecessary force. Be sure to lubricate the scope and tubes that are passed over the scope. For more information, see Chap. 11.

Option C: Extubation with Video Laryngoscopic Guidance

With the patient's airway topically anesthetized, a video laryngoscope can be used to evaluate the supraglottic and glottic anatomy, prior to extubation. The scope can be left in place to observe the airway after extubation. It can act as a guide for reintubation. If an airway catheter has been left in the trachea, the scope can confirm its placement and also help guide a tube back into the trachea, should that contingency be indicated. Peral et al.[11] reported the use of the Glidescope© to direct an endotracheal tube exchange. They described a direct endotracheal intubation and an intubation over an airway catheter. Both techniques were visually directed by the video laryngoscope.

COOK AIRWAY EXCHANGE CATHETER

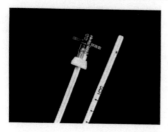

Used for uncomplicated, atraumatic endotracheal tube exchange.

• Use of removable Rapi-Fit® Adapter permits use of ventilatory device if necessary during exchange procedure.

• Through-lumen design of catheter with distal sideports ensures adequate air flow.

• Blunt tip of catheter is atraumatic to internal structures.

• Centimeter marks facilitate accurate placement with shortened endotracheal tubes.

Supplied sterile in peel-open packages. Intended for one-time use.

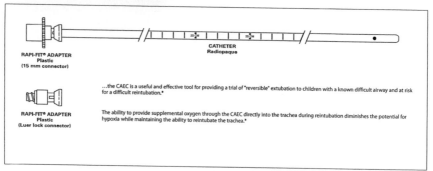

RAPI-FIT® ADAPTER
Plastic
(15 mm connector)

CATHETER
Radiopaque

RAPI-FIT® ADAPTER
Plastic
(Luer lock connector)

...the CAEC is a useful and effective tool for providing a trial of "reversible" extubation to children with a known difficult airway and at risk for a difficult reintubation.*

The ability to provide supplemental oxygen through the CAEC directly into the trachea during reintubation diminishes the potential for hypoxia while maintaining the ability to reintubate the trachea.*

Global Product Number	Order Number	French Size	Length	Inner Diameter	Use in Replacement of Endotracheal Tube with Inner Diameter
FOR USE WITH SINGLE LUMEN ENDOTRACHEAL TUBES					
G07833	C-CAE-8.0-45	8.0	45 cm	1.6 mm	3 mm or larger
G06732	C-CAE-11.0-83	11.0	83 cm	2.3 mm	4 mm or larger
G07873	C-CAE-14.0-83	14.0	83 cm	3 mm	5 mm or larger
G05880	C-CAE-19.0-83	19.0	83 cm	3.4 mm	7 mm or larger

*Wise-Faberowski L, Nargozian C: "Utility of Airway Exchange Catheters in Pediatric Patients with a Known Difficult Airway," *Pediatr Crit Care Med, 2005; 6:454-56.*
Patent Number 5,052,386

Fig. 14.5 Cook Medical makes a variety of AECs in various lengths and diameters

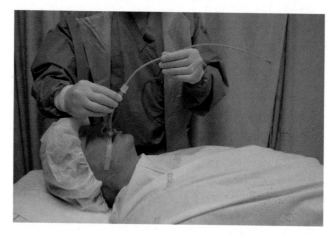

Fig. 14.6 A gum elastic Bougie can be used as an extubation guide

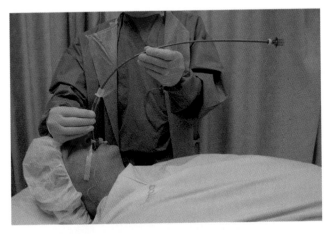

Fig. 14.7 The first step to extubate over an AEC or airway guide is to place the lubricated catheter into the trachea through the endotracheal tube

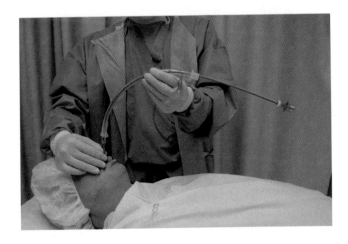

Fig. 14.8 Step two is to remove the endotracheal tube over the exchange catheter

Combined Extubation Options

The literature supports the recommendation of using an AEC or guide when extubating the difficult airway. Using a catheter or guide in conjunction with fiberoptic or a video laryngoscopic observation of the airway might offer more control under certain circumstances. When the extubation strategy is formulated, combined extubation options should be considered.

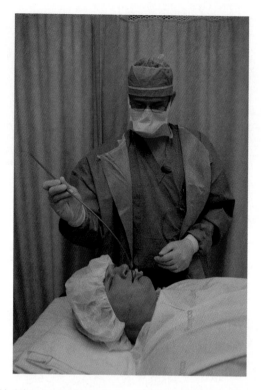

Fig. 14.9 The AEC is left in the trachea until the clinician determines that the patient is oxygenating and ventilating adequately and that the airway will remain patent. At this point, the catheter is removed

Summary

The A.S.A. difficult airway algorithm has proven to be a very useful clinical tool. Anesthesiologists and other airway management specialists use it to prepare to deal with patients who have a difficult airway. The algorithm addresses both anticipated and unanticipated difficult airway scenarios. An algorithm is a schematic way of organizing the steps that lead to a defined endpoint. An algorithm lists instructions that are based on prudent thought, practice, and research. The extubation algorithm presented in this chapter, like the Hagberg et al. algorithm, represents one author's attempt to present an extubation schema that is applied to the difficult airway. Future algorithms will be based on data obtained after testing the validity of the algorithms presented in this chapter and will include new instrumentation options and airway management techniques. When it comes to extubating the difficult airway, an old saying offers a lot of advice:

Don't burn your bridges after you pass.

References

1. Hagberg CA, Benumof JL. *Benumof's Airway Management.* 2nd ed. Philadelphia: Mosby-Elsevier; 2007:238–239.
2. Hagberg CA, Lam NC, Brambrink AM. Current concepts in airway management in the operating room. *Curr Rev Clin Anesth.* 2007;28(7):75–84.
3. Wilson WC. Trauma: airway management. *ASA Newsl.* 2005;69:11.
4. Wolfram Math World. Algorithm. http://mathworld.wolfram.com/Algorithm.html; 2009. Accessed 3.02.09.
5. Mort TC. Strategies for extubation of the difficult airway. *Anesthesiology News Guide to Airway Management.* 2008; 100–107.
6. American Society of Anesthesiologists. Task Force on the Management of the Difficult Airway. *Anesthesiology.* 2003; 98(5):1269–1277.
7. Baraka A, Salem MR. *Benumof's Airway Management.* 2nd ed. Philadelphia: Mosby-Elsevier; 2007:303–318.
8. Mort TC. Continuous airway access for the difficult extubation: the efficacy of the airway exchange catheter. *Anesth Analg.* 2007;105(5):1357–1362.
9. Biro P, Priebe HJ. Editorial: staged extubation strategy: is an airway exchange catheter the answer? *Anesth Analg.* 2007;105(5):1182–1185.
10. Schulte TE, Tinker JH. Snapping of Cook Exchange catheter with subsequent dislodgement in a Double-Lumen endotracheal tube. *Anesth Analg.* 2007;105(4):1174–1175.
11. Peral D, Porcan E, Bellver J, et al. Glidescope video laryngoscope is useful in exchanging endotracheal tubes. *Anesth Analg.* 2006;103(4):1043–1044.

Chapter 15
Complications of Airway Management

Contents

B.T. Finucane et al., *Principles of Airway Management*,
DOI 10.1007/978-0-387-09558-5_15, © Springer Science+Business Media, LLC 2011

Introduction

The routine use of endotracheal tubes in anesthesia occurred following the introduction of the neuromuscular blocking drugs by Griffith and Johnson.[1] Few will
dispute the importance of endotracheal anesthesia; however, the technique is associated with a myriad of complications, ranging from minor injuries to lips and teeth
to permanent brain damage and death. The process of endotracheal intubation
involves bag/valve/mask ventilation, insertion of airways, the use of various aids,
laryngoscopy, and endotracheal intubation. Complications can occur at any stage of
the process, but the majority of serious complications occur in association with the
insertion or failure to insert an endotracheal tube. Therefore, most of the emphasis
is placed on complications arising from endotracheal intubation. Complications
related to LMA insertion have been addressed in Chapter 6.

    We attempt to address the various complications of tracheal intubation in a
sequential and logical fashion and it should be understood from the outset that only
the most common complications are discussed. We first discuss complications that
occur during the performance of tracheal intubation. We then discuss complications
that occur immediately after the insertion of an endotracheal tube. Next, we discuss
complications that occur upon removal of the endotracheal tube. We address complications specifically associated with nasotracheal intubation. Finally, we briefly
allude to complications associated with long-term intubation and present data from
the most recent airway morbidity and mortality studies from around the world.

Complications Arising During Intubation

Trauma

Eyes

Occasionally during intubation attempts, a watch strap or ring may graze the cornea,
leading to a corneal abrasion. Intraocular pressure rises significantly during endotracheal intubation, especially in patients who are improperly anesthetized.
Succinylcholine, a depolarizing neuromuscular blocking agent, is also associated
with increases in intraocular pressure.[2] However, bucking and coughing during
attempts at intubation are the most common causes of significant increases in intraocular pressure. Sudden surges in intraocular pressure may be associated with extrusion
of the lens or vitreous in patients presenting for anesthesia with open-eye injuries.

Upper Lip

Careless laryngoscopy often results in damage to the upper lip in the form of hema-
tomas, lacerations, and teeth marks. During laryngoscopy, the upper lip tends to

become trapped between the laryngoscope blade and the teeth. This problem is best avoided by manually clearing the upper lip from the laryngoscope blade before advancing the blade deep into the oropharynx. Such trauma is usually self-limiting, but its disfigurement can be annoying to the patient. Artificial airways are frequently placed in the oropharynx prior to extubation. Semiconscious patients emerging from anesthesia sometimes vigorously bite down on these airways, and if the airway has not been properly positioned, self-inflicted and unsightly bite marks to the lips occur.

Mucous Membranes of the Oropharynx

During laryngoscopy, the blade may inadvertently tear the mucous membranes in the region of the tonsillar bed. This is a common complication, most often seen on the right side, and is usually associated with inexperience. It is self-limiting and may be partly responsible for the sore throat often reported in the postintubation period. Trauma to mucous membranes in the region of the larynx, however, is more serious and may result in subcutaneous air or, worse, tension pneumothorax and pneumomediastinum. Subcutaneous air is an ominous sign and should alert the clinician to the possibility of tension pneumothorax and mediastinal air. A chest X-ray must be obtained as soon as possible and systemic antibiotics administered immediately. Positive-pressure ventilation is extremely hazardous in these patients. In elective situations, intubation and positive-pressure ventilation should be deferred if possible.

Koh and Coleman[3] recently reported a 5-mm ulceration in the oropharynx most likely caused by an overheated laryngoscope lightbulb. The laryngoscope was in the "cocked" position for several minutes before laryngoscopy. This anecdotal report reminds us of the importance of an equipment check before attempted intubation.

Teeth

Dental damage remains the single most common complication resulting in litigation against anesthesiologists. It is difficult to obtain accurate information about all aspects of dental damage associated with airway management. Most of the data we have access to are retrospective and involve small numbers of patients. However, there are two recent publications on this topic, involving large numbers of patients, and the first of these is from the Mayo Clinic[4]; even though this was a retrospective study, it was well designed, had good controls and surveillance rates at 24 h and 7 days, and was carried out in a single, large, reputable institution. The study involved 598,904 anesthetics and there were 132 cases of dental injury. The overall risk of dental damage in that study was 1:4,500 cases and the risk was much greater in those patients requiring tracheal intubation. The upper incisors were most vulnerable. The most frequent injuries were crown fractures and partial dislocations. More than one tooth was involved in 13% of cases. The median cost of repair was $782 (range, $88–$8,200).

The second large study, and the more recent one, took place at the University of Nebraska and involved 161,687 anesthetics.[5] This was a 1:2 case study designed to reveal the frequency, risk factors, and outcomes of dental injury, and took place over a 14-year period. Seventy eight patients sustained dental damage or 1:2,073 anesthetics. Patients with poor dentition and whose tracheas were moderately difficult, or difficult to intubate, were at a 20-fold increased risk of dental damage. The anesthesia provider discovered the injury in 86% of cases. The patterns of injury reported in the previous study were quite similar.

The introduction of supraglottic devices, predictably, should reduce the incidence of dental damage associated with anesthesia as the insertion of these devices usually does not involve instrumentation. It is best to avoid direct laryngoscopy in patients who present with multiple crowns, if possible. In many cases intubation can be readily achieved using blind techniques; for example, the lighted stylet. The simple message here is to avoid laryngoscopy in those with dental risk factors, if at all possible.

Restorative dentistry has become quite sophisticated in recent years,[6] and a number of innovative techniques have been introduced to replace missing teeth. Some patients present with removable bridgework. These appliances are held in place by retainers and can be easily removed by the patient. Butterfly bridges are now being used with increasing frequency. They lack the durability of a fixed bridge, and the "wings" are bonded to adjacent teeth and are easily broken. Titanium implants are now frequently used by dentists. If dental trauma is anticipated, these appliances may be removed by the dentist before the procedure and replaced postoperatively.

Despite the frequency of claims against anesthesiologists for dental damage, insufficient attention has been paid to this problem. Evaluation of the airway should always include a thorough assessment of dental risk. If a patient is particularly vulnerable, alternative methods of anesthesia must be considered. Protective dental guards are available and may be inserted prior to laryngoscopy; however, few clinicians use these protective devices. Oral airways, which account for a large percentage of injuries, should be avoided whenever possible in those at risk. When dental damage occurs, the incident must be recorded in the patient's chart and the patient informed as soon as possible. Undiscovered dental debris may be aspirated. Recovery room personnel sometimes discover fractured teeth during the recovery period and sometimes dental damage is reported by the patients upon regaining consciousness.

Laryngeal Injuries

Some laryngeal injuries occur at the time of intubation but are usually not evident until the patient regains consciousness or even later. In the "Closed Claims Study" by Domino et al.,[7] 34% of laryngeal injuries involved paralysis of the vocal cords; granuloma occurred in 17% of cases and arytenoid dislocation in 8%. The vast majority of traumatic injuries (80%) were associated with routine tracheal intubation that was short term.

Pharyngeal Injuries

As with many of these complications, the best source of information is Domino's paper in the Closed Claims Study.

The most common pharyngeal injuries in this study were:

- Pharyngeal perforation (37%)
- Lacerations and contusions (31%)
- Localized infection (12%)
- Sore throat (no obvious injury) (12%)
- Miscellaneous injury (8%)

More than 50% of all pharyngeal injuries and 68% of pharyngeal perforations were associated with difficult intubation. Pharyngeal perforations were attributed to nasogastric tubes, jet ventilation, and suction catheters in equal number and the cause was not determined in 50% of cases. Death occurred in 81% of pharyngeal perforations (5/6) and was caused by mediastinitis.

Esophageal Trauma

Esophageal perforation was the most common esophageal injury in the Closed Claims Study (90%) and was clearly linked with difficult intubation in the majority of cases (62%). Esophageal perforation was strongly linked with female gender and in those aged more than 60 years. Instruments causing esophageal perforation included nasogastric tubes, esophageal dilators, esophageal stethoscopes, and laryngoscopes. Nineteen percent of patients presenting with esophageal injury died as a result of the complication.

The problem with both pharyngeal and esophageal perforation is that they are difficult to diagnose. Early signs of perforation include pneumothorax or subcutaneous emphysema. These signs were present in only about 50% of the cases. In many cases, there was no history of difficult intubation. A chest X-ray must be performed in all cases of difficult intubation and perhaps should be repeated 24 h later. Typical symptoms of pharyngo-esophageal perforation include severe sore throat, deep cervical or chest pain, and fever; and patients presenting with these symptoms following difficult intubation or nasogastric tube placement are prime candidates for mediastinitis, especially if aged 60 or older and female.

Tracheal/Bronchial Injuries

The majority of tracheal injuries reported in the "Closed Claims Study" were in association with injuries that occurred following tracheostomy for difficult intubation. These injuries included tracheal perforation and infection.

Marty-Ané et al.[8] recently described six cases of membranous tracheal rupture, following endotracheal intubation. Overinflation of the endotracheal tube cuff was deemed to be the cause of this problem in some of the cases. The diagnosis was suspected on the basis of the following signs: subcutaneous emphysema, respiratory distress, pneumomediastinum, and pneumothorax.

A number of reports, mostly letters to the editor, discuss the concern about increased endotracheal tube cuff pressures when nitrous oxide is used. In some of these reports, it is suggested that we monitor intracuff pressures in intubated patients.

Tu et al.[9] showed that cuff pressure changes due to N_2O could be minimized by using the same mixture of gases in the cuff that is used to anesthetize the patient.

Karasawa et al.[10] showed that when N_2O is used in the cuff of the endotracheal tube, serious cuff leaks occurred on withdrawal of N_2O. Fewer and fewer anesthesiologists are using nitrous oxide as an adjuvant to other inhalation anesthetics in modern anesthesia; therefore, this issue will be solved when nitrous oxide is no longer used.

Lung

Pneumothorax may occur as a result of overzealous manual or mechanical ventilation in normal lungs, or normal manual or mechanical ventilation in diseased lungs. Endobronchial intubation is a risk factor for barotrauma in normal and diseased lungs. We need to pay much more attention to the tidal volumes we select when we place patients on mechanical ventilation. There is a tendency to prescribe larger tidal volumes than are necessary and we recommend erring on the side of lower tidal volumes, at least initially.

Hypoxemia

Hypoxemia is an abnormally low tension of oxygen in arterial blood. In normal individuals who are breathing room air, the tension of oxygen in arterial blood is between 90 and 100 mmHg. When the quantity of oxygen delivered to the tissues falls below metabolic demand, hypoxia occurs despite adequate perfusion.

Acute Hypoxic Encephalopathy

Acute hypoxic encephalopathy is a global insult to the brain from lack of oxygen that results in an arrest of aerobic metabolic activity, which is necessary to sustain the function of the Krebs cycle and the hydrogen ion transport system. The degree of permanent damage is variable and unpredictable, but, generally, oxygen deprivation for more than 3 minutes in normothermic conditions is likely to result in permanent brain damage. Every effort should be made to prevent hypoxic episodes because damaged brain cells take a long time to recover and, in many cases, do not recover at all. If a significant hypoxic insult occurs, every effort should be made to minimize the damage. The patient's circulation and oxygenation must be restored as soon as possible. Hyperventilation and steroids are recommended to reduce cerebral edema. Anticonvulsants should be used if seizure activity occurs. Barbiturates reduce the cerebral metabolic rate and have been recommended by some authorities. In Haldane's words, "oxygen lack not only stops the machine, but wrecks the machinery."

Failure of Oxygen at the Source

Very rarely, there may be failure of the oxygen supply at the central source. These central banks are usually situated in a remote part of the hospital in the open air. Severe weather conditions may cause excessive buildup of ice on the piping, which may interfere with oxygen delivery. Historically but, fortunately, rarely, serious plumbing errors have occurred whereby oxygen lines have been interchanged with nitrous oxide lines – with serious consequences. Defects such as these can be readily detected by using oxygen analyzers. If oxygen has failed at the source, the safety officer, the chiefs of anesthesiology and respiratory therapy, and the executive director of the hospital should all be contacted immediately.

Failure of Oxygen at the Delivery Site

The inability to deliver oxygen when needed is an emergency. The inability to deliver oxygen to patients who are apneic is a dire emergency. The most common cause of this problem is a breach in the delivery system close to the patient (e.g., a ventilator disconnect or an actual leak). Decreased oxygen concentration can also occur if the oxygen flowmeters are faulty. Furthermore, because of inexperience or inattention, the clinician may select a hypoxic mixture. Modern anesthesia machines are now designed so that it is next to impossible to deliver a hypoxic mixture.

In case of oxygen failure, remember the basics: If an endotracheal tube is not in place already, begin mouth-to-mouth or mouth-to-mask ventilation immediately. If an Ambu bag is available, use it. If an endotracheal tube is in place, deliver a tidal volume directly into it. In an operating room, each anesthesia machine should be equipped with two E-cylinders of oxygen that will allow a 10-L flow of oxygen for 2 h.

Improper Procedure

Because of failure to ventilate and oxygenate patients before and during attempts at intubation, hypoxemia may occur in the course of an intubation. Prevention of hypoxemia should always be your *main* priority when attempting endotracheal intubation.

Inability to Intubate or Ventilate

There are occasions when, for one reason or another, you will be unable to intubate or ventilate a patient. These patients are at great risk of hypoxemia and aspiration of acid gastric contents. Risk factors for difficult mask ventilation (DMV) include: obesity, age, macroglossia, beard, edentulous state, short thyromental distance, history of snoring, and Mallampati class III or IV.[11] (For a more detailed discussion of DMV please refer to Chap. 2.).

Vomiting and Aspiration

Aspiration of gastric contents into the tracheobronchial tree is one of the most feared complications in anesthesia, and a number of preventative strategies are routinely used to prevent this complication.

Blitt et al.[12] suggested that for every 1,000 patients undergoing elective surgery, six would aspirate, and that the presence of a cuffed endotracheal tube was no guarantee against aspiration. Engelhardt et al.[13] published a very comprehensive review of this important topic in 1999, and in that learned treatise, they challenged a number of the accepted medical doctrines that we have been practicing for years. While the true incidence of aspiration pneumonitis is difficult to determine, it is clear from recent reports that the incidence of this malady is low and mortality following pulmonary aspiration in surgery is rare (Table 15.1).

These data should not encourage us to be complacent. We should still continue to take precautions to prevent aspiration. There are no data demonstrating that there is improved outcome following the use of antacids, H_2 receptor blocking agents or proton pump inhibitors. However, serious side effects, though rare, occur with their use. So we must question the routine use of these agents in at-risk groups. The critical volume and pH of gastric aspirant triggering a serious pneumonitis was established by Roberts and Shirley[14] almost 40 years ago (pH 2.5 and volume 0.4 ml/kg). Those values have recently been challenged. Schwartz et al.[15] have shown that serious pneumonitis can occur in animals when the pH is as high as 7. They also suggested that the critical volume required to trigger a serious pneumonitis is 1 ml/kg. There are three pathophysiologic processes associated with aspiration of gastric contents:

1. Particle-related complication – Patients might develop acute airway obstruction, severe hypoxemia, or be at risk for death. Particles must be rapidly cleared from the airway to prevent acute asphyxiation.
2. Acid-related complications – These occur in two phases: (a) immediate tissue injury, and (b) a later inflammatory response. Most cases of aspiration are a combination of particle- and acid-related injuries that, when combined, have a synergistic effect on pulmonary capillary leaks.
3. Bacterial-related complications – Gastric and pharyngeal contents usually contain bacteria; however, prophylactic antibiotics are not routinely recommended as a preventative measure following aspiration of gastric contents.

Table 15.1 Incidence of aspiration

References	Period of assessment	Method of assessment	Patient group	Number of anesthetics	Number of aspirations	Incidence of aspiration per 10,000	Factors thought to contribute to the risk of aspiration
Olsson 1986	1967–1970 1975–1985	Retrospective study from database at Karolinska Hospital, Sweden	Children and adults	185,358	87	4.7	Emergency; abdominal surgery; history of delayed gastric emptying; pregnancy; obesity; pain; stress; raised intracranial pressure
Warner 1993	1985–1991	Retrospective study from database at Mayo Clinic, Rochester, New York	Adults	215,488	67	3.1	Emergency; lack of coordination of swallowing; depressed conscious level; previous esophageal surgery; recent meal; laryngoscopy; tracheal extubation
Brimacombe 1995	1988–1993	Meta-analysis of 101 publications on the Laryngeal Mask Airway	Children and adults	12,901	3	2.3	Emergency; Trendelenberg position; bronchospasm and light anesthesia
Mellin-Olsen 1996	1989–1993	Prospective study from database at Trondheim University Hospital, Norway	Children and adults	85,594	25	2.9	Emergency; general anesthesia

Study	Years	Study type	Population	N	No.	Rate	Comments
Borland 1998	1988–1993	Retrospective study from database at Children's Hospital of Pittsburgh, Pennsylvania	Children	50,880	52	10.2	Increased severity of illness; intravenous induction; ages 6–11; emergency
Ezri 2000	1979–1993	Retrospective study from a hospital database	Adult females Peripartum period, except Cesarean Sections	1,870	1	5.3	
Warner[4]	1985–1997	Prospective study from database at Mayo Clinic, Rochester, New York	Children	63,180	24	3.8	Emergency; depressed conscious level; gastrointestinal problems such as gastroesophageal reflux, ileus, bowel obstruction, hemoperitoneum, recent meal; sepsis; shock
Lockey 1999	1999	Prospective study of the London Helicopter Emergency Medical Service	Adults Severe trauma from road traffic accidents and falls from heights	53	18	3396.2	Emergency

Source: From Engelhardt et al.[13]

Preventative Measures

The use of antacid therapy, endotracheal intubation, rapid sequence induction, and Sellick's maneuver is now standard of care in anesthesia, even though we do not have robust data to support these measures. However, common sense tells us that some of these preventative measures do not need definitive proof. However, the risk/benefit ratio of routine antacid therapy must be challenged.

For treatment of pulmonary aspiration, the following measures are recommended:

1. Administer 100% oxygen by mask. Place the patient in 30° Trendelenburg and lateral if possible.
2. Thoroughly suction all gastric material from the oropharynx.
3. The clinician must decide whether the patient needs intubation or not.
4. Mild cases do not require intubation.
5. In many situations aspiration occurs during an attempt at intubation.
6. However, in some cases aspiration occurs after extubation and the clinician has a small window of time to decide whether the patient should be intubated or not, and that decision is based on clinical signs and objective measures, e.g., oxygen saturation.
7. Intubated patients should be suctioned immediately.
8. Apply positive pressure ventilation (PPV) with PEEP.
9. Administer 100% oxygen initially.
10. Bronchodilator therapy.
11. Insert an arterial catheter and obtain serial blood gas measurements.
12. Arrange for admission to an ICU.

Steroids or antibiotics are not routinely recommended as prophylactic measures.

When intubating patients on the ward, be mindful of the fact that they are at considerable risk for aspiration. In a number of these cases, aspiration of gastric contents is frequently the reason for tracheal intubation. Unlike patients presenting for routine surgery, few of these patients are prepared. Many will have ingested food recently. Furthermore, their reflexes may be impaired to some degree through illness, infirmity, and old age. Always be prepared to deal with this emergency. Oxygen and suction must be immediately at hand. In patients who are particularly at risk, do not hesitate to conscript a bystander to apply cricoid pressure (Sellick's maneuver).[16] However, be sure to give clear instructions as to how this should be done. Cricoid pressure is performed most effectively by placing the thumb and index finger of either hand on the cricoid cartilage, in the midline, and pressing firmly downward. Patients should be in the supine position. Also, the person applying cricoid pressure must not release it until instructed to do so, i.e., until correct tube placement has been confirmed and the cuff inflated. It seems ironic that the very procedure that is implemented to prevent aspiration and regurgitation (intubation) is often associated with this serious complication. On rare occasions, a tooth, laryngoscope lightbulb, or other foreign body will enter the pharynx during attempted intubation. Be sure that teeth or foreign bodies lost in this manner are not aspirated or swallowed by the patient.

Complications Arising Immediately After Intubation

Hypoxemia

Accidental Esophageal Intubation

Despite advances in monitoring technology during the past 20 or 30 years, intubation of the esophagus is still a major cause of cerebral damage or death in anesthesia. Adverse respiratory events accounted for 27% of all cases in one Closed Claims Study[17] (p1) and these were invariably associated with either brain damage or death. About one fifth were due to esophageal intubation (conservative estimate).

One of the most disturbing aspects about esophageal intubation is that it frequently occurs in relatively young, healthy patients. Data from the Closed Claims Study[18] indicated that the mean age of those who died or who were injured was 39 years and the median American Society of Anesthesiologists (ASA) score was 2.

Endotracheal intubation is readily performed in a large number of patients undergoing anesthesia, and esophageal intubation seldom occurs. It can be considered a forgivable mistake provided it is detected in time, before cerebral damage occurs. But do not become complacent about this seemingly simple procedure, and definitely do not rely solely on the usual clinical means to verify correct placement of an endotracheal tube. When a tube is correctly placed in the trachea, you cannot guarantee it will remain there. The consequences of failure to detect esophageal intubation are so grave that every effort must be made both to verify correct placement initially and to monitor placement continuously while the tube is in the trachea. The most reliable method of continuously monitoring tracheal intubation and tracheal tube placement is by using *capnometry*. Capnometry has become the standard for use during endotracheal intubation in most parts of the developed world, and though it is not foolproof, it is the most reliable technology available today in the developed world.

Details about the principles of capnometry/capnography are beyond the scope of this text, so only the basics will be mentioned. The key to capnometry is the presence or absence of carbon dioxide. Carbon dioxide concentrations in exhaled air are usually around 5%, and in inhaled air they are about 0.04%. There are many ways to detect carbon dioxide. You should be able to not only detect the presence or absence of the gas, but to also quantitate it numerically (see a wave form via capnography). The use of capnometry, however, does not relieve you of the responsibility of performing the usual clinical chores associated with endotracheal intubation. Although capnometry clearly verifies the presence of an endotracheal tube in the trachea in all but exceptional circumstances, it does not verify appropriate tube placement. Thus, one still needs to use clinical means to verify both, that the tube is in the tracheobronchial tree and that it is correctly placed in the trachea, above the carina. This is best done by listening with a stethoscope over the axillae and the epigastrium. And yet, even the presence of breath sounds at auscultation is not foolproof evidence that the tube has been correctly placed. For example, breath sounds over the epigastrium may be absent in a patient who has had a major gastric resection, despite the fact that the tube is in the esophagus. The consequences of an incorrectly placed endotracheal tube usually become evident within 1–2 min.

However, there are numerous anecdotal reports about delayed diagnoses of esophageal intubation. We are aware of a situation in which 40 minutes elapsed after the initial intervention before esophageal intubation was diagnosed. A number of factors may delay the diagnosis:

- A preoxygenated patient with good respiratory function may recover from paralysis and breathe spontaneously for several minutes before hypoxia becomes evident. Some authors have even suggested that for this very reason, routine preoxygenation should be avoided. The logic of avoiding preoxygenation to make an earlier diagnosis of esophageal intubation, however, is difficult to accept.
- An accidental extubation may occur with movement of the patient, especially movement of the head or neck.
- An endotracheal tube may slide up and down in the trachea (by as much as 5 cm according to radiologic studies).[19]
- A patient may be accidentally extubated during attempts to place a nasogastric tube.

If the vital signs of a recently intubated patient suddenly deteriorate, esophageal intubation must first be ruled out. There may be great reluctance to remove an endotracheal tube in some cases, especially when the initial intubation was difficult or when the patient has a full stomach or is morbidly obese. Nevertheless, the best advice to give under these circumstances is "if in doubt, take it out," and the sooner this decision is made the better.

The consequences of esophageal intubation include asphyxia (especially if the patient is paralyzed), regurgitation of gastric contents (enormously increased and a frequent cause of death), and acute gastric and intestinal distension (which becomes very obvious after several minutes of delivering about 5 L of gas per minute into the stomach).

Esophageal intubation is a preventable complication. Ideally, capnometry/capnography should be performed on every patient who is intubated because there is no guarantee that an endotracheal tube correctly placed initially will remain in position after intubation.

Accidental deglutition of endotracheal tubes is well documented in the neonatal and pediatric literature, but rarely seen in adults. Block et al.[20] reported such a case in a 28-year-old patient with head trauma. Attempts at intubation in the field by paramedics were unsuccessful. He was later intubated in the hospital. He made a full recovery and was discharged soon thereafter. Two years later, an incidental chest X-ray revealed an endotracheal tube in the stomach, which was surgically removed.

Ingestion of Laryngoscope Lightbulb

Ince et al.[21] reported an accidental ingestion of a lightbulb during laryngoscopy. The infant vomited a few hours later and the lightbulb was retrieved from the vomitus.

This complication would have been far more serious if the lightbulb was aspirated into the airway. Part of the equipment check before intubation should include scrutiny of all the detachable parts of the laryngoscope.

Accidental Endobronchial Intubation

In the early stages of learning the technique of endotracheal anesthesia, most students have a natural tendency to advance the tube too far into the tracheobronchial tree. Because of the anatomical layout of the trachea and mainstem bronchi, there is a greater tendency to advance the tube into the right mainstem bronchus particularly in adults (Fig. 15, Chap. 8). The right upper lobe bronchus arises, in most cases, about 2.5 cm from the carina. Thus, right mainstem intubations are quite often associated with collapse of both the left lung and the right upper lobe.

This complication is easily detected provided one follows the basic instructions of auscultation of the chest after placing an endotracheal tube. Notice also whether compliance of the lungs is significantly diminished. With a keen eye, one can detect asymmetrical movement of the chest wall. In addition, endobronchial intubation is often associated with "bucking" and straining by the patient and some become cyanotic. With the tube in the right mainstem bronchus, one is attempting to deliver the complete tidal volume into one lung, causing a significant increase in peak inspiratory pressure, and thus alerting one to the diagnosis. Also look at the centimeter marking on the tube. In an adult patient, it should be about 25 cm at the level of the nose during nasotracheal intubation, and about 22 cm at the level of the teeth during orotracheal intubation. However, these numbers should only be used as a guide. In some cases, the distance from the teeth to the carina may be only 20 cm, in others it may be 25 cm. For these reasons, auscultation of the chest is of paramount importance. One may also notice that it requires higher concentrations of inhalational anesthetics to keep the patient anesthetized. Finally, pulse oximetry and end-tidal CO_2 monitoring can be used to detect misplacement of the tube in a more timely fashion.

Bronchospasm

Asthmatic patients are very sensitive to any type of airway manipulation and, unless properly handled, will develop bronchospasm that is sometimes so severe that it causes life-threatening hypoxemia. Bronchospasm may be described as an increased tone in the bronchial smooth muscles, leading to narrowing of the bronchi and bronchioles. The diagnosis is made when high-pitched rhonchi are detected upon auscultation of the chest. The etiology is not clearly known, but may be related to an excessive discharge from the nerves that supply the smooth muscles of the bronchi. It may also be chemically mediated. These patients are a particular challenge to those responsible for airway management. If there is even a hint of bronchospasm, elective surgery must be postponed because invariably the bronchospasm will become more intense during anesthesia, possibly due to an increased production of bronchial secretions and increased bronchomotor tone. Preoperative preparation is optimally facilitated by priming patients with aerosolized bronchodilators, anticholinergics, and in severe cases, steroids. Endotracheal intubation should be performed only after the patient is deeply anesthetized. Bronchospasm may be the first manifestation of pneumonitis following aspiration of acidic material from the stomach.

Difficulty with Ventilation

Successfully placing an endotracheal tube in the glottis does not guarantee successful ventilation. If, after connecting the oxygen source, you are unable to effectively ventilate a patient, you must evaluate the situation systematically. First deliver 100% oxygen and auscultate the chest. The most common problems are endobronchial tube placement, bronchospasm, and undiagnosed pathology (e.g., pleural effusions or pneumothorax). Difficulty with ventilation may occur following esophageal intubation, especially in the later stages, and the aspiration of gastric contents may go unnoticed, though it usually presents with signs of bronchospasm. In the delivery room, you may encounter a neonate with diaphragmatic hernia. In these cases pulmonary compliance is so poor that ventilation is almost impossible.

When confronted with difficulty ventilating a patient, one must ask four questions:

- Is the problem related to disease process in the patient?
- Is it related to tube placement?
- Is it due to obstruction of the tube?
- Is it caused by the oxygen delivery system?

Time permitting, each of these questions should be answered satisfactorily. Obstruction of the endotracheal tube may occur secondary to any of the following:

- Kinking
- Biting
- Cuff herniation
- Foreign body in the lumen
- A small-diameter tube
- Blood and secretions
- Manufacturing defects

Laryngeal Intubation

This is not strictly a complication, but it could become one. Typically, one is called to the ward to replace an endotracheal tube because of excessive air leak around the cuff. Before doing so, however, one should investigate further. It is always a good idea to note the centimeter marking on the tube at the level of the teeth, which gives a reasonable clue as to the depth of the tube. In situations such as this, the tip of the tube is indeed below the vocal cords, but the cuffed portion may be partly outside and partly inside the larynx. Thus, large volumes of air are required to seal the leak. The nurse may inform you that as much as 30 cc have already been injected, but it is always a good idea to perform simple laryngoscopy. If the diagnosis is correct, a large globular, transparent (balloon like) object is evident in the oropharynx. A timely laryngoscopy at this stage may save the day and spare the patient the inconvenience of an unnecessary repeat intubation. If the problem is not corrected, the patient is at risk for regurgitation and aspiration of gastric contents into the pulmonary tree as well as complete extubation.

Accidental Extubation

Failure to secure the endotracheal tube properly may result in an untimely extubation, which could be serious in an anesthetized patient undergoing surgery, especially when the patient is in the prone position.

Rupture of the Trachea or Bronchus

Rupture of the trachea or bronchus in association with endotracheal or endobronchial intubation is a rare and devastating complication. Most of the problems seem to arise in association with endobronchial tubes.[22-24] Sakuragi et al.[25] reported a case of rupture of a mainstem bronchus during insertion of a double lumen (DL) tube. Rupture occurred in the membranous portion of the DL tube, which was advanced too far into the left mainstem. The patient was a very small, elderly female. Even though very little force was used, the tracheal portion of the DL tube was too large for the bronchus and ruptured it at its weakest point. In many instances, the etiology is poorly understood. Predisposing factors include:

- Trauma
- Age
- Preexisting disease
- Nitrous oxide diffusion
- Tissue fragility
- Excessive force

The diagnosis may be suspected when patients present with:

- Subcutaneous emphysema
- Decreased pulmonary compliance
- Tension pneumothorax
- Hemorrhage
- Unexplained air leak
- Surgical exposure

To avoid such complications, the following guidelines should be used when placing endotracheal or endobronchial tubes:

- Never use force
- Be careful with stylets and bougies and always apply lubricant to both the tube and the stylet
- Do not overinflate the cuff
- When using nitrous oxide, be sure to intermittently deflate the cuff
- When performing esophagoscopy, always deflate the cuff during insertion of the esophagoscope
- Use fiberoptic bronchoscopy to verify tracheal placement of endobronchial tube

Tension Pneumothorax

Tension pneumothorax is a life-threatening complication that may occur in association with endotracheal intubation. The diagnosis is made clinically, and one rarely has time to obtain radiologic confirmation. The cardinal signs are:

1. Marked cyanosis
2. Deteriorating vital signs
3. Tracheal deviation
4. Diminished breath sounds
5. A marked decrease in pulmonary compliance

Immediate treatment consists of inserting a large-bore needle into the affected side of the chest beneath the second rib. Most patients improve dramatically within a matter of seconds.

Hypertension, Tachycardia, and Arrhythmias

Laryngoscopy and intubation are powerful stimuli to patients even in the anesthetized state. The most significant stimulus occurs when the endotracheal tube enters the trachea. A marked surge in blood pressure and heart rate may occur in the hypertensive patient unless he or she is deeply anesthetized or unless a vasodilator is used. Arrhythmias may also occur during and following intubation. ST segment changes may be evident on the ECG.

Persistent changes of this nature must be treated aggressively. Fortunately, ischemic changes are usually transient. Hypertension and tachycardia in the setting of intubation are likely due to systemically mediated vasomotor center stimulation. Hemodynamic responses to intubation in children are quite different from those in adults, especially those in the younger age groups. They frequently experience bradycardia during intubation, which is probably vagally mediated.

Elevated Intracranial Pressure

Endotracheal intubation often provokes a significant increase in intracranial pressure, which could be dangerous in an individual who has an intracranial aneurysm, cerebral edema, intracranial bleeding, or raised intracranial pressure. Every effort, therefore, must be made to control intracranial pressure in susceptible patients. Changes in intracranial pressure can be minimized with hyperventilation and blood pressure control and by the prevention of coughing and straining. Anesthetic drugs (e.g., thiopental and lidocaine) reduce intracranial pressure and may be useful in this situation.

Complications Arising upon Removal of Endotracheal Tube

Hypoxemia

Laryngospasm

Laryngospasm is a functional form of airway obstruction that, to date, has defied definition. It is poorly understood and often mislabeled. A physiologic mechanism has not yet been elucidated. The term *laryngospasm* has been loosely connected with any "crowing" sound emanating from the larynx. Fink,[26] who has shed more light on this interesting condition than most others, suggests that crowing emanating from the airway is due to apposition of the "true" vocal cords (which are readily separated by positive pressure ventilation). This phenomenon is otherwise known as "shutter spasm" and is often a harbinger of true laryngospasm. Fink suggests that true laryngospasm is a form of airway obstruction caused by contraction of the extrinsic muscles of the larynx, which encroach on the airway in a ball valve-like fashion (Fig. 15.1). He maintains that the extrinsic muscles of the larynx come together much like a closed accordion, and in contrast to shutter spasm or stridor, the application of positive pressure may make the obstruction worse by forcing air into the piriform fossae (Fig. 15.2).

Incidence

Laryngospasm has a predilection for younger individuals.[27] The incidence in all age groups has been estimated to be 8.7/1,000 persons studied and 17.4/1,000 between the ages of 0 and 9 years. The highest incidence seemed to be in infants between 1 and 3 months of age. While most anesthesiologists view it as a self-limiting condition devoid of serious morbidity, the literature reveals that 5/1,000 patients who develop laryngospasm have a cardiac arrest.

The following factors influence its development:

- Inadequate anesthesia
- Premature extubation
- Semicomatose states
- Aspiration of materials into the tracheobronchial tree
- Presence of a nasogastric tube

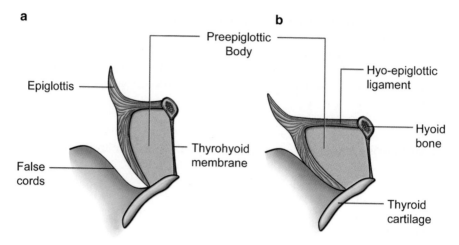

Fig. 15.1 Sagittal section showing the action of a laryngeal ball valve. (**a**) Open; (**b**) closed. During laryngeal closure, the preepiglottic body (*PB*) is squeezed between the hyoid bone (*H*) and the thyroid cartilage (*T*). The paraglottis buckles and is forced against the upper surface of the false cords (*FC*)

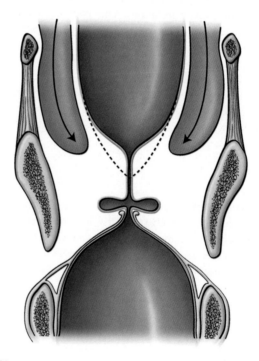

Fig. 15.2 Effect of bag pressure on the closed larynx. Attempted inflation of the lungs distends the piriform fossae (*arrows*) and reinforces the closure

The highest incidence has been reported in children with upper respiratory tract infections (95.8/1,000).

Clinical Features

The onset of laryngospasm is usually quite sudden. It may occur in any age group, but children are especially vulnerable. Premature extubation is the usual offending stimulus. Typically, there is very little warning and the patient rapidly desaturates. Effective positive-pressure ventilation is rarely possible until either a neuromuscular blocking drug is administered or profound hypoxia ensues. Premature application of a tourniquet or a rectal examination in a lightly anesthetized patient may be sufficient to induce it. Light anesthesia may sensitize laryngeal reflexes to develop spasm.

Laryngospasm typically occurs with unusual rapidity following stimulation of the airway in a lightly anesthetized patient. In contrast to stridor, which is characterized by a crowing sound of varying pitch, laryngospasm is a relatively silent phenomenon characterized by strenuous respiratory efforts similar to those observed in a choking victim. There is no obvious movement of air and O_2 saturation falls rapidly. Positive-pressure ventilation (PPV) is generally ineffective under these circumstances. Laryngospasm usually breaks when profound hypoxia occurs; however, most anesthesiologists intervene before allowing this to occur. Although PPV is probably ineffective under these circumstances, few authors would argue with its use because, when the spasm eventually does abate, O_2 may be immediately delivered to the lungs. Small doses of neuromuscular blocking drugs intravenously (succincylcholine 10 mg/70 kg) are usually rapidly effective in breaking the spasm. An anticholinergic is recommended when Succinylcholine is administered under these circumstances especially in children. (An intramuscular [IM] injection may be necessary in the absence of IV access.) Fink has suggested that laryngospasm may be relieved by performing the triple airway maneuver (which serves to disengage the supraglottic body from its locked position on the glottis).

Larson[28] published a letter to the editor in *Anesthesiology* describing the most effective treatment of laryngospasm. The author's description of the maneuver is as follows: "The technique involves placing the middle finger of each hand in what I call the laryngospasm notch. This notch is behind the lobule of the pinna of each ear. It is bounded anteriorly by the ascending ramus of the mandible adjacent to the condyle, posteriorly by the mastoid process of the temporal bone, and cephalad by the base of the skull. The therapist presses very firmly inward toward the base of the skull with both fingers, while at the same time lifting the mandible at a right angle to the plane of the body (i.e., forward displacement of the mandible or "jaw thrust"). Properly performed, it will convert laryngospasm within one or two breaths to laryngeal stridor and in another few breaths to unobstructed respirations" (Fig. 15.3).

The author convincingly reported the high degree of success experienced with this maneuver in cases of laryngospasm, but was unable to explain the mechanism and gave credit to a former mentor for this important "pearl."

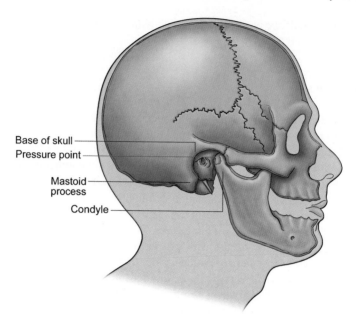

Base of skull
Pressure point
Mastoid process
Condyle

Fig. 15.3 Schematic illustration of laryngospasm notch bounded anteriorly by the condyle of the mandible, posteriorly by the mastoid process, and superiorly by the base of the skull. Digital pressure is applied firmly inwardly and anteriorly on each side of the head at the apex of the notch (see *pressure point arrow*), which is slightly cephalad to the plane of the earlobes (not shown)

Laryngospasm may be life-threatening in patients with limited cardiorespiratory reserve and should be avoided in all patients, not just those who are particularly vulnerable. It is impossible to quantitate the long-term effects of brief episodes of hypoxemia, but common sense suggests that one should strive to maintain good oxygenation in any patient who has entrusted one with this responsibility. Therefore, every effort should be made to prevent laryngospasm. Negative pressure pulmonary edema may develop in spontaneously breathing patients following laryngospasm. Extubation should be carefully timed especially in children and all external stimuli should be avoided in a child who is emerging from anesthesia. Ideally, the child should be able to open his eyes and make purposeful movements before extubation. And, if deep extubation is required, be sure that the child is indeed deep. Lidocaine 2 mg/kg IV within 2–3 min of extubation may reduce the tendency toward laryngospasm. If a child is bucking on the endotracheal tube or has a conjugate gaze, it is advisable to allow him to wake up before extubation. It is also important to allow regular respirations to occur before extubation.

In summary, laryngospasm is a relatively common clinical situation in pediatric anesthesia. Serious morbidity rarely occurs, but healthy patients may become profoundly hypoxic for brief periods. The problem can be prevented by following some simple rules when the patient is emerging from anesthesia.

Airway Obstruction

Airway obstruction may occur immediately upon removal of the endotracheal tube if done prematurely. For example, a patient may not have recovered fully from anesthesia, narcotic and sedative drugs, or neuromuscular blocking agents. Inadequate tone in the muscles of the jaw and tongue allows the tongue to approach the posterior pharyngeal wall, causing obstruction of the airway. Patients who develop airway obstruction following extubation should be given high O_2 concentrations; bag/valve/mask ventilation may be required, and occasionally patients may require reintubation. This issue is discussed in much greater detail in Chap. 14.

Vomiting and Aspiration

If a patient's reflexes are impaired upon removal of the endotracheal tube, vomiting and regurgitation can result in aspiration.

Sore Throat

Sore throat is probably the most common complaint that patients have following intubation, especially in association with anesthesia. The incidence varies somewhere between 5 and 100%, depending on the author.[29] There have been some interesting observations in the literature. First, the incidence is doubled in patients who are intubated during anesthesia vs. those who are not. Second, it is greater in patients who have a nasogastric tube in place. Third, it is greater in female than in male patients. And fourth,[30] the incidence and severity are proportional to the internal diameter of the endotracheal tube that was used.

Abrasions and lacerations of the oropharynx and nasopharynx can occur, especially lacerations of the palatopharyngeal and the palatoglossal folds, when intubation is attempted by inexperienced personnel.

Steward[31] reviewed the problem in children undergoing outpatient anesthesia and reported a 59% incidence. He also found that the incidence was proportional to the duration of surgery: 24% when an oral airway was in place and 8.5% when neither an oral airway nor an endotracheal tube was used. A more recent study by Monroe et al.[32] in adults showed that the presence of a hard, plastic, oropharyngeal airway did not appear to influence the incidence of sore throat, although the incidence of sore throat was increased relative to the incidence of pharyngeal trauma from any cause. Vigorous suctioning of the oropharynx may contribute significantly to the incidence of postoperative sore throat.

Temporomandibular Joint Dysfunction

Temporomandibular joint dysfunction following the administration of an anesthetic is quite unusual. Etiologic factors include prolonged mouth opening and forcible advancement of the mandible during airway maneuvers. Subluxation with dislocation has been reported.[33] Upon awakening, the patient notices the inability to close the mouth. Subluxation and dislocation may occur during intubation when patients are profoundly relaxed. Although the mandible can be manually manipulated, it is quite painful in the conscious state. Do not hesitate to consult an oral surgeon when the problem arises. The temporomandibular joint is quite complicated and must be handled carefully.

Vocal Cord Injury

Postintubation Croup

Postintubation croup occurs in association with edema of the true vocal cords and is most commonly seen in children. A barking cough is diagnostic. The smaller the child, the higher the risk. It is usually self-limiting, and treatment consists of humidified oxygen, racemic epinephrine, and dexamethasone (2 mg/kg IV). Caution should be used before discharging a child from outpatient facilities when stridor is present; if in doubt, admit the patient overnight for observation. As it progresses, the treatment presents the physician with a real dilemma because the very instrument that caused the problem may also be the one needed to deal with it.

Difficult Extubation

Volumes have been written about the "difficult" intubation; however, it is interesting to note that extubation may also be difficult, for a variety of reasons. Clearly, pathology within the larynx can interfere with one's ability to withdraw an endotracheal tube. Occasionally, and not always easily explained, the cuff of an endotracheal tube remains inflated. This complication has occurred with the Laser-Flex tube, but may also occur with regular endotracheal tubes. Sometimes an endotracheal tube will become inadvertently fixed to surrounding structures by an unsuspecting surgeon operating in the vicinity of the oropharynx or neck. The inability to deflate the cuff is easily remedied by piercing the balloon under direct vision, or by inserting a needle through the cricothyroid ligament. The number of anecdotes about endotracheal tubes being accidentally fixed in place with Kirschner wires, screws, and sutures increases with the passage of time.

Arytenoid Dislocation

Dislocation of an arytenoid cartilage is an unusual injury that can occur following blunt trauma to the neck, or medical instrumentation of the larynx (Fig. 15.4). The symptoms and signs include hoarseness, aphonia, stridor, sore throat, a "lump in the throat," and unilateral or bilateral vocal cord paresis or paralysis. This condition has been reported in adults, children, and neonates. Older patients and women may be more susceptible, and left-sided dislocation appears to be more common. There are only about 80 cases reported in the anesthesia literature.[34] The problem may become evident immediately upon recovering from anesthesia or later, although the diagnosis is usually made clinically (direct laryngoscopy) or by CT scan. The dislocation

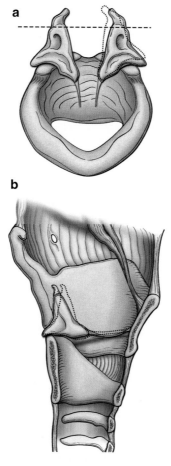

Fig. 15.4 Position of a displaced arytenoid (*solid line*) compared to normal (*dotted line*). (**a**) Anterior view showing the left arytenoid displaced anteriorly, medially, and inferiorly with bowing of the true vocal fold. (**b**) Sagittal view showing anteroinferior displacement of the arytenoid with paradoxical posterior displacement of the superior process

may be corrected by manipulating the arytenoid cartilage with a spatula, which is done under local anesthesia and requires the expertise of an otolaryngologist. Postoperative vocal cord paralysis may be a manifestation of arytenoids dislocation; however, a neurogenic cause of these symptoms must be ruled out. Arytenoid dislocation has been reported in two patients following the use of the lighted stylet.[35] Usui et al.[36] reported a case following the use of the McCoy laryngoscope. Common sense would suggest that the incidence might be higher following traumatic intubation. For more complete details about this interesting condition, refer to a treatise on the topic published in the *Archives of Otolaryngology* by Quick and Merwin.[37]

Cord Avulsion

Avulsion of the vocal cords is a rare form of traumatic injury associated with endotracheal intubation that occurs in association with unsuccessful blind attempts at intubation using a styletted endotracheal tube. If suspected at any time, an ENT surgeon should be consulted regarding further treatment.

Neural Injury

Recurrent Laryngeal Nerve Injury

Unilateral or bilateral vocal cord paralysis or paresis is a rare occurrence following intubation and the etiology is not well understood.[38-40] It may occur following prolonged intubation or intubation for a brief period.[41] Symptoms may be immediately evident or delayed. Patients usually present with stridor and dyspnea and tracheostomy may be necessary. The etiology is not well understood, but it has been suggested that the cuff of the endotracheal tube exerts pressure on one or both recurrent laryngeal nerves. Ellis and Pallister[42] have suggested that the anterior branch of the recurrent laryngeal nerve can be compressed against the lamina of the thyroid cartilage by the inflated cuff of the endotracheal tube. Whited[43] has suggested that traumatic cricoarytenoid joint arthritis is the mechanism of this malady. The prognosis depends upon whether the recurrent laryngeal nerves recover spontaneously or not, which is dependent upon the degree of scarring and fibrosis in the cricoarytenoid joints. Tracheostomy is the initial front line treatment for this problem and arytenoidectomy may be necessary later if decannulation cannot be achieved.

The authors recollect one case of vocal cord paralysis in our combined years' experience. The patient developed bilateral vocal cord paresis following a relatively short surgical procedure. The anesthesiologist reported an uneventful laryngoscopy and intubation and even recorded the amount of air that was used to inflate the cuff. Fortunately, this patient did not require a tracheostomy and recovered fully after several days.

Although neuropraxia is the most likely explanation, other possibilities must also be considered. The random nature of Bell's palsy, for example, is well known; perhaps some recurrent laryngeal nerve injuries are caused by a viral neuritis. The recurrent laryngeal nerve can be injured during attempts to place a central venous catheter. Surgical trauma during thyroid surgery or thoracotomy should also be considered. Hyperextension of the neck may exert traction on the recurrent laryngeal nerve. Vocal cord paralysis has also been linked with nasogastric tube insertion. The mechanism is thought to be due to erosion or ulceration of the posterior cricoid plate followed by diffuse inflammation, eventually involving the recurrent laryngeal nerves.[44-46] In a way, this condition is a bit of a medical curiosity, though not a pleasant experience for the person afflicted. Therefore, be meticulous when performing endotracheal intubation. Select the correct-sized tube and inject the minimum amount of air required to create a seal into the cuff. Also, be aware that nitrous oxide can diffuse into the cuff and add significantly to the pressure applied to the tracheal mucosa. When the cuff pressure on the mucosa exceeds normal capillary pressure (25–30 mmHg), ischemia may occur.

Lingual, Hypoglossal, and Mental Nerve Damage

Neurological deficits over the distribution of the lingual and hypoglossal nerves have been reported[47,48] (p72-73). These deficits are probably related to traction during routine airway management or direct laryngoscopy, and the patient usually recovers with time. Lingual nerve injury is a rare complication of laryngoscopy and airway management, which may occur as an isolated event or in association with hypoglossal nerve injury. Although the etiology is not clearly delineated, it is likely due to compression of the nerve during forceful laryngoscopy. A recent report by Venkatesh and Walker[49] (p74) describes a case of hypoglossal nerve injury following an unplanned extubation of a patient while the cuff of the endotracheal tube remained inflated. They suggested that the inflated cuff may have compressed the hypoglossal nerve up against the hyoid bone (see Fig. 15.15 in Chap. 1) and that traction during extubation may have stretched the nerve. Cricoid pressure and vigorous mandibular maneuvers may be contributing factors. As many as eight cases have been reported in the world literature so far. Similar to other neuropraxic injuries, the condition is usually temporary and recovery is complete.

Mental Nerve

Montoya Pelaez et al.[50] recently reported a case of mental nerve compression, secondary to pressure exerted on the chin by a Ring Adhere Elwin (RAE) tube.

Complications Arising from Long-Term Intubation

With advances in technology, materials used for endotracheal intubation have become less injurious to the tissues. However, long-term complications still occur.

Ulceration of the Mouth, Pharynx, Larynx, and Trachea

Ulcers are uncommon following endotracheal intubation and heal spontaneously after the offending agent is removed.

Granuloma Formation

Polypoid growths occur on the vocal cords of some patients who have been intubated and are most likely the result of trauma. The incidence varies between 1/1,000 and 1/20,000 cases and is more common in women. Surgical removal may be required.

Formation of Synechiae and Webs

Trauma to the vocal cords may lead to loss of mucous membrane, causing the vocal cords to adhere to one another. This condition, called synechiae formation, is a rare occurrence. Membrane or web formation may occur in the larynx or trachea following intubation and is also rare, usually an incidental finding at autopsy.

Tracheal Stenosis

Tracheal stenosis occurs because of damage to the mucous membrane and cartilaginous framework of the trachea. It is most often associated with prolonged intubation. In recent years, however, cuffs have been designed to minimize the amount of pressure exerted on the tracheal wall, and the current materials used to manufacture endotracheal tubes are less irritating to tissues.

When the pressure exerted laterally on the tracheal wall exceeds capillary pressure (approximately 25 mmHg in a healthy patient), ischemia to the mucous membrane may occur. This can be minimized by using more compliant cuffs and injecting the minimal amount of air required. The cuff should be deflated at intervals in any patient undergoing prolonged ventilation to allow perfusion of the mucous membrane at the cuff site.

The length of time an endotracheal tube should be allowed to remain in place before a tracheostomy is a controversial issue. There are two schools of thought. The traditional approach is to perform tracheostomy after 2 weeks of endotracheal intubation unless the patient is ready to be extubated in the near future. The other, more liberal approach is to allow intubation for several months before a tracheostomy is considered. There are no hard-and-fast rules about which school is correct. Each should be assessed on its own merits. Patients requiring chronic airway care are rarely accepted by chronic care institutions unless a tracheostomy is performed. This is one of the more common indications for tracheostomy in a hospital setting today. More outcome studies are needed to make a decision on this very important issue.

Complications Occurring Specifically in Relation to Nasotracheal Intubation

Epistaxis

Bleeding is common during nasal intubation. Sometimes it occurs as a result of nasal polyps or trauma to Little's area (or Kiesselbach's area). Endotracheal tubes should be well lubricated, and a decongestant should be used whenever possible. When introducing a nasal tube, be sure to align the bevel parallel to the septum to avoid disruption of the turbinates. On attempting to pass a tube through the nose, direct it at a right angle to the horizontal in a supine patient. The tube selected should be a half to one whole size less than that commonly used for orotracheal intubation. It is also a good idea to place the tube in warm saline before use as it softens the texture of the tube.

Submucosal Dissection

Occasionally, an endotracheal tube may be forcibly passed submucosally into the nasopharynx. This complication manifests itself by creating an elongated bulge just above the tonsillar area of the oropharynx on either side. The operator usually complains of not being able to find the tip of the tube in the oropharynx. This complication is self-limiting, unless the tube is hooked to an oxygen source. In that event, massive subcutaneous emphysema and airway obstruction may develop.

Middle Turbinectomy

Middle turbinectomy is a reported complication of nasotracheal intubation. Dislocation of the middle turbinate has also been reported following nasotracheal intubation. These complications can also follow the passage of nasopharyngeal airways. The authors observed an unusual case of airway obstruction following passage of a nasopharyngeal airway. The patient developed complete airway obstruction following passage of a nasopharyngeal airway. Direct laryngoscopy revealed a large polyp completely occluding the airway. The polyp was removed with a McGill forceps and the obstruction was immediately relieved.

Baumann et al.[51] recently reported airway obstruction following the passage of a "trumpet" nasopharyngeal airway into the nose that entered the submucosal space and eventually the retropharyngeal space, causing serious airway obstruction.

Trauma to the Posterior Pharyngeal Wall

As with oral intubation, when nasotracheal intubation is being done, the endotracheal tube may encroach on the posterior pharyngeal wall and cause bleeding.

Trauma to the Adenoids

Bleeding during either nasotracheal or orotracheal intubation may occur secondary to trauma to the adenoids, especially in children.

Pressure Necrosis in the Nose

Ischemia of and necrosis within the nose may occur following nasotracheal intubation, but it can be prevented by proper stabilization of the tube and by using a specially designed connector. Necrosis may eventually lead to stricture of a nostril.

Obstruction of the Eustachian Tube

The eustachian tube may become obstructed secondary to prolonged nasotracheal intubation.

Maxillary Sinusitis

Sinusitis[52] is a complication of nasotracheal intubation caused by blockage of the opening into the maxillary sinus. It may be a hidden source of sepsis in a critically ill patient on an intensive care ward.

Complications of Laser Surgery

Laser surgery has now been in vogue for several years for the treatment of many conditions, including laryngeal tumors.[53] A number of precautions must be taken when it is performed on the larynx. First, the exposed part of the endotracheal tube must be wrapped with metallic foil to prevent the tube from igniting. Specially designed tubes are also available for this purpose. Second, nitrous oxide and oxygen both support combustion. Therefore, a combination of oxygen and helium is preferable in these situations because the mixture is less likely to flare and helium is capable of dissipating the heat at a faster rate. Furthermore, because of its physical properties, helium may enhance the flow of gases through the tube. Finally, personnel should wear protective glasses when laser treatment is in progress.

Summary

Although the list of complications associated with endotracheal intubation is lengthy and imposing, most of them can be avoided by paying attention to a few details. Many are associated with hypoxemia and thus every effort must be made to maintain adequate oxygenation at all times. If difficulties are anticipated, preoxygenate the patient for 2 or 3 min. Traumatic complications are quite common and some can be disfiguring and annoying to the patient; others, such as tension pneumothorax, are life-threatening.

Never use force when placing an endotracheal tube. Dental damage, though common, is often avoidable and is a great source of annoyance to patients. Esophageal intubation is a major cause of serious morbidity and mortality. You can never be too sure about placing an endotracheal tube, and there is no guarantee that once placed correctly, it will remain in place. Even experienced clinicians have failed to detect esophageal intubation. Finally, remember that there is no greater responsibility than that of oxygenating patients who are unable to do so themselves.

Airway Management Complications Summarized from Anesthesiology Morbidity Studies

Over the years, anesthesiologists have sought to catalog the types of airway-related injuries, as well as to establish causes. Understanding the problems and causes and implementing changes of technique, pharmacology, and equipment have led to improved patient safety. Guidelines and protocols are published to disseminate information and to standardize and improve care.

Anesthesiologists have led the way in establishing safer airway management practices. Worldwide, professional organizations, researchers, and teachers dedicate a very large portion of their time, expense, and effort toward improving airway management practices. Organizations such as the Society of Airway Management (USA) and the Difficult Airway Society (DAS) in UK were founded, in part, to establish a forum dedicated to this aspect of medicine, which is important to all practitioners, not just anesthesiologists.

In the past, morbidity studies have been rather limited in scope, anecdotal, and even biased. Poor outcomes implied blame. A litigious social environment did not encourage the practitioner to broadcast shortcomings. Because poor anesthesia-related outcome is so rare, large, prospective, controlled, randomized studies would be very expensive to conduct. None has been undertaken to date.

Recently, several ongoing studies have been reporting morbidity statistics that are gathered utilizing different methods. Some of the studies are large and investigators have been retrieving and analyzing data for many years. Other studies are unique because of methodology or more focused scope. While many aspects of anesthesia morbidity are dealt with in these studies, only complications related to airway management will be described in this section. Hopefully, the lessons learned by anesthesiologists will be useful to other practitioners of airway management.

American Society of Anesthesiologists Closed Claims Study

The ASA Closed Claims Study was initiated in 1985 by the ASA Committee on Professional Liability.[17] The study analyzes closed insurance claims. A *claim* is a financial demand made to an insurance company by a person alleging injury sustained from medical care. Once the claim is resolved, it is *closed*. Through the years, the ASA has gained the cooperation of 35 medical liability insurance companies and has gathered close to 8,000 claims into its database. Dental claims are not included in the study. A closed claim file typically includes the hospital and anesthesia records, narratives from involved personnel, "expert and peer reviews, deposition summaries, outcome reports, and the cost of settlement or jury awards."[54] The file is examined on site at the insurance company office by volunteer practicing anesthesiologists using standardized forms with specific instructions. The claims are further reviewed by project investigators and other anesthesiologists to establish reliability of the review process. The study characterizes claims according to two basic features: *damaging events* and *adverse outcomes*. There are more adverse outcomes than damaging events "because some patients display injuries for which a specific damaging event cannot be identified in the records."

The project managers and authors reporting data from the study admit that there are limitations to the study's design that must be considered when reviewing the published findings. Most notably, these limitations include the following:

Limitations of the Closed Claims Study

1. The study does not provide a denominator for calculating the risk of injury.
2. The study is voluntary.
3. The insurance carriers do not cover all of the practicing anesthesiologists in the country.
4. The study is retrospective.
5. Some injured patients do not submit claims.
6. Data may be conflicting or incomplete.

Despite these limitations, the study can be used to define specific types of morbidity and to establish hypotheses concerning the mechanism and prevention of anesthetic injuries.

Following are various findings from the Closed Claims Study relating to *airway management complications.*

Respiratory System

Since the study began, damaging events related to respiration have been the single leading source of injury. These accounted for 27%[17] (p1) of the total claims reported in 2000 and 38% of the claims for death and brain damage[54] (p555) reported in 1999. The three most common mechanisms of injury, accounting for 75% of all respiratory claims involved, are as follows[54] (p4):

1. Inadequate ventilation (38% of cases)
2. Esophageal intubation (18% of cases)
3. Difficult intubation (17% of cases)

Respiratory-related claims were associated with severe outcomes (85% death or brain damage) and costly payments (median $200,000)[54] (p4).

An interesting conclusion of the study published in 2000 states that "most adverse respiratory outcomes were considered preventable with pulse oximetry, capnometry, or a combination of these two monitors"[54] (p4). A recent paper that addressed this hypothesis demonstrated that, while there was a significant decrease in the proportion of claims for death or brain damage from 1975 through 2000, the investigators were unable to demonstrate that the increased use of capnometry and pulse oximetry in recent years had any influence on this trend.[55] Since the introduction of these monitors, there has been a significant decline in the proportion of respiratory events and an increase in the number of cardiovascular damaging events leading to death or brain damage. It is clearly difficult to prove such a hypothesis, but, at the same time, common sense tells us that these monitors should reduce the risk of respiratory-related damaging events. However, there have been some other major changes in practice since 1986. One can speculate that the introduction of the laryngeal mask and other supraglottic devices has also had a significant influence on the incidence of respiratory events. If there are fewer attempts at intubation overall, there will be fewer adverse respiratory events. These devices have also become an important part of the "Difficult Airway Algorithm". Also difficult to measure is the impact of education on these outcomes. The number of airway management-related publications has increased exponentially in the last 30 years. Those responsible for airway management are now far more up-to-date about how to diagnose and manage the problem airway in modern times.

Management of the Difficult Intubation in Closed Malpractice Claims

A report published in 2000 analyzed 4,459 claims and deals specifically with the management of difficult intubation.[56] The most common *damaging events* reported in the study were difficult intubation (6.4%), esophageal intubation (4.5%), inadequate ventilation/oxygenation (7%), and the wrong drug or dose (4%).

Brain damage or death was the outcome of 57% of the claims involving difficult intubation, compared to 43% of the claims concerning other *damaging events*.

Demographically, the claims involving difficult intubation tended to represent older, sicker, and more obese patients.

Disconcertingly, the study revealed that in nearly half of the claims involving difficult intubation, *difficulty was not anticipated*. In fact, a preoperative airway history was not taken and a preoperative airway physical examination was not conducted in 25 and 22% of the claims, respectively. *When airway difficulty was anticipated, 28% of the claims contained no information concerning airway management strategy.*

This report also introduced a new "difficult airway" subset generated from data gathered on a collection form based on the ASA Difficult Airway Algorithm. Ninety-eight claims fell into this category. (These claims were collected before the LMA was commonly used in difficult airway scenarios).

Analysis of these 98 claims revealed that the "cannot intubate and cannot ventilate" situation occurred in nearly half of the reports. Hopefully, the "Closed Claims Project" will expand this subset's database and report more findings in the future.

Aspiration in Closed Malpractice Claims[57]

A report published in 2000 reviewing 4,459 claims states, "Of the total database, aspiration was either the primary or secondary *damaging event* (mechanism of injury) in 158 claims (3.5%). Aspiration was noted as the primary cause of the adverse event in about ½ of the 158 patients"[57] (p5).

The incidence of death and brain damage in aspiration-related claims is 60%, compared to 43% of the remainder of the claims in the database. This high percentage of severe morbidity of aspiration-related claims may reflect the fact that most aspiration complications are readily treatable and that only in those cases in which extremely poor outcome ensues is legal action instigated.

Gas Delivery Equipment and Closed Malpractice Claims[58]

Gas delivery equipment in the operating room, the recovery room, and the ICU was associated with 72 of 3,791 closed claims analyzed and reported in 1997. Problems with the breathing circuit accounted for the majority of equipment-based problems.

Misuse of the equipment rather than failure was implicated in 75% ($n=54$) of the claims.

The three most common damaging events identified were: breathing circuit misconnects (19%), breathing circuit disconnects (15%), and supply tank problems, most notably, oxygen switches (10%).

The reviewers judged that 78% of the claims could have been prevented if better monitoring had been used. Overall, 38% of the claims were deemed preventable if capnography, pulse oximetry, or both monitors had been used.

Ambulatory and Office-Based Anesthesia and Closed Claims[59,60]

Claims involving ambulatory surgery and office-based anesthesia practices are increasing as the database incorporates more recently gathered information. As of 2001, 14 office-based claims and 666 ambulatory surgery anesthesia claims in which damaging events could be identified have been recorded. Damaging events involved the respiratory system in 22% of the ambulatory claims and 50% of the office-based claims. Damaging events associated with ambulatory claims included difficult intubation, inadequate oxygenation or ventilation, and airway obstruction. In the office, damaging events included airway obstruction, bronchospasm, inadequate oxygenation-ventilation, and esophageal intubation. While the numbers are small, it was judged that in the office setting, 50% of the claims involved substandard care, while 46% of the claims were judged preventable if better monitoring had been utilized.

Airway Injury During Anesthesia

A review of 4,460 closed claims found 266 (6%) to be associated with airway injury (including injuries to the pharynx, esophagus, and TM joint). The most common sites of airway-related injury were the larynx (33%), the pharynx (19%), the esophagus (18%), and the trachea (15%).[7]

Laryngeal injuries included vocal cord paralysis (34%), granuloma (17%), arytenoid dislocation (8%), and hematoma (3%). Most laryngeal injuries were associated with short-term intubation.

Pharyngeal injuries included perforation (37%), lacerations and contusions (31%), localized infection (12%), sore throat without physical evidence of injury (12%), and miscellaneous (8%). Pharyngeal perforations were also caused by other equipment such as the nasogastric tube, suction catheter, and jet ventilator.

The most common esophageal injury was perforation (90%). Esophageal perforations were also caused by a nasogastric tube, esophageal dilator, esophageal stethoscope, and surgical manipulation of a laryngoscope.

Tracheal injuries included injury from the creation of a tracheotomy (64%), perforation (33%), and infection (3%).

With respect to the perforation claims, early signs (pneumothorax and subcutaneous emphysema) were present 51% of the time. Late signs (retropharyngeal abscess and mediastinitis) were present 63% of the time.

The payment for esophageal injuries (median: $138,975) was higher than for any other class of injury.

"Injuries to the esophagus and trachea were more frequently associated with difficult intubation. Injuries to the temporomandibular joint and the larynx were more frequently associated with routine intubation"[7] (p1703).

In conclusion, the ASA Closed Claims Study has been a very useful instrument to help anesthesiologists understand the types and mechanisms of airway-related morbidity. The information generated from the study will help researchers design prospective studies that could establish cause and effect relationships between specific injuries and the mechanisms leading to the injuries. Information reported by the study has guided anesthesiologists to propose protocols and guidelines designed to promote safer patient care.

Australian Incident Monitoring Study (AIMS)

The AIMS began in 1988. The study is administered by the Australian Patient Safety Foundation. The purpose of AIMS is to collect data documenting incidents that could or did cause patient injury in the practice of anesthesia in Australia. The anesthesiologist involved in the incident voluntarily submits a confidential form concerning the incident to the AIMS staff, who then process the data. While the methodology of the study shares some of the limitations of the ASA Closed Claims Study, the AIMS design may offer more clinically relevant and accurate data for a few noteworthy reasons. First, the clinician involved with the incident personally and promptly submits the data. The data are supplied firsthand. Second, investigators do not have to wait for an alleged victim to instigate data collection either through a malpractice suit or an insurance claim. Third, the form submitted in the proper fashion is complete. It is designed to minimize incomplete data collection. Fourth, reviewers are not biased by narratives from self-proclaimed medical experts, or confused by trying to interpret court proceedings; nor are they influenced by financial awards.

In 1993, the first 2,000 incidents of the AIMS were reported in a landmark symposium in the journal *Anaesthesia and Intensive Care*.[61,62] The following is a summary of the information reported in the symposium that is related to airway management complications. Information concerning equipment and monitors has been included, since the proper use and maintenance of both types of devices help to insure safe airway management. Updates to the 1993 data are made where available. Many incidents involved problems with the airway circuitry. These are listed in Table 15.2.

Table 15.2 Circuitry incidents, AIMS

Type of incident	1993 (2,000 Incidents)	2000 (6,000 Incidents)
Leak	129	474
Disconnect	148	437
Rebreathing	0	130
Misconnection	36	115
Disruption of gases	0	77
Overpressure	0	71
Other	6	404
Total	319[a]	1,708

Source: Russell et al.[62]; Petty[63]

[a]In two cases, more than one circuitry component was involved

Table 15.3 documents which circuitry component was involved in the incident reported.

Table 15.4 summarizes information from multiple studies related to difficult intubation, esophageal intubation, and endotracheal tube problems.[61,63-66]

The classification nomenclature was slightly different for the 2 years reported. In 1993, a subset of "difficult intubation" was described. In 2000, only a "failed intubation" category of incidents was presented. By implication, difficult intubations are included in this group.

Table 15.3 Circuitry involved in the incident, AIMS

Component	1993 (2,000 Incidents)	2000 (6,000 Incidents)
Endotracheal tube	4	550
Tubing or connection	5	392
Vaporizer	4	231
Ventilator	32	218
Absorber	4	159
Patient circuit valve (unidirectional valve)	46	144
Common gas outlet	0	112
Gas supply	6	74
Flowmeter	0	73
Humidifier	0	50
Scavenging system	0	43
Patient relief valve	0	24
Oxygen bypass	0	15
Laryngoscope	2	0
Other	6	225
Total	109	2,310

Source: Petty[63]; Webb et al.[64]

Table 15.4 Airway incidents, AIMS

Type of incident	1993 (2,000 Incidents)	2000 (6,000 Incidents)
Obstruction	35	686
Nonventilation	12	408
Endobronchial intubation	79	203
Difficult intubation	85	–
Failed intubation	17	174
Extubation	0	130
Esophageal intubation	35	104
Trauma	0	70
Misplaced tube (not in trachea or esophagus)	7	0
Inappropriate tube choice	5	0
Other	0	606
Total	275	2,381

The paper entitled "Difficult Intubation"[61] will be discussed in more detail. The authors analyzed 2,000 incidents and reported 85 (4%) cases of difficult intubation. One cardiac arrest was reported in this subset of cases, while there were no deaths. Of the 85 cases reported, in 27 (32%) difficult intubation was not predicted. In 22 (26%) preoperative evaluation of the airway predicted difficulty. In 17 (20%) of the cases intubation failed. A switch to regional anesthesia was made in 6 of the failures, surgery was canceled in 5 cases, and in 6 cases an emergency airway procedure was instituted. Various aids to intubation were utilized to help secure the difficult airway (Table 15.5).

Many factors contributed to the intubation's classification as difficult. These are listed in Table 15.6.

Finally, the complications that were associated with the 85 cases of difficult intubation are listed in Table 15.7.

Table 15.5 Aids to intubation, AIMS, 1993 (2,000 incidents)

Aid used	Number of cases
Gum elastic bougie	24
Introducer	15
Fiberoptic endoscope	11
Magill forceps	3
Rigid bronchoscope	1
Blind nasal intubation (all failed)	7

Source: Williamson et al.[61] with permission

Table 15.6 Factors contributing to difficult intubation, AIMS, 1993 (2,000 incidents)

Contributing factor	Number of reports
Obesity	14
Limited neck mobility	12
Limited mouth opening	11
Inadequate assistance	9
Teeth limiting access	5
Equipment deficiencies	5
Inexperienced intubator	4
Beard	2
Incorrect cricoid pressure	2
Wrong drug administered	2
Laryngeal tumor	1
Facial carcinoma	1
Masseter spasm	1
Ruptured trachea	1

Source: Williamson et al.[61] with permission

Table 15.7 Complications reported in association with difficult intubation, AIMS, 1993 (2,000 incidents)

Complication	Number of reports
Esophageal intubation	18
Arterial desaturation	15
Central cyanosis	7
Esophageal reflux	7
Bronchospasm	5
Laryngospasm	4
Intubation right mainstem bronchus	2
Loosened tooth	2
Epistaxis	1
Ruptured tube cuff	1
ECG ischemic signs	1
Esophageal tear	1
Lacerated tongue	1
Cardiac arrest	1
Annoyed theater staff	1

Source: Williamson et al.[61] with permission

The authors of the study suggested that a more thorough preoperative assessment of the airway and more readily available emergency airway equipment would be appropriate steps to help avoid and to manage difficult airways. Finally, the authors presented an algorithm that could be used to deal with difficult airway situations.

Monitors and the AIMS (1993: 2,000 Incidents)[67-69]

Of the 2,000 incidents under consideration, in 1,256 (63%) the authors signified that the role of the device used to monitor the patient undergoing general anesthesia was applicable to the study. They determined that the monitor detected the incident in 52% of the cases. The oximeter detected the incident in 27% of the cases, the capnography in 24% of the cases; this was followed by the ECG (19%), the blood pressure monitor (12%), low pressure (circuit) alarm (8%), and the oxygen analyzer (4%). The authors predicted that the oximeter used alone would have detected 82% of the incidents, 65% before organ damage occurred. Subsequent studies vindicate the guideline that both an oximeter and a capnograph be used on all patients undergoing any type of anesthetic. Oximeters should also be used to monitor sedated patients preoperatively as well as patients admitted to the recovery room after surgery.

AIMS and Obstetric Anesthesia[70]

An analysis of the first 5,000 AIMS incidents was published in 1999 which explored obstetric patients undergoing anesthesia and analgesia. There were 203 reports of 226 incidents related to anesthesia. Seven groups of incidents were reported.

Twenty-six reports were related to equipment problems (12.8%), 18 related to difficult or failed intubation (8.9%), and 16 related to problems with the endotracheal tube (7.8%). Equipment failure included problems with the anesthesia machine, circuit disconnects, central gas (oxygen) system failure, and one case of laryngoscope blade breakage. Difficult intubation was reported in 18 cases; intubation failed completely in 12 of these cases. Nine of the 12 cases occurred in the emergency setting. Other airway-related incidents dealt with single cases of aspiration, bronchospasm and hypoventilation, and desaturation of oxyhemoglobin to 89%.

In conclusion, the AIMS is an ongoing, large-scale study that continues to gather and report studies related to patient safety.

Deaths Attributed to Anesthesia in New South Wales: 1984–1990[71]

A study published in 1996 concerning anesthesia-related deaths from the years 1984 to 1990 reported data collected under more stringent methodological conditions than those imposed by the ASA Closed Claims Study or the AIMS. Under government mandate, all deaths that occurred under, as a result of, or within 24 h of an anesthetic had to be reported to the coroner. The coroner then notified the specialty committee investigating each death. The secretary of the committee would write the anesthetist to request that a questionnaire concerning details of the case be completed. The response rate for the years involved in the study was 93%. The New South Wales Special Committee Investigating Deaths Under Anaesthesia analyzed and reported the data. During this period, it was estimated that 3.5 million anesthetics had been performed in New South Wales. Confidentiality regarding the committee's activities has been legally guaranteed.

When considering the results of the study, the reader should recall that the data represent, at least in part, rather old findings. Many of the drugs, the equipment (such as the LMA), and the techniques (such as fiberoptically guided intubation) were not available or widely used in the early years of the study. Popular airway management protocols had not been published. However, since entry into the study was mandatory and a reasonable denominator had been established, the risk of mortality associated with anesthesia could be estimated. Unfortunately, the types and causes of less severe morbidity were not analyzed in the study.

The committee identified 1,503 deaths occurring in the years 1984–1990. The overall mortality rate per 10,000 anesthetics was calculated to be 4.4 (6.6 for males, 2.8 for females). Sixty percent of the deaths were considered inevitable, while 4% were considered accidental. The committee classified 172 deaths as "wholly or partly attributable to anaesthesia"[71] (p66). The airway-related conclusions of the study are reported here.

The first manifestation of crisis was respiratory in 22% of the deaths. Interestingly, the respiratory problem was first detected either in the recovery room or at another postoperative location in three quarters of the cases. Problems with the airway were the first indicators of crisis in 10 of the 172 cases. Most frequently, these airway problems occurred during surgical anesthesia, but 4 of these 10 cases occurred in the recovery room or in another postoperative location. The types and causes of the respiratory and airway problems were not specified in the study.

An important conclusion of the study was that postoperative care of the patient should include more vigilant airway and ventilation monitoring[71] (p73).

This study is unique for its methodological design. Hopefully, in the future, the study will be updated and the types and causes of injury will be more specifically reported. Perhaps less morbid outcomes could also be defined and analyzed.

The Pediatric Perioperative Cardiac Arrest Registry (POCA)[72]

In an attempt to determine factors and outcomes associated with cardiac arrest in anesthetized children, the POCA Registry was established in 1994. Institutions that provide anesthesia to children (patients 18 years or younger) voluntarily provide data to the Registry. Cardiac arrest is "defined as the need for chest compressions or as death"[72] (p6).

In the year 2000, data from the Registry's first 4 years of collection were published. There were 289 cases of cardiac arrest reported. Thirty of these deaths were respiratory-related, and the majority of these respiratory-related cardiac arrests were caused by laryngospasm, airway obstruction, or difficult intubation.[73]

The POCA Registry represents a new vehicle to collect, analyze, and report data related to one outcome of anesthesia practice. Its limitations are similar to those of the ASA Closed Claims Study. However, as more cases are reported, more insights into the airway-related causes of pediatric cardiac arrest and anesthesia will be gleaned.

NCEPOD (National Confidential Enquiry into Perioperative Deaths)

In the United Kingdom, an ongoing study has been updated and published since 1990. It is known as the NCEPOD. "The National Confidential Enquiry into Perioperative Deaths is a registered charity whose aim is to review clinical practice and identify potentially remediable factors in the practice of anaesthesia, surgery and other invasive medical procedures."[74] NCEPOD is an independent body with executives, a steering group, clinical coordinators, and local reporters in each of the participating hospitals. The steering group is composed of representatives from medical associations, colleges, and faculties in England, Wales, and Northern Ireland. Scotland conducts its own enquiry. All hospitals in the National Health Service and Defense Secondary Care Agency and public hospitals in Guernsey, Jersey, and the Isle of Man are included in the Enquiry, as well as many hospitals in the independent health care sector. Confidentiality is guaranteed.

The authors of the report specifically state that NCEPOD is "not a research study based on differences against a control population and does not produce any kind of comparison between clinicians or hospitals." The Enquiry does not look at the causation of death.

For the 2000 report, all deaths that occurred within 30 days of a surgical procedure between 1 April, 1998 and 31 March, 1999 were included in the present Enquiry. Ten percent (10%) of the cases were randomly selected for analysis. A questionnaire was sent to each surgeon or anesthesiologist with whom a case was identified. The physician had until 31 December, 1999 to return the questionnaire. Since April 1999, the government has made it mandatory for physicians in the National Health Service (NHS) to return the questionnaires. Enquiry staff members try to assure full compliance. In the present study, anesthetists returned 85% of the questionnaires, while surgeons returned 83%.

Because of the Enquiry's design, no specific airway-related information was reported with respect to causation of morbidity. The study listed "critical events" during anesthesia or recovery and compared these to events reported in the 1990 report (Table 15.8).

Other data documented that the recent trend was toward increased utilization of oxygenation and ventilation monitoring both in the operating room and especially in the recovery room.

NCEPOD 1996/1997 Report

Two airway-related recommendations published in a previous NCEPOD report are the following:

1. "A fiberoptic intubating laryngoscope should be readily available for use in all surgical hospitals. Several anesthetists working in a department should be trained for, and competent at, awake fiberoptic intubations."
2. "The technique of tracheostomy should be taught to trainee surgeons. The indications for performing this procedure under local or general anaesthesia should also be taught."[74]

Table 15.8 Critical events during anesthesia or the immediate recovery period, (airway-related), NCEPOD,[75] number of cases: 431

Critical event
Airway obstruction
Bronchospasm
Hypoxemia (<90% sat)
Misplaced tracheal tube
Pneumothorax
Pulmonary aspiration
Respiratory arrest (unintended)
Ventilatory inadequacy

NCEPOD, 2000

The NCEPOD is a very large study in which participation is mandatory. Perhaps the steering group should change the aim of the study and begin to ask questions that are included in the ASA Closed Claims Study and the AIMS. Then, specific mechanisms of injury as well as clinical practice patterns that lead to morbidity could begin to be defined in a population with a known denominator. This would be a very important step toward understanding anesthetic (and airway-related) morbidity and mortality.

SAMS (Scottish Audit of Surgical Mortality)

In Scotland, a mortality report similar in scope and design to NCEPOD is published annually. While "adverse factors"[76] are discussed and there is an "anaesthetics overview"[76] (p31–32) section in the latest report reviewed (1999), no specific mechanisms of injury are documented. This is not a criticism of the report, as its aims were not to define causative factors related to surgical mortality. However, as with the NCEPOD, should the future goals of the study be changed to include more detailed questions concerning the mechanisms of injury, another significant step toward understanding airway-related morbidity and mortality would have been taken.

Danish Morbidity Study: 1994–1998[77]

The Danish National Board of Patients' Complaints (NBPC) was founded in 1988. The board receives complaints from patients or relatives against personnel employed by the Danish Health Care System. The board collects and reviews information concerning the complaint through a regional medical officer, expert reviews, comments from the involved parties, and a review of the medical records. The board reaches a final decision concerning the complaint after review by a committee consisting of a chairman, a judge, two laymen, and two professional members. The board may issue a reprimand, may turn the case over to the police or medical–legal council, or it may decide that the person or persons named in the complaint were not guilty of any violation of the standards of care.

From 1994 to 1998, the NBPC received 8,869 complaints. Three percent ($n=284$) involved anesthesia or intensive care personnel. Complaints involving dental damage not associated with difficult intubation were excluded from analysis in a study that summarized the Danish morbidity findings.

Of the 284 complaints, 60 involved the respiratory system. They are summarized in Table 15.9.

Table 15.9 Danish National Board of Patients' complaints: 1994–1998, total complaints: 8,869, respiratory complaints: 60

Category	Number
Misuse of anesthetic equipment	5
Neonatal resuscitation	8
Pulmonary aspiration	7
Uncomplicated intubation	8
Difficult intubation	15
Miscellaneous causes	17
Total	60

Outcomes

Of the 60 respiratory complaints reported by the NBPC, "Thirty patients died, thirteen suffered permanent damage, and nine patients had temporary minor damage." In 32% of the complaints, treatment was ruled to have been substandard.

Difficult Endotracheal Intubation

Ten of fifteen difficult intubations were not anticipated. Nine patients died. Two cases were associated with cesarean section. Poor communication and inadequate assessment of existing medical records in the preoperative period contributed to poor outcome.

Complaints Related to Uncomplicated Endotracheal Intubation

Many different complaints involving the airway were lodged. These included hoarseness, temporomandibular joint pain, tracheal stenosis, and neurological symptoms involving the cervical spinal cord. No criticism was made about the anesthetic treatment in this subgroup of complaints.

Conclusions

The Danish study shares many design features with the American Closed Claims Study. However, the Danish study has confirmed, once again, that adverse respiratory events occur in the anesthesia–intensive care setting. The mechanisms of the different types of injuries are documented in this study. Finally, the study should lead to the establishment of educational strategies and programs that are designed to improve patient care.

Summary

The information presented in this section of the book clearly establishes the fact that airway management complications associated with the practice of anesthesia are myriad. Many complications are serious. Many problems involve the most basic airway maneuvers, such as ventilation, intubation, and observation of the patient. Many difficult airways are not predicted. Moreover, studies report that even when difficulty is predicted, strategies to deal with the anticipated difficulty are not documented. Problems with equipment and monitors are more likely to result from misuse rather than failure.

As a result of the lessons learned, anesthesiologists have established protocols, guidelines, and training strategies that are designed to improve patient safety. Hopefully, practitioners in other fields of medicine who are involved with airway management will learn from their anesthesia colleagues.

References

1. Griffith HR, Johnson GE. The use of curare in general anesthesia. *Anesthesiology*. 1942;3:418.
2. Pandey K, Badola R, Kumar S. Time course of intraocular hypertension produced by suxamethonium. *Br J Anaesth*. 1974;44:191.
3. Koh THHG, Coleman R. Oropharyngeal burn in a newborn baby: new complication of light-bulb laryngoscopes. *Anesthesiology*. 2000;92:277–279.
4. Warner ME, Benenfeld SM, Warner MA, Schroeder DR, Maxson PM. Perianesthetic dental injuries. *Anesthesiology*. 1999;90(5):1302–1305.
5. Newland M, Ellis S, Peters K, et al. Dental injury associated with anesthesia: a report of 161, 687 anesthetics given over fourteen years. *J Clin Anesth*. 2007;19:339–345.
6. Klokie C, Metcalf I, Holland A. Dental trauma in anaesthesia. *Can J Anaesth*. 1989;36(6): 675–680.
7. Domino KB, Posner PL, Caplan RA, Cheney FW. Airway injury during anesthesia. *Anesthesiology*. 1999;91(6):1703–1711.
8. Marty-Ane CH, Picard E, Jonquet O, Mary H. Membranous tracheal rupture after endotracheal intubation. *Ann Thorac Surg*. 1995;60(5):1367–1371.
9. Tu HN, Saidi N, Leiutand T, Bensaid S, Menival V, Duvaldestin P. Nitrous oxide increases endotracheal cuff pressure and the incidence of tracheal lesions in anesthetized patients. *Anesth Analg*. 1999;89(1):187–190.
10. Karasawa F, Mori T, Kawatani Y, Ohshima T, Satoh T. Deflationary phenomenon of the nitrous oxide-filled endotracheal tube cuff after cessation of nitrous oxide administration. *Anesth Analg*. 2001;92:145–148.
11. Langer O, Masso E, Huraux C, Guggiari M, Bianchi A, et al. Prediction of difficult mask ventilation. *Anesthesiology*. 2000;19:209–216.
12. Blitt CD, Gutman HL, Cohen DD, Weisman H, Dillon JB. Silent regurgitation and aspiration during general anesthesia. *Anesth Analg*. 1970;49:707.
13. Engelhardt T, Webster NR. Pulmonary aspiration of gastric contents in anaesthesia. *Br J Anaesth*. 1999;83(3):453–460.
14. Roberts RB, Shirley MA. Reducing the risk of acid aspiration during cesarean section. *Anesth Analg*. 1974;53(6):859–868.

15. Schwartz DJ, Wynne JW, Gibbs CP, Hood CI, Kuck EJ. The pulmonary consequences of aspiration of gastric contents at pH values greater than 2.5. *Am Rev Respir Dis.* 1980;121: 119–126.

16. Sellick BA. Cricoid pressure to control regurgitation of stomach contents during induction of anesthesia. *Lancet.* 1961;2:404.

17. Caplan RA. The ASA Closed Claims Project: lessons learned. *ASA Refresher Course #265.* 2000;1–7.

18. Caplan RA, Posner KL, Ward RJ, Chaney SW. Adverse respiratory events in anaesthesiology: a closed claims analysis. *Anesthesiology.* 1990;72:828–833.

19. Conrardy TA, Goodman LR, Lainge F, Singer MM. Alteration of endotracheal tube position. Flexion and extension of the neck. *Crit Care Med.* 1976;4:7–12.

20. Block EFJ, Cheatham ML, Parrish GA, Nelson LD, Beam N. Ingested endotracheal tube in an adult following intubation attempt for head injury. *Am Surg.* 1999;65:1134–1136.

21. Ince Z, Tu cu D, Çoban A. An unusual complication of endotracheal intubation: ingestion of a laryngoscope bulb. *Ped Emerg Care.* 1998;14(4):275–276.

22. Kumar MS, Pandey SK, Cohen PJ. Tracheal laceration associated with endotracheal anesthesia. *Anesthesiology.* 1977;47:298.

23. Wagener DL, Gamage GW, Wong ML. Tracheal rupture following the insertion of disposable double lumen endotracheal tube. *Anesthesiology.* 1985;63:700.

24. Foster JMG, Lao OJ, Alimo ED. Ruptured bronchus following endobronchial intubation. *Br J Anaesth.* 1983;55:697.

25. Sakuragi T, Kumano K, Yasumoto M, Dan K. Rupture of the left mainstem bronchus by the tracheal portion of a double-lumen endobroncheal tube. *Acta Anaesthesiol Scand.* 1997;41:1218–1220.

26. Fink BR. The etiology and treatment of laryngospasm. *Anesthesiology.* 1956;17:569.

27. Roy WL, Lerman J. Laryngospasm in paediatric anaesthesia. *Can J Anaesth.* 1988;35(1):93–98.

28. Larson CP. Laryngospasm – the best treatment. *Anesthesiology.* 1998;89:1293–1294.

29. Hartsell CJ, Stevens CR. Incidence of sore throat following endotracheal intubation. *Can Anaesth Soc.* 1964;111:307.

30. Stout D, Bishop MJ, Dwersteg JF, Cullen BF. Correlation of endotracheal tube size with sore throat and hoarseness following general anesthesia. *Anesthesiology.* 1987;67:419–421.

31. Steward DJ. Experience with an outpatient anesthesia service for children. *Anesth Analg.* 1973;52:877.

32. Monroe MC, Gravenstein N, Saga-Rumley S. Postoperative sore throat: effect of oropharyngeal airway in orotracheally intubated patients. *Anesth Analg.* 1990;70:512–516.

33. Kinbbe MA, Carter JB, Frokjer GM. Postanesthetic temporomandibular joint dysfunction. *Anesth Prog.* 1989;36:21–25.

34. Castella X, Gilabert J, Perez C. Arytenoid dislocation after tracheal intubation: an unusual cause of acute respiratory failure. *Anesthesiology.* 1991;74:615–618.

35. Szigeti CL, Beauerle JJ, Mongan PD. Arytenoid dislocation with lighted stylet intubation: a case report and retrospective review. *Anesth Analg.* 1994;78:185–186.

36. Usui T, Saito S, Goto F. Arytenoid dislocation while using a McCoy laryngoscope. *Anesth Analg.* 2001;92:1347–1348.

37. Quick CA, Merwin GE. Arytenoid dislocation. *Arch Otolaryngol.* 1978;104:267–270.

38. Hahn FW, Martin JT, Lillie JC. Vocal cord paralysis with endotracheal intubation. *Arch Otolaryngol.* 1970;92:226.

39. Holley HS, Gildea JE. Vocal cord paralysis after tracheal intubation. *JAMA.* 1971;214:281.

40. Lim EK, Schia KS, Ng BK. Recurrent laryngeal nerve palsy following endotracheal intubation. *Anaesth Intensive Care.* 1987;15:342–345.

41. Dalton C. Bilateral vocal cord paralysis following endotracheal intubation. *Anesth Intensive Care.* 1995;23:350–351.

42. Ellis PDM, Pallister WK. Recurrent laryngeal nerve palsy and endotracheal intubation. *J Laryngol Otol.* 1975;89:823–826.

43. Whited RE. Laryngeal dysfunction following prolonged intubation. *Ann Otol*. 1979;88: 474–478.

44. Sofferman RA, Hubbell RN. Laryngeal complications of NG tubes. *Ann Otol Rhinol*. 1981;90:465.

45. Friedman M, Baim H, Shelton V, et al. Laryngeal injuries secondary to NG tubes. *Ann Otol Rhino Laryngol*. 1981;90:469–474.

46. Tichner RL. Lingual nerve injury: a complication of oral tracheal intubation. *Br J Anaesth*. 1971;43:413.

47. Tichner RL. Lingual nerve injury: a complication following laryngoscopy. *Anesthesiology*. 1991;76:650–665.

48. Silva DA, Colingo KA, Miller R. Lingual nerve injury following laryngoscopy. *Anesthesiology*. 1991;76:650–651.

49. Venkatesh B, Walker D. Hypoglossal neuropraxia following endotracheal intubation. *Anesth Intensive Care*. 1997;25:699–700.

50. Montoya Pelaez LF, du Toit PW, Norlund DM, et al. Mental nerve neuropraxia associated with tracheal intubation using a RAE tube. *Br J Anaesth*. 1999;82:650–651.

51. Bauman RC, McGregor DA. Dissection of the posterior pharynx resulting in acute airway obstruction. *Anesthesiology*. 1995;82:1516–1518.

52. Deutschman CS, Wilton P, Sinow J, Dibbell D Jr, Konstantinides FN, Cerra FB. Paranasal sinusitis associated with nasotracheal intubation: a frequently unrecognized and treatable source of sepsis. *Crit Care Med*. 1986;14:111–114.

53. Hermens JM, Bennett MJ, Hirshman CA. Anesthesia for laser surgery. *Anesth Analg*. 1983;62:218.

54. Cheney FW. The American Society of Anesthesiologists Closed Claims Project. *Anesthesiology*. 1999;91(2):552–556.

55. Cheney FW, Posner KL, Lee LA, Caplan RA, Domino KB. Trends in anesthesia-related death and brain damage. A Closed Claims Analysis. *Anesthesiology*. 2006;105:1081-1086.

56. Miller CG. Management of the difficult intubation in closed malpractice claims. *ASA Newsl*. 2000;64(6):13–19.

57. Cheney FW. Aspiration: a liability hazard for the anesthesiologist? *ASA Newsl*. 2000;64(6):5–26.

58. Caplan RA, Vistica MF, Posner KL, Cheney FW. Adverse anesthetic outcomes arising from gas delivery equipment. *Anesthesiology*. 1997;87(4):741–748.

59. Domino KB. Office-based anesthesia: lessons learned from the Closed Claims Project. *ASA Newsl*. 2001;65(6):9–15.

60. Posner KL. Liability profile of ambulatory anesthesia. *ASA Newsl*. 2000;64(6):5–12.

61. Williamson JA, Webb RK, Szekely S, Gillies ER, Dreosti AV. Difficult intubation: an analysis of 2000 incident reports. *Anaesth Intensive Care*. 1993;21(5):602–607.

62. Russell WJ, Web RK, Van der Walt JH, Runciman WB. Problems with ventilation: an analysis of 2000 incident reports. *Anaesth Intensive Care*. 1993;21(5):617–620.

63. Petty WC. Anesthesia critical incidents: ASA and AIMS (part II). *Curr Rev Clin Anesth Lesson 23*. 2000;20:(Miami).

64. Webb RK, Russell WJ, Klepper ID, Runciman WB. Equipment failure: an analysis of 2000 incident reports. *Anaesth Intensive Care*. 1993;21(5):673–677.

65. Holland R, Webb RK, Runciman WB. Oesophageal intubation: an analysis of 2000 incident reports. *Anaesth Intensive Care*. 1993;21(5):608–610.

66. Szekely SM, Webb RK, Williamson JA, Russell WJ. Problems related to the endotracheal tube: an analysis of 2000 incident reports. *Anaesth Intensive Care*. 1993;21(5):611–616.

67. Webb RK, Van Der Walt JH, Runciman WB, et al. Which monitor? an analysis of 2000 incident reports. *Anaesth Intensive Care*. 1993;21(5):529–542.

68. Runciman WB, Webb RK, Barker L, Curriie M. The pulse oximeter: applications and limitations – an analysis of 2000 incident reports. *Anaesth Intensive Care*. 1993;21(5): 543–550.

69. Williamson JA, Webb RK, Cockings J, Morgan C. The capnograph: applications and limitations – an analysis of 2000 incident reports. *Anaesth Intensive Care.* 1993;21(5): 551–557.
70. Sinclair M, Simmons S, Cyna A. Incidents in obstetric anaesthesia and analgesia: an analysis of 5000 incident reports. *Anaesth Intensive Care.* 1999;27(3):275–281.
71. Warden JD, Horan BF. Deaths attributed to anaesthesia in New South Wales, 1984–1990. *Anaesth Intensive Care.* 1996;24(1):66–73.
72. Morray JP, Geiduschek JM, Ramamoorthy C, Haberkern CM, Hackel A, Caplan RA. Anesthesia-related cardiac arrest in children. *Anesthesiology.* 2000;93(1):6–14.
73. Gray AJG, et al. NCEPOD. *Anaesthesia.* 2000:37.
74. NCEPOD. Executive summary. 2000.
75. NCEPOD. Report summary; recommendations. 1996/1997.
76. *Scottish Audit of Surgical Mortality.* 1999:19–20.
77. Rosenstock C, Moller J, Hauberg A. Complaints related to respiratory events in anaesthesia and intensive care medicine from 1994 to 1998 in Denmark. *Acta Anaesthesiol Scand.* 2001;45:53–58.

Suggested Reading

American Heart Association standards and guidelines for cardiopulmonary resuscitation (CPR) and emergency cardiac care (ECC). *JAMA.* 1986;255:2905.
Blanc VF, Tremblay NAG. The complications of tracheal intubation: a new classification with a review of the literature. *Curr Res Anesth Analg.* 1973;53:202.
Cowley RA, Trump BF, eds. *Pathophysiology of Shock, Anoxia, and Ischemia.* Baltimore: Williams & Wilkins; 1982.
Harrison TR et al., eds. *Harrison's Principles of Internal Medicine.* 6th ed. New York: McGraw-Hill; 1970.

Index

Printed in the United States of America